Harsh Vyas • Nikhita Gune • Pooja Balgi

Dental Caries and Traumatic Injuries in Pediatric Dentistry

Current Concepts in Clinical Practice

Springer

Harsh Vyas
Pediatric and Preventive Dentist
Dr Vyas's Pediatric Dentistry
Mumbai, Maharashtra, India

Nikhita Gune
Pediatric and Preventive Dentist
Mumbai, Maharashtra, India

Pooja Balgi
Pediatric and Preventive Dentist
Mumbai, Maharashtra, India

ISBN 978-3-031-98928-5 ISBN 978-3-031-98929-2 (eBook)
https://doi.org/10.1007/978-3-031-98929-2

This Springer imprint is published by the registered company Springer Nature Switzerland AG
The registered company address is: Gewerbestrasse 11, 6330 Cham, Switzerland

To all,
dedicated to the dental care of children.
If the content helps to improve the treatment
of children in the smallest of ways,
it would give us immense satisfaction to have
contributed to Pediatric Dentistry in a
meaningful way.

Harsh Vyas *Nikhita Gune* *Pooja Balgi*

Foreword

It is my honor and pleasure to introduce readers to *Dental Caries and Traumatic Injuries in Pediatric Dentistry: Current Concepts in Clinical Practice*, the latest Pediatric Dentistry textbook, and one dedicated to contemporary oral health care of children and the clinicians who strive to provide the most current, evidence-based care. This text accomplishes several "firsts" in practical clinical dental literature.

First and foremost, it is a clinician's text, focused on direct clinical care, making the jump from evidence and emerging science to chairside application. By doing so, authors focus Pediatric and General dentists caring for children on the best possible care, removing ambiguity, but at the same time, allowing us to meld recommendations into individualized care for our patients. Secondly, the text focuses on two of our most challenging problems as clinicians—meaningful precision management of dental caries, and treatment of what is most parents' worst dental experience, and often as stressful for us, traumatic injury. Perhaps the most important for clinicians is the author's algorithmic approach to patient clinical presentations, thus taking some of the guesswork and randomness out of two clinical situations often clouded with social, emotional, and other nondental issues.

The authors deal with caries, our predominant daily clinical challenge, with consideration of caries risk, disease progression and choices for care that reflect the "big picture" of a child's needs. It should escape no reader that the authors—clinicians themselves—have worked hard to meld the tooth, child, family, and social characteristics into an algorithmic approach to the disease's prevention and management. This micro-/macrocosmic approach to dental caries provides clinicians with a refreshing and optimistic approach to successful immediate and long-term management! The treatment aspects of caries management in this text provide the latest approaches to both definitive and palliative care, another real-world view of caries management in diverse populations across age spans. The text's materials and technique offerings are the most up-to-date. When reading the caries management chapters in this text, it is hard not to reflect and recall many children not only with obvious disease but the challenges we face trying to provide sustainable care and prevention. The authors' roadmap should be a benefit to both clinicians and educators.

Traumatic injuries are everyone's worst nightmare and ambiguity in management can make matters worse! This text offers systematic, realistic, and contemporary management of dentoalveolar trauma, using the same comprehensive, short- and long-term considerations that the authors have made the hallmark of caries management. Pivotal to trauma management is the dental pulp and its susceptibility to frank or subtle injury and this text addresses that aspect of trauma well. Like the caries section of this book, the authors have provided an algorithmic view of the continuum of dental trauma, and for those general dental clinicians, this roadmap reference tool should be in the operatory at hand when these children need our help. Finally, the authors have provided a view of advanced imaging for trauma, an area not well-described by clinicians who deal with diagnosis and management, so a welcome addition to the literature!

In summary, for the two topics of dental caries and dentoalveolar trauma, this book offers the education many of us wish we'd had in our earlier training on our two greatest challenges. Take the time to read through this text to make you current and keep it at chairside for ready reference!

Professor Emeritus, The Ohio State University
Columbus, OH, USA
Paul S. Casamassimo

Conflict of Interest Statement

The authors declare no conflict of interest. In line with the content of this book, an attempt has been made to include a broad range of commercially available dental products worldwide. Any omission of specific commercial product(s) is unintentional and purely coincidental. The authors and their immediate families have no financial interests or affiliations that could be perceived as influencing the content of this publication. Due permission has been taken where needed as per the publisher's guidelines.

Contributors

Dr. Manini Shah
Dr. Abhishek Soni
Dr. Mayur Bhattad
Dr. Gopika Sharma

Preface

Why another book on Dental Caries and Traumatic Dental Injuries? The management of dental caries is second nature to Pediatric Dentistry and not a day goes by, when we are not forced to confront a mouth full of decay. In comparison, Traumatic Dental Injuries can be a rarity, but when a case is suddenly thrust upon us, we sometimes find ourselves caught off guard. There has been a significant shift in the approach to managing dental caries, moving away from the traditional restorative methods to the more preventive, minimally invasive strategies. This shift is still being assimilated into everyday clinical practice and many practitioners are navigating the learning curve as they adjust. Dental trauma presents with a wide spectrum of injuries and permutations that often leads to unpredictable consequences, requiring careful evaluation and management. Despite their differences, both conditions highlight a shared reliance on sound clinical judgment to ensure consistent, favorable outcomes.

I have always believed that understanding the scientific rationale and significance behind each step in a treatment workflow is key to good clinical practice, as it minimizes the risk of missteps that can compromise treatment results. This book presents procedures through visual narratives and clinical cases, uses mind maps to simplify complex decision-making, and discusses evidence-based protocols in a way that is easy to apply in everyday clinical practice.

The idea to write this book first emerged through a conversation with Dr. Ujwal Kontham. That initial spark led to the coming together of our dream team during the Covid-19 pandemic: Dr. Nikhita Gune and Dr. Pooja Balgi. These two young, extremely well-read, and knowledgeable Pediatric Dentists matched my years of experience with their deft ability to draw upon and contextualize relevant clinical literature. They challenged and collaborated with me, dedicating countless hours both virtually and in person, molding this manuscript into what it is today. Their hard work and brilliance made these three years incredibly enriching and memorable.

I am deeply grateful to the mentors who have shaped my journey in Pediatric Dentistry. Dr. Pankaj Mehra taught me how to simplify procedures by providing a visual narrative, a concept that I have tried to implement throughout this book. The opportunities he provided helped me understand that a good speaker is one who shows the audience what *they* can do.

During the short but meaningful time I spent with Dr. Paul Casamassimo and Dr. Dennis McTigue, they generously shared their knowledge and clinical expertise.

Their humility and the way they engage with residents and colleagues taught me the importance of staying grounded. I am especially thankful for the time they took to review our draft and offer valuable feedback.

This project would not have been possible without Dr. Manini Shah, the bedrock of our Pediatric Dentistry practice. Her exceptional documentation skills and remarkable memory for noteworthy cases we've treated made her the go-to person during the development of this book.

Dr. Gopika Sharma has been a fellow traveler on my journey of gaining and sharing knowledge, both in academics and clinical practice. She has been an invaluable sounding board, helping me over the years, on how best I could benefit my intended audience.

I owe special thanks to my wife, Dr. Anuradha, who has been my silent yet unwavering support since my initiation into the world of Pediatric Dentistry. Her wholehearted encouragement and patience gave me the freedom to devote countless non-practicing hours to the development of this manuscript.

Lastly, the children I treat have taught me everything I know—through failures and successes, tears and laughter- fueling my passion for this speciality that continues to bring me immense joy and fulfilment.

Mumbai, India Harsh Vyas
Mumbai, India Nikhita Gune
Mumbai, India Pooja Balgi

Acknowledgments

Dr. Paul Casamassimo
Dr. Dennis McTigue
Dr. Vineet Dhar
Dr. Manini Shah
Dr. Gopika Sharma
Dr. Shreyas Gupte
Dr. Ajit Kalia
Dr. Prachi Sengupta

Contents

Abbreviations

AAE	American Association of Endodontists
AAP	American Association of Pediatrics
AAPD	American Academy of Pediatric Dentistry
ACP	Amorphous Calcium Phosphate
ADA	American Dental Association
APC	Autologous Platelet Concentrate
APF	Acidulated Phosphate Fluoride
BCR	Blood clot revascularization
Bis-GMA	Bis-glycidyl methacrylate
CAMBRA	Caries Management by Risk Assessment
CBCT	Cone Beam Computed Tomography
CCR	Complete Caries Removal
CDC	Centre for Disease Control
CH	Calcium Hydroxide
CHX	Chlorohexidene Gluconate
CIRR	Cervical Inflammatory Root Resorption
CPP-ACP	Casein Phosphopeptide-Amorphous Calcium Phosphate
CRA	Caries Risk Assessment
CT	Computed Tomography
DAP	Double Antibiotic Paste
DOM	Dental Operating Microscope
DPC	Direct Pulp Capping
EAL	Electronic Apex Locator
EAPD	European Academy of Pediatric Dentistry
EIRR	External Inflammatory Root Resorption
ENT	Ear Nose Throat
EPT	Electric Pulp Test
FDA	Food and Drug Administration
FHA	Fluorhydroxyapatite
FOV	Field of View
GIC	Glass Ionomer Cement
HBSS	Hank's Balanced Salt solution
IADT	International Association of Dental Traumatology
IAPD	International Association of Pediatric Dentistry

ICCC	International Caries Consensus Collaboration
ICCMS	International Caries Classification and Management System
IIRR	Internal Inflammatory Root Resorption
IOPA	Intraoral Periapical Radiograph
IPT	Indirect Pulp Treatment
IRM	Intermediate Restorative Material
IRR	Inflammatory Root Resorption
ISO	International Organization of Standardization
MID	Minimal Intervention Dentistry
MIH	Molar Incisor Hypomineralization
MRI	Magnetic Resonance Imaging
NaF	Sodium Fluoride
NaOCL	Sodium Hypochlorite
NiTi	Nickel titanium
NRCC	Non-Restorative Cavity Control
NS	Normal Saline
OPG	Orthopantomogram
PATF	Professionally Applied Topical Fluorides
PRF	Platelet-Rich Fibrin
PRP	Platelet-Rich Plasma
PTD	Probable Toxic Dose
REP	Regenerative Endodontic Procedures
RI	Resin Infiltration
RRR	Replacement Root Resorption
SCR	Selective Caries Removal
SDCEP	Scottish Dental Clinical Effectiveness Program
SDF	Silver Diamine Fluoride
SES	Socioeconomic Status
SMART	Silver Modified Atraumatic Restorative Technique
SSC	Stainless Steel Crown
SWR	Stepwise Caries Removal
TAB	Transient Apical Breakdown
TAP	Triple Antibiotic Paste
TCP	Crystalized Calcium Phosphate-β Tricalcium Phosphate
TDI	Traumatic Dental Injuries
TMJ	Temporo-Mandibular Joint
UK	United Kingdom
VPT	Vital Pulp Therapy
WSL	White Spot Lesions
ZOE	Zinc Oxide Eugenol

Integrating Caries Risk Assessment in Clinical Practice

1

1.1 Introduction

The last two decades have led to a gradual change in our understanding of the pathophysiology of dental caries. Consequently, this has had a cascading effect on how caries is diagnosed, prevented, and treated in clinical practice. Earlier, dental caries was considered synonymous with cavitated carious lesions which were treated by routine restorative procedures. Today, dental caries is more than just a "cavity," rather it is a "disease process" characterized by the presence of factors linked to active demineralization on tooth surfaces. It is now understood that a "cavity" is only a symptom of the caries process [1, 2].

Contemporary caries management in children requires the clinician to identify and eliminate those factors that are believed to put a child at an increased risk of tooth surface demineralization, i.e., caries risk factors such as

- Poor oral hygiene
- Presence of non-cavitated and cavitated carious lesions
- Increased frequency of fermentable carbohydrate ingestion
- Reduced salivary function
- Presence of acidogenic bacteria
- Deep retentive pits and fissures

and promote those which are known to cause remineralization (cario-protective) such as [3–5]:

- Exposure to systemic and topical fluoride sources
- Child has a dental home

  (a) Professional preventive regime
  (b) Recall/follow-up program
  (c) Anticipatory guidance

H. Vyas et al., *Dental Caries and Traumatic Injuries in Pediatric Dentistry*,
https://doi.org/10.1007/978-3-031-98929-2_1

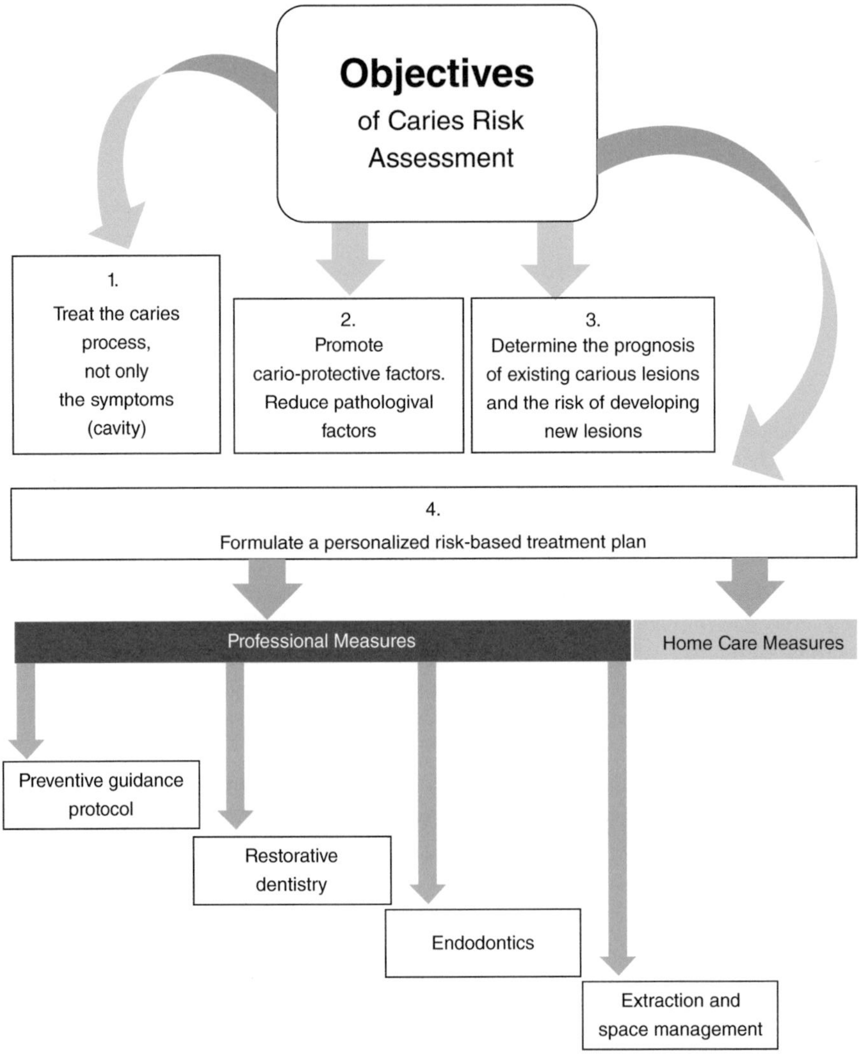

Fig. 1.1 Objectives of caries risk assessment

The concept of "*Caries Risk Assessment*" enables clinicians to identify caries risk factors and customize a treatment plan that can prevent new lesions and treat existing lesions (Fig. 1.1) [6].

1.2 Classification of Risk Factors

International Caries Risk Assessment systems use categories such as socio-demographic, microbiological, dietary, and clinical indicators of disease in their protocol. From a clinical standpoint, there are only certain caries risk factors which

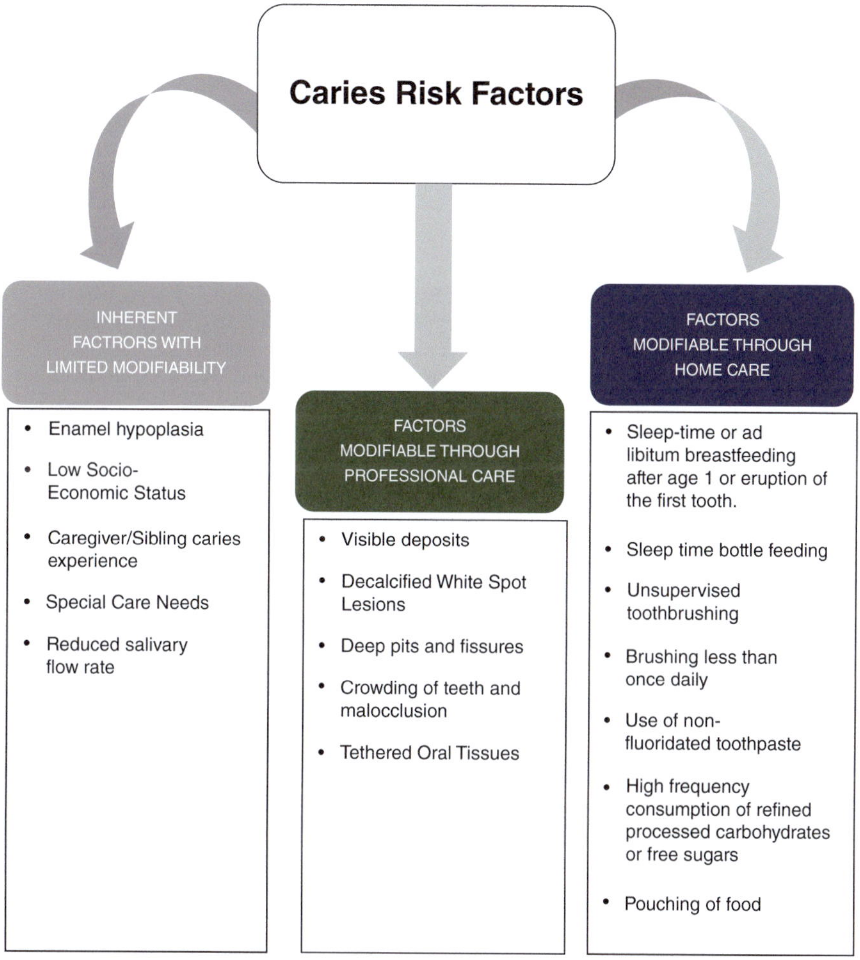

Fig. 1.2 Classification of caries risk factors based on the ease of modification by professional or home care measures

can be effectively modified by the dentist using evidence-based preventive methods, and by parental and child counseling. Therefore, it is beneficial to concentrate on those factors which lie within our control. These have been detailed below (Fig. 1.2) [6–11].

The table below is a compilation of the risk factors from the following (Table 1.1) [7–11]:

1. IAPD (International Association of Pediatric Dentistry) Caries Care Pathway [7]
2. AAPD (American Academy of Pediatric Dentistry) [8]
3. CAMBRA (Caries Management by Risk Assessment) [9, 10]
4. ICCMS™ (International Caries Classification and Management System) [11]

Table 1.1 Compilation of caries risk factors taken from the International Association of Pediatric Dentistry (IAPD) Caries Risk Assessment and Care Pathway, American Academy of Pediatric Dentistry (AAPD), Caries Management by Risk Assessment (CAMBRA), and The International Caries Classification and Management System (ICCMS™)

Low risk	Moderate	High risk
Clinical indicators Child has no caries. No new lesions in 1 year. No white spot lesions.	*Clinical indicators* Child has/had one or more lesions. One or more new lesions/year. Infrequent white spot lesions. Deep pits and fissures. Orthodontic appliances. Child with visible plaque.	*Clinical indicators* Child has/had one or more proximal lesions. More than two new lesions/year. Multiple white spot lesions. Child has heavy plaque on teeth. Child presents with dental enamel defects. Patient has low salivary flow. Recent restorations in the last 2 years (new patient) or the last year (patient of record). New cavities or lesions into dentin (radiographically).
General indicators Child has teeth brushed daily with fluoridated toothpaste. Child receives topical fluoride from health professional. Presence of background fluoride exposure. Child has dental home/regular dental care. High socioeconomic status (SES).	*General indicators* Child has special health care needs. Middle SES.	*General indicators* Mother/primary caregivers have active dental caries. Child has frequent exposure (more than 3 times/day) between-meal sugar-containing snacks or beverages per day. Child uses bottle or non-spill cup containing natural or added sugar frequently, between meals and/or at bedtime. Low SES.

Based on these risk factors, the practitioner must categorize patients into low, moderate, or high-risk at the first dental visit and subsequent follow-ups. After determining the child's caries risk, an age-appropriate Preventive Guidance Protocol can be implemented.

1.3 Preventive Guidance Protocol

The Preventive Guidance Protocol (Table 1.2) is an easy-to-follow regimen in clinical practice and is an adaptation of home and professional care recommendations by the IAPD [7, 12], AAPD [8], SDCEP [13] (Scottish Dental Clinical Effectiveness Program), CAMBRA [9, 10], and ICCMS™ [11]. While most guidelines restrict fluoride application to moderate and high caries risk children only, this protocol recommends fluoride application even in children with low caries risk. In countries with no community water fluoridation or poor availability of optimally fluoridated toothpastes, this may be particularly significant.

Table 1.2 Preventive Guidance Protocol recommending home care and professional measures to prevent dental caries based on the child's age and caries risk status

	6 months-3 years	3–6 years	Above 6 years
Home care (low risk)	Supervised brushing twice/day. Use of a smear or rice grain size of 1000 ppm fluoridated toothpaste. Avoidance of ad libitum breastfeeding and sleep-time bottle feeding. Wiping teeth after every feed. Gradual weaning of the child and introduction of age-appropriate complementary foods. Avoid introduction of sugar in any form in the diet till age two	Supervised brushing twice/day. Use of a pea-sized amount of 1000 ppm to 1450 ppm fluoridated toothpaste Restriction on consumption of processed refined carbohydrates/free sugars. Flossing once daily.	
Home care (moderate and high risk)	In addition to the home care measures given in the low-risk group. Twice-daily application of Casein Phosphopeptide-Amorphous Calcium Phosphate (CPP-ACP) for 3 months. Use can be extended after examination at follow-up visits.		In addition to the home care measures given in the low-risk group. In children above 6 years of age, twice-daily application of Casein Phosphopeptide-Amorphous Calcium Phosphate (CPP-ACP) for 3 months. Use can be extended after examination at follow-up visits. 0.12% chlorhexidine mouthrinse daily for 1 week followed by 0.05% (900 ppm) fluoride mouth rinses daily for other 3 weeks of the month. Brushing with a high fluoride toothpaste (5000 ppm) twice daily, for adolescents who are in the high caries risk group.

(continued)

Table 1.2 (continued)

	6 months-3 years	3–6 years	Above 6 years
Professional Care (low risk)	12-monthly dental examinations and parental counseling as soon as the first tooth erupts. 12- to 24-monthly radiographic evaluation (if contacts are closed). Sealing of stained pits and fissures in primary teeth.	6-monthly dental examinations. 12- to 24-monthly radiographic evaluation (if contacts are closed). Sealing of stained pits and fissures in primary teeth. Oral prophylaxis and 6-monthly 5% sodium fluoride varnish application.	6-monthly dental examinations. 12- to 24-monthly radiographic evaluation. Sealing of first and second permanent molars after eruption. Oral prophylaxis and 6-monthly 5% sodium fluoride varnish application.
Professional Care (Moderate to high risk)	Dental examination, oral prophylaxis, and 5% sodium fluoride varnish applications 6-monthly (moderate risk) and 3-monthly (high risk) after the first tooth erupts. 12-monthly radiographic examination if contacts are closed. Sealing of stained pits and fissures in primary teeth.	Dental examination, oral prophylaxis, and 5% sodium fluoride varnish applications 6-monthly (moderate risk) and 3-monthly (high risk). 12-monthly radiographic examination if contacts are closed. Sealing of first and second permanent molars after eruption. Sealing of stained pits and fissures in primary teeth.	

1.4 Concluding Remarks

Caries Risk Assessment must be adopted in routine clinical practice as part of the first consultation. Based on the assigned caries risk status, customized professional and home care recommendations must be explained to the parents and child. Professional care recommendations should be focused on 6-monthly applications of topical fluorides in low and moderate caries risk children and 3-monthly fluoride application in high caries risk children and placement of sealants in susceptible fissures. Home care protocols must center around providing age-appropriate anticipatory guidance regarding feeding habits, consumption of refined processed carbohydrates, toothbrushing, and routine use of fluoridated toothpastes and remineralizing agents.

References

1. Kidd E. The implications of the new paradigm of dental caries. J Dent. 2011;39:S3–8.
2. Fejerskov O. Concepts of dental caries and their consequences for understanding the disease. Community Dent Oral Epidemiol. 1997;25:5–12.

3. Twetman S, Fontana M. Patient caries risk assessment. In: Detection, assessment, diagnosis and monitoring of caries. Monogr Oral Sci, vol. 21. Basel: Karger; 2009. p. 91–101.
4. Featherstone JDB. Prevention and reversal of dental caries: role of low-level fluoride. Community Dent Oral Epidemiol. 1999;27:31–40.
5. Featherstone JD. The caries balance: the basis for caries management by risk assessment. Oral Health Prev Dent. 2004;2(Suppl 1):259–64.
6. Harris R, Nicoll Kirthiga M, Murugan M, Saikia A, Kirubakaran R. Risk factors for early childhood caries: a systematic review and meta-analysis of case control and cohort studies. Pediatr Dent. 2019;41(2):95–112.
7. IAPD Foundational articles and consensus recommendations: caries risk assessment and care pathways,2022.
8. American Academy of Pediatric Dentistry. Caries-risk assessment and management for infants, children, and adolescents. The reference manual of pediatric dentistry. Chicago: American Academy of Pediatric Dentistry; 2024. p. 306–12.
9. Featherstone JDB, et al. An updated CAMBRA caries risk assessment tool for ages 0 to 5 years. J Calif Dent Assoc. 2019;47(1):37–47.
10. Featherstone JD, Adair SM, Anderson MH, Berkowitz RJ, Bird WF, Crall JJ. Caries management by risk assessment: consensus statement. J Calif Dent Assoc. 2002;31(3):257–69.
11. Martignon S, Pitts NB, Goffin G, Mazevet M, Douglas GV, Newton JT, Twetman S, Deery C, Doméjean S, Jablonski-Momeni A, Banerjee A. Caries care practice guide: consensus on evidence into practice. BDJ. 2019 Sep;227(5):353–62.
12. Tinanoff N, Baez RJ, Diaz Guillory C, Donly KJ, Feldens CA, McGrath C, Phantumvanit P, Pitts NB, Seow WK, Sharkov N, Songpaisan Y, Twetman S. Early childhood caries epidemiology, aetiology, risk assessment, societal burden, management, education, and policy: global perspective. Int J Paediatr Dent. 2019 May;29(3):238–48.
13. Scottish Dental Clinical Effectiveness Programme. Prevention and management of dental caries in children: dental clinical guideline. Dundee: Scottish Dental Clinical Effectiveness Programme; 2010.

2 Professional Regimes for Caries Prevention

2.1 Introduction

Preventive Dentistry is widely practiced by pediatric dentists across the world due to the high global prevalence of dental caries [1, 2] and the deep reaching effects it has on the oral and general health of children [3]. With the contemporary understanding of the caries process, preventive dentistry is no longer limited to strengthening or protecting the enamel surface (primary prevention) but has extended its role to reversing the initial white spot lesions and arresting frank carious lesions (secondary prevention). To this effect, primary and secondary caries preventive strategies that have been around for decades and are well supported by published literature, continue to be relevant in today's practice [4, 5].

Primary preventive strategies are directed at preventing the development of a carious lesion. They include full mouth application of Professionally Applied Topical Fluoride (PATF) on healthy teeth, placement of pit and fissure sealants on caries-free teeth with deep fissures and anticipatory guidance [4].

Anticipatory guidance is integral to the success of all preventive dentistry techniques as it ensures improved oral care at home and involves counseling the parent and child on good oral hygiene and dietary habits specific to the caries risk. The caries preventive strategies performed in the dental office will be effective only if equal time and effort are spent on delivering anticipatory guidance to the child and parent at each dental visit [6]. Secondary preventive strategies are directed at arresting or reversing the progression of an existing carious lesion. They include application of fluoride varnish on surfaces with white spot lesions to remineralize them, sealing carious pits and fissures [4, 5], and applying Silver Diamine Fluoride (SDF) on cavitated dentinal lesions to arrest the caries progression [7].

H. Vyas et al., *Dental Caries and Traumatic Injuries in Pediatric Dentistry*,
https://doi.org/10.1007/978-3-031-98929-2_2

2.2 Professionally Applied Topical Fluoride (PATF): Recommendations and Technique

The epidemiological studies conducted by Dr. Trendley Dean and coworkers between 1901 and 1942 established that the presence of 1 ppm of fluoride in drinking water reduced caries prevalence by 50% [8]. This discovery highlighted the *pre-eruptive effect of fluoride* and led to the development of artificial water fluoridation programs. In the 1940s, Arnold et al. suggested that periodic or continuous renewal of the fluoride content of tooth enamel is required to maintain the maximum caries-inhibiting effect [9]. By the 1970s and 1980s, it was demonstrated that primary teeth in fluoridated areas remained protected against caries, even though prenatal incorporation of fluoride in them was insignificant [10]. This established the importance of the *post-eruptive effects of fluoride* and resulted in the development of different topical fluoride delivery systems, that exert a cario-protective action by maintaining consistent intraoral levels of fluoride on the enamel surface [11].

At present, topical fluorides are classified as Professionally Applied Topical Fluoride (PATF) and home-use topical fluorides based upon the fluoride content and delivery system. PATF mainly include fluoride gels and varnishes. Essentially, the general mechanism of action of both is the same and they are more effective in preventing dental caries on smooth surfaces than the occlusal surfaces [12]. The commonly used professionally applied fluorides are sodium fluoride/NaF (varnish and gels), Acidulated Phosphate Fluoride/APF (gel), and stannous fluoride (liquid).

2.2.1 How Does Professionally Applied Topical Fluoride (PATF) Work?

The ability of fluoride to prevent dental caries is because of the chemical interaction between the fluoride molecule and enamel–plaque–saliva interface that results in the formation of fluorhydroxyapatite (FHA) which is more resistant to demineralization [13, 14]. Also, there are auxiliary benefits of periodic PATF that gives the clinician an opportunity to evaluate the child's oral health (Fig. 2.1).

2.2.2 Composition

Fluoride Gels

Sodium fluoride and APF are commonly used fluoride gels of which APF is more popular. APF is an aqueous solution of sodium fluoride dissolved in phosphoric and hydrofluoric acid to prepare a fluoride ion concentration of 1.23% at pH 3. For the preparation of APF gel, methylcellulose or hydroxyethyl cellulose is added to the

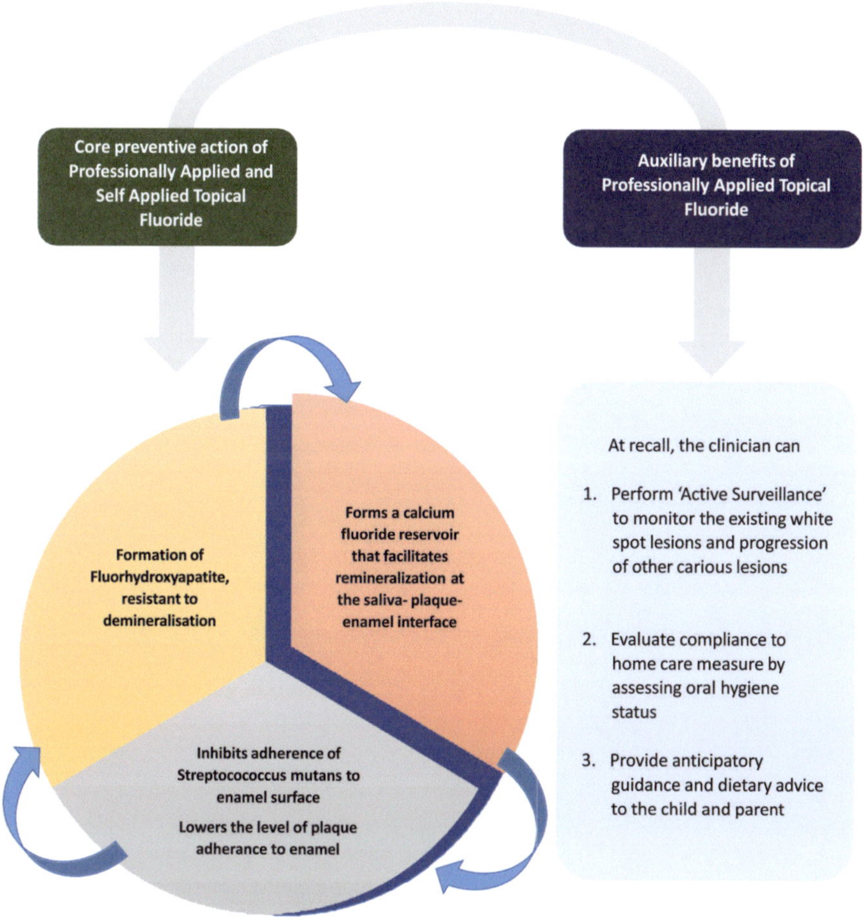

Fig. 2.1 Core and auxiliary preventive actions of professionally applied topical fluoride (PATF)

solution to make it thixotrophic. Commercially available products incorporate additional sugar-free flavoring agents or xylitol [15].

Fluoride Varnish

The oldest commercially available fluoride varnishes are Duraphat® (5% Sodium Fluoride or 22,500 ppm F) and Fluorprotector (0.9% difluorosilane or 7000 ppm F). Both varnishes are effective in preventing the incidence of dental caries even though they differ in the availability of fluoride ions and viscosity [16]. Many of the present-day 5% Sodium Fluoride (NaF) varnishes incorporate newer caries preventive and remineralizing compounds such as Xylitol, Casein Phosphopeptide-Amorphous Calcium Phosphate, Tri Calcium Phosphate, Amorphous Calcium Phosphate, and Nanohydroxyapatite (Table 2.1).

Table 2.1 Commercially available fluoride varnishes

No	Product	Concentration of sodium fluoride	Additional anticaries/ remineralizing agents	Dose available	Manufacturer	Flavors
1	Duraphat®	5% sodium fluoride		0.4 ml	Colgate	No added flavor
2	Colgate PreviDent® varnish	5% sodium fluoride	Xylitol	1 ml	Colgate	Raspberry, grape, bubblegum, mint
3	Fluorprotector	0.9% difluorosilane		1 ml	Ivoclar Vivadent	No added flavor
4	Fluorprotector S	1.5% ammonium fluoride		0.4 ml	Ivoclar Vivadent	No added flavor
5	Duraflor®	5% sodium fluoride	Xylitol	0.5 ml	Medicom	Caramel, strawberry, mint
6	Embrace varnish®	5% sodium fluoride	Xylitol coated calcium and phosphate	0.4 ml	Pulpdent	Bubblegum
7	Profluorid varnish	5% sodium fluoride	Xylitol	0.25 ml/0.4 ml	VOCO	Mint, melon, cherry, caramel
8	MI varnish®	5% sodium fluoride	Casein Phosphopeptide-amorphous calcium phosphate	0.4 ml	GC	Fresh strawberry, fresh mint
9	3 M vanish white varnish™	5% sodium fluoride	Xylitol and tri calcium phosphate	0.25 ml/0.4 ml/0.5 ml	3 M	Mint, melon, cherry
10	3 M fast release varnish™	5% sodium fluoride	Xylitol	0.4 ml	3 M	Strawberry, mint, caramel
11	NUPRO white varnish®	5% sodium fluoride		0.4 gm	Dentsply	Mint, bubblegum, grape, raspberry, caramel
12	Enamelast™	5% sodium fluoride	Xylitol	0.4 ml unit dose 1.2 ml syringe	Ultradent	Coolmint, bubblegum, Walterberry, Orange cream
13	Enamel pro varnish®	5% sodium fluoride	Amorphous calcium phosphate	0.25 ml and 0.4 ml	Premier	Vanillamint, strawberry n cream, bubblegum
14	Kolorz ClearShield varnish®	5% sodium fluoride	Xylitol	0.4 ml	DMG America	Mint, cookie dough, watermelon, bubblegum
15	Fluorimax®	2.5% sodium fluoride		0.3 ml 12 ml bottle	Elevate oral care	Bubblegum
16	Acclean varnish®	5% sodium fluoride	Xylitol	0.4 ml	Henry Schein	Bubblegum
17	Vella varnish®	5% sodium fluoride	Xylitol	0.5 ml	Preventech	Spearmint, strawberry, melon, bubblegum

These commercial products have been listed after visiting the manufacturers' websites on 7th May 2025. The availability of these products may vary across different regions

2.2.3 What Is the Application Schedule for Professionally Applied Topical Fluoride (PATF) in a Clinical Setup?

The International Association of Pediatric Dentistry (IAPD) and the American Academy of Pediatric Dentistry (AAPD) recommend a fluoride application protocol that is based on the caries risk assessment [17, 18]. Children must be identified as having a low, moderate, or high risk status depending on the following factors taken from IAPD caries care pathway [17], AAPD [18] and Caries Management by Risk Assessment (CAMBRA) [19], and The International Caries Classification and Management System (ICCMS™) [20] (Table 2.2).

A child can have multiple clinical and general indicators that may fall under different risk categories. The identification of any one indicator from the highest category will decide the risk status of the child. For example, a caries free (low-risk indicator) child showing the presence of enamel defects (high-risk indicator) will be assigned a *high caries risk status.*

Studies conducted in both high and low caries risk populations show that there are no additional health gains achieved by fluoride varnish application in low-risk populations and the cost–benefit ratio is also found to be more supportive of such

Table 2.2 Compilation of caries risk factors taken from the International Association of Pediatric Dentistry (IAPD) caries care pathway, American Academy of Pediatric Dentistry (AAPD), Caries Management by Risk Assessment (CAMBRA), and The International Caries Classification and Management System (ICCMS™)

Low risk	Moderate	High risk
Clinical indicators Child has no caries. No new lesions in 1 year. No white spot lesions.	*Clinical indicators* Child has/had 1 or more lesions. 1 or more new lesions/year. Infrequent white spot lesions. Deep pits and fissures. Orthodontic appliances. Child with visible plaque.	*Clinical indicators* Child has/had 1 or more proximal lesions. More than 2 new lesions/year. Multiple white spot lesions. Child has heavy plaque on teeth. Child presents with dental enamel defects. Patient has low salivary flow. Recent restorations in the last 2 years (new patient) or the last year (patient of record). New cavities or lesions into dentin (radiographically).
General indicators Child has teeth brushed daily with fluoridated toothpaste. Child receives topical fluoride from health professional. Presence of background fluoride exposure. Child has dental home/ regular dental care. High socioeconomic status (SES).	*General indicators* Child has special health care needs. Middle SES.	*General indicators* Mother/primary caregivers have active dental caries. Child has frequent exposure (>3 times/day) between-meal sugar-containing snacks or beverages per day. Child uses bottle or non-spill cup containing natural or added sugar frequently, between meals and/or at bedtime. Low SES.

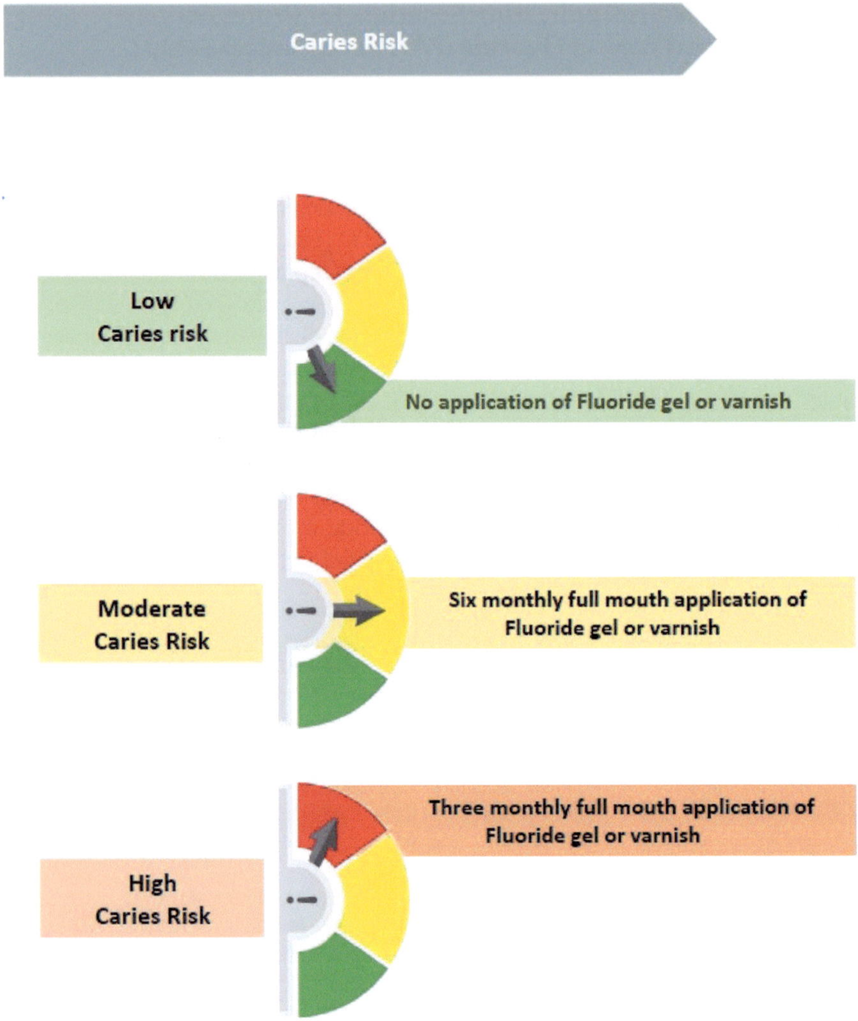

Fig. 2.2 Recommended schedule for fluoride application based on the child's caries risk status

applications in moderate and high-risk populations [21]. Health-oriented organizations such as the Centre for Disease Control (CDC), American Association of Pediatrics (AAP), and the US Preventive Task Force Services recommend that primary care clinicians apply fluoride varnish to infants and children starting at the age of first tooth emergence in low- and high-risk categories [22, 23]. A 3- to 6-monthly fluoride varnish application is advised for the low caries risk and a 3-monthly application is advised for the high caries risk group that also includes the moderate risk group (Fig. 2.2). There may be advantages of biannual fluoride applications even in low-risk populations in areas, where there is high caries prevalence and access to systemic fluoride is limited.

2.2.4 Technique of Fluoride Application

Gel Application

5 ml (1/3rd of tray volume) of APF gel should be dispensed in two Styrofoam disposable trays, which can be placed simultaneously in the maxillary and mandibular arches. The trays are available in different sizes and the selected tray must not extend posteriorly beyond the teeth as it stimulates the gag reflex. The patient is asked to bite on the trays to take advantage of the thixotropic nature of the gel, which will cause it to flow into the proximal contact areas due to the masticatory load. A saliva ejector should be placed inside the oral cavity and the patient seated upright during application to reduce swallowing of the fluoride gel. Leave the gel in contact with the teeth for 4 min. On completion, remove the trays and instruct patients to expectorate the excess gel. The child is instructed to refrain from consumption of food and water for an hour after application [15].

Varnish Application

Perform quadrant wise isolation with cotton rolls and saliva ejector and air dry the teeth. Apply a thin layer of fluoride varnish on the tooth surfaces with a disposable brush or applicator tip. Varnish can be applied in the interproximal areas with help of an interdental floss (Fig. 2.3). The teeth need to be isolated and kept dry only till the varnish is being applied as it sets on contact with saliva. A full mouth application should take 3–4 min. The correct dosages for fluoride varnish application in children with only deciduous dentition is 0.25 ml. For children with mixed dentition, it is 0.4 ml. For permanent dentition, 0.5 ml is recommended [24].

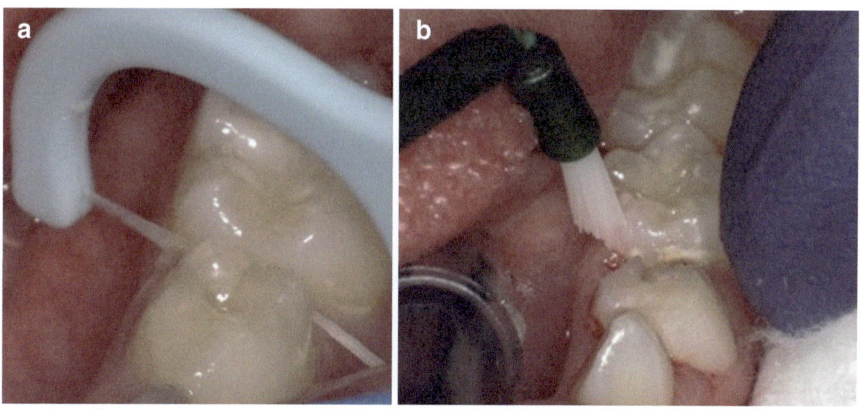

Fig. 2.3 Interproximal application of fluoride varnish with dental floss (**a**) and interpoximal brush (**b**)

2.2.5 What Are Post Application Instructions for Gels and Varnish?

Patients should avoid eating and drinking for 1 h post application as the action of fluoride is seen to reach its peak at that time. They should be advised to rinse prior to consuming any food or water to remove excess varnish and improve taste. To allow for the varnish to adhere to the tooth surface, the patient is advised to eat a soft semisolid diet and avoid brushing for 8 h post application [24].

2.2.6 Is Oral Prophylaxis Recommended Prior to Fluoride Application?

The mechanism of fluoride uptake from varnishes or gels is unaffected by the presence of organic integuments. A professional prophylaxis is not mandatory before every varnish or gel application unless a significant amount of visible plaque and calculus is seen that would interfere with the fluoride exchange between the source and enamel surface [25, 26]. Below is the list of different brands of varnish and the manufacturer's recommendations for the protocol to be followed for isolation (Table 2.3).

2.2.7 Fluoride Gels or Varnish?

Fluoride gels may cause nausea or gagging and may be less acceptable among children due to the bitter taste. Fluoride varnishes are safer to use in the younger age groups due to their adherent nature, whereas gels have a higher chance of ingestion

Table 2.3 Categorization of commercially available fluoride varnishes based on the amount of moisture control and isolation recommended by manufacturers during application

Isolation and moisture control required	Minimal isolation and application in the presence of moisture
Colgate duraphat®	3 M Vanish white varnish™
Colgate Prevident varnish®	Fluorimax® varnish
Fluorprotector	
Voco profluorid	
Duraflor®	
3 M Fast release varnish™	
NUPRO white Varnish®	
Enamelast™	
Enamel Pro Varnish®	
Kolorz ClearShield Varnish®	
Acclean Varnish®	
Vella Varnish®	

These commercial products have been listed after visiting the manufacturers' websites on 7th May 2025. The availability of these products may vary across different regions

Table 2.4 Age-wise recommendations by international dental organizations on application of fluoride varnish and gel

American Academy of Pediatric Dentistry (AAPD) [18]	Unit dose of only 5% NaF varnish for children below 6 years. Above 6 years, 5% NaF varnish or 1.23% APF gel recommended.
European Academy of Pediatric Dentistry (EAPD) [28]	5% NaF varnish can be used in preschool children and older age groups.
International Association of Pediatric Dentistry (IAPD) [17]	5% NaF varnish and 1.23% APF gels can be used for children of any age at risk of dental caries.
Scottish Dental Clinical Effectiveness Program (SDCEP) [29]	5% NaF varnish recommended for children aged 2 years and above.

during application. On the other hand, the tooth discoloration, stickiness, and the remnants of the varnish can be a deterrent to some children. The efficacy of caries prevention for both, gels and varnishes, are similar [27] and the decision to choose between the two depends on the operator's preference and age of the child (Table 2.4) [12].

2.2.8 Should an Intensive Fluoride Regimen Be Performed in Children?

Certain studies have recommended different intensive fluoride regimens in children, which are as follows:

1. Three fluoride varnish applications within 2 weeks [30]
2. Three weekly applications of fluoride varnish [31]
3. Three fluoride varnish applications within 2 weeks and additional applications at 1 and 3 months [32]
4. Three applications within a week (after every 2 days) [33]
5. Three applications of fluoride at an interval of 2 weeks each [34]

Presently, there is limited evidence to support an intensive fluoride regimen in children. This approach has been employed empirically on decalcified white spot lesions where visible signs of remineralization have been appreciated (Fig. 2.4) [35, 36]. Anticipatory guidance reinforced at the frequent dental visits may also have improved the home care regimen facilitating remineralization.

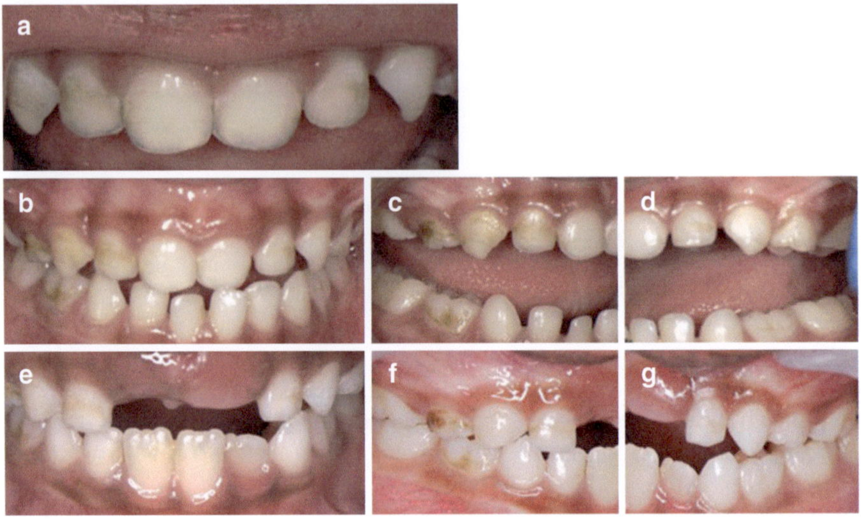

Fig. 2.4 Initial stage lesions on the labial surfaces of maxillary anterior teeth. High-intensity fluoride regimen was initiated once a week for three weeks and followed by three monthly fluoride varnish application (**a**). One-year follow-up showed signs of remineralization of the initial stage lesions on the primary maxillary incisors and primary molars. Fluoride varnish application was continued once in three months (**b–d**). The two-year follow-up shows further remineralization and non-progression of the initial stage lesions (**e–g**). (Image Courtesy: Dr Manini Shah, India)

2.3 Silver Diamine Fluoride: Recommendations and Technique

The use of silver compounds to treat carious lesions dates to the 1800s. Modern-day commercially available Silver Diamine Fluoride (SDF), which evolved from these compounds was pioneered by Drs Nishino and Yamaga in Japan in 1970. It was first marketed as "Saforide" [37, 38]. In the last decade, there has been renewed global interest in the use of SDF, an inexpensive, alkaline, caries-arresting liquid that combines the antimicrobial properties of silver and the remineralizing properties of fluoride (Fig. 2.5). In 2014, the US Food and Drug Administration (FDA) approved the use of SDF as a desensitizing agent [39]. While the manufacturer's instructions are limited to its use as a dentin desensitizer in adults, a document published by the American Academy of Pediatric Dentistry (AAPD) on SDF recommends the off-label adoption of this solution for caries arrest, much as fluoride varnish is used for caries prevention [40].

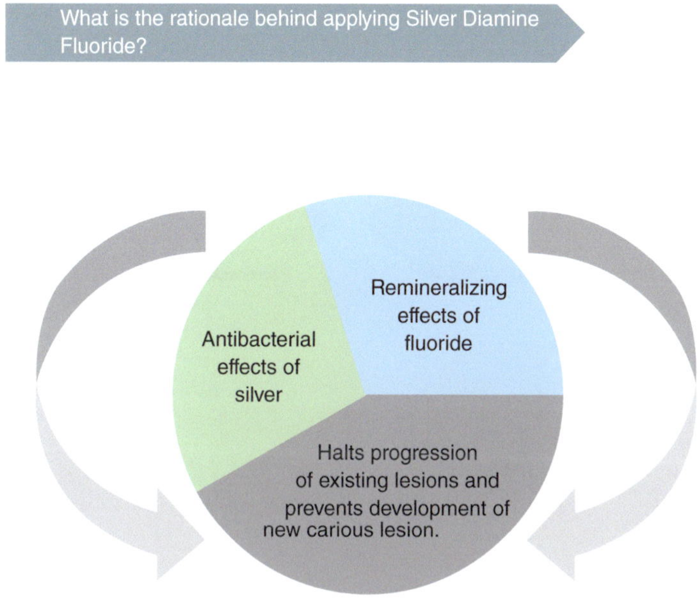

Fig. 2.5 Rationale behind application of Silver Diamine Fluoride (SDF)

2.3.1 What Is the Rationale Behind Applying SDF?

2.3.2 How Does SDF Work?

The dead bacteria in the superficial layers act as a conduit for carrying the silver ions to living bacteria in the deeper layers, effectively killing them too (Fig. 2.6). This is known as the "zombie effect." In addition, silver phosphate complexes with the organic components of the tooth penetrating much deeper into dentin (150 μm) as compared to enamel (30 μm). Consequently, a higher arrest rate is seen in dentinal lesions with SDF applications [37].

2.3.3 What Is the Composition of Silver Diamine Fluoride?

Silver Diamine Fluoride with concentration ranging between 12% and 55% are available globally (Tables 2.5 and 2.6). A 38% solution of SDF (44,800 ppm of fluoride) has been proven to better inhibit collagenase activity and degradation of dentin compared to the lower concentration solutions [41–43]. 38% SDF is also available in gel form enclosed in unit dose ampoules that make material handling easier for the clinician.

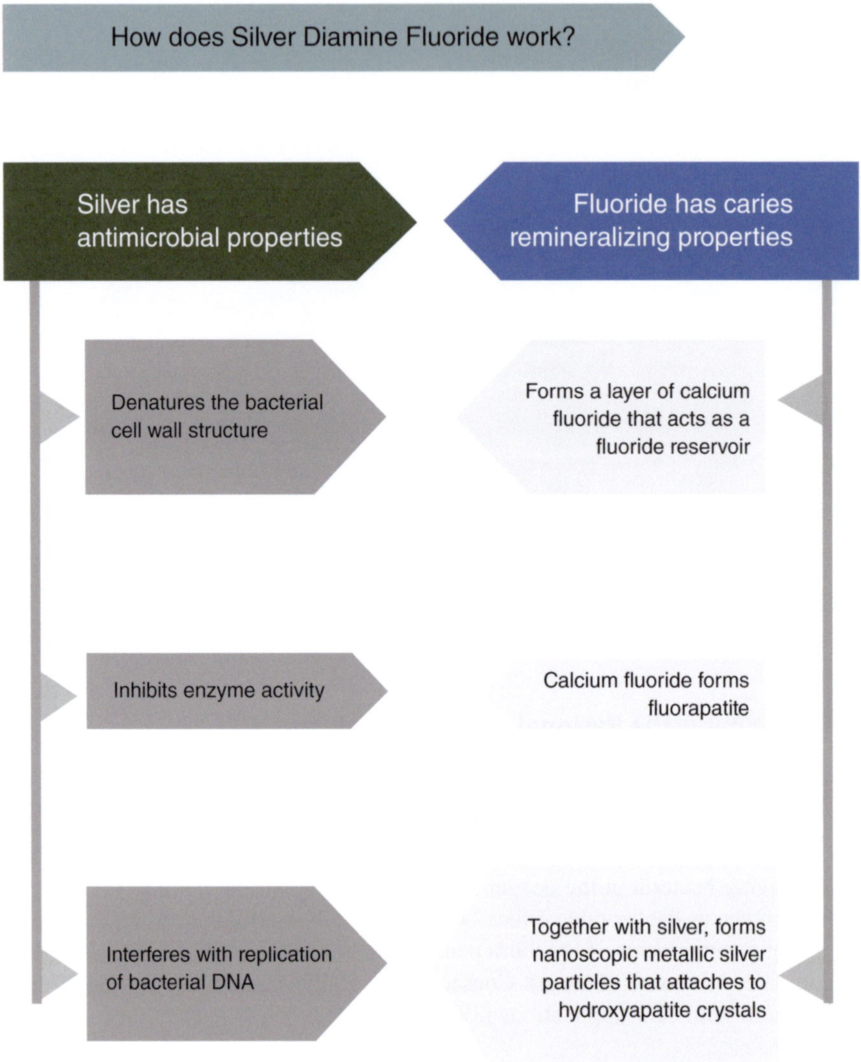

Fig. 2.6 Mechanism of action of Silver Diamine Fluoride in arresting caries progression

Table 2.5 Composition of Silver Diamine Fluoride (SDF)

24%–27%	Silver
7.5%–11%	Ammonia
5%–6%	Fluoride (approximately 44,800 ppm)
<62.5%	Deionized water

Table 2.6 Commercial formulations of Silver Diamine Fluoride

Concentration	Product	Manufacturer	Country
38%	Advantage Arrest™	Elevate Oralcare	USA
38	Riva Star	SDI	Australia
38%	Kids-e-SDF®	Kids-e-Dental	India
38%	FAgamin®	Tedequim	Argentina
10%	Cariostatic	Inodon Laborotório	Brazil
12%	SDF	PROBEM Laboratório de Produtos Farmacêuticos Odontológicos	Brazil
30%	Cariestop	Biodinâmica	Brazil
38%	Saforide	Bee Brand Medical/Toyo Seiyaku Kasei	Japan
38%	Topamine	DentaLife	Australia
38%	Advantage Arrest® Gel	Elevate Oralcare	USA
38%	Kedo SDF Gel	Kedo Dental	India
38%	NuNamel™	NuSmile	USA

These commercial products have been listed after visiting the manufacturers' websites on 7th May 2025. The availability of these products may vary across different regions

2.3.4 When Are Silver Diamine Fluoride Applications Indicated?

SDF acts as an interim caries-arresting medicament and preserves tooth vitality till sequential definitive treatment is rendered. It can be applied in a child with multiple carious lesions that cannot be treated in a single visit. It can also be performed on carious lesions in children displaying behavioral challenges and, in those with special healthcare needs who may not cooperate for invasive procedures and in whom the risks of general anesthesia outweigh the benefits. It forms a component of Non Restorative Cavity Control (NRCC) and Silver Modified Atraumatic Restorative Technique (SMART). While the AAPD recommends the use of 38% SDF for arresting only cavitated carious lesions [44, 45], the International Association of Pediatric Dentistry (IAPD) recommends application of 38% SDF for both, cavitated and non-cavitated carious lesions [46].

2.3.5 When Should Silver Diamine Fluoride Not Be Applied?

SDF should not be applied in extensive carious lesions, where the patient history, the clinical or radiographic appearance of the tooth indicates the presence of a pulpal exposure or signs of irreversible pulpitis. It should be avoided in patients with oral mucositis, desquamative gingivitis, apthous ulcers, ulcerative gingival lesions as SDF may exacerbate the existing lesions. SDF should not be applied in individuals reporting a history of true silver allergy [45].

2.3.6 Application Technique

While selecting lesions for SDF application, ensure they are accessible with a microbrush. Orthodontic separators may be used to gain access to proximal lesions. Alternatively, interdental or expandable floss (Oral B superfloss, G.U.M® expanding floss) can be used to apply SDF in these areas (Fig. 2.7). The gross debris should be removed and minimal caries excavation can be performed. The soft tissues (lip, labial mucosa, gingiva) and perioral region are protected with petroleum jelly and the tooth isolated with cotton rolls and/or saliva ejector. A drop of SDF is taken on a microbrush and the excess is dabbed. 1 drop is effective for up to 5 teeth. SDF is scrubbed into the lesion for a 1 min followed by air drying for 3 min. The child is recalled after 1 week to check the color of the lesion. The lesion color should have changed to dark brown or black and must be leathery (Fig. 2.8). If desired results are not obtained, the procedure is repeated. If the presence of debris and plaque is seen due to the retentive nature of the lesion, place a Glass Ionomer Cement (GIC) restoration and if the lesion is self-cleansing, repeat SDF as per guidelines [44, 45].

2.3.7 How Frequently Should Silver Diamine Fluoride Be Applied?

It is recommended to perform biannual applications of SDF to sustain the caries arrest rate. The AAPD has given a few recommendations, which are outlined below:

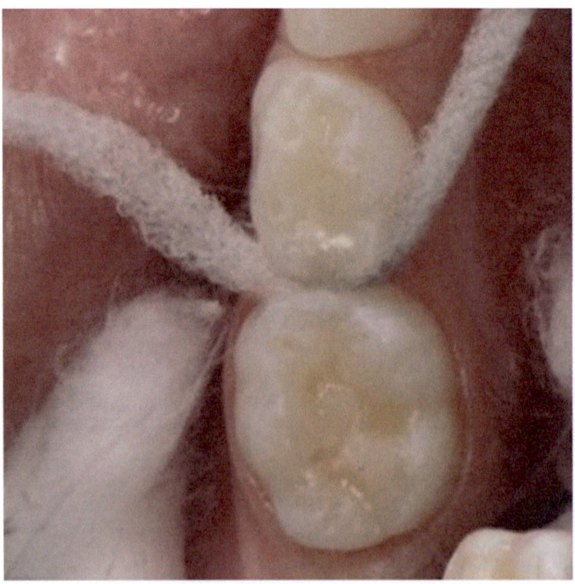

Fig. 2.7 38% SDF applied interproximally with superfloss. (Image Courtesy: Dr Abhishek Soni, India)

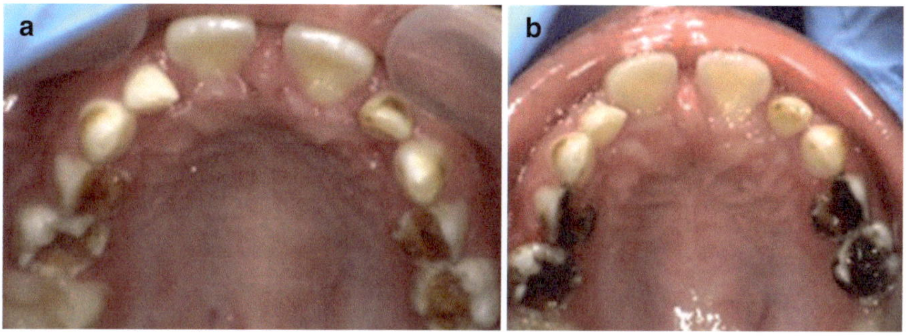

Fig. 2.8 Carious lesions on occlusal surfaces of primary maxillary molars (**a**). SDF was applied as an interim measure. Caries arrest seen and patient recalled for restorations (**b**). (Image Courtesy: Dr Manini Shah, India)

A. First application at baseline followed by next application after 3 months. Thereafter, apply SDF every 6 months for 2 years.
B. In patients at high risk, AAPD recommends application of SDF and fluoride varnish alternately every 3 months to bolster the preventive effects [44].

2.3.8 Favorable Results After Silver Diamine Fluoride Application

1. *Color of lesion*: SDF tends to discolor soft dentin more than normal healthy dentin. Likewise, partially excavated dentin will discolor lesser than unexcavated lesions. The color of lesion may appear brown to black and this change may take 24 h to 7 days (Figs. 2.8b and 2.9c, d).
2. *Consistency of lesion*: During follow-up appointment, the dentin ideally must feel leathery to firm. Though the dentin may still flake and yield under the pressure of a spoon excavator, this does not necessitate reapplication, particularly if the lesion appears not to have progressed or appears inactive.
3. *Oral hygiene status*: There should be minimal debris and visible plaque in and around the lesion as this dictates success and therefore, maintenance of oral hygiene must be reinforced at every follow-up. Lesions with visible plaque and retentive areas are less likely to arrest and need to be restored as soon as possible (Fig. 2.10) [47].

While the immediate discoloration due to SDF mimics an arrested carious lesion, the actual hardening and lesion arrest is seen over time with quarterly and biannual SDF application, in combination with maintenance of good oral hygiene that reduces biofilm formation (Fig. 2.9).

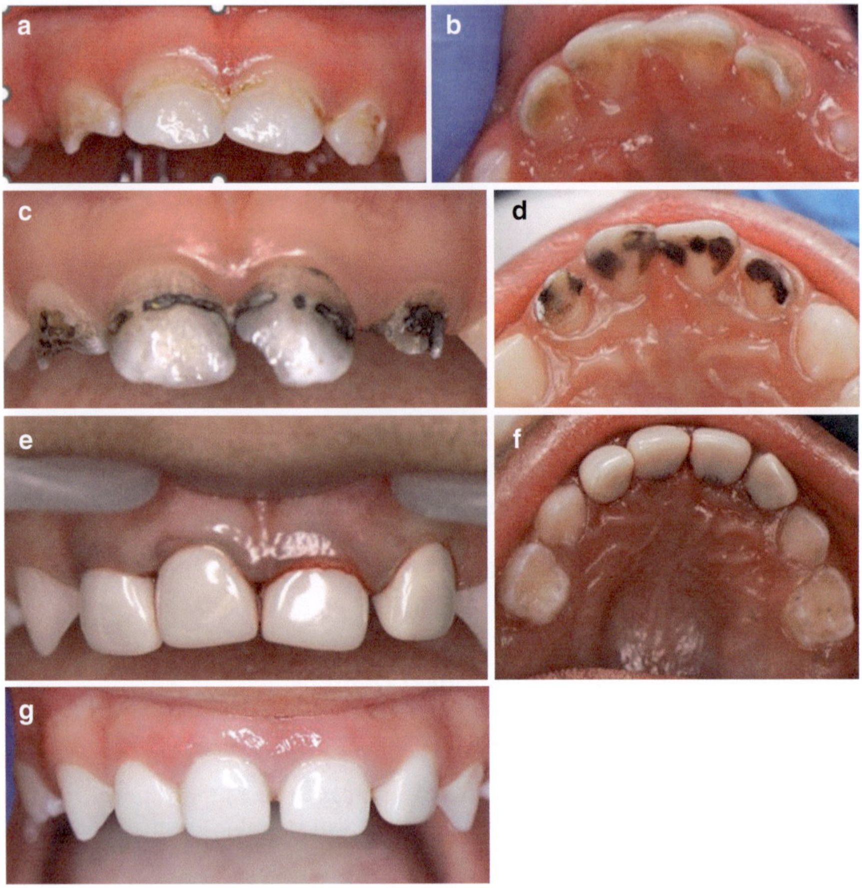

Fig. 2.9 Carious lesions on the labial and palatal surfaces of maxillary anterior teeth in a 14-month pre-co-operative child. SDF application was advised biannually (**a**, **b**). At the six-month follow-up, caries arrest seen in labial and palatal view (**c**, **d**). Zirconia crowns placed at age 2.5 years, to restore aesthetics and function (**e**, **f**). Two-year follow-up shows good gingival health and aesthetics (**g**)

2.3.9 Adverse Effects of SDF?

The most common adverse effect is brown to black staining of the carious lesion due to precipitation of silver phosphate and silver sulphide. This is more limiting when applied on carious anterior teeth. Excavating the carious lesion as much as possible would help in reducing the extent of discoloration and the overall unesthetic appearance. The application of saturated solution of potassium iodide as a separate preparation following SDF application has also been suggested. Studies assessing the efficacy of potassium iodide were mostly in vitro and short term and

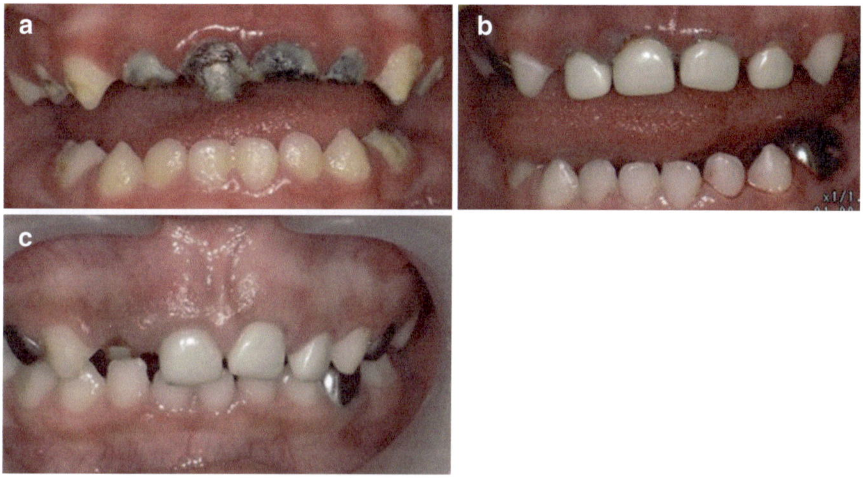

Fig. 2.10 Plaque deposits on the labial surface of SDF applied maxillary anterior teeth causing caries progression (**a**). Child was treated under general anesthesia, and anterior zirconia crowns (NuSmile® ZR, USA) were placed which successfully masked the SDF (**b**). Two-year follow-up showing good gingival health and improved oral hygiene. Remineralization of white spot lesion on the maxillary right canine. Loss of preformed zirconia crown from the maxillary right lateral incisor shows arrested dentin and an intact post-endodontic restoration (**c**)

carried out before restoring the tooth. Currently, the views on potassium iodide (KI) reducing long-term staining are inconclusive [48].

While staining of the tooth with SDF application is expected, inadvertent staining of oral and perioral tissues of the patient must be avoided by coating the oral mucosa and lips with petroleum jelly. Accidental staining of oral mucosa appears like a "henna tattoo." It disappears within 48–72 h owing to the turnover rate of oral mucosal cells. However, SDF stains on the skin may take between 7 and 14 days to disappear. Any SDF stain appearing on clothes will be permanent. Gingival inflammation, gingival pain, and erosion are transient uncommon findings which disappear within 48 h [49, 50].

2.3.10 How Effective Is Silver Diamine Fluoride?

Primary anterior teeth treated with 38% SDF solution has demonstrated caries arrest rate around 77% after a 6 to 30 months follow-up [51]. Anterior teeth have a higher chance of caries arrest than posterior teeth. Children with visible plaque and non-self-cleansing lesions had lesser likelihood of caries arrest [52]. An increased frequency of SDF application according to the above protocols and placing a restoration to prevent plaque accumulation in retentive lesions will ensure caries arrest.

2.3.11 Silver Diamine Fluoride in Molar Incisor Hypomineralization (MIH)

The treatment of MIH-affected teeth remains a clinical challenge for practitioners due to the fragile tooth structure and the hypersensitivity experienced by patients. Recent evidence recommends the use of SDF as a desensitizing application to relieve hypersensitivity in hypomineralized molars (Fig. 2.11). Depending on the severity of MIH, SDF application alone or prior to a restoration is a viable treatment alternative. SDF helps reduce sensitivity, arrests the caries process, and possibly remineralize early lesions. The use of SDF in MIH-affected teeth has the potential to improve treatment outcomes in terms of both clinical success and patient satisfaction [53].

2.3.12 Response of Pulp Dentin Complex to SDF

When SDF is applied to moderately cavitated lesions, the response of the pulp dentin complex was seen to be favorable with deposition of tertiary dentin and a mild inflammatory reaction localized to the subodontoblastic region. At present, there is insubstantial evidence of a similar favorable pulpal response in deep carious lesions approaching the pulp.

In cases, where SDF is accidentally applied on an exposed pulp, there are concerns regarding fluoride toxicity, due to the high fluoride content present in it. However, studies conducted are inconclusive regarding the passage of fluoride ions from pulpal to systemic circulation. SDF should not be applied on pulpally exposed teeth and those lesions approaching the pulp, where a clear band of dentin is not seen on the radiograph [54].

2.3.13 Can SDF Be Light-Cured?

There may be some benefits to light curing the SDF after application on the tooth. Light curing oxidizes the SDF, inducing silver ion precipitation out of the solution. This improves the binding of silver ions with oxygen, phosphorus, and sulfur groups to form silver oxide, silver phosphate, and silver sulfide. While the silver ions stay superficially in the infected dentin and penetrate lesser into the deeper layers, the silver sulfide increases the hardness of the dentin under a carious lesion. This may be considered as a favorable outcome [55]. On the downside, it results in blackish discoloration immediately after curing.

2.3.14 Should Fluoride Varnish Application Be Done Over the SDF?

After SDF application, the treated area can be covered with a thin layer of fluoride varnish [56]. This will create a barrier keeping the silver in contact for as long as possible and may also mask the metallic taste of SDF. While there is no scientific

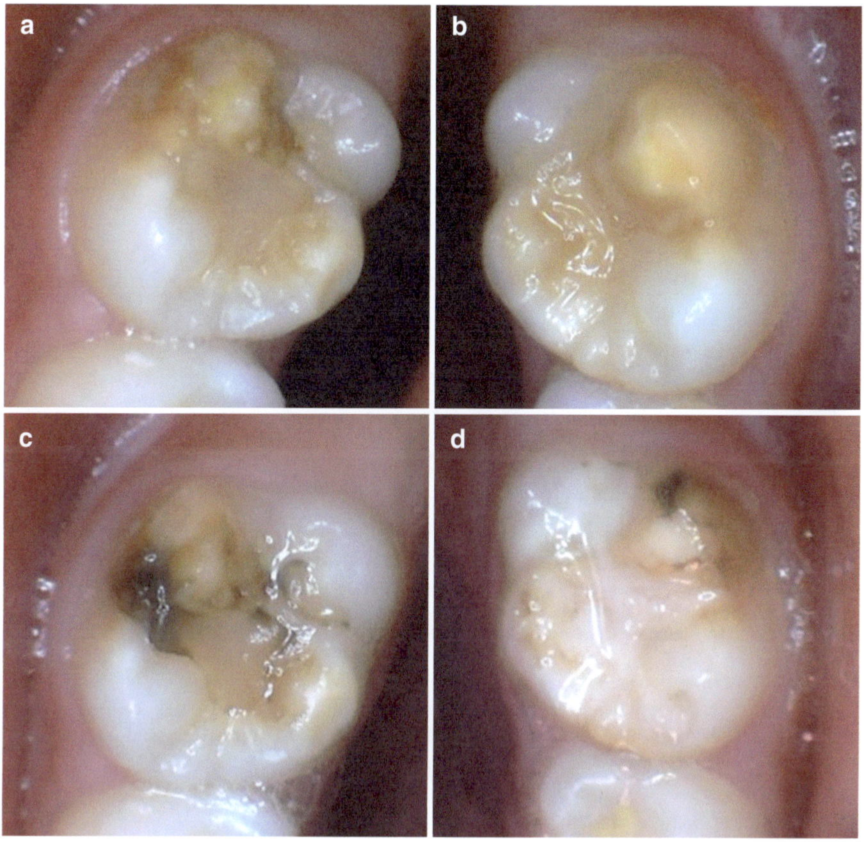

Fig. 2.11 Dentin hypersensitivity with hypomineralized maxillary permanent right and left first molars, previously restored with Glass Ionomer Cement. 38% Silver Diamine Fluoride was applied on the occlusal surface of both teeth and a pit and fissure sealant placed on the maxillary left molar (**a**, **b**). At 2 weeks, black staining seen at the hypomineralized areas. Dentin hypersensitivity had subsided (**c**, **d**)

evidence supporting augmented benefits of applying fluoride varnish over SDF during the same appointment, the AAPD recommends applying 5% sodium fluoride varnish to sites not treated by the SDF solution [41].

2.3.15 Prognosis of Teeth Treated Only by SDF Application

While the immediate benefits of SDF in causing caries arrest is firmly established, there is little evidence regarding the long-term prognosis of teeth treated purely by SDF application. Most trials at present have a follow-up of only 24–36 months. In recognition of the same, the ADA came out with a Current Dental Terminology (CDT) code D1354 that recognized SDF as an "interim caries arrest medicament" [57]. A few are of the opinion that there is no need to restore a tooth after SDF

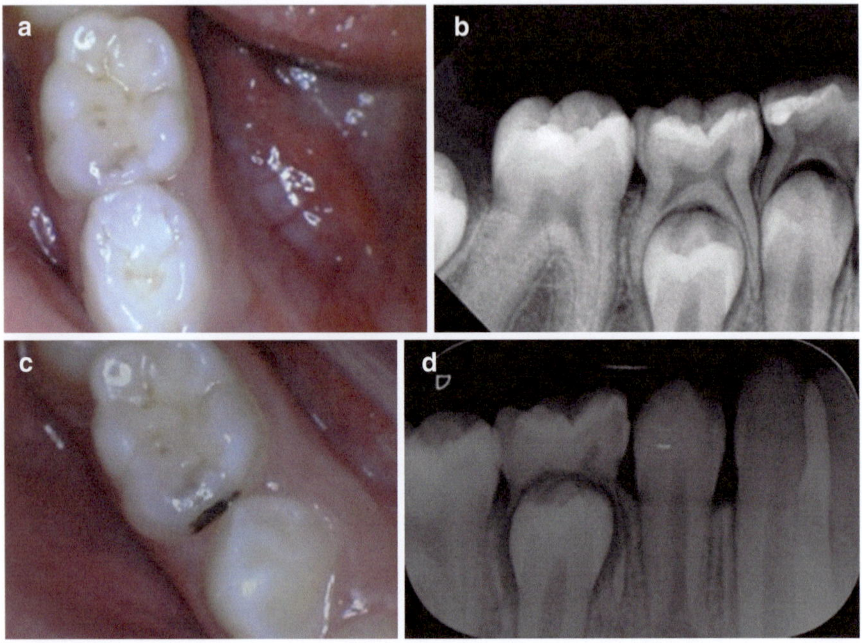

Fig. 2.12 Discoloration seen mesially in the mandibular primary right second molar (**a**). Radiograph shows radiolucency in the outer enamel. SDF applied and child recalled every 6 months (**b**). At 3-year follow-up, the lesion had not progressed clinically (**c**) and on the radiographic (**d**). (Image Courtesy: Dr Manini Shah, India)

application. However, there are no clear guidelines on the necessity of reapplying SDF beyond 2 years, or to continue SDF application till exfoliation if the decision to not restore the tooth is made (Fig. 2.12). While SDF application halts the caries process, it does not restore the tooth anatomy and function which is a requisite of good restorative dentistry.

2.3.16 Does Silver Diamine Fluoride Influence the Choice of Restoration?

Masking the black discoloration is a challenge and may show through the restoration as greyish hue. This is of greater concern in anterior teeth and hence, full coverage zirconia crowns are preferred over composites or strip crowns (Figs. 2.9 and 2.10). Studies show that the bonding of GIC to SDF is superior to resin-bonded composite systems [58]. Hence, crowns luted with a glass ionomer cement will have better retention on SDF-treated teeth as compared to bonded crowns. In posterior teeth, the type of restoration depends upon on the extent of lesion involvement. For only occlusal lesions within the confines of line angles, a glass ionomer restoration can be done. In proximal cavitated lesions or occlusal lesions involving the cusps, a full coverage restoration should be placed.

2.3.17 Chances of Toxicity with SDF

Fluoride content of SDF is 2.24 mgF/drop and the probable toxic dose for a child is 5 mgF/kg body weight. A child needing full-mouth SDF application will need 4 drops of SDF to be applied on 20 teeth. This would approximately be 9 mgF (4 drops × 2.24 mgF), well below the probable toxic dose of 50 mgF for a child weighing 10 kg (10 × 5 mgF/kg bodyweight) [39].

2.4 Pit and Fissure Sealants: Recommendations and Technique

The incorporation of topical fluorides in home care and professional preventive protocols has shown a decrease in caries prevalence. This decline was seen more with respect to smooth surface caries than occlusal caries [59, 60]. In children and adolescents, occlusal surfaces are most likely to develop caries from the time the tooth erupts. The teeth exhibiting the highest caries experience on occlusal surfaces are the first permanent molars followed by the second permanent molars [61]. This can be primarily attributed to the tooth morphology that easily retains food and harbors bacteria leading to the formation of a carious lesion. An effective way to prevent pit and fissure caries is by applying a physical barrier in the form of sealants which severs the nidus of retentive pits and fissures from the oral environment [62].

Historically, methods like prophylactic odontomy and the application of different chemicals were used to prevent pit and fissure caries. Many of these approaches were invasive in nature and had a poor long-term prognosis. The pathbreaking discovery of enamel etching by Buonocore in 1955 eventually led to the development of pit and fissure sealants, a preventive measure that has revolutionized the way we practice dentistry. The earliest sealants were composed of methyl cyanoacrylate and zinc oxide which was later replaced by Bis-glycidyl methacrylate (Bis-GMA), as it was seen to be more stable to bacterial breakdown [63]. In 1974, McLean and Wilson first reported the use of Glass Ionomer-based sealant (GI sealant) that could be successfully applied on selected teeth. The material chemically bonded to the tooth and was known for its ability to release fluoride ions [64]. Since then, resin based and glass ionomer sealants have been continuously evolving to materials with superior mechanical and chemical properties.

2.4.1 Rationale of Sealant Placement

The occlusal surfaces, particularly the pit and fissure systems of newly erupted teeth, are highly susceptible to dental caries as they possess a thinner enamel with a relatively higher organic content and increased permeability, which make them vulnerable to demineralization (Fig. 2.13a). Also, they show the presence of deep, narrow, and tortuous pit and fissure morphology that provides an environment conducive to plaque retention and bacterial proliferation. The above-mentioned factors

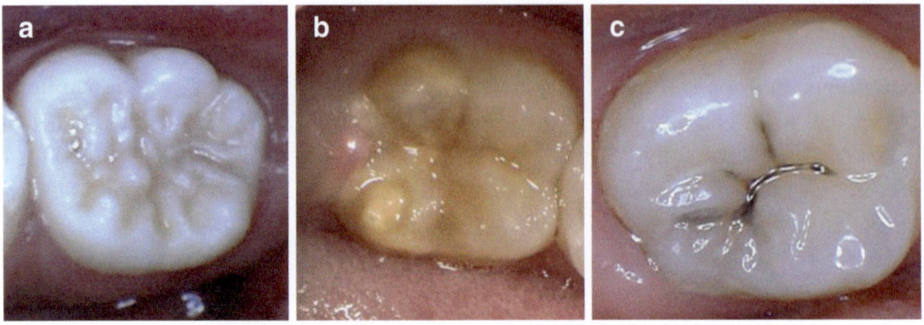

Fig. 2.13 Caries susceptible fissures in mandibular permanent first molar (**a**). Erupting hypomineralized molar (**b**). Stained fissures in mandibular primary second molar (**c**)

coupled with the prolonged eruption periods of the permanent molars may cause dental plaque to mature undisturbed in these deep pits and fissures [65]. Hence, targeting preventive efforts at the occlusal surfaces of molars with fissure sealants is appropriate for attempting to decrease the caries experience.

2.4.2 Clinical Decision for Sealant Placement

Sealants can be placed on

1. All healthy permanent molars and premolars irrespective of the individual's caries risk.
2. On permanent molars and premolars showing developmental defects such as hypoplasia (Fig. 2.13b).
3. On susceptible lingual/palatal fissures present on the permanent incisors.
4. On healthy primary molars in children with a high caries risk.
5. On primary molars exhibiting stained fissures (Fig. 2.13c).
6. On initial-stage lesions in both permanent and primary molars.

There are no absolute contraindications for the placement of dental sealants. Resin sealant placement on partially erupted teeth must be avoided, as moisture control and placement of sealant under the operculum is difficult. The clinician must defer sealant placement until the entire occlusal surface of the tooth is completely exposed [66]. Conversely, the presence of an operculum on partially erupted teeth may encourage food lodgment and increase caries risk. In such cases, glass ionomer sealants can be placed in actively erupting molars and premolars, when they present with white spot lesions or developmental enamel defects. While placing sealants on partially erupted teeth, the clinician must ensure that the sealant which extends below the operculum should be flush with the tooth surface. Once the tooth has erupted, a sealant must be placed in the remaining unsealed fissures.

2.4.3 Sealant Placement Based on Caries Risk Assessment (CRA)

There are some variations among the recommendations given by internationally validated Caries Risk Assessment (CRA) Systems and accredited dental organizations regarding the same, which have been outlined below (Tables 2.7 and 2.8).

Considering that a number of organizations are in favor of sealing teeth even in children who have a low caries risk status, clinicians should consider placing sealants on all permanent molars soon after eruption. Sealants should be placed on the primary molars of children who are susceptible to caries (i.e. those with a history of caries) or show the presence of stained fissures.

2.4.4 Composition and Classification of Sealants

The sealant materials used in contemporary pediatric dental practice are predominantly resin sealants (Table 2.9) and Glass Ionomer (GI) sealants (Table 2.10). A major difference between them is the nature of their bonding to the tooth enamel. Resin sealants form a micromechanical bond with the tooth, while GI sealants form a chemical bond with it. At present, GI sealants and a few resin sealants release fluoride [73]. The fluoride released by a resin sealant is lesser than that of a GI sealant. Also, GI sealants have better fluoride recharging ability than resin sealants [74].

The generic formulation of a resin sealant shows the presence of different multifunctional monomers such as urethane trimethyl acrylate and a light cure initiator system based on camphorquinone. With respect to the filler content, both filled (Filler content—up to 58%) and unfilled sealants are currently available. Filler particles increase sealant viscosity and metal oxides impart color to the material. GI

Table 2.7 Sealant recommendations by validated CRA systems

Sr no	Age	Recommendations
CAMBRA [67, 68]		
1	0–5 years	It is recommended to seal deep pits and fissures after 2 years of age with high fluoride conventional glass ionomer cements in children having moderate, high, or extreme high risk of dental caries. Sealant placement can be optional in patients having low caries risk.
2	6 years and older	It is recommended to seal all teeth in those children having high or extreme high caries risk status. While in children with moderate caries risk, it is recommended only on those teeth showing a distinct visual change on examination with or without air drying. Sealant placement is optional in children with low caries risk.
CRA [69]		
Studies report unfavorable cost–benefit ratios for sealant placement in children with low caries risk. Expert opinion is in favor of sealant placement in permanent molars even in low caries risk. The decision to seal primary and permanent molars should take the individual level and tooth level risk into account.		

Table 2.8 Recommendations on sealant placement by International Dental Organizations

Sr no	Organization	Recommendations
1	AAPD/American Dental Association (ADA) [70, 71]	Recommends the use of sealants in primary and permanent molars with both sound occlusal surfaces and non-cavitated occlusal carious lesions in children and adolescents.
2	EAPD/United Kingdom(UK) National Guidelines [72]	Recommends sealing of all susceptible pits and fissures in: Special needs patients Children with caries in the primary dentition Children having even one carious permanent molar Children with individual tooth characteristics such as deep fissures or hypoplastic molars
3	IAPD Care Pathway [17]	Sealant placement is recommended in all children irrespective of their caries risk status.
4.	SDCEP [29]	Recommends sealing of all permanent molars in children at an increased risk of caries. Also recommends sealing second primary molars, premolars, and palatal fissures of permanent lateral incisors.

Table 2.9 Commercially available resin-based sealants

Product	Manufacturer	Filled/ unfilled	Fluoride releasing	Clear/ opaque/ other	BPA free	Country
Conseal F pit and fissure sealant	SDI	Filled (7% submicron 0.04 microns)	Yes	Clear, light gray, opaque	Yes	Australia
Beautisealant	Shofu	S-PRG fillers Self-etch	Yes	Opaque	Yes HEMA free	USA
Helioseal®	Ivoclar Vivadent					Liechtenstein
Helioseal® Clear	Ivoclar Vivadent					Liechtenstein
Helioseal® F plus	Ivoclar Vivadent	Filled	Yes	White-pigmented	Yes	Liechtenstein
Clinpro sealant™	3 M ESPE	Unfilled	Yes	Opaque	Yes	USA
Fissurit F	Voco		Yes	Opaque	No	Germany
Fissurit FX	Voco	Filled (55% micro fillers)	No	Clear	No	Germany
Grandio Seal	Voco	Filled (70% nano fillers)	Yes	Opaque	No	Germany
Delton sealant®	Dentsply Sirona	Unfilled	Yes	White	No	USA
Biocoat®	Premier	Filled bioactive	Yes	Opaque	Yes	USA
Embrace wetbond™	Pulpdent	Hydrophilic	Yes	Off white and natural shade	Yes	USA
Ultraseal XT Plus™	Ultradent	Filled (58%) Hydrophilic	Yes	Opaque, Clear, A1, A2	Yes	USA
Ultraseal XT Plus™	Ultradent	Filled (53%)	Yes	Opaque, natural	Yes	USA

These commercial products have been listed after visiting the manufacturers' websites on 7th May 2025. The availability of these products may vary across different regions

Table 2.10 Commercially available Glass Ionomer Sealants

Product	Manufacturer	Fluoride releasing	Color	Country
Fuji VII	GC	Yes	Pink and white	Japan
Fuji triage	GC	Yes	Pink and white	Japan
Fuji triage EP	GC	Yes with RECALDENT (CPP-ACP)	Pink and white	Japan
Riva protect	SDI	Along with ACP	Pink and white	Australia
Ionoseal	VOCO	Yes	White	Germany

These commercial products have been listed after visiting the manufacturers' websites on 7th May 2025. The availability of these products may vary across different regions

sealants set by an acid–base reaction between a fluoroaluminosilicate glass powder and an aqueous solution of polyacrylic acid [75].

2.4.5 Application Protocol of Resin Sealant

After cleaning the occlusal fissures with pumice/fluoride-free polishing paste and prophy brushes, the tooth must be isolated with rubber dam or saliva ejector and cotton roll. This is followed by etching of the occlusal surface with 37% phosphoric acid for 15–20 s. The etchant is washed thoroughly for 30 s followed by airdrying for 10 s. The bonding agent is then applied with a microbrush for 10 s followed by air drying for 5 secs. The bonding agent can be cured separately or co-cured later along with the sealant.

The sealant is dispensed directly from the syringe through the disposable tips and is flowed into the pits and fissures with applicator tips or explorer. A thin layer of sealant should be confined to the pits and fissures only and not extend to the cuspal inclines (Figs. 2.14 and 2.15). The excess material may be removed with an applicator tip. After checking for air bubbles, the sealant and bonding agent can be co-cured together. An explorer should be run over the cured sealant to check smoothness, presence of air bubbles, or deficient sealant. Occlusal adjustment is usually not required after sealant placement.

2.4.6 Application Protocol for GI Sealant

After cleaning the occlusal fissures with pumice/fluoride-free polishing paste and prophy brushes, the tooth must be isolated with rubber dam or saliva ejector and cotton roll. The surface is conditioned with cavity conditioner (10 s) or dentin conditioner (20 s). The tooth is washed away thoroughly for 10 s. Sealants are available as powder liquid or capsule and accordingly can be carried with an applicator tip or capsule on the tooth surface. The sealant must be flown into the pits and fissures with an explorer. Excess material may be removed with the applicator tip. Light curing is optional and should be followed according to manufacturer's instructions. The sealant is adjusted for occlusion and a protective coating (as recommended by the manufacturer) applied on the surface (Fig. 2.16).

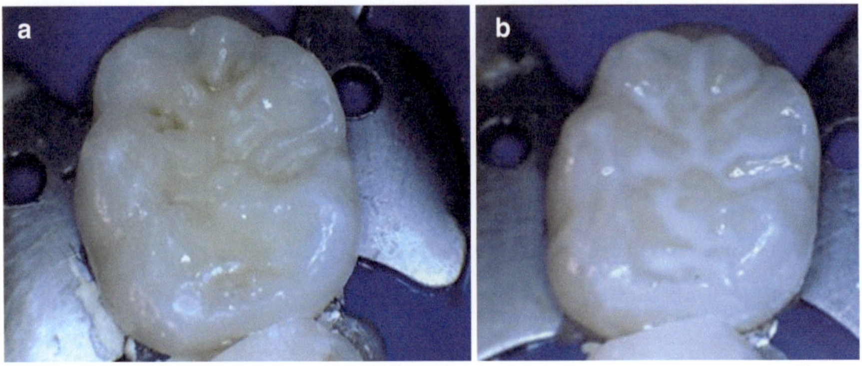

Fig. 2.14 Susceptible fissures seen on the mandibular primary right second molar, which were cleaned and prepared to receive a sealant (**a**). Pit and fissure sealant placed (**b**). (Image Courtesy: Dr Manini Shah, India)

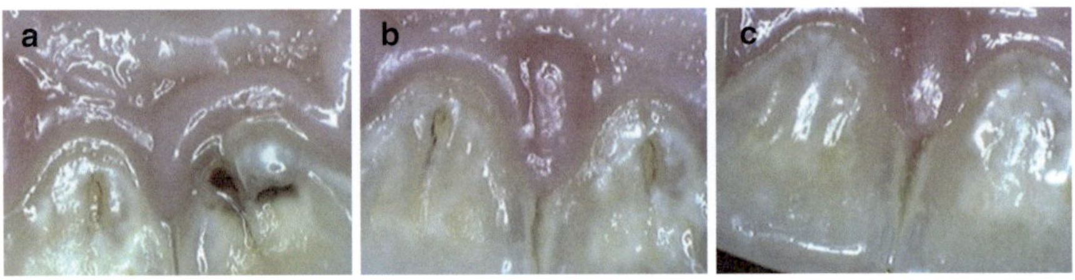

Fig. 2.15 Carious lingual fissures on the maxillary permanent incisors (**a**). Fissures prepared to receive a sealant (**b**). Pit and fissure sealant placed (**c**)

2.4.7 Post Application Instructions

Patients must be informed that the chewing surfaces of their teeth might feel hard and uneven, just after sealant placement. However, the occlusion will settle down in a few hours to a day. If GI sealants are placed, the patient should be advised to avoid eating for 2 h and maintain a soft diet for the rest of the day. Brushing and oral hygiene regimen can be resumed the same day. Parents must be informed that if a regular oral hygiene regimen is not followed, caries is likely to develop around sealants. The importance of follow-up to recognize potential loss of sealant must be stressed. Sealants usually last between 2 and 5 years. The decision to replace or repair a sealant should be taken during recall appointments.

2.4.8 Clinical Strategies that Influence Sealant Retention

2.4.8.1 Adequate Isolation and Four-Handed Dentistry

Isolation is critical to ensure proper placement of sealants and can be achieved in different ways. While the use of a rubber dam is the ideal way to achieve optimum moisture control, it may not always be possible in young children. The other commonly used methods of achieving isolation are cotton rolls, dry shield, and buccal dry pads with saliva ejector. This requires four-handed dentistry. A few studies have shown no statistical difference between the retention rates of sealants placed under rubber dam or with the use of cotton rolls and saliva ejector [76]. Another alternative to rubber dam is the Isolite system® (a hands-free vacuum suction that also allows for illumination and retraction) that provides sealant retention rates comparable to rubber dam and cotton roll–saliva ejector isolation [77]. Literature suggests that four-handed delivery, compared to two-handed delivery, increases sealant retention by 9% [78]. Thus, sealants should be placed only with the help of at least one trained dental assistant.

2.4.8.2 Pretreatment of Enamel to Improve Sealant Retention?

Though performing the acid-etch technique is a requisite for the preparation of pits and fissures before sealant application, it might not entirely be able to remove the pellicle and remaining debris from the base of the deeper fissures. An adjunctive method of tooth preparation that can be used with the acid-etch technique is enameloplasty. In this technique, the fissures are opened up using fissurotomy burs (Original, Shallow Tapered Fissure, and Narrow Tapered Fissure burs by SS White® Dental, USA) or one quarter round carbide bur with a high- or slow-speed handpiece (Fig. 2.16). This method of preparation improves enamel surface energy and penetration of sealant material. It also removes the prismless layer on newly erupted permanent teeth that can potentially influence retention of the sealant.

One major disadvantage of this technique is that if the fissurotomy bur is not used in light brush stroke motions, it can open the fissures much wider at the entrance. Besides removing sound tooth structure, it will lead to the tooth developing caries if the sealant is lost. The other methods that have been suggested for tooth preparation prior to the acid-etch technique are toothbrush prohylaxis, handpiece prophylaxis with prophy paste, air abrasion, and lasers. Toothbrush prophylaxis and use of prophy pastes can be considered in school-based or community-based sealant program where other methods are not feasible. Preparation with air abrasion and laser was seen to improve sealant retention similar to enameloplasty. However, they are not as cost-effective and easily adaptable to clinical practice as compared to

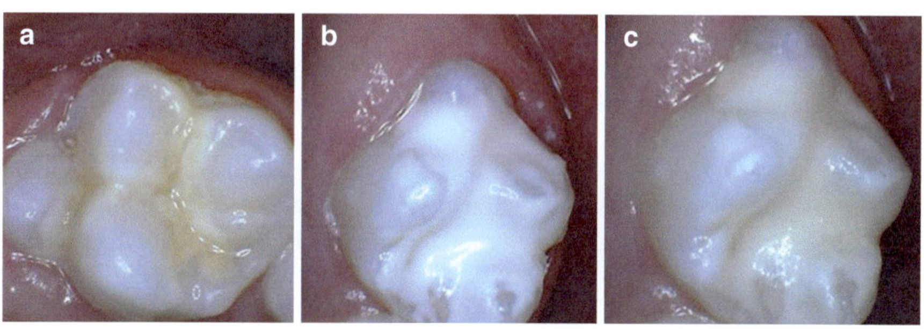

Fig. 2.16 Hypomineralized fissure on maxillary permanent left first molar (**a**). Glass Ionomer sealant placed (**b**). One-year follow-up showing good retention of the sealant (**c**)

enamleoplasty [79]. Evidence shows that the above preparation methods increase sealant retention when used in conjunction with acid etching.

2.4.8.3 Etch and Rinse Versus Self-etch?

Self-etch adhesives have reported lower enamel bond strengths compared to those obtained with 37% phosphoric acid. Total etch systems are still considered to be the gold standard when comes it to enamel bond strengths [79].

2.4.8.4 Does the Use of Bonding Agents Improve Sealant Retention?

The use of an intermediate adhesive system has been shown to enhance the retention of resin sealants. In deep fissures, the presence of moisture residue is commonly seen due to the exposure of dentinal tubules. Dentinal fluid can leach out of these tubules and may not allow the hydrophobic resin to penetrate to the bottom of the fissure. The use of a hydrophilic bonding agent can improve the wettability and penetration of the sealant even in the presence of slight moisture [80].

2.4.8.5 Filled Versus Unfilled Sealants?

Unfilled sealants can flow easily into tortuous pits and fissures owing to their consistency and low viscosity. This not only improves their penetrability but also their retention rate. Their wear resistance is lower compared to resin sealants containing fillers. These sealants do not require occlusal adjustment after sealant placement. Filled resin sealants contain filler particles up to 58% and despite their higher filler content have a viscosity low enough to penetrate pits and fissures unimpeded. Incorporation of fillers also ensures lesser polymerization shrinkage and higher wear resistance compared to unfilled sealants. These sealants may need adjustments if they interfere with occlusion. The studies comparing retention rates of unfilled and filled sealants have shown mixed results. Thus, the clinician could consider using an unfilled sealant in deep, narrow pits and fissures and prefer filled sealants in those which have wider pits and fissures [81, 82].

2.4.8.6 Hydrophobic Sealants Versus Hydrophilic Sealants?

Hydrophilic sealants are fluoride releasing, light-cure resin materials, which are claimed by manufacturers to be moisture tolerant in contrast to conventional hydrophobic sealants. While applying a hydrophilic sealant, the tooth need not be dried to appear white frosted after etching, as the area to be sealed should have slight moisture to facilitate their setting reaction. Also, manufacturers of hydrophilic sealants do not recommend the use of a bonding agent after etching and rinsing. The clinician should consider using hydrophilic sealants particularly in deeper fissures likely to have a higher residual moisture content. While these sealants are hydrophobic and can tolerate some moisture within the tooth, their integrity will be compromised if there is salivary contamination during placement. Hence, isolation measures should be optimal regardless of the type of resin sealant being placed. Presently, studies comparing hydrophilic sealants with hydrophobhic sealants have shown them to be comparable in terms of retention rates and marginal integrity [83, 84].

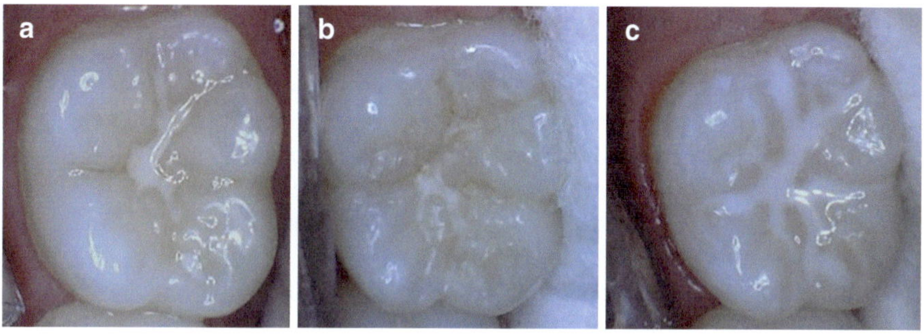

Fig. 2.17 Loss of sealant seen on mandibular permanent molar (**a**). The existing sealant was left untouched (**b**). The surrounding fissures were resealed (**c**). (Image Courtesy: Dr Manini Shah, India)

2.4.9 Comparison of Resin-Based Sealants vs GI Sealants

The clinical success of a sealant is measured by its retention rate and caries preventive effects. There is a significant difference between the retention rate of resin based (83.8%) and GI sealants (5.2%) at 5 years in permanent teeth. The mean retention rates of resin based and glass ionomer sealants in primary molars over an 18-month period were 85.94% and 23.18%, respectively.

Resin sealants are effective as they mechanically obliterate the fissures preventing the buildup of food or plaque debris. Hence, the retention of a resin sealant is critical to its caries preventive effect. The caries preventive action conferred on teeth by GI sealants is due to the fluoride release to the tooth. The chemical bond of the GI sealant prevents complete sealant loss, and a part of the sealant is seen remaining at the base of the fissures. Despite significant differences in retention rates, both materials show comparable caries preventive effects up to 4 years. Molars with partially lost resin and GI sealants were still seen to have a lower caries risk than the teeth that did not receive sealants. While the partial loss of both GI and resin sealants may confer some caries-preventive benefits on the tooth, the duration of their effect is questionable. Therefore, the decision to replace a sealant following loss should be taken based on the patient's caries risk status [85–88].

Sealants, whether partially or completely lost, must be replaced at the earliest, especially in children with high caries risk in whom maintenance of sealants will confer prolonged caries preventive effect (Fig. 2.17). The only clinical situation in which replacement of the sealant can be deferred is in patients with a low caries risk status, who have permanent molars exhibiting well, coalesced fissures that do not retain food.

2.5 Concluding Remarks

PATF remain an indispensable tool to prevent dental caries and remineralize early lesions. Among the currently marketed PATF, varnishes are recommended to a wider age group and have been shown to have better acceptability among patients.

In children showing carious lesions where dentinal involvement is present, fluoride varnish alone may not be effective and SDF applications have proven to be effective in arresting dentinal caries, particularly in primary teeth. For preventing caries on occlusal surfaces in permanent molars, sealants are an evidence-based method and should be advised in all children irrespective of their caries risk. While resin sealants have better retention than GI sealants, the latter are seen to have better caries preventive ability. Resin sealants must be placed in pits and fissures, where moisture control can be maintained. For hypomineralized molars or erupting molars, where moisture control may be suboptimal, GI sealants are advised. Regular recalls are advocated to check the integrity of previously placed sealants and ensure the child follows the recommended fluoride application schedule as per caries risk.

References

1. Kassebaum NJ, Smith AGC, Bernabé E, et al. Global, regional, and national prevalence, incidence, and disability-adjusted life years for oral conditions for 195 countries, 1990–2015: a systematic analysis for the global burden of diseases, injuries, and risk factors. J Dent Res. 2017;96(4):380–7.
2. Global burden of disease 2019. (GBD 2019) results [online database]. Seattle: Institute of Health Metrics and Evaluation(IHME); 2020. https://vizhub.healthdata.org/gbd-results/. Accessed 18 April 2024.
3. Sheiham A. Oral health, general health and quality of life. Bull World Health Organ. 2005;83:644.
4. Veiga N, Figueiredo R, Correia P, Lopes P, Couto P, Fernandes GVO. Methods of primary Clinical Prevention of dental caries in the adult patient: an integrative review. Healthcare (Basel). 2023;11(11):1635.
5. Twetman S. The evidence base for professional and self-care prevention – caries, erosion and sensitivity. BMC Oral Health. 2015;15(Suppl 1):S4.
6. Nowak AJ, Casamassimo P. Using anticipatory guidance to provide: early dental intervention. JADA. 1995;126(8):1156–63.
7. Inshiya Alazhar Contractor, Girish MS, Indira MD. Silver diamine fluoride: extending the spectrum of preventive dentistry, a literature review. Pediatr Dent J. 2021;31(1):17–24.
8. Dean HT. Distribution of mottled enamel in the United States. JADA. 1933;20(2):319–33.
9. Arnold FA, Dean HT, Singleton DE. The effect on caries incidence of a single topical application of a fluoride solution to the teeth of young adult males of a military population. JDR. 1944;23(3):155–62.
10. Lemke CW, Doherty JM, Arra MC. Controlled fluoridation: the dental effects of discontinuation in Antigo, Wisconsin. J Am Dent Assoc. 1970;80(4):782–6.
11. Hellwig E, Lennon ÁM. Systemic versus topical fluoride. Caries Res. 2004;38(3):258–62.
12. Hawkins R, Locker D, Noble J, Kay EJ, Prevention. Part 7: professionally applied topical fluorides for caries prevention. Br Dent J. 2003;195:313–7.
13. Tencate JM. Mechanistic aspects of the interactions between fluoride and dental enamel. Crit Rev Oral Biol Med. 1991;2(2):283–96.
14. Featherstone JDB. Prevention and reversal of dental caries: role of low level fluoride. Community Dent Oral Epidemol. 1999;27(1):31–40.
15. Marinho VCC, Higgins JPT, Logan S, Sheiham A. Fluoride gels for preventing dental caries in children andadolescents. Cochrane Database Syst Rev. 2002;1:CD002280.
16. Beltrán-Aguilar E, Goldstein J, Lockwood S. Fluoride varnishes: a review of their clinical use, cariostatic mechanism, efficacy and safety. JADA. 2000;131(5):589–96.

17. IAPD Foundational articles and consensus recommendations: caries risk assessment and care pathways, 2022. http://www.iapdworld.org/2022_13_caries-risk-assessment-and-care-pathways.
18. American Academy of Pediatric Dentistry. Fluoride therapy. The reference manual of pediatric dentistry. Chicago: American Academy of Pediatric Dentistry; 2020. p. 288–91.
19. Featherstone JDB, Crystal YO, Alston P, Chaffee BW, Doméjean S, Rechmann P, Zhan L, Ramos-Gomez F. Evidence-based caries management for all ages-practical guidelines. Front Oral Health. 2021;2:657518.
20. Ismail AI, Pitts NB, Tellez M, et al. The international caries classification and management system (ICCMS™) an example of a caries management pathway. BMC Oral Health. 2015;15(Suppl 1):S9.
21. Schwendicke F, Splieth CH, Thomson WM, Reda S, Stolpe M, Foster Page L. Cost effectiveness of caries-preventive fluoride varnish applications in clinic settings among patients of low, moderate and high risk. Community Dent Oral Epidemiol. 2017;46(1):8–16.
22. Final update summary: dental caries in children from birth through age 5 years: screening. U.S. Preventive Services Task Force; 2016. https://www.uspreventiveservicestaskforce.org/Page/Document/UpdateSummaryFinal/dental-caries-in-children-frombirth-through-age-5-years-screening.
23. Clark MB, Slayton RL. Section on oral health. Fluoride use in caries prevention in the primary care setting. Pediatrics. 2014;134:626–33. https://www.cdc.gov/oralhealth/basics/childrens-oral-health/index.html.
24. Miller EK, Vann WF Jr. The use of fluoride varnish in children: a critical review with treatment recommendations. J Clin Pediatr Dent. 2008;32(4):259–64.
25. Ripa LW. Need for prior tooth cleaning when performing a professional topical fluoride application: review and recommendations for change. JADA. 1984;109(2):281–5.
26. Seppa L. Effect of dental plaque on fluoride uptake by enamel from sodium fluoride varnish in vivo. Caries Res. 1983;17:71–5.
27. Marinho VC, Worthington HV, Walsh T, Clarkson JE. Fluoride varnishes for preventing dental caries in children and adolescents. Cochrane Database Syst Rev. 2013;11(7):CD002279.
28. Toumba KJ, Twetman S, Splieth C, et al. Guidelines on the use of fluoride for caries prevention in children:an updated EAPD policy document. Eur Arch Paediatr Dent. 2019;20:507–16.
29. Scottish Intercollegiate Guidelines Network: SIGN 138: dental interventions to prevent caries in children; 2014.
30. Weinstein P, Spiekerman C, Milgrom P. Randomized equivalence trial of intensive and semiannual applications of fluoride varnish in the primary dentition. Caries Res. 2009;43(6):484–90.
31. Duangthip D, Wong MCM, Chu CH, Lo ECM. Caries arrest by topical fluorides in preschool children: 30-month results. J Dent. 2018;70:74–9.
32. Paek AE, et al. Caries outcome following an intensive fluoride varnish treatment regimen for children at high risk for early childhood caries. IJPD. 2018;28(3):291–9.
33. Gugwad SC, Shah P, Lodaya R, Bhat C, Tandon P, Choudhari S, Patil S. Caries prevention effect of intensive application of sodium fluoride varnish in molars in children between age 6 and 7 years. J Contemp Dent Pract. 2011;12(6):408–41.
34. Mekky AI, Dowidar KML, Talaat DM. Casein phosphopeptide amorphous calcium phosphate fluoride varnish in remineralization of early carious lesions in primary dentition: randomized clinical trial. Pediatr Dent. 2021;43(1):17–23.
35. Lenzi TL, Montagner AF, Soares FZ, de Oliveira RR. Are topical fluorides effective for treating incipient carious lesions?: a systematic review and meta-analysis. J Am Dent Assoc. 2016;147(2):84–91.e1.
36. Gao SS, Zhang S, Mei ML, et al. Caries remineralisation and arresting effect in children by professionally applied fluoride treatment – a systematic review. BMC Oral Health. 2016;16:12.
37. Nishino M, Yoshida S, Sobue S, et al. Effect of topically applied ammoniacal silver fluoride on dental caries in children. J Osaka Univ Dent Sch. 1969;9:149–55.
38. Yamaga R, Nishino M, Yoshida S, et al. Diamine silver fluoride and its clinical application. J Osaka Unic Dent Sch. 1972;12(20):1–10.

39. Horst JA, Ellenikiotis H, Milgrom PL. UCSF protocol for caries arrest using silver diamine fluoride: rationale, indications and consent. J Calif Dent Assoc. 2016;44(1):16–28.
40. American Academy of Pediatric Dentistry. Policy on the use of silver diamine fluoride for pediatric dental patients. In: The reference manual of pediatric dentistry. Chicago: American Academy of Pediatric Dentistry; 2024. p. 104–6.
41. Gotjamanos T, Afonso F. Unacceptably high levels of fluoride in commercial preparations of silver fluoride. Aust Dent J. 1997;42:52–3.
42. Gao SS, Zhao IS, Hiraishi N, et al. Clinical trials of silver diamine fluoride in arresting caries among children: a systematicreview. JDR Clin Transl Res. 2016;1(3):201–10.
43. Fung MHT, Duangthip D, Wong MCM, et al. Randomized clinical trial of 12% and 38% silver diamine fluoride treatment. J Dent Res. 2018;97(2):171–8.
44. AAPD Clinical Practice Guideline, Crystal YO, Marghalani AA, Ureles SD, et al. Use of silver diamine fluoride for dental caries management in children and adolescents, including those with special health care needs. Pediatr Dent. 2017;39(5):E135–45.
45. Crystal YO, Marghalani AA, Ureles SD, et al. Use of silver diamine fluoride for dental caries management in children and adolescents, including those with special health care needs. Pediatr Dent. 2017;39(5):E135–45.
46. IAPD. Foundational articles and consensus recommendations: use of fluoride for caries Prevention; 2022.
47. Seifo N, Robertson M, MacLean J, et al. The use of silver diamine fluoride (SDF) in dental practice. Br Dent J. 2020;228:75–81.
48. Roberts A, Bradley J, Merkley S, Pachal T, Gopal JV, Sharma D. Does potassium iodide application following silver diamine fluoride reduce staining of tooth? A systematic review. Aust Dent J. 2020;65(2):109–17.
49. Seifo N, Cassie H, Radford JR, Innes NP. Silver diamine fluoride for managing carious lesions: an umbrella review. BMC Oral Health. 2019;19:1.
50. Duangthip D, Fung MH, Wong MC, Chu CH, Lo EC. Adverse effects of silver diamine fluoride treatment among preschool children. J Dent Res. 2018;97(4):395–401.
51. Oliveira, et al. The effect of silver diamine fluoride in preventing caries in the primary dentition: a systematic review and meta-analysis. Caries Res. 2018;53:24–32.
52. Llodra JC, Rodriguez A, Ferrer B, Menardia V, Ramos T, Morato M. Efficacy of silver diamine fluoride for caries reduction in primary teeth and first permanent molars of schoolchildren: 36-month clinical trial. J Dent Res. 2005;84(8):721–4.
53. Ballikaya E, Ünverdi GE, Cehreli ZC. Management of initial carious lesions of hypomineralized molars (MIH) with silver diamine fluoride or silver-modified atraumatic restorative treatment (SMART): 1-year results of a prospective, randomized clinical trial. Clin Oral Investig. 2022 Feb;26(2):2197–205.
54. Zaeneldin A, Yu OY, Chu CH. Effect of silver diamine fluoride on vital dental pulp: a systematic review. J Dent. 2022;119:104066.
55. Min SN, Duangthip D, Detsomboonrat P. Effects of light curing on silver diamine fluoride-treated carious lesions: a systematic review. PLoS One. 2024;19(8):e0306367.
56. Yan IG, Zheng FM, Gao SS, Duangthip D, Lo ECM, Chu CH. A review of the protocol of SDF therapy for arresting caries. Int Dent J. 2022;72(5):579–88.
57. https://www.ada.org/-/media/project/ada-organization/ada/ada-org/files/publications/cdt/d1354_guideto_v1_2017jul.pdf?rev=a#:~:text=D1354%20application%20of%20caries%20arresting,removal%20of%20sound%20tooth%20structure.
58. Fröhlich TT, Botton G, Rocha RO. Bonding of glass-ionomer cement and adhesives to silver diamine fluoride-treated dentin: an updated systematic review and meta-analysis. J Adhes Dent. 2022;24:29–38.
59. Macek MD, Beltrán-Aguilar ED, Lockwood SA, Malvitz DM. Updated comparison of the caries susceptibility of various morphological types of permanent teeth. Public Health Dent. 2003;63:174–82.

60. Wright JT, et al. Evidence-based clinical practice guideline for the use of pit-and-fissure sealants: a report of the American Dental Association and the American Academy of Pediatric Dentistry. J Am Dent Assoc. 2016;147:672–82.
61. Carvalho JC, Dige I, Machiulskiene V, Qvist V, Bakhshandeh A, Fatturi-Parolo C, Maltz M. Occlusal caries: biological approach for its diagnosis and management. Caries Res. 2016;50:527–42. https://doi.org/10.1159/000448662.
62. Simonsen RJ. Clinical applications of the acid etch technique, vol. 96. 1st ed. Hanover Park: Quintessence Publishing; 1978. Pit and Fissure Sealants. p. 977.
63. Naaman R, El-Housseiny AA, Alamoudi N. The use of pit and fissure sealants-a literature review. Dent J (Basel). 2017;5(4):34.
64. McLean JW, Wilson AD. Fissure sealing and filling with an adhesive glass ionomer cement. Br Dent J. 1974;136:136269–76.
65. Carvalho JC. Caries process on occlusal surfaces: evolving evidence and understanding. Caries Res. 2014;48:339–46.
66. Azarpazhooh A, Main PA. Pit and fissure sealants in the prevention of dental caries in children and adolescents: a systematic review. J Can Dent Assoc. 2008;74(2):171–7.
67. Ramos-Gomez FJ, Crall J, Gansky SA, Slayton RL, Featherstone JD. Caries risk assessment appropriate for the age 1 visit (infants and toddlers). J Calif Dent Assoc. 2007;35(10):687–702.
68. Featherstone JD, Domejean-Orliaguet S, Jenson L, Wolff M, Young DA. Caries risk assessment in practice for age 6 through adult. J Calif Dent Assoc. 2007;35(10):703–13.
69. American Academy of Pediatric Dentistry. Caries-risk assessment and management for infants, children, and adolescents. The reference manual of pediatric dentistry. Chicago: American Academy of Pediatric Dentistry; 2024. p. 306–12.
70. Wright JT, Crall JJ, Fontana M, et al. Evidence-based clinical practice guideline for the use of pit-and-fissure sealants. American Academy of Pediatric Dentistry, American Dental Association. Pediatr Dent. 2016;38(5):E120–E36.
71. Beauchamp J, Caufield PW, Crall JJ, Donly K, Feigal R, Gooch B, Ismail A, Kohn W, Siegal M, Simonsen R, American Dental Association Council on Scientific Affairs. Evidence-based clinical recommendations for the use of pit-and-fissure sealants: a report of the American Dental Association Council on Scientific Affairs. J Am Dent Assoc. 2008;139(3):257–68.
72. Welbury R, Raadal M, Lygidakis NA, European Academy of Paediatric Dentistry. EAPD guidelines for the use of pit and fissure sealants. Eur J Paediatr Dent. 2004;5(3):179–84.
73. Babu G, Mallikarjun S, Wilson B, Premkumar C. Pit and fissure sealants in pediatric dentistry. SRM J Res Dent Sci. 2014;5:253–7.
74. Bayrak S, Tunc ES, Aksoy A, Ertas E, Guvenc D, Ozer S. Fluoride release and recharge from different materials used as fissure sealants. Eur J Dent. 2010;4(3):245–50.
75. Bandi M, Mallineni S, Nuvvula S. Influence of isolation methods on retention of pit and fissure sealants in young permanent teeth based on simonsen's criteria: a randomised clinical trial. JCDR. 2021;15(4):ZC06–9.
76. Alhareky M, Mermelstein D, Finkelman M, Alhumaid J, Loo C. Efficiency and patient satisfaction with the Isolite system versus rubber dam for sealant placement in pediatric patients. Pediatr Dent. 2014;36:400.
77. Griffin SO, Jones K, Gray SK, Malvitz DM, Gooch BF. Exploring four-handed delivery and retention of resin-based sealants. J Am Dent Assoc. 2008;139:281–9.
78. Bagherian A, Sarraf Shirazi A. Preparation before acid etching in fissure sealant therapy: yes or no? J Am Dent Assoc. 2016;147(12):943–95.
79. Aman N, Khan FR, Salim A, Farid H. A randomized control clinical trial of fissure sealant retention: self etch adhesive versus total etch adhesive. J Conserv Dent. 2015;18:20–4.
80. Bagherian A, Sarraf Shirazi A, Sadeghi R. Adhesive systems under fissure sealants: yes or no?: a systematic review and meta-analysis. J Am Dent Assoc. 2016;147(6):446–56.
81. Bagheri E, Sarraf Shirazi A, Shekofteh K. Comparison of the success rate of filled and unfilled resin-based fissure sealants: a systematic review and meta-analysis. Front Dent. 2022;19:10.
82. Colombo S, Beretta M. Dental sealants part 3: which material? Efficiency and effectiveness. Eur J Paediatr Dent. 2018;19(3):247–9.

83. Kapoor V, Kumar A, Manjunath BC, et al. Comparative evaluation of retention and cariostatic effect of glass ionomer, hydrophobic & hydrophilic resin-based sealants: a systematic review and meta-analysis. Evid Based Dent. 2023;24:41–2.
84. https://live-pulpdent.pantheonsite.io/wp-content/uploads/2023/06/XP-EMS-IN-15w_REV-02.23.pdf. Accessed 10 May 2024.
85. Ahovuo-Saloranta A, Forss H, Walsh T, Nordblad A, Mäkelä M, Worthington HV. Pit and fissure sealants for preventing dental decay in permanent teeth. Cochrane Database Syst Rev. 2017;7(7):CD001830.
86. Kuhnisch J, Mansmann U, Heinrich-Weltzien R, Hickel R. Longevity of materials for pit and ssure sealing – results from a meta-analysis. Dent Mater. 2012;28:298–303.
87. Mickenautsch S, Yengopal V. Validity of sealant retention as surrogate for caries prevention – a systematic review. PLoS One. 2013;8:e77103.
88. Lam PPY, Sardana D, Ekambaram M, Lee GHM, Yiu CKY. Effectiveness of pit and fissure sealants for preventing and arresting occlusal caries in primary molars: a systematic review and meta-analysis. J Evid Based Dent Pract. 2020;20(2):101404.

3 Fluoride Regimes for Home Use

3.1 Introduction

The onus for preventing the occurrence of new carious lesions in children lies both on the clinician, as well as on the parents. Dental practices that schedule regular follow-up appointments, provide anticipatory guidance to parents and the child, perform three to six monthly applications of fluoride and place pit and fissure sealants are more effective in preventing dental caries in children. For continued long-term success, these clinical efforts must be complemented by a home care regime curated for the child based on their age and caries risk status. Home-use fluoride products like toothpastes, mouth rinses, and dietary supplements form an integral part of this regime. Fluoridated toothpastes and mouthrinses have a synergistic action of preventing plaque buildup due to their cleansing action and deliver fluoride ions to the enamel subsurface promoting remineralization. Dietary fluoride supplements have both systemic and topical caries preventive actions and are recommended in children residing in areas with low concentration of fluoride in water [1].

3.2 Fluoridated Toothpastes

Fluoridated toothpastes are one of the most important and cost-effective home-use fluoride delivery systems available, as they help to maintain constant low levels of fluoride in the oral environment. Since the time of their introduction, they have shown to cause substantial decrease in the global prevalence of dental caries. Their widespread use has changed the character of dental caries with there being a decrease in the number of smooth surface lesions, as topical fluoride action is more effective on these surfaces compared to occlusal lesions. An important factor determining the effectiveness of the caries preventive action of fluoridated toothpastes is the fluoride concentrations used in different formulations. It is established that a

H. Vyas et al., *Dental Caries and Traumatic Injuries in Pediatric Dentistry*,
https://doi.org/10.1007/978-3-031-98929-2_3

dose–response relationship does exist and toothpastes containing higher concentration of fluorides are more effective in preventing dental caries [2].

3.2.1 What Should Be the Ideal Concentration of Fluoride in a Toothpaste for Preventing Dental Caries?

Based on fluoride concentration, the fluoridated toothpastes can be classified as

- Low fluoride toothpastes (less than 1000 ppm fluoride, contain 450–500 ppm fluoride).
- Standard toothpastes (1000–1500 ppm fluoride).
- High fluoride toothpastes (more than 1500 ppm fluoride, contain 2000–5000 ppm fluoride).

Toothpastes containing 1450 to 1500 ppm fluoride have been shown to reduce the number of new carious lesions, as compared to toothpastes containing 1000 to 1250 ppm F. In caries-free individuals, there are no additional benefits found on using toothpastes containing fluoride between 1700 and 5000 ppm. These high-concentration fluoride toothpastes have a role to play in remineralization in individuals with white spot lesions. Most pediatric dental organizations recommend the use of an age-appropriate dose of 1000 ppm fluoridated toothpaste by children from the time of eruption of the first tooth, while toothpastes containing 1450 ppm fluoride should be given to children aged 6 years and above (Table 3.1). While there are non-fluoridated toothpastes available, the current guidelines do not mention its use in any age group [3, 4].

3.2.2 What Are the Age-Wise Recommendations for Use of Fluoridated Toothpastes in Children?

3.2.3 Fluorosis Concerns on Use of Fluoride Toothpastes

A 1000 ppm fluoride toothpaste is used to brush the child's teeth from the time of eruption of the first tooth. Young children may not spit out effectively and can ingest 80–100% of the fluoride dispensed at each brushing [10]. Consequently, toothpastes may become a significant source of ingested fluoride during the critical period of permanent tooth development [11], raising concerns on the possibility of dental fluorosis. However, the evidence associating the ingestion of fluoride toothpastes with incidence of fluorosis is weak and unreliable [4]. Additionally, high concentration fluoride toothpastes have shown fluorosis to be of a very mild grade and not aesthetically compromising [12]. To reduce ingestion of the fluoridated toothpaste, limit the amount to a "smear" or to the size of a grain of rice. The toothpaste can be squeezed into the bristles to avoid licking of the paste by the child. Parents or the caregiver should supervise the brushing till the age of 7 to ensure appropriate use of toothpaste.

Table 3.1 Recommendations by internationally accredited dental organization on the use of fluoridated toothpastes

	6 months-2 years	3–6 years	Above 7 years
International Academy of Pediatric Dentistry (IAPD) [5]	Use of a smear or rice grain size of 1000–1500 ppm fluoridated toothpaste	Use of a pea size amount of 1000–1500 ppm fluoridated toothpaste	Use of a 1000–1500 ppm fluoridated toothpaste Use of prescription-strength 1.1% NaF (0.5% F) pastes in high caries risk children
European Academy of Pediatric Dentistry (EAPD) [6]	Use of a smear or rice grain size of 500 ppm F	Use of a pea size amount of 1000 ppm F	Use of 1450 ppm fluoridated toothpaste
Scottish Dental Health Clinical Effectiveness Programme (SDCEP) [7]	Age under 3 years (smear amount) 3 years and above (pea-sized amount)		Age 10 +
	Standard risk 1000–1500 ppm F	Enhanced risk 1350–1500 ppm F	Standard risk (1000–1500 ppm F) Enhanced risk (2800 ppm F)
American Academy of Pediatric Dentistry (AAPD) [8]	Age under 3 years (smear amount/0.1 mg) 3–6 years (pea-sized amount/ 0.25 mg) Over-the-counter toothpaste approved by the American dental association that contains at least 1000 ppm F and less than 1500 ppm F		
World Health Organization (WHO) [9]	Recommends the use of 1000–1500 ppm fluoridated toothpastes		

3.2.4 Clinical Tips to Enhancing the Effectivity of Fluoridated Toothpastes

A key factor influencing the effectivity of fluoridated toothpastes is the intraoral retention of fluoride. This can be enhanced by the following evidence-based rinsing protocols, post brushing.

- *Spit, do not rinse*—Patients should be advised to spit after brushing and not to rinse with water. This will help maintain the intraoral fluoride levels. This is also a practical way to teach the child how to expectorate [13].
- *Modified toothpaste technique*—Take a sip of water (approximately 10 ml) and with the remaining toothpaste foam in the mouth, use the toothpaste slurry as a mouthrinse and filter it between the teeth by active cheek movements for 1 min before carefully spitting out [14].
- *Combining toothbrushing with the use of a Fluoride mouthrinse*—The mouthrinse can be used immediately after toothbrushing and is only advised for children who have developed spitting and swallowing reflex.
- *Avoid eating or drinking for 2 hours post brushing* as this has shown to reduce the salivary fluoride level by 12–15 times. Thus, children should be advised to brush after breakfast in the morning and after sleeping at night to enhance intraoral fluoride levels [15].

Table 3.2 Recommendations by internationally accredited dental organizations on the use of fluoride mouthrinses

	International Body	Concentration of fluoride mouthrinse	Usage frequency
1	EAPD [6]	0.05% sodium fluoride mouthrinse (225 ppm)	Twice daily
		0.2% sodium fluoride mouthrinse (900 ppm)	Weekly
2	AAPD [8]	0.09% fluoride rinse (900 ppm)	

3.3 Fluoride Mouthrinses

These are home-use topical fluorides advised to children who have a high caries risk. Fluoride mouthrinses are of two types, those which contain fluoride in the range of 100–500 ppm and those containing 900 ppm fluoride.

Based on the concentration of fluoride in the mouth rinse, *two dosage schedules* can be prescribed. The low potency/high-frequency schedule involves using mouthrinses containing 100-500 ppm fluoride once or twice daily. The high-potency/low-frequency schedule involves using mouthrinses containing 900 ppm fluoride only once weekly. The 900 ppm fluoride mouthrinse is also used in weekly or fortnightly school-based mouthrinsing programs in non-fluoridated areas with high caries prevalence [16].

International dental organizations have made the following recommendations for fluoride mouthrinses in children (Table 3.2).

It is recommended that children should use undiluted 10 ml of any of the above formulations and rinse for 1 minute. For younger children, prescribe a lower volume of the undiluted mouth rinse. The use of fluoride mouthrinse is not recommended to children below the age of 6 as they lack the ability to spit out effectively [6, 8].

There is no danger of acute toxicity if the child swallows 10 ml mouthrinse of a 225–450 ppm F or even a 900 ppm F as the margin of safety is high. For example, a 10 ml of 900-ppm fluoride mouthrinse contains 9 mg F, which is almost 10 times lower than the Probable Toxic Dose (PTD) for a 6-year-old child weighing 20 kg (PTD = 5 mg/kg × 20 kg = 100 mg F) [17].

3.4 Dietary Fluoride Supplements

Fluoride supplements were shown to be effective in children with high caries risk and were first introduced in areas where optimally fluoridated water was not available. The presence of a fluoride-rich layer in close contact with enamel has more preventive and remineralizing effects than systemic fluoride. Dietary fluoride supplements must be used as they have both, topical and systemic effect. The fluoride tablets that are available are flavored and chewable, so that they contact the tooth enamel exerting a topical effect. The AAPD and EAPD recommend use of dietary supplements only in areas deficient in fluoridated water (less than 0.6 ppm) [6, 8].

Following is the daily dietary fluoride supplement schedule recommended by the AAPD [8] based on age of the child and the fluoride content in the water of the region, they reside in.

- *Birth to 6 months of age*: The AAPD does not recommend any dietary fluoride supplements for infants living in areas where the fluoride present in water is less than 0.3 ppm.
- *6 months to 3 years*: A dietary fluoride supplement of 0.25 mg is recommended in areas where the fluoride present in water is less than 0.3 ppm.
- *3 to 6 years*: Dietary fluoride supplements of 0.50 mg and 0.25 mg are recommended in areas where fluoride present in the water is less than 0.3 ppm or between 0.3 and 0.6 ppm, respectively.
- *6 years and above*: Dietary fluoride supplements of 1 mg and 0. 50 mg are recommended in areas where fluoride present in the water is less than 0.3 ppm or between 0.3 and 0.6 ppm, respectively.

Dietary fluoride supplements are not recommended for children living in areas having water sources containing more than 0.6 ppm fluoride.

3.5 Concluding Remarks

Home-use topical fluorides and dietary supplements are effective caries prevention methods. While they act as an adjunct to professional treatment to stabilize dental caries, their success largely depends on parent and patient compliance. The operator should consider factors such as patient demographics, background fluoride exposure, caries risk status, and compliance with home oral care to tailor the recommendations for each patient.

Fluoridated toothpastes containing 1000 ppm fluoride should be recommended to children with low caries risk between 0 and 3 years of age. Children above 6 years of age with low caries risk status should be recommended to use toothpastes containing 1450 ppm fluoride. Prescription-based high fluoride toothpastes containing 5000 ppm fluoride and the use of fluoride mouthrinses are recommended in children above 6 years of age with a high caries risk status. Dietary fluoride supplements are recommended only in areas with suboptimal fluoride content in drinking water.

References

1. Featherstone JD. Prevention and reversal of dental caries: role of low level fluoride. Community Dent Oral Epidemiol. 1999;27(1):31–40.
2. Mullane DM, Baez RJ, Jones S, et al. Fluoride and oral health. CDH. 2016;33(2):69–99.
3. Marinho VC, Higgins JP, Sheiham A, Logan S. Fluoride toothpastes for preventing dental caries in children and adolescents. Cochrane Database Syst Rev. 2003;1:CD002278.

4. Walsh T, Worthington HV, Glenny AM, Appelbe P, Marinho VC, Shi X. Fluoride toothpastes of different concentrations for preventing dental caries in children and adolescents. Cochrane Database of Syst Rev. 2010; Issue 1. Art. No.: CD007868
5. IAPD Foundational articles and consensus recommendations: use of fluoride for caries prevention, 2022. http://www.iapdworld.org/2022_05_use-of-fluoride-for-caries-prevention.
6. Toumba KJ, Twetman S, Splieth C, et al. Guidelines on the use of fluoride for caries prevention in children: an updated EAPD policy document. Eur Arch Paediatr Dent. 2019;20:507–16.
7. Scottish Dental Clinical Effectiveness Programme (SDCEP) achieves NICE accreditation. Evid Based Dent 2016;17(2):62.
8. American Academy of Pediatric Dentistry. Fluoride therapy. The reference manual of pediatric dentistry. Chicago: American Academy of Pediatric Dentistry; 2024. p. 351–7.
9. https://cdn.who.int/media/docs/default-source/essential-medicines/2021-eml-expert-committee/applications-for-addition-of-new-medicines/a.14_fluoride-toothpaste.pdf?sfvrsn=4eb40f4c_4
10. Cochran JA, Ketley CE, Duckworth RM, van Loveren C, Holbrook WP, Seppa L, Sanches L, Polychronopoulou A, O'Mullane DM. Development of a standardized method for comparing fluoride ingested from toothpaste by 1.5-3.5-year-old children in seven European countries. Part 2: ingestion results. Community Dent Oral Epidemiol. 2004;32(Suppl 1):47–53.
11. Buzalaf MAR, Levy SM. Fluoride intake of children: considerations for dental caries and dental fluorosis. In: Fluoride and the oral environment. Monogr Oral Sci. 2011;22:1–19.
12. Wong MC, Zhang R, Luo BW, Glenny A-M, Worthington HV, Lo EC. Topical fluoride as a cause of dental fluorosis in children. Cochrane Database of Syst Rev.2024; Issue 6. Art. No.: CD007693.
13. Sjögren K, Birkhed D. Effect of various post-brushing activities on salivary fluoride concentration after toothbrushing with a sodium fluoride dentifrice. Caries Res. 1994;28:127–31.
14. Sjögren K, Birkhed D, Rangmar B. Effect of a modified toothpaste technique on approximal caries in preschool children. Caries Res. 1995;29:435–41.
15. Parnell C, O'Mullane D. After-brush rinsing protocols, frequency of toothpaste use: fluoride and other active ingredients. Monogr Oral Sci. 2013;23:140–53.
16. Marinho VC, Higgins JP, Logan S, Sheiham A. Fluoride mouthrinses for preventing dental caries in children and adolescents. Cochrane Database Syst Rev. 2003;3:CD002284.
17. Whitford GM. Fluoride in dental products: safety considerations. J Dent Res. 1987;66(5):1056–60.

4 Remineralizing Agents for Initial Stage Lesion

4.1 Introduction

Dental caries is initiated due to cyclic periods of demineralization and remineralization at the enamel–plaque interface. If the process of demineralization dominates, it can lead to the formation of White Spot Lesions (WSL) that proceed to frank cavitation unless an environment conducive to remineralization is created. The process of remineralization occurs when the local environment is supersaturated with calcium and phosphate ions resulting in their deposition into the crystal voids of the demineralized tooth structure. The presence of free fluoride (F–) ions from topical fluoride use helps drive the Ca2+ and PO4 3– into the crystal lattice to form Fluorhydroxyapatite (FHA), which is more resistant to a subsequent acid challenge. This has prompted researchers to develop remineralizing agents that could deliver calcium and phosphate ions to the oral environment which along with topical fluorides would help in reversal of the WSL [1–3].

4.2 Are the Salivary Stores of Calcium and Phosphates Sufficient to Remineralize White Spot Lesions?

At physiological pH, saliva is supersaturated with phosphoprotein-stabilized Ca2+ and PO4 3– ions, ensuring that these ions remain available to diffuse into mineral deficient lesions (initial-stage lesions). However, studies following the progress of white spot lesions in the absence of artificial remineralizing technologies have reported that most of these lesions are not reversed by natural remineralization

H. Vyas et al., *Dental Caries and Traumatic Injuries in Pediatric Dentistry*,
https://doi.org/10.1007/978-3-031-98929-2_4

mechanisms even after 2 years. Moreover, since net salivary remineralization is a slow process, there is a tendency for mineral gain only on the surface of the WSL due to the ion concentration gradient decreasing from saliva into the lesion. The remineralization action of topical fluorides is restricted to the outer 30 μm of the enamel surface. This kind of surface-only remineralization does not improve the aesthetics and the structural properties of the subsurface lesion. The presence of additional extrinsic sources of Ca2+ and PO4 3– ions could augment the natural remineralization potential of saliva by favoring faster and deeper subsurface remineralization. Further, while natural remineralization mechanisms may be effective in patients with a low caries risk, they possibly would be inadequate in high caries risk populations [2].

4.3 Classification of Non-fluoride Remineralizing Agents

Non-fluoride remineralizing agents can be broadly categorized based on their mechanism of action as follows:

- Agents that supply Calcium and Phosphate.
  (a) Calcium phosphate systems.
  These include stabilized Calcium Phosphate (Casein Phosphopeptide–Amorphous Calcium Phosphate), Crystalline Calcium Phosphate (Functionalized β-Tricalcium Phosphate), and Unstabilized Calcium Phosphate (Amorphous Calcium Phosphate).
  (b) Polyphosphate systems.
  Polyphosphate systems include Sodium Trimetaphosphate, Sodium hexametaphosphate, and Calcium lycerophosphate.
- Biomimetic agents such as Nanohydroxyapatite and Self-assembling Peptides.

While currently many different remineralizing technologies are being developed and tested by researchers, only those agents whose commercial formulations (Table 4.1) are being marketed will be discussed.

Table. 4.1 Commercial formulations of remineralizing agents

No	Chemical compound name	Product name	Flavor	Manufacturer	Country
1.	Casein phosphopeptide–amorphous calcium phosphate	GC Tooth Mousse® GC Tooth Mousse Plus® (contains fluoride) MI Paste® MI Paste plus® (contains fluoride) MI Paste ONE® MI varnish™ Trident White sugar-free gum	Mint, strawberry, vanilla, melon, Tutti frutti Mint, strawberry, vanilla Mint, strawberry, vanilla, melon, Tutti frutti Mint, strawberry, vanilla, melon, Tutti frutti Mint Fresh strawberry, fresh mint Peppermint, spearmint, minty bubble, microcrystals, wintergreen, cool rush	GC Trident	Japan USA USA
2.	Functionalized β-tricalcium phosphate	Clinpro Crème toothpaste (950 ppm) ClinPro Crème Toothpaste (5000 ppm fluoride) Clinpro XT™ varnish	Vanilla mint	3 M	USA
3.	Calcium sodium phosphosilicate	Sensodyne Repair and Protect Oravive® toothpaste		Haleon	UK
4.	Amorphous calcium phosphate	Enamelon® toothpaste (0.45% Stannous fluoride) EnamelPro® Varnish	Mint Vanillamint, strawberry and cream, bubblegum	Premier	USA
5.	Sodium hexametaphosphate	Oral-B pro expert toothpaste	Mild mint	Oral B	USA
6.	Nanohydroxyapatite	Apagard® toothpaste		Sangi Co Ltd.	Japan
7.	Self-assembling P11-4 peptides	Curodont Repair™ Curodont Protect™		Credentis	Switzerland

These commercial products have been listed after visiting the manufacturer's website on 7 May 2025. The availability of these products may vary across different regions

4.4 Casein Phosphopeptide–Amorphous Calcium Phosphate Complexes (CPP–ACP)

CPP–ACP is a milk-based product, which has been developed to aid in the remineralization of initial-stage lesions. It was conceptualized by Dr. Eric Reynolds at the University of Melbourne, Australia, in 1987. It is composed of a protein, Casein Phosphopeptide (CPP), which is used to deliver and bind the Amorphous Calcium Phosphate (ACP) to the tooth enamel [4].

4.4.1 Mechanism of Action

Milk-derived casein stabilizes nanoclusters of calcium and phosphates to form a bioactive complex called Casein Phosphopeptide–Amorphous Calcium Phosphate (CPP–ACP). The CPP–ACP complex can traverse through the plaque as a whole or the CPP component dissolves in the presence of saliva releasing calcium, phosphate, and fluoride ions into the oral environment. When in proximity to the tooth enamel, the minerals diffuse down the concentration gradient into the subsurface white spot lesion to form fluorapatite. Along with facilitating the delivery of ACP to the tooth enamel, CPP can also decrease the Streptococcus mutans count [4, 5].

4.4.2 Indications and Contraindications

It is advised in patients with multiple white spot lesions as an adjunct to preventive home care measures and professional application of fluoride gels or varnishes (Fig. 4.1). Patients undergoing orthodontic treatment should be encouraged to apply CPP–ACP around brackets to stabilize white spot lesions (Fig. 4.2). In patients with developmental defects of enamel such as hypomineralization, CPP–ACP can be used as an adjunct to topical fluoride.

Its use is contraindicated in children who are intolerant to milk protein—Casein. Commercial home care formulations of CPP–ACP which also incorporate fluoride are not recommended in children below the age of 6, to prevent inadvertent swallowing.

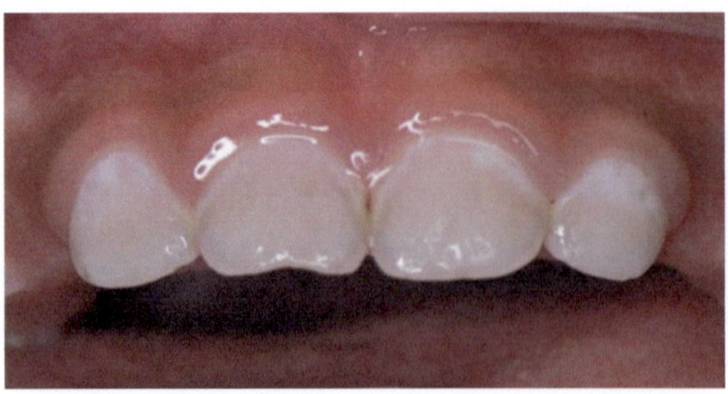

Fig. 4.1 White spot lesions on maxillary primary incisors

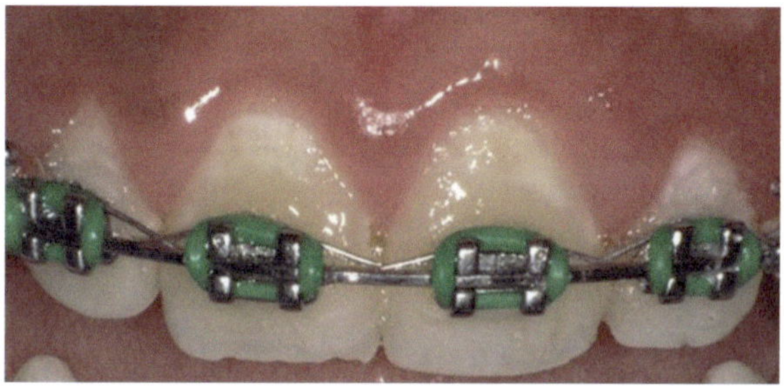

Fig. 4.2 Cervical white spot lesions in a patient undergoing orthodontic treatment

4.4.3 Method of Application

CPP–ACP paste (GC Tooth Mousse®, USA /MI paste®, Australia) must be applied on the tooth surface using a clean finger, after brushing in the morning and evening. The quantity of paste should be sufficient to cover all the teeth. The paste must be held in the mouth for as long as possible (at least 5 minutes) without expectorating or swallowing [6]. It is essential for the saliva to contact the paste to facilitate the release of calcium and phosphate ions. Hence, it should not be applied using a custom-fabricated tray. In a professional setting, varnishes containing CPP–ACP along with 5% sodium fluoride (MI varnish) can be applied at 3 monthly or 6 monthly intervals depending upon the caries risk status. If the patient reports any allergic symptoms such as rashes, itching, and angioedema, its use should be immediately discontinued.

4.4.4 Efficacy of CPP–ACP in Prevention and Remineralization

4.4.4.1 Caries Prevention in Primary and Permanent Dentition

There is limited evidence demonstrating the efficacy of CPP–ACP in *preventing caries in the primary dentition*. Existing evidence shows no significant difference in caries prevention between the use of CPP–ACP and 1000 ppm F toothpaste [7–10].

The efficacy of CPP–ACP in *preventing white spot lesions in orthodontic patients* has been documented in few trials. A systematic review showed no benefits of CPP–ACP over brushing with 1000 ppm F toothpaste. It is still not clearly established if the use of CPP–ACP along with a fluoridated toothpaste can confer additional preventive benefits to patients compared to when fluoridated toothpaste is used alone [11].

4.4.4.2 Caries Remineralization in Primary and Permanent Dentition

It has been reported that the three-monthly use of CPP–ACP was more effective than a placebo in remineralizing white spot lesions in primary dentition. When the remineralization efficacy of CPP–ACP was compared to 1000 ppm fluoridated toothpaste, the results of a trial did not show it to be superior, as both agents reduced the severity of white spot lesions and decreased the occurrence of new lesions. On

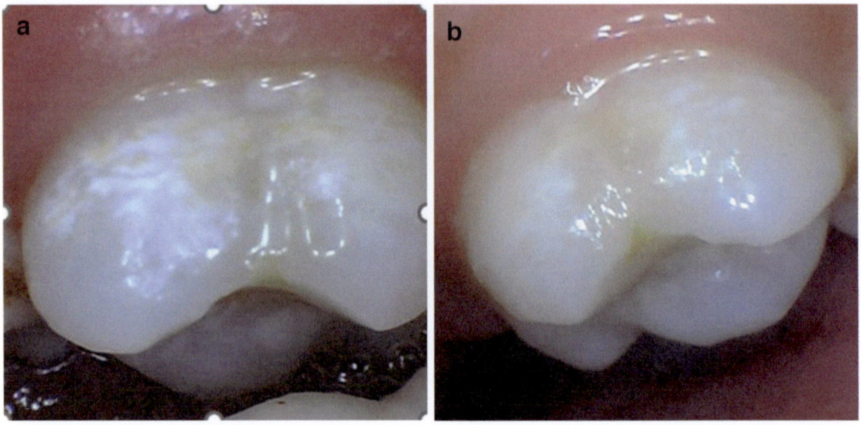

Fig. 4.3 White spot lesion on the buccal surface of maxillary primary right second molar. Home use of CPP–ACP application was recommended twice daily along with the use of fluoridated toothpaste (**a**). Two-year follow-up shows remineralization of the lesion (**b**). (Image Courtesy: Dr. Manini Shah, India)

the other hand, when it was compared to low fluoride toothpaste (500 ppm), another study showed that CPP–ACP performed better in reducing white spot lesions in primary dentition (Fig. 4.3) [7–10].

Regression of white spot lesions was seen when CPP–ACP was used with 1000–1450 ppm F toothpaste in the *permanent dentition* [11, 12]. Though CPP–ACP/ACPF is seen to remineralize white spot lesions, it cannot act as a replacement for home care and professional care fluoride therapy. The clinician can recommend that patients regularly use the CPP–ACP formulations once or twice a day for three to six months. Based on the progression of the earlier detected white spot lesions, patients could be asked to continue or stop application.

Besides CPP–ACP, there are two other remineralizing agents, whose commercial formulations are currently being marketed. They are:

4.5 Crystalized Calcium Phosphate-β-Tricalcium Phosphate (TCP)

The application of β-tricalcium phosphate in toothpastes and other remineralizing systems such as varnishes was implemented by combining fluoride and functionalized *TCP*. Functionalized TCP is a tailored, low-dose calcium phosphate system that is incorporated into a topical fluoride formulation such as dentifrice, gel, rinse, or varnish. Functionalization of TCP serves two major roles: first, it provides a barrier that prevents premature TCP–fluoride interactions, and second, it provides targeted delivery of TCP when applied to the teeth. Although this is a relatively new approach, evidence for the benefits of TCP has begun mounting. When compared to fluoride alone, the combination of fluoride plus functionalized TCP is shown to improve remineralization by building stronger, more acid-resistant mineral in both white-spot lesions as well as eroded enamel. It is available commercially as 3 M Clinpro XT™ varnish and 3 M Clinpro crème toothpaste (950 ppm F) or 3 M Clinpro Crème (5000 ppm F) [13, 14].

4.6 Amorphous Calcium Phosphate (ACP)

Commercial formulations of ACP deliver a calcium salt (e.g., calcium sulphate) and phosphate salt (e.g., ammonium phosphate) intraorally that dissolve to release calcium and phosphate ions. These ions are transiently available to promote enamel remineralization before precipitating to form ACP or amorphous calcium fluoride phosphate (ACFP), in the presence of fluoride ions. Intraorally, ACP and ACFP are extremely unstable and transform into the stable, hydroxyapatite and fluorhydroxyapatite, when near the enamel. Alternatively, they may get precipitated in the form of undesirable calculus deposits (octacalcium phosphate and brushite) on the tooth surface. ACP is available commercially as Enamelon toothpastes® or gels or varnishes [15]. Along with ACP, the Enamelon® toothpaste contains 5000 ppm Stannous fluoride. Enamel Pro is another fluoride varnish containing ACP, which is currently available in the market.

4.7 Comparison of Different Remineralization Agents

4.7.1 Professionally Applied Products

Professionally applied remineralizing agents available commercially are MI™ varnish (CPP–ACP), Clinpro XT™ varnish (TCP), and Enamel Pro® varnish (ACP). Studies have compared 5% NaF varnishes with those containing CPP–ACP, TCP, and ACP. While a few studies demonstrated the superiority of fluoride varnish containing CPP–ACP over the others, most of them concluded that all the above varnishes were comparable to each other. The choice of fluoride varnish with remineralizing agent depends on the product availability and operator preference [16–22].

4.7.2 Home Care Products

In vitro studies showed that fluoridated toothpaste with TCP (970 ppm F) and ACP (970 ppm F) did not have a superior remineralizing efficacy over conventional fluoridated toothpastes (1000 ppm–1450 ppm F). A toothpaste containing TCP along with 5000 ppm fluoride has shown better results than fluoridated pastes (with or without ACP and CPP–ACP) in remineralizing white spot lesions. While the results could be due to higher fluoride concentration, it can be advised in individuals undergoing orthodontic treatment or post orthodontic treatment to remineralize white spot lesions [23–25].

4.8 Concluding Remarks

Commercially available remineralizing agents are beneficial for reversing the White Spot Lesions. Fluoride available from toothpastes or formulations containing 5% sodium fluoride work alongside CPP–ACP, TCP, and ACP facilitating remineralization to a greater lesion depth. These remineralizing agents are the choice for preventive home care and professionally applied regimens for individuals who have high caries risk and demonstrate White Spot Lesions.

References

1. Willmot DR. White lesions after orthodontic treatment: does low fluoride make a difference? J Orthod. 2004;31:235–42.
2. Philip N. State of the art enamel remineralization systems: the next frontier in caries management. Caries Res. 2019;53:284–95.
3. Cochrane NJ, Reynolds EC. Calcium phosphopeptides—mechanisms of action and evidence for clinical efficacy. Adv Dent Res. 2012;24(2):41–7.
4. Reynolds EC, Cai F, Cochrane NJ, Shen P, Walker GD, Morgan MV, Reynolds C. Fluoride and casein phosphopeptide- amorphous calcium phosphate. J Dent Res. 2008;87(4):344–8.
5. Farooq I, Moheet I, Imran Z, Farooq U. A review of novel dental caries preventive material: casein phosphopeptide–amorphous calcium phosphate(CPP–ACP) complex. King Saud University. J Dental Sci. 2013;4:47.
6. https://www.gc.dental/australasia/sites/australasia.gc.dental/files/products/downloads/gctoothmousse/ifu/ifu-tooth-mousse.pdf. Last Accessed on 18th April, 2025.
7. Sitthisettapong T, Phantumvanit P, Huebner C, Derouen T. Effect of CPP-ACP paste on dental caries in primary teeth: a randomized trial. J Dent Res. 2012;91(9):847–52.
8. Sitthisettapong T, Doi T, Nishida Y, Kambara M, Phantumvanit P. Effect of CPP-ACP paste on enamel carious lesion of primary upper anterior teeth assessed by quantitative light-induced fluorescence: a one-year clinical trial. Caries Res. 2015;49(4):434–41.
9. Kargul B, Durmus B, Bekiroglu N. Effect of CPP-ACP on remineralisation of early caries lesions in primary teeth. OHDM. 2017;16:1–4.
10. Memarpour M, Fakhraei E, Dadaein S, Vossoughi M. Efficacy of fluoride varnish and casein Phosphopeptide-amorphous calcium phosphate for remineralization of primary teeth: a randomized clinical trial. Med Princ Pract. 2015;24:231–7.
11. Raphael S, Blinkhorn A. Is there a place for Tooth Mousse® in the prevention and treatment of early dental caries? A systematic review. BMC Oral Health. 2015;15:113.
12. Imani MM, Safaei M, Afnaniesfandabad A, Moradpoor H, Sadeghi M, Golshah A, Sharifi R, Mozaffari HR. Efficacy of CPP-ACP and CPP-ACPF for prevention and Remineralization of white spot lesions in orthodontic patients: a systematic review of randomized controlled clinical trials. Acta Inform Med. 2019;27(3):199–204.
13. Karlinsey RL, Pfarrer AM. Fluoride plus functionalized β-TCP: a promising combination for robust remineralization. Adv Dent Res. 2012;24:48–52.
14. Amaechi BT, Ramalingam K, Mensinksai PK, Narjibfard K, Mackey AC, Karlinsey RL. Remineralization of eroded enamel by a NaF rinse containing a novel calcium phosphate agent in an in situ model: a pilot study. Clin Cosmet Invest Dent. 2010;2:93–100.
15. Reynolds EC. Calcium phosphate-based remineralization systems: scientific evidence? Aust Dent J. 2008;53(3):268–73.
16. Varma V, Hegde KS, Bhat SS, Sargod SS, Rao HA. Comparative evaluation of Remineralization potential of two varnishes containing CPP-ACP and Tricalcium phosphate: an in vitro study. Int J Clin Pediatr Dent. 2019;12(3):233–6. https://doi.org/10.5005/jp-journals-10005-1629.

17. Radha S, Kayalvizhi G, Adimoulame S, et al. Comparative evaluation of the Remineralizing efficacy of fluoride varnish and its combination varnishes on white spot lesions in children with ECC: a randomized clinical trial. Int J Clin Pediatr Dent. 2020;13(4):311–7.
18. Jain A, Suprabha BS, Shenoy R, Natarajan S, Rao A. Remineralising effectiveness of two fluoride varnishes containing additives: an in vitro study. Oral Health Prev Dent. 2019;17(4):385–93.
19. Shah M, Paramshivam G, Mehta A, Singh S, Chugh A, Prashar A, Chugh VK. Comparative assessment of conventional and light-curable fluoride varnish in the prevention of enamel demineralization during fixed appliance therapy: a split-mouth randomized controlled trial. Eur J Orthod. 2018;40(2):132–9.
20. Majithia U, Venkataraghavan K, Choudhary P, Trivedi K, Shah S, Virda M. Comparative evaluation of application of different fluoride varnishes on artificial early enamel lesion: an in vitro study. Indian J Dent Res. 2016;27:521–7.
21. Virupaxi SG, Roshan NM, Poornima P, Nagaveni NB, Neena IE, Bharath KP. Comparative evaluation of longevity of fluoride release from three different fluoride varnishes – an in vitro study. J Clin Diagn Res. 2016;10(8):ZC33–6.
22. Shen P, Bagheri R, Walker GD, Yuan Y, Stanton DP, Reynolds C, Reynolds EC. Effect of calcium phosphate addition to fluoride containing dental varnishes on enamel demineralization. Aust Dent J. 2016;61(3):357–65.
23. Kau CH, Wang J, Palombini A, Abou-Kheir N, Christou T. Effect of fluoride dentifrices on white spot lesions during orthodontic treatment: a randomized trial. Angle Orthod. 2019;89(3):365–71.
24. Lippert F, Gill KK. Carious lesion remineralizing potential of fluoride- and calcium-containing toothpastes: a laboratory study. J Am Dent Assoc. 2019;150(5):345–51.
25. Pinto de Souza SCT, Araújo KC, Barbosa JR, Cancio V, Rocha AA, Tostes MA. Effect of dentifrice containing fTCP, CPP-ACP and fluoride in the prevention of enamel demineralization. Acta Odontol Scand. 2018;76(3):188–94.

Minimal Intervention Dentistry in Contemporary Practice

5

5.1 Introduction: Understanding How Minimal Intervention Dentistry (MID) Came About

Until the early 1990s, clinicians relied on a purely surgical approach for the management of dental caries that was based on the traditional principles of cavity preparation by the "Father of Modern Dentistry," G.V. Black, who recommended the "extension for prevention" philosophy wherein a clinician performed complete removal of carious tissue from a lesion [1]. Consequently, dentists for many years practiced an invasive form of dentistry that involved the removal of healthy tooth structure. However, with time, substantial development in the field of dental research resulted in a shift in the understanding of how dental caries is initiated, progresses, and is treated. This changed thought process even led to Dr. Black himself, remarking that "the day is surely coming, when we will be engaged in practicing preventive, rather than reparative dentistry." [1] Considerations like these have paved the way for the development of the Minimal Intervention Dentistry (MID) philosophy.

5.2 Rationale of Minimal Intervention Dentistry

The recognition of the post-eruptive effects of systemic fluoride and the application of topical fluorides demonstrated that in the early stages of dental caries, fluoride ions promoted remineralization [2, 3]. In the 1960s, histological studies by Fusayama identified two separate layers of carious dentin, an outer "infected layer" and an inner "affected layer." This led to a more cautious approach to caries removal

H. Vyas et al., *Dental Caries and Traumatic Injuries in Pediatric Dentistry*,
https://doi.org/10.1007/978-3-031-98929-2_5

targeting only the outermost infected dentin layer, which has a disrupted collagen structure and was considered incapable of remineralization. Simultaneously, researchers began to believe that the inner, partially demineralized affected layer retains its original collagen framework and can be remineralized, therefore it should be left behind [4, 5].

Studies by Shovelton showed that softening of dentin generally precedes the organisms causing it. Furthermore, Edwina Kidd's work on permanent teeth showed that leaving small amounts of infected dentine in a cavity does not seem to result in caries progression, pulpitis, or pulp death, provided the overlying restoration has a good seal. Also, studies on carious dentin of primary teeth showed that the microorganisms colonizing the deep carious layer did not contain significant bacterial count [6–8].

In 1994, Dr. Phillip Marsh developed the "Ecological Plaque Hypothesis," wherein dental caries began to be perceived as a disease that is driven by the dental plaque and the oral environment in which it matures [9]. This led researchers to conclude that the management of dental caries should not focus on eliminating bacteria by complete excision of carious tissue, but it is important to transform the oral environment into a cario-protective environment.

Along with these landmark papers that led to the development of the MID philosophy; the advancement of adhesive restorative materials such as Resin Composites (RC) and Glass Ionomer Cement (GIC), and the emergence of bioactive materials such as Mineral Trioxide Aggregate (MTA) and Biodentine™ (Septodont, France) added a new dimension to MID [10]. The use of GIC was shown to be favorable in the practice of MID due to its ability to bond to carious dentin, stimulate remineralization, and promote healing. Additionally, these adhesive materials allowed clinicians to opt for cavity designs that preserved tooth structure, which increased the chance of maintaining tooth vitality and function. The reintroduction of Silver Diamine Fluoride (SDF) further aided in the arrest of caries progression and improved the chances of pulpal preservation [11, 12]. Based on the above, the philosophy of MID as we know it today, came into practice.

Its core principles are:

To implement MID effectively, each of these four elements (Fig. 5.1) must be integrated into patient examination and treatment process [13].

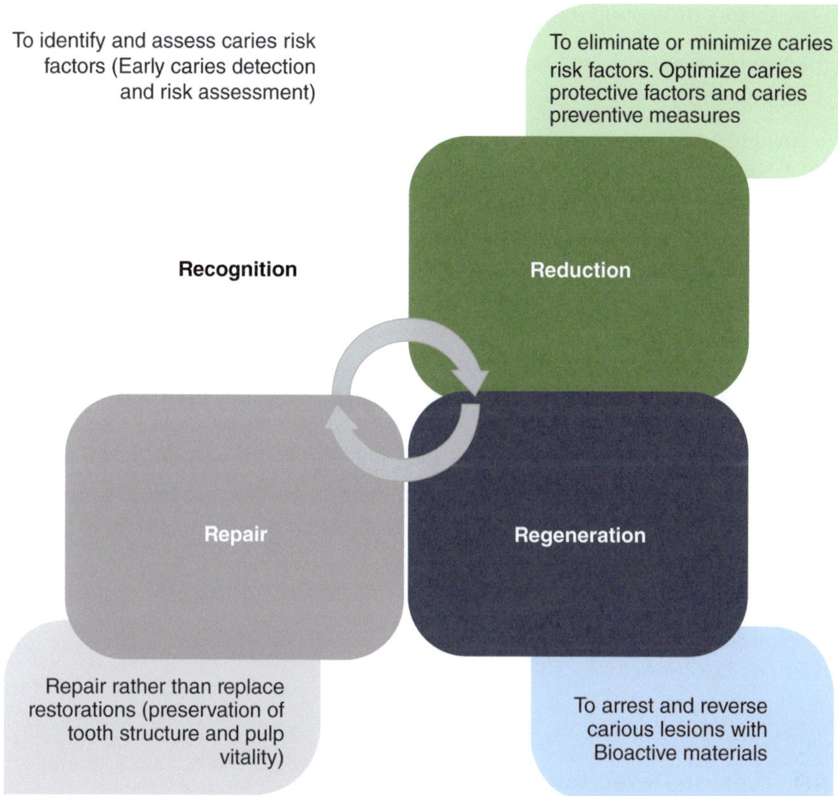

Fig. 5.1 The 4Rs—core principles of Minimal Intervention Dentistry

5.3 The Caries Process

For a long time, dental caries- the disease was synonymous with its signs and symptoms such as the presence of a carious lesion or the complaint of pain and swelling. However, dental caries is more than just a "cavity." It is a cyclic disease process characterized by periods of demineralization and remineralization occurring at the tooth–plaque interface [14].

The factors responsible for demineralization are

- Poor oral hygiene.
- Presence of carious lesions (non-cavitated and cavitated).
- Increased frequency of ingestion of fermentable carbohydrates.
- Reduced salivary function.
- Presence of acidogenic bacteria.

The factors promoting remineralization are

- Exposure to systemic and topical fluoride sources.
- Child having a Dental Home that includes.
  - Anticipatory guidance.
  - Professional preventive dental program.
  - Recall or follow-up program.

When the periods of demineralization dominate, dental caries visibly manifests, initially, as an innocuous carious lesion, which can later progress to pulpal and periapical infection [14].

5.4 Carious Detection and Diagnosis for the Clinician

In the context of the modern definition of dental caries, the carious lesion must be detected and assessed with the use of an internationally validated system, the International Caries Classification and Management System (ICCMS™), that includes the following: [15–17]

- Lesion detection.
- Lesion staging.
- Carious Lesion Activity.

5.4.1 Lesion Detection

While the most accepted methods for the detection of caries by clinicians are the visual, visuo-tactile examination, and radiographic examination, pediatric patients show the highest acceptance to visual examination and that is why it is the first caries detection method that is introduced to them. It should include the use of a good lighting source, mouth mirror, and three-way syringe. Every tooth should ideally be dried before examination, and in cases where the patient exhibits apprehension or anxiety at the appearance of any new stimulus, blot drying can be performed with a cotton pellet. Earlier, in a visual examination, clinicians used to limit themselves to identifying carious lesions that exhibited frank cavitation. Today, we know that caries presents not just in the form of lesions showing significant involvement of enamel and dentin, but also in the form of early white spot lesions. Thus, a clinician can expect to detect carious lesions at different stages in the same individual. Even where carious lesions are not suspected, a clinical examination must be complemented with a radiographic examination (Table 5.1). Along with detecting a "hidden" carious lesion, radiographs provide a baseline record and help to assess the progression or regression of a lesion and the effectiveness of primary and secondary preventive measures.

Table 5.1 Organizational recommendations for radiographic examination

Organization	Recommendation
International Association of Pediatric Dentistry (IAPD) [18]	A radiographic examination should be conducted at an interval of 6–12 months in children with low or moderate caries risk. It should be conducted at 6-month intervals in children with high caries risk.
American Academy of Pediatric Dentistry (AAPD) [19]	A bitewing radiograph should be taken every 6 to 12 months for children and adolescents at increased caries risk or those with closed proximal contacts. Patients with no caries or low caries risk radiographs are indicated at an interval of 12 to 24 months if proximal surfaces cannot be examined visually or with a probe.
European Academy of Paediatric Dentistry (EAPD) [20]	The clinical indicator for prescribing bitewing radiographs is the presence of active, non-cavitated as well as manifested caries lesions in the primary, mixed, or permanent dentition. Intervals for repeating bitewing radiographs should be justified on the basis of the latest documented caries extent. The younger the patient and more extended/active the caries the higher seems to be the probability to progress which may indicate shorter monitoring intervals, i.e., 24 months.
Scottish Dental Clinical Effectiveness Programme (SDCEP) [21]	Bitewing radiographs advised for all children who do not have previous radiographs taken as baseline. For those with increased caries risk, bitewing radiographs advised at 6–12 months interval. For other children, bitewing radiographs taken at 24 months interval.

5.4.2 Lesion Staging

The International Caries Classification and Management System (ICCMS)™ stages carious lesions as [17]

- Initial-stage lesions.
- Moderate-stage lesions.
- Extensive-stage lesions.

5.4.2.1 Initial-Stage Lesions

Initial-stage lesions or white spot lesions as they are known, appear as opacities or visible discoloration of enamel. They show no evidence of surface breakdown or an underlying dentin shadow after air drying. These lesions are often seen around the cervical third, along the gingival margin (Fig. 5.2). On *occlusal surfaces*, the entrance of pits and fissures appear opaque, and are usually seen harboring plaque.

The presence of a lesion is suspected in *proximal areas* where plaque stagnation and food debris are seen. Visual examination of proximal surfaces can be done directly in case of open contacts or by the placement of elastic separators between suspected teeth (Fig. 5.3).

While examining initial-stage lesions, all surfaces should be gently air dried for 5s to inspect for roughness or areas of pitting or initial cavitation. In case of the presence of excessive plaque on the tooth surface, it should be removed with the flat end of an explorer, or by lightly cleaning the surface with moist cotton or gauze or

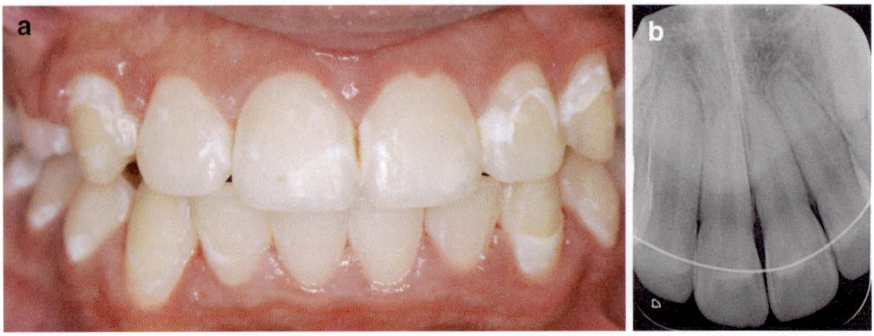

Fig. 5.2 Initial-stage lesions on labial and interproximal surfaces of maxillary anterior teeth (**a**). Radiolucency on mesial surfaces of maxillary permanent central incisors limited to outer third of dentin (**b**)

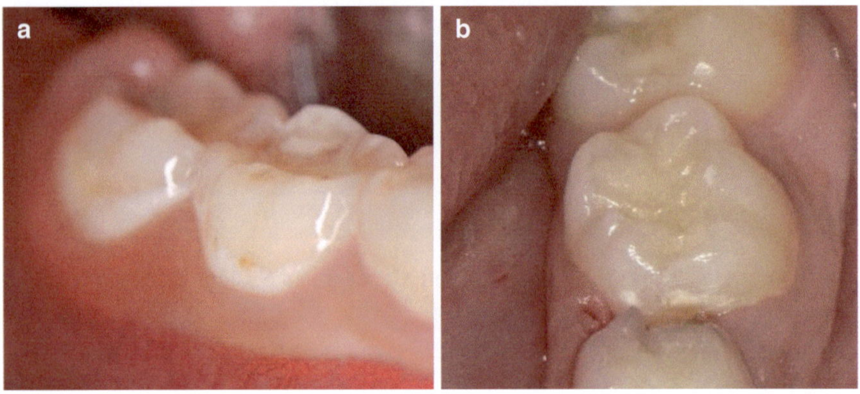

Fig. 5.3 Initial-stage lesions on cervical third of buccal surface (**a**) and proximal surface (**b**) of mandibular molars

by using a soft bristle toothbrush or microbrush, particularly on occlusal surfaces. One must avoid probing suspected early lesions, as there is a risk of causing iatrogenic damage to the enamel.

On a radiograph, initial-stage lesions may show no radiolucency if there is insufficient mineral loss. Radiolucency, if detected, is limited to the outer third of dentine (Fig. 5.4). The bitewing radiograph remains by far the best method for detecting initial-stage proximal lesions whereas the initial-stage occlusal lesions may not always be detected.

Enamel breakdown must be considered as a threshold to render restorative therapy. As there is no breakdown in initial stage lesions, treatment involving any surface must be limited to remineralization by home care and professional preventive measures. If there is any doubt regarding the surface integrity of the enamel, it is prudent to err on the side of caution. Use of topical fluoride (Fig. 5.5), SDF, and

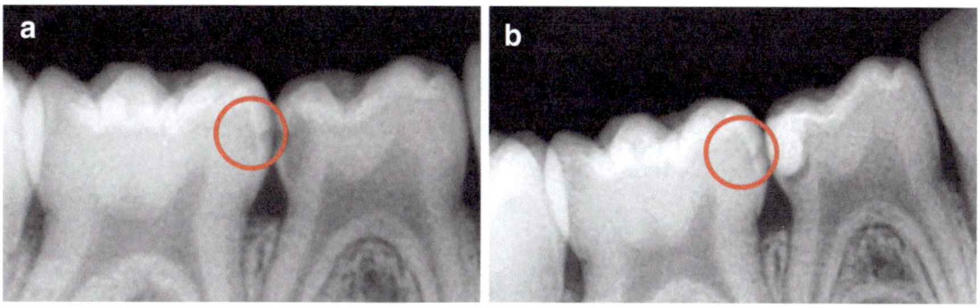

Fig. 5.4 Proximal surface of mandibular primary right second molar showing radiolucency extending to the dentino-enamel junction (**a**). Initial-stage lesion must not be prepared for a restoration as there is no enamel breakdown. In this case, the lesion was treated with three monthly application of fluoride varnish, while the adjacent mandibular primary first molar was restored (**b**)

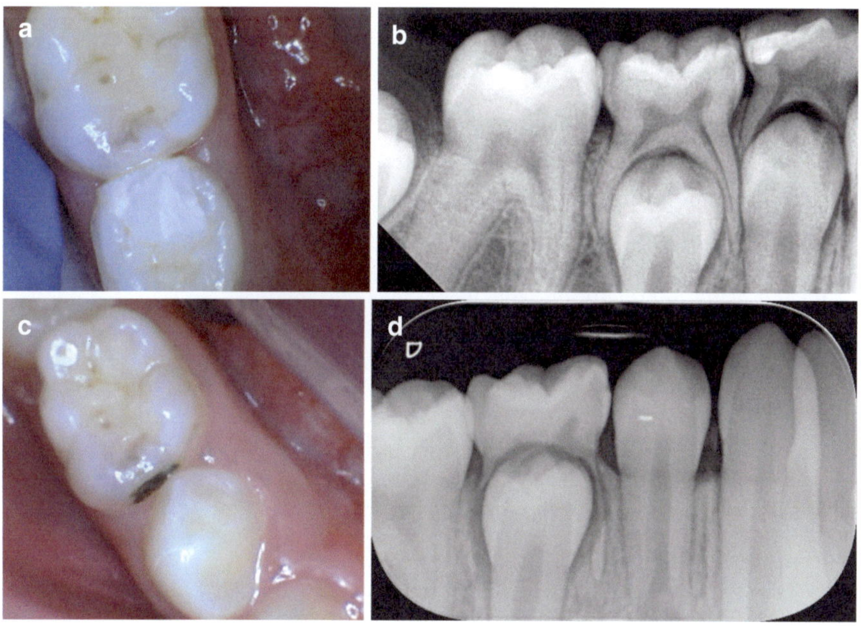

Fig. 5.5 Initial-stage proximal lesion on mandibular primary right second molar (**a**). Radiolucency extending to the dentino-enamel junction (**b**). 38% Silver Diamine Fluoride was applied at the initial visit (**c**) and recalled in six months. Application was continued six monthly for four years to keep the lesion arrested and without progression. Radiolucency has not progressed at a four-year recall (**d**)

sealants even in the presence of enamel microcavitation will help in remineralizing or arresting the lesion, which is a preferred treatment than preparing the tooth for restoration. The proximal lesions must also be longitudinally monitored on a radiograph to detect progression.

5.4.2.2 Moderate-Stage Lesion

Moderate-stage lesions show the presence of enamel breakdown without underlying dentinal exposure (Fig. 5.6a). At times, they may be mistaken for initial-stage carious lesions when there is an occurrence of microcavitation of enamel, which is not easily discernible on visual examination. In such situations, they are detected at a relatively later stage when the discoloration of dentin shines through the enamel (Fig. 5.6b).

Proximal surface lesions are characterized by the presence of subsurface discoloration of the marginal ridge (Fig. 5.7a), plaque accumulation, food lodgment, and enamel breakdown. *On radiographic examination*, moderate-stage lesions show radiolucency that extends to the middle third of dentine on both occlusal and proximal surfaces. These lesions are less likely to be missed on a radiographic examination unlike many initial-stage lesions [17] (Fig. 5.7b).

Moderate-stage lesions are managed by the placement of conventional restorations or with the use of minimally invasive techniques such as the Hall technique, Non-Restorative Cavity Control (NRCC), and Silver Modified Atraumatic Restorative Technique (SMART).

5.4.2.3 Extensive-Stage Lesions

Extensive-stage lesions present with frank cavitation revealing underlying dentin. *On a radiograph*, these lesions extend to the inner third of dentin or show pulpal involvement (Fig. 5.8).

To preserve pulpal integrity, extensive-stage lesions approaching the pulp should be treated using minimally invasive techniques that involve "No Caries Removal" such as the Hall technique or "Selective Caries Removal" that forms the basis of Indirect Pulp Treatment. The tooth should show no clinical and radiographic signs

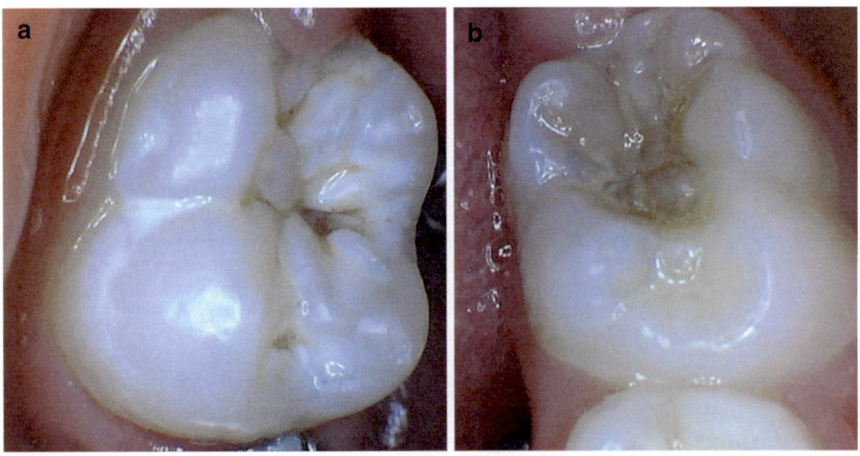

Fig. 5.6 Moderate-stage lesions on occlusal surface, with enamel breakdown (**a**). Moderate-stage lesions on occlusal surface without enamel breakdown but underlying dentinal shadow showing through (**b**)

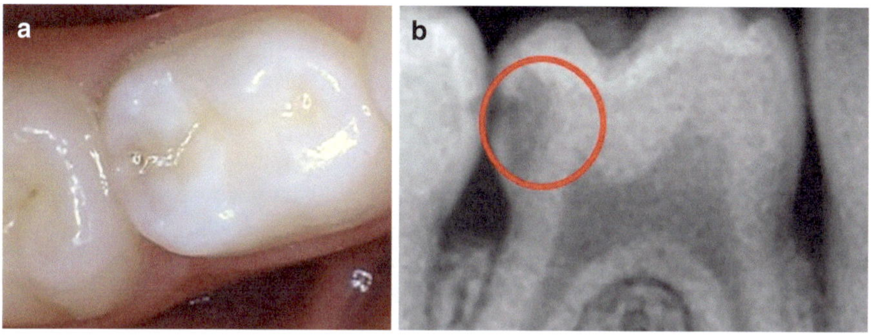

Fig. 5.7 Moderate-stage proximal lesion on mandibular primary first molar showing marginal discoloration (**a**). Radiolucency is seen extending to middle third of dentin (**b**)

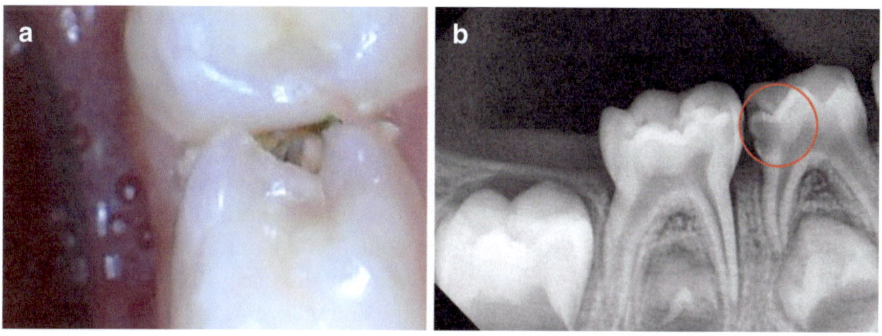

Fig. 5.8 Extensive-stage lesions on the proximal surface of mandibular primary first molar showing underlying dentin (**a**). Radiolucency into the inner third of dentin (**b**)

and symptoms of irreversible pulpitis or frank pulpal exposure. Endodontic therapy should be performed in cases where the tooth shows clear pulpal involvement, on both clinical and radiographic examination [17].

5.4.3 Carious Lesion Activity

Once caries is detected and staged, clinicians should assess the activity of a lesion with the use of indicators such as visual appearance, tactile examination, the potential for plaque accumulation, and gingival health. An active enamel lesion appears whitish or yellowish in color. On air drying it looks opaque, lacks luster and feels rough when gently probed with the ball end of an explorer or any non-sharp, flat instrument [22].

The lesion is covered with plaque and is often seen

- At the entrance of pits and fissures.
- Cervical third of smooth surfaces, typically near the gingival margin.
- Above or below the contact area on proximal surfaces.

On tactile exploration, the dentin feels soft or leathery.

An inactive enamel lesion is shiny and hard when felt with the ball end of an explorer or any non-sharp, flat instrument is moved gently across the surface. The dentin is hard and shiny on probing (Fig. 5.9). An active lesion is more likely to progress than an inactive lesion. Differentiating between an active and inactive carious lesion is important, as it determines the pulpal status, treatment approach, and prognosis [17, 22].

5.4.4 What Are the Adjunct Methods of Caries Detection?

There are supplemental tools developed to assist in detecting early lesions. One such tool which has been commonly available to the clinician is the DIAGNOdent™ pen (KaVo Dental Technologies LLC, USA). The laser energy emitted by the device is absorbed by the surrounding tooth material causing fluorescence within the infrared spectrum. The underlying mechanism is that carious tissue emits stronger fluorescence than sound tissue and is expressed as a higher numerical readout by the device [23]. Other caries detection systems based on the principles of Fiberoptic Transillumination (FOTI), Digital Fiberoptic Transillumination (DIFOTI), Electrical Conductance Measurement (ECM), and Artificial Intelligence (AI) are being extensively researched across the world. Despite the emergence of advanced diagnostic aids, clinical and radiographic examination still remains the standard of practice for detecting carious lesions.

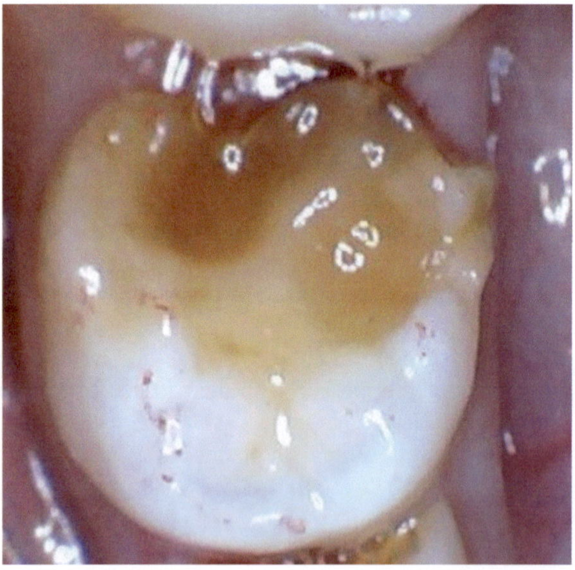

Fig. 5.9 An inactive open lesion showing hard shiny dentin

5.5 Differentiating Layers of Carious Dentin

Earlier, it was customary to remove all carious tissue from a tooth, while treating a lesion. Contemporary strategies of caries management have introduced the concept of "Selective Caries Removal" which is in accordance with the principles of MID. However, the primary dilemma faced by the clinician is—*How much carious tissue should be removed or not removed at all?*

To answer the above question, the clinician must first be able to reasonably identify the types of carious dentinal tissue, which one may encounter based on a simple visual and tactile examination. To help clinicians with the same, the International Caries Consensus Collaboration (ICCC) [24] has developed terminologies for carious tissue removal (Fig. 5.10).

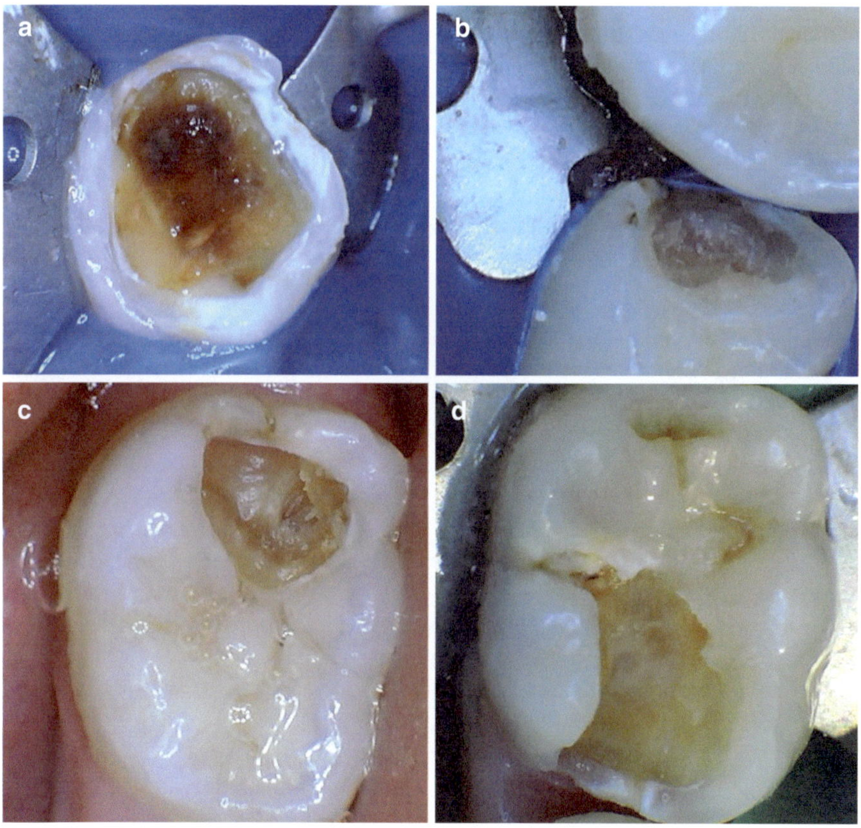

Fig. 5.10 *Hard dentin* is the part that requires a pushing force "with a hard instrument to engage the dentin, and only a sharp cutting edge or a bur will lift it. A scratchy sound or 'cri dentinaire' can be heard when a straight probe is taken across the dentin" (**a**). *Firm dentine* is physically resistant to hand excavation, and "some pressure needs to be exerted through an instrument to lift it" (**b**). *Leathery dentine* "does not deform when an instrument is pressed onto it but can still be easily lifted without much force being required" (**c**). *Soft dentine* will deform when a hard instrument is "pressed onto it and can be easily scooped up (with a sharp hand excavator) with little force being required" (**d**)

There may be little difference between leathery and soft dentine, with leathery being a transition on the spectrum between soft and firm dentine [24]. A distinguishing feature between the two layers is that firm dentin appears dry and soft or leathery dentin appears moist.

5.6 Carious Tissue Removal Methods

- *Non-Selective Caries Removal (previously known as Complete Caries Removal or CCR)*

This is the traditional approach that involves complete removal of caries from the walls and floor of the lesion. This approach can be followed for cavitated lesions that have sufficient healthy tooth structure and radiographically extend up to the middle third of dentin (moderate-stage lesions), where there is minimal to no risk of pulp exposure (Fig. 5.11) [25]. This also allows for a sufficient bulk of the direct restorative material.

However, CCR is not recommended in extensive-stage lesions, as pulp preservation is the key (Fig. 5.12). The operator should ensure minimal tooth structure is removed, which is also in accordance with the principles of MID [13, 26, 27]. In line with this approach, Complete Caries Removal is being replaced by the strategies described below.

- *Stepwise Caries Removal (SWR)* (Fig. 5.13)

At the first appointment, the carious lesion is excavated to healthy tooth structure peripherally, while caries on the pulpal floor is excavated to soft dentin. Calcium Hydroxide or Calcium Silicate Cement is placed as a liner or base over which a Glass Ionomer Cement restoration is done to last up to 12 months. This maintains a coronal seal to allow reparative changes in the dentin and pulp to take place [27–29]. The reasoning for the first step is that the altered environment within the tooth will allow dentin to remineralize, harden, and reduce the number of viable bacteria [30, 31]. At the second visit, when the operator reenters, the restoration is removed, and there is an opportunity to reevaluate changes in lesion color and hardness. However, the disadvantage of attempting a reentry is that the operator risks causing damage to the remineralized dentinal tissue or even causing a pulpal exposure at this stage. Secondarily, this also leads to additional costs, increased treatment duration, and possible discomfort to the patient [27–29, 32].

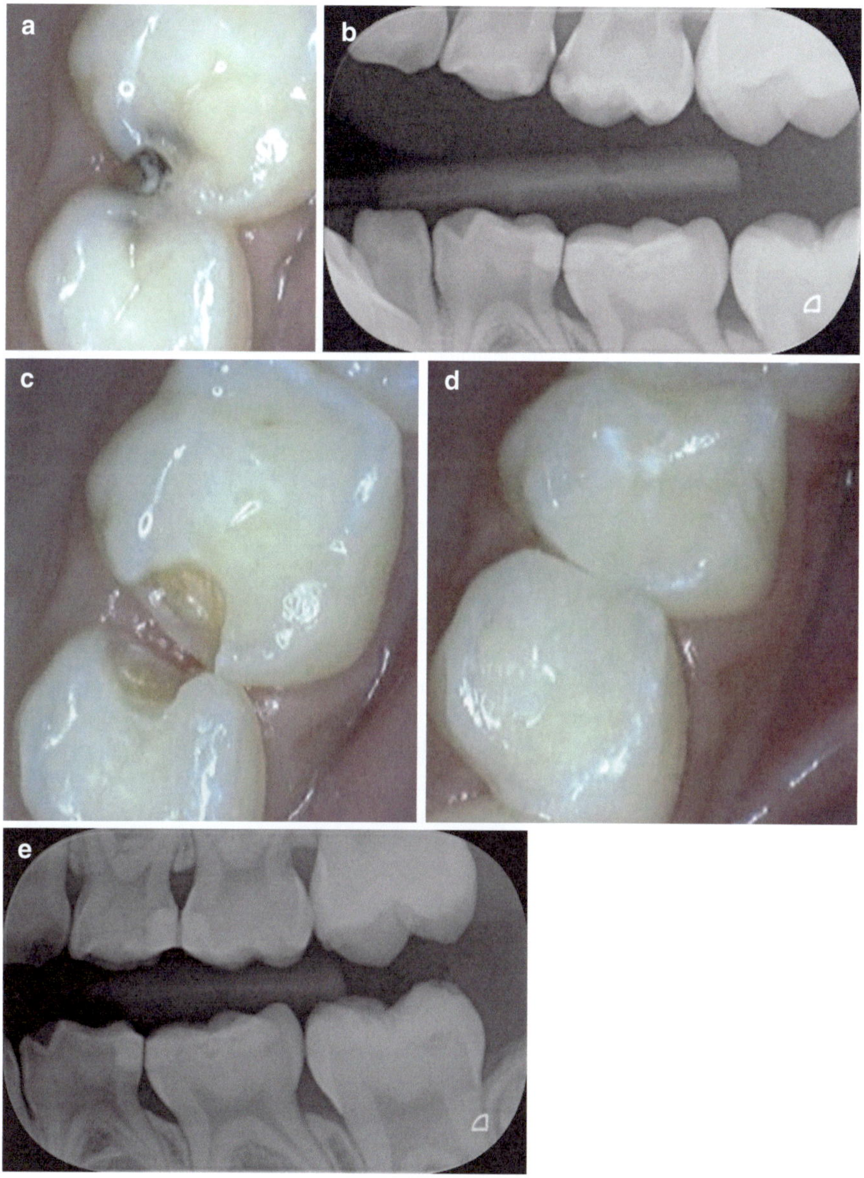

Fig. 5.11 Moderate-stage proximal lesions in maxillary primary left first and second molars (**a**). Radiograph showing radiolucency extending to middle third in both molars (**b**). Complete Caries Removal done from walls and floor of the lesion (**c**). Teeth restored with Resin-Modified Glass Ionomer Cement (**d**). There must be no residual caries or restoration overhangs on the radiograph (**e**)

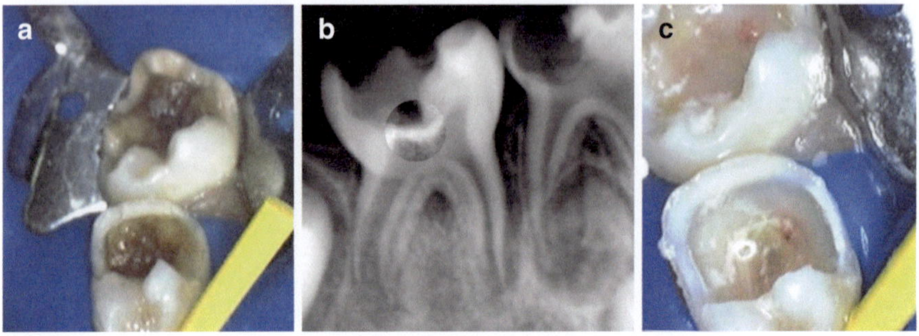

Fig. 5.12 Extensive-stage lesions in mandibular primary right first and second molars (**a**). Radiolucency extending to inner third of dentin. A band of remaining dentin overlying the pulp may not always be visible (**b**). Complete Caries Removal resulted in pin point pulp exposure in both molars (**c**)

- *Selective Caries Removal (SCR)*

  Selective Caries Removal (SCR) involves excavating the peripheral walls of the cavity to healthy tooth structure, leaving behind a thin layer of firm or soft dentin on the pulpal floor, to avoid a pulp exposure (Fig. 5.14). The tooth is restored with a definitive direct or full coverage restoration. It is the treatment of choice for moderate and extensive-stage lesions in primary and permanent teeth, provided there are no signs and symptoms of irreversible pulpitis [25, 28, 29, 33–35]. SCR approach forms the basis of Indirect Pulp Treatment.

  In primary teeth, SWR and SCR present a lower risk of pulp exposure when compared with complete caries removal. SWR requires a second visit which adds to the risk of pulp exposure and cost of treatment while reentering the lesion. While the success of SCR and SWR are comparable, the operator may choose to perform a single-visit SCR over SWR in children [36–38]. Caries removal approaches in permanent teeth is discussed in Chap. 10 (Managing the Immature Tooth: Apexogenesis, Apexification, and Regenerative Endodontics).

- *No Removal of Carious Tissue*

  The principle here is to modify the environment without the removal of carious tissue by making the lesion self-cleansing such as the Non-Restorative Cavity Control (NRCC) or sealing in caries to arrest the lesion progression, like the Hall technique.

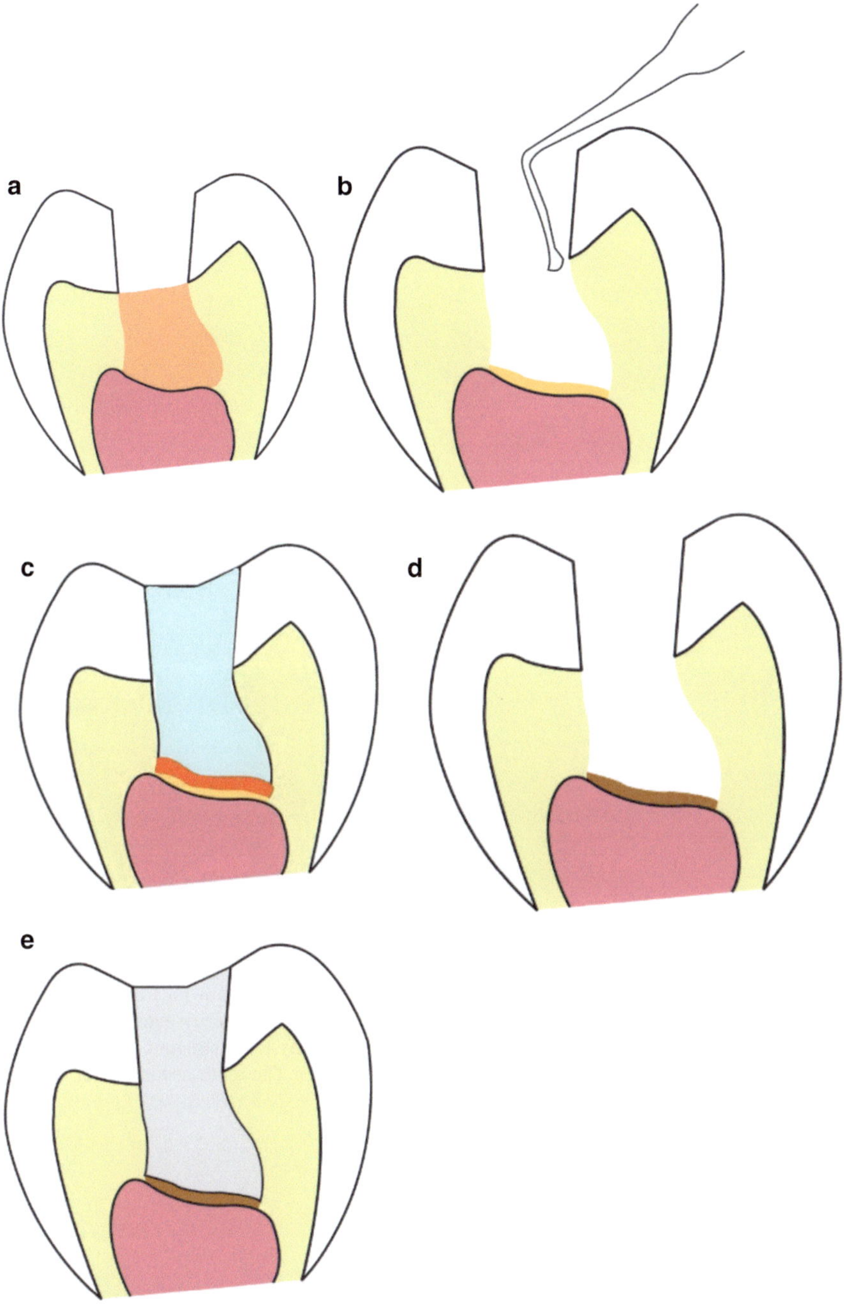

Fig. 5.13 Extensive-stage lesion showing soft dentin from superficial to deeper layers, overlying the pulp (**a**). The lesion is excavated completely from the peripheral walls to healthy tooth structure, and a layer of soft dentin is left overlying the pulp (**b**). A liner is placed over the remaining soft dentin and tooth sealed with an interim restoration for 6 to 12 months (**c**). The interim restoration is removed and lesion is reentered. The remaining carious dentin is evaluated for change in color and hardness. The tooth is not excavated further so as to avoid a pulp exposure (**d**). A definite or permanent restoration is placed (**e**)

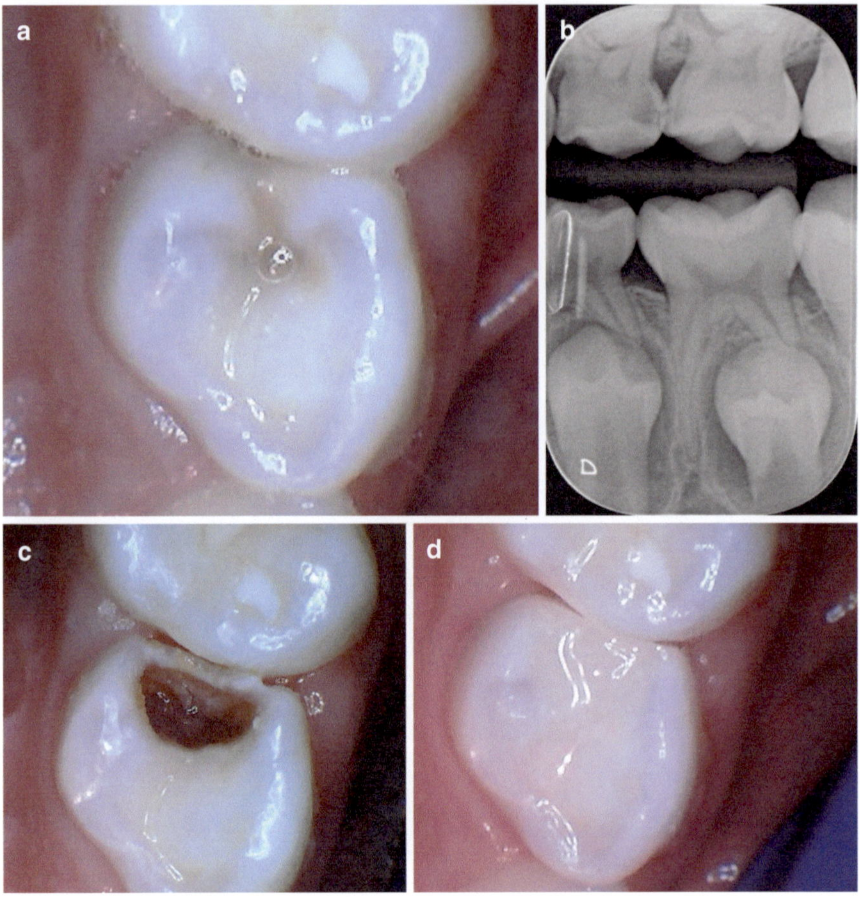

Fig. 5.14 Carious lesion suspected due to interproximal dark shadow showing through enamel on maxillary primary left first molar (**a**). The radiograph shows radiolucency extending to middle third of dentin (**b**). The walls of the lesion excavated to healthy tooth structure, while Selective Caries Removal done to firm dentin on floor of the lesion (**c**). The tooth restored with a Resin-Modified Glass Ionomer Cement (**d**)

5.7 Application of MID in Practice (Figs. 5.15, 5.16, and 5.17)

5.7.1 Non-Restorative Cavity Control (NRCC)

NRCC is a causal or etiological or biological approach first advocated by G.V. Black to treat dental caries [39]. NRCC treatment has been proposed based on the understanding that the clinician can reverse or arrest a carious lesion by modifying the cariogenic oral environment. [40–42] As NRCC involves both professional and homecare preventive routines, it will achieve the dual goals of improving the

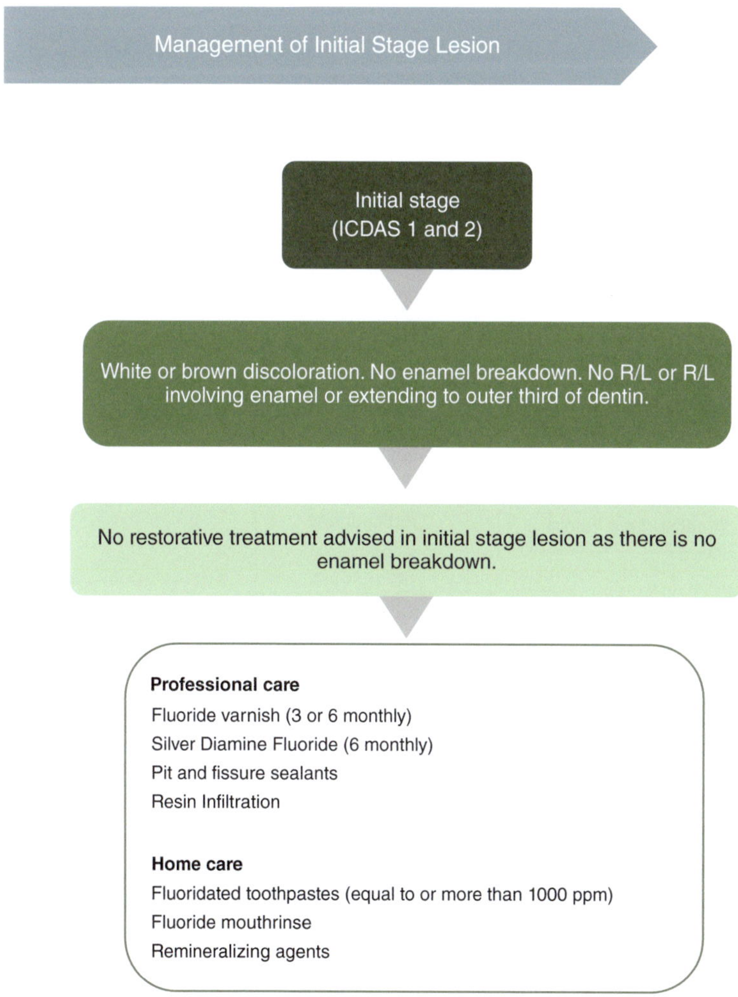

Fig. 5.15 Management of initial-stage lesion

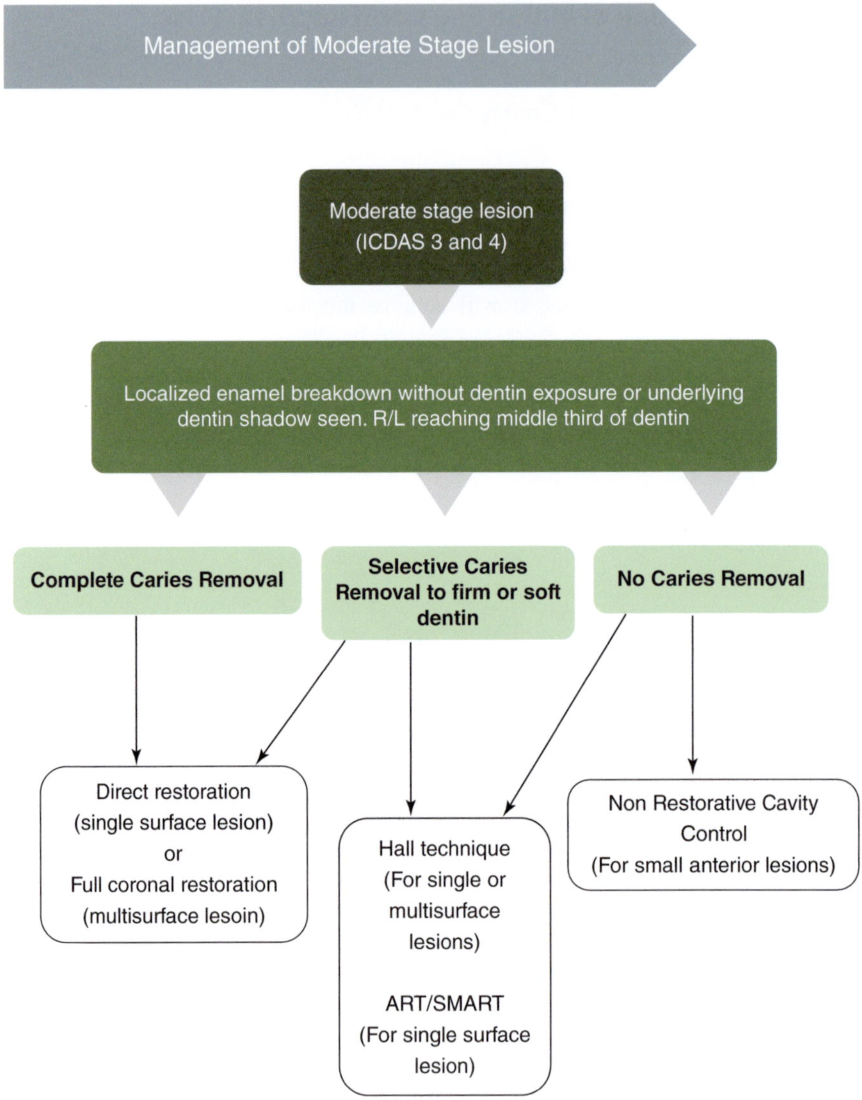

Fig. 5.16 Management of moderate-stage lesion

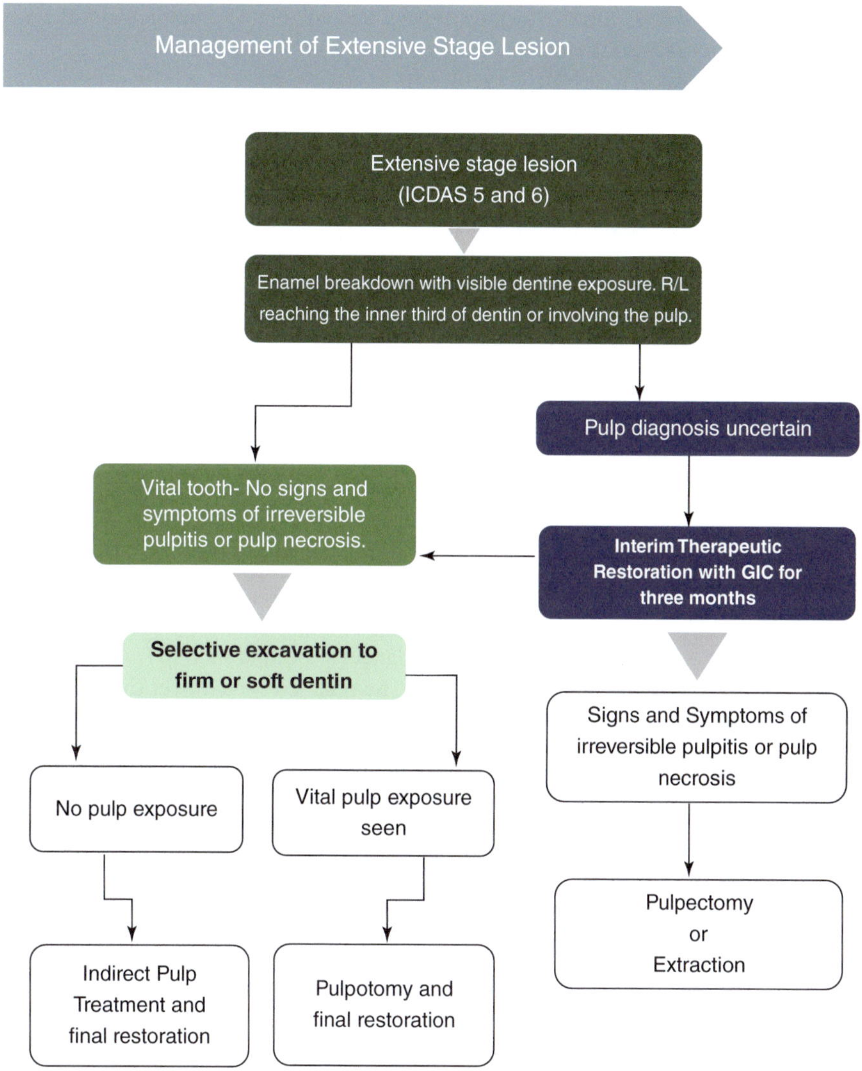

Fig. 5.17 Management of extensive-stage lesion

parents or care giver's attitude toward oral hygiene and create a favorable oral environment for succedaneous teeth.

The clinical protocol of NRCC involves.

- Making the lesion cleansable by removing weak enamel or enamel overhangs in proximal lesions in anterior teeth and occlusal lesions in posterior teeth.
- Application of 5% NaF or 38% Silver Diamine Fluoride (SDF) or a layer of GIC to slow down the lesion progression.

The clinician can undertake this approach in pre-cooperative children or those with special needs who may not be able to cooperate for restorative dental procedures, and are contraindicated or do not wish to receive treatment under General Anesthesia. It can be designated as an interim solution in children requiring extensive chairside dental treatment till these teeth receive definitive restorations. Stringent home care measures that will help in improving cario-protective factors must be reinforced to the child and parents. They must be advised on restricting consumption of refined processed carbohydrates. Additionally, a toothpaste containing at least 1000 ppm fluoride must be prescribed for daily use.

5.7.1.1 When Must NRCC Not Be Performed?

NRCC must not be used in patients showing clinical signs and symptoms of irreversible pulpitis or where agenesis of the succedaneous tooth is seen [41, 42]. In these cases, where the primary teeth are required to be retained for a longer time, a definitive procedure must be chosen. A relative contraindication is parents and caregivers who show poor compliance, as the success of NRCC depends on how well the patient and care giver are acquiescent with the oral hygiene and follow-up regimen. During follow-up appointments of NRCC-treated lesions, if they seem active, an alternate intervention must be rendered for managing them [42–44].

5.7.1.2 On Which Tooth Surfaces Can NRCC Be Done?

NRCC is best indicated in anterior teeth for treating carious lesions on labial or lingual and proximal surfaces without removal of caries (Figs. 5.18 and 5.19). NRCC involves the application of fluoride varnish on lesions restricted to enamel (white spot lesions) or 38% SDF for lesions exposing underlying dentin. Alternatively, a layer of GIC can also be applied to dentinal lesions. In cases of proximal surfaces, where the contacts are closed or the child has a crowded dentition, the operator will need to slice these surfaces to make them self-cleansing. Post-slicing, the operator must check that the surfaces are smooth, and all undercuts are removed to avoid creating a plaque stagnation area (Figs. 5.20 and 5.21).

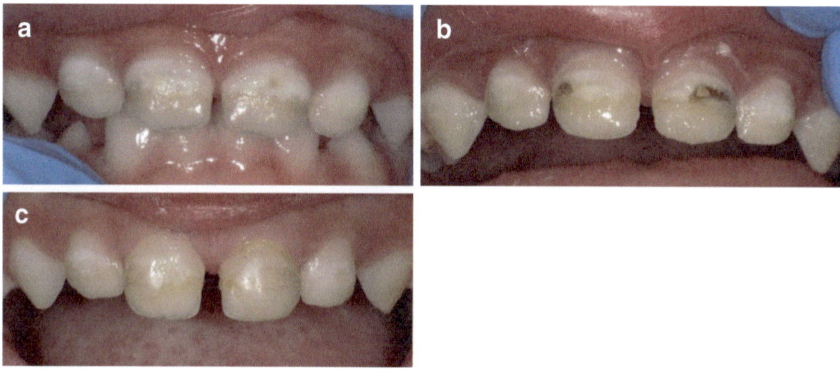

Fig. 5.18 Initial-stage lesions on maxillary primary incisors. Fluoride varnish applied every three months for one year (**a**). The central incisors showed cavitation at 12-month follow-up and fluoride varnish application was continued (**b**). The central incisors were restored subsequently. Two-year follow-up shows remineralization of initial-stage lesions on lateral incisors. Fluoride varnish application was continued every three months (**c**). (Image courtesy: Dr. Manini Shah, India)

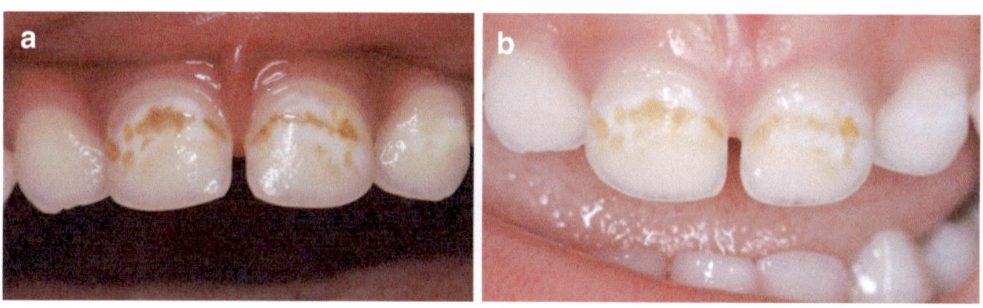

Fig. 5.19 Initial-stage lesions and enamel hypoplasia on maxillary primary central incisors. Fluoride varnish was applied every three months for two years (**a**). Two-year follow-up shows inactivation or non-progression of initial-stage lesions (**b**). (Image courtesy: Dr. Manini Shah, India)

5.7.1.3 Can NRCC Be Used on Posterior Teeth?

Application of 38% SDF on occlusal surfaces showing initial-stage lesions has shown to be more successful than 5% sodium fluoride varnish. The cavitated occlusal lesions must be made self-cleansing prior to SDF application, to prevent the formation of a biofilm that can reactivate the lesion. A thin layer of GIC can also be placed with or without SDF to slow down lesion progression. For cervical lesions, 38% SDF may be used as an interim treatment only. The tooth must be restored at subsequent visits. Initial-stage lesions on proximal surfaces of posterior teeth can be treated with 5% sodium fluoride varnish or 38% SDF along with stringent home care measures. NRCC is not advised in cavitated proximal lesions, as there is a risk of space loss and food retention, leading to caries progression (Fig. 5.22).

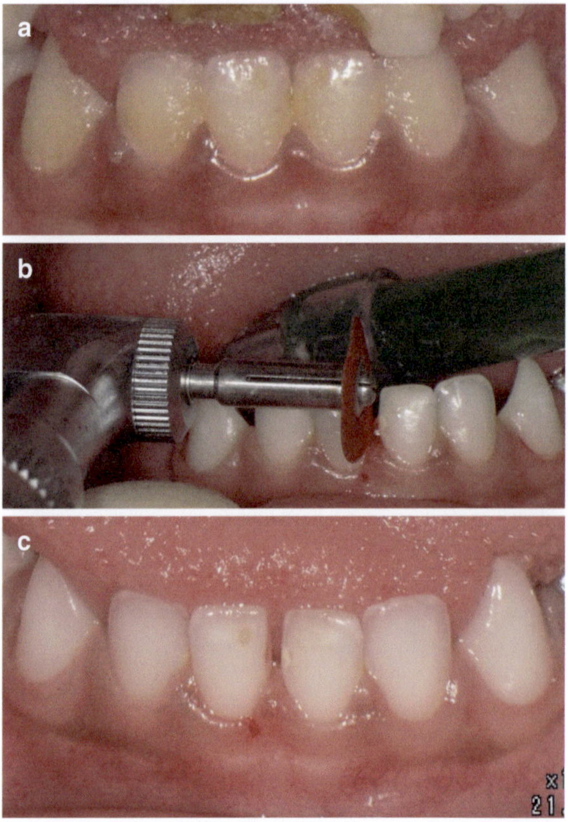

Fig. 5.20 Initial-stage proximal lesions on mandibular primary incisors (**a**). Proximal slicing was done with abrasive discs and fluoride varnish applied (**b**). Interproximal gap created to allow better cleaning (**c**)

While this approach is used often in pre-cooperative children and those with special needs, the clinician must emphasize to the care giver that the treatment success is dependent upon the adherence to good oral hygiene measures. Though NRCC has been shown to perform better in anterior teeth, a major drawback is that it does not restore the esthetics of the child. Similarly, when performed on posterior teeth, it does not restore the form and function of the tooth. Regardless of the above, the minimalistic yet highly effectual nature of the treatment in teeth that are easily accessible to brushing makes it a valuable addition to the MID toolkit.

5.7.2 Hall Technique

Among all the techniques included in the practice of MID, the Hall technique is backed by a large body of high-quality evidence which stands as a testament to its

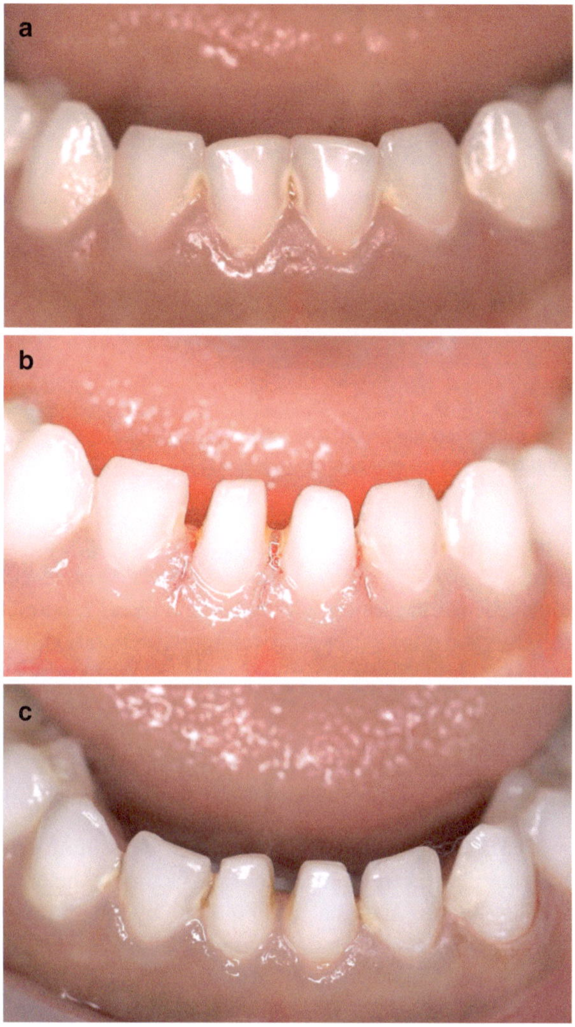

Fig. 5.21 Carious proximal lesions on mandibular primary incisors (**a**). Proximal slicing was done with abrasive discs and fluoride varnish applied every three months (**b**). Follow-up at two years shows non-progression of the lesions (**c**)

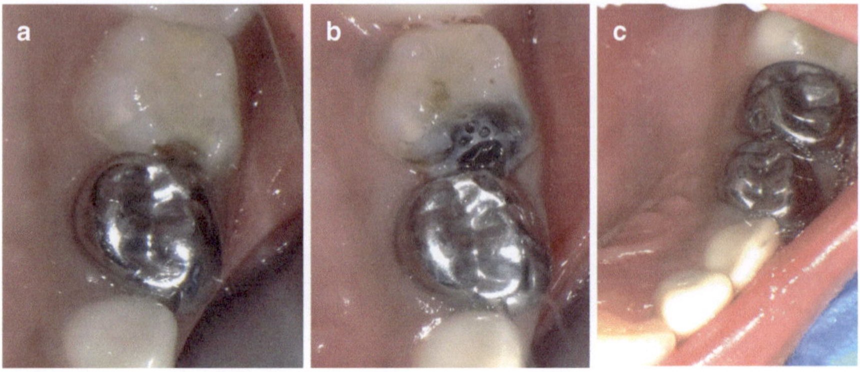

Fig. 5.22 Extensive-stage proximal lesion in maxillary primary left second molar (**a**). 38% SDF applied to arrest the lesion. The lesion was retentive and harbored food debris (**b**). Stainless-Steel Crown was placed as a definite restoration (**c**)

long-term clinical success and patient-friendly nature. It involves the seating of a correctly sized preformed Stainless-Steel Crown (SSC) over a carious primary molar to seal the lesion within, using a Glass Ionomer luting cement, without performing any prior caries removal, tooth preparation, or administering local anesthesia to the child. It was developed in the mid-1990s by Dr. Norna Hall from Scotland, who used this technique for 15 years in her practice [45].

5.7.2.1 How Does the Hall Technique Work?

The underlying principle behind no caries removal is that:

- The preformed stainless-steel crown will cut off the carious lesion and the overlying biofilm from the cariogenic factors in the oral environment.
- The superior marginal seal provided by the preformed SSC and the remineralizing properties of the Glass Ionomer Cement (GIC) used to lute it can arrest the carious lesion and prevent its further progression.

The Hall technique is quick and noninvasive, and does not necessitate the administration of local anesthesia, as the painful stimuli generated during caries removal or tooth preparation is avoided.

5.7.2.2 When Can the Clinician Choose to Do the Hall Technique?

The Hall technique is indicated in primary posterior teeth with:

- Moderate- and extensive-stage lesions either on occlusal surfaces or proximal surfaces.
- Multisurface cavitated or non-cavitated lesions.
- Hypoplastic molars.

The tooth should not show signs and symptoms of irreversible pulpitis which must be confirmed after thorough clinical and radiographic evaluation. The ease of this procedure as compared to placing conventional restorations makes it useful for young and/or borderline cooperative children.

5.7.2.3 The Hall Technique (Figs. 5.23 and 5.24)

- Assess the tooth shape, contact areas, and points of occlusion to ensure these parameters are not significantly altered post crown cementation.
- In case the contacts appear tight such that a crown may not pass through, separators are placed on proximal sides of the tooth at the first appointment.
- In the second appointment, food debris is removed from the lesion, without any caries removal.
- Attempt seating the selected crown on the tooth using finger pressure. The crown should cover all the cusps and approach the contact points with a slight feeling of spring back. Choose the smallest crown that can fit.
- During trial placement, avoid seating the crown fully through the contact points, as this can be difficult to remove.
- Prior to cementation, the area around the tooth should be isolated with cotton rolls. Fill two/thirds of the crown with Glass Ionomer luting cement and place the crown on the tooth. Once it is completely seated, ask the patient to bite on a cotton roll to seat the crown.
- Remove the excess cement and check the fit of the crown and occlusion.

5.7.2.4 How Does the Hall Technique Affect the Occlusion?

Since the traditional Hall technique involves no occlusal preparation, it can cause the vertical dimension to be raised after crown placement. As the primary dentition is in a state of dynamic occlusion, the change in bite is resolved in 7 to 14 days without affecting the Temporomandibular joint [46–48].

5.7.2.5 Can Two Adjacent Primary Molars Be Placed Using the Hall Technique at the Same Time?

It would be difficult to seat crowns on adjacent primary molars using the Hall technique, even after placing separators. Similarly, seating crowns on opposing primary molars at the same visit increases the vertical dimension causing discomfort to the child, necessitating separate appointments. In cases where space loss has occurred due to proximal lesions, the clinician can consider minimal tooth reduction in addition to the space created by the elastic separators to allow placement of the preformed SSC, while observing the rationale of "no caries removal."

5.7.2.6 Is It Advisable to Perform the Hall Technique in General Anesthesia?

In the true sense, the Hall technique may not be feasible under General Anesthesia as multiple crowns may need to be placed on adjacent and opposing teeth and the child would require placement of elastic separators on a prior appointment. The rationale of "no caries removal" of the Hall technique can be adopted as it will

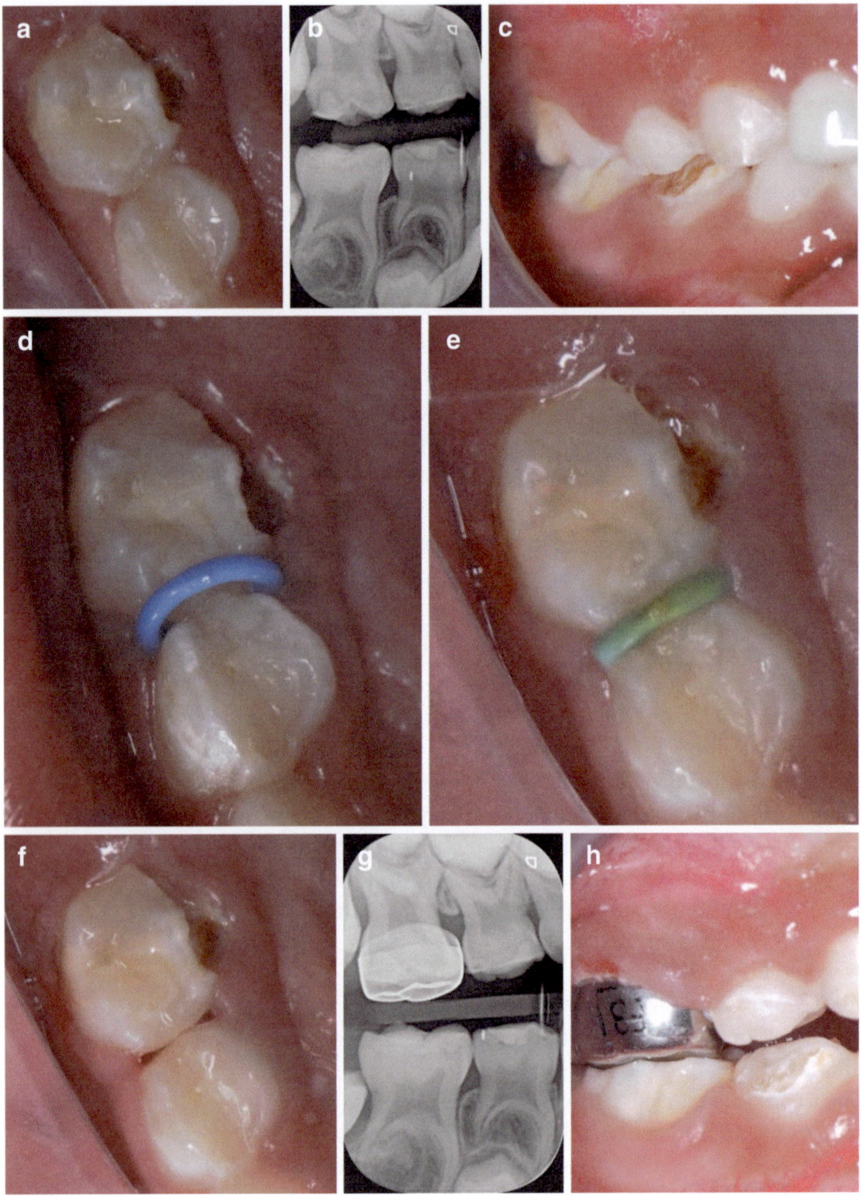

Fig. 5.23 Extensive-stage lesion on palatal surface of maxillary primary right second molar (**a**). Radiograph shows a buccal carious lesion restored previously (**b**). Occlusion is checked before placing separators (**c**). Elastic separator placed (**d**). Child is recalled in two days to remove separators (**e**). Tooth separation seen (**f**). A pre-cementation radiograph is taken to check the distal margin of the crown. The margin should flush with the distal tooth surface to prevent impeding the eruption of the first permanent molar (**g**). Crown is cemented and bite opened by 2–3 mm post crown placement (**h**)

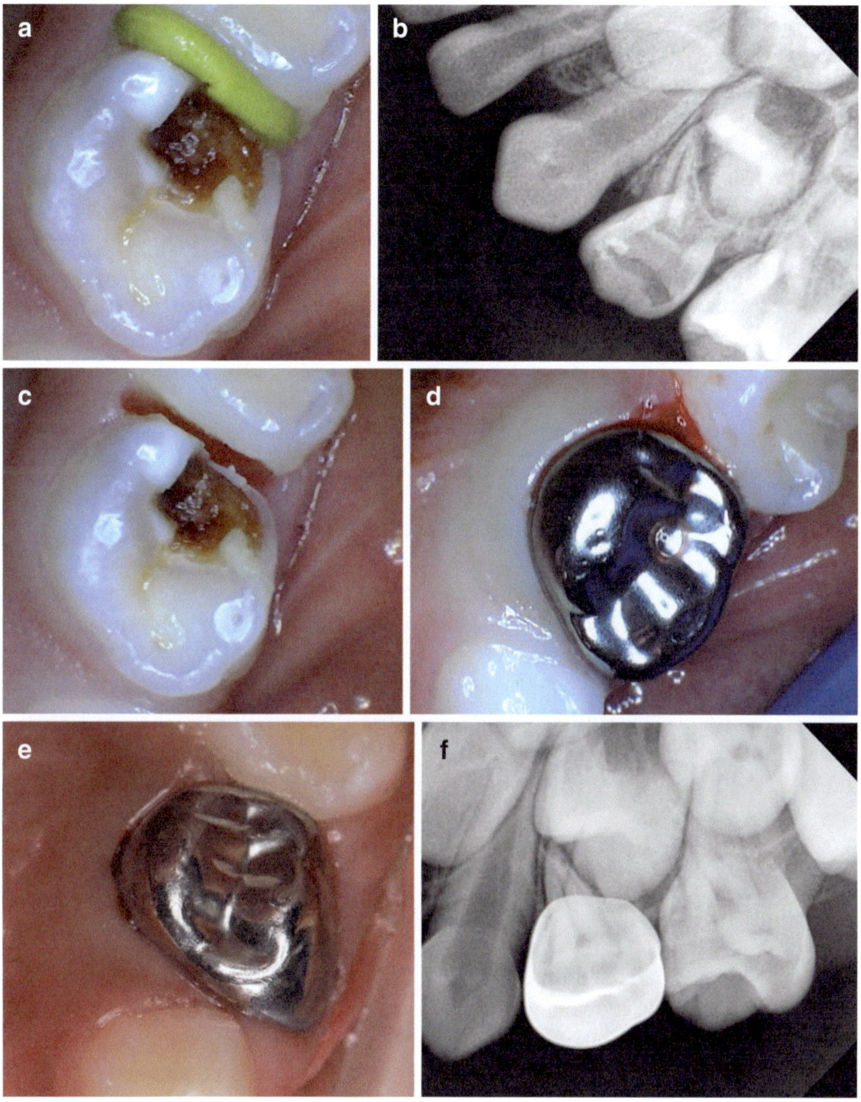

Fig. 5.24 Extensive-stage proximal lesion on maxillary primary left first molar. Elastic separator placed and child recalled in two days (**a**). Preoperative radiograph taken to rule out periapical changes (**b**). Tooth separation noted after removal of separator (**c**). Stainless-Steel Crown cemented (**d**). Clinical (**e**) and radiographic (**f**) follow-up at two years

ensure pulpal preservation. One must keep in mind that in case the patient develops post-operative complications following the Hall technique, it may be difficult to re-treat the tooth without administering General Anesthesia again to the patient. Therefore, while treating an extensive-stage lesion under General Anesthesia, it is advisable to excavate the carious lesion to firm dry dentin or even lower the treatment threshold and perform a pulpotomy, to ascertain pulp vitality.

5.7.2.7 Are There Any Additional Advantages of Applying SDF Before the Hall Technique?

The placement of a crown with the Hall technique itself ensures caries arrest; as this technique isolates the tooth from the oral environment and hence, application of SDF on a tooth before crown cementation may not yield any additional advantage to the clinician. However, when multiple carious lesions are seen, 38% SDF can be applied on lesions as an interim medicament before crowns are placed at subsequent visits.

5.7.2.8 Can the Hall Technique Be Attempted with Zirconia and Flexible Crowns?

To cement a crown without any preparation, the crown material must have certain ductility and elasticity, so that it can pass over the cervical bulge of a primary molar without fracturing or permanently deforming, a quality that the Stainless Steel Crown possess. The low flexural strength of zirconia crowns renders them unsuitable for the traditional Hall technique. Flexible crowns (BioFlx®, Kids-e-Dental®, India; Bioflx®, NuSmile® USA) cannot be left high in occlusion as per the manufacturer. Hence, they are not recommended for use with the Hall technique.

5.7.2.9 What Are the Common Failures That May Be Seen with the Hall Technique?

- Improper case selection resulting in pulpal pathology.

After clinical and radiographic examination of the tooth showing pulpal pathology following the Hall technique, the clinician may consider performing endodontic treatment through the crown and restoring the access area with a Resin Composite restoration or replacing the crown, if required. In teeth that show poor prognosis, the clinician may decide to extract the tooth followed by space management, if needed.

- Wear of the occlusal surface of the crown.

This may occur in cases in which the crown's orientation does not coincide with the anatomy of the tooth surface, or the crown is too high in occlusion. In such cases, the defect may be repaired with a Resin Composite restoration, or the crown can be removed and replaced.

- Crown is impeding the eruption of permanent teeth.

While an oversized crown may be placed as part of the Hall technique, the distal margin must be contoured and crimped such that there is no overhang that could impede the eruption of the first permanent molar. If required, a radiograph can be taken pre-cementation to ensure the crown is well adapted to the distal surface of the tooth.

One must note that despite these possible complications, studies have shown the Hall technique to outperform conventional restorations [49, 50]. The success rate in studies with a follow-up of 5 years was shown to be 5 times that of conventional methods (conventional SSC and intracoronal restorations). The success rates (retention of tooth, no signs of pain and infection) shown in trials examined individually are as high as 92% (Scotland trial) and 92.5% (Germany trial) at three years and, 94% (New Zealand trial), 73.4% (Scotland trial), and 97% over five years (USA trial) [49–55].

5.7.3 Silver-Modified Atraumatic Restorative Technique (SMART)

In the last few years, the increasing evidence on the effectiveness of Silver Diamine Fluoride (SDF) applications in causing caries arrest has led researchers to recommend a new restorative technique called the Silver-Modified Atraumatic Restorative Technique or SMART restorations. SMART is an extension of the Atraumatic Restorative Treatment (ART), which uses only hand instruments to remove carious tissue, followed by restoration and sealing of adjacent enamel fissures with a High-Viscosity Glass Ionomer Cement (HVGIC). When SDF is applied directly to the carious tissue, it causes lesion arrest due to its antimicrobial and remineralizing properties. The accumulation of food debris and plaque on an SDF-treated tooth can cause lesion reactivation. Placing a Glass Ionomer Cement (GIC) prevents the formation of the biofilm, allowing the caries-arresting properties of SDF to continue unhindered, while restoring the tooth's form and function. This synergistic action of SDF and GIC to prevent lesion reactivation forms the basis of the SMART technique [56, 57].

5.7.3.1 When Should an Operator Choose SMART?

The SMART technique is most suited for occlusal surface lesions where the restoration is supported by healthy tooth structure. On proximal surfaces, it should be used only for small lesions in which a Glass Ionomer restoration is expected to withstand the masticatory load. On clinical and radiographic examination, the tooth selected for SMART should not exhibit any signs and symptoms of irreversible pulpitis.

5.7.3.2 How Much Caries Should Be Excavated Before SMART?

There is no established protocol for the SMART technique, yet. Based on published case reports, it is suggested that:

1. The clinician can gain access to the lesion, using a hand excavator, high-speed airotor, or a slow-speed micromotor handpiece with a carbide bur. The choice of armamentarium used should be decided based on the accessibility of the lesion, the amount of enamel overhang present, the child's cooperation, and the clinician's preference (Figs. 5.25 and 5.26).

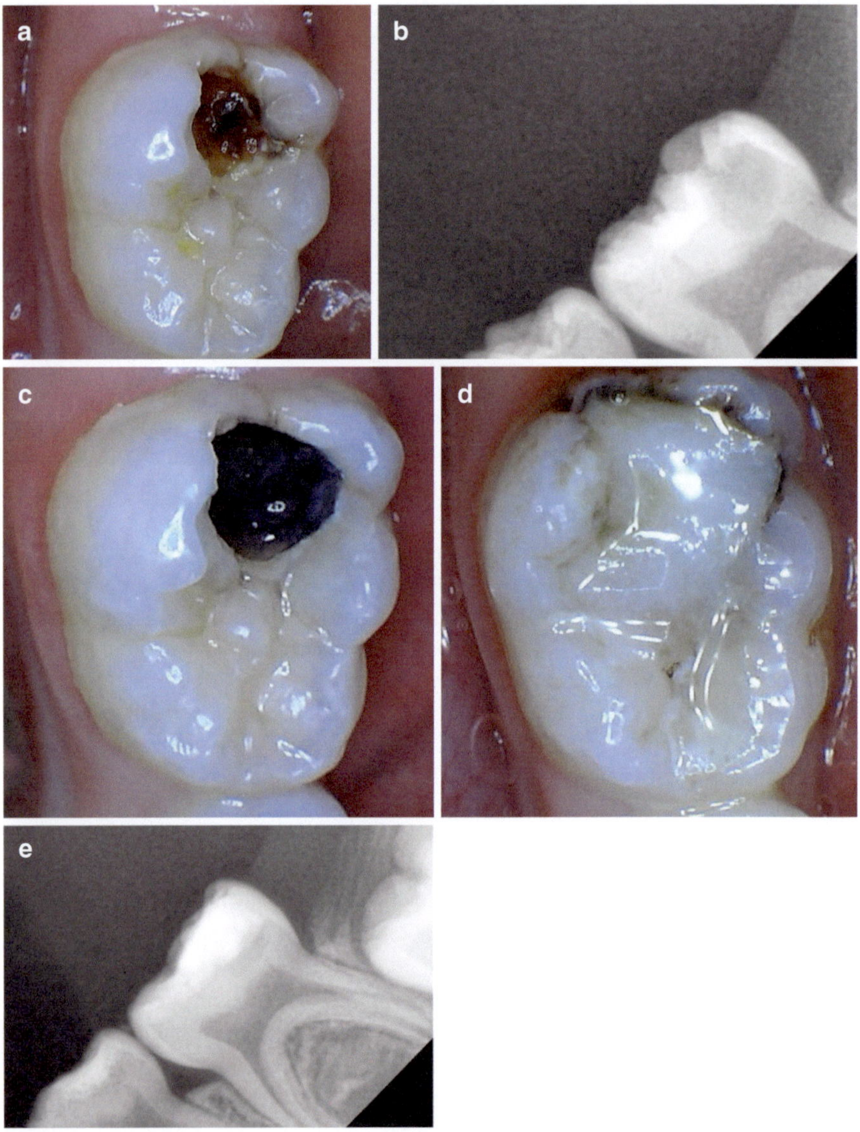

Fig. 5.25 Extensive-stage lesion in mandibular primary left second molar (**a**). Child was pre-cooperative and did not allow for an appropriate radiograph (**b**). Minimal excavation done to retain restorative material bulk and 38% SDF scrubbed for a minute on the lesion (**c**). Tooth restored with High-Viscosity Glass Ionomer Cement (**d**). Radiograph taken at one-year follow-up (**e**)

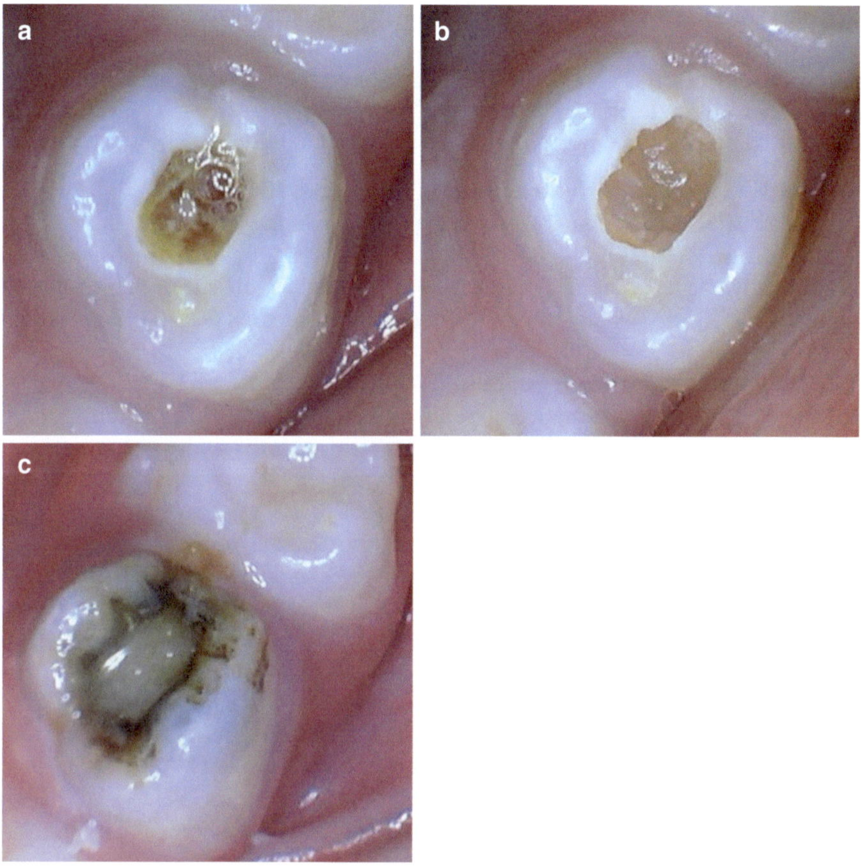

Fig. 5.26 Extensive-stage lesion in maxillary primary left first molar (**a**). Minimal excavation of the lesion done (**b**). 38% SDF applied and tooth restored with Resin-Modified Glass Ionomer Cement. The discoloration of the restoration is accentuated with the curing light (**c**)

2. Once the lesion has been completely exposed, all plaque and debris must be removed from the walls and floor of the lesion.
3. The walls of the lesion must be excavated to healthy tooth structure to ensure optimal bonding with the GIC.
4. A "no caries removal" approach is advised on the floor of the lesion, however selective excavation to firm or soft dentin may be done to achieve optimal depth for the restorative material.
5. After protecting the surrounding soft tissues with cocoa butter, the tooth must be dried and isolated with cotton rolls, and if the child's cooperation permits, a high vacuum suction should be used.
6. 38% SDF solution should be scrubbed into the lesion for 1 minute followed by air drying. The tooth must then be kept isolated for another 3 minutes, to allow the SDF to penetrate the lesion.

7. Once SDF is applied, a self-curing hand-mixed or capsulated HVGIC (3 M™ESPE™Ketac™ Molar, GC Fuji IX GP®) should be placed.
8. A coat of varnish is applied on the restoration to prevent desiccation of the GIC due to exposure to oral fluids (Table 5.2).

5.7.3.3 Which Restorative Material Is Advisable for SMART?

High-Viscosity Glass Ionomer Cements have shown better bond strengths to SDF-treated dentin, followed by Resin-Modified GIC and Resin Composites [58]. Additionally, the remineralizing properties of GIC and its self-curing nature make it the material of choice when placing an intracoronal restoration post SDF application.

5.7.3.4 Can Discoloration Following SMART Be Reduced?

It is inevitable that the application of SDF will result in blackish discoloration of the carious lesion. Similar discoloration is seen with RMGIC and the conventional Glass Ionomer Restoration when the cement or the protective varnish is light cured while doing a SMART restoration (Table. 5.2). The use of potassium iodide (KI) solution (Riva Star, SDI Australia; Kedo SDF, Kedo Dental, India) is seen to reduce the immediate discoloration that occurs after the application of SDF. As per the manufacturer, KI solution must be rubbed onto the SDF-treated tooth, until the creamy white precipitate turns clear. The tooth is then blot dried and restored. Even after the application of KI, some staining may still occur while doing SMART.

5.7.3.5 Are there Additional Benefits of Placing a Crown Over a SMART Restoration in the Same Appointment?

Certain case reports have suggested the placement of Stainless-Steel Crowns over a SMART restoration at the same appointment based on the rationale that the marginal seal provided by a crown is significantly superior to that of a GIC restoration. When a full-coverage restoration itself can ensure lesion arrest, the clinician does not need to place a SMART restoration prior to the Hall technique.

Presently, there is a paucity of published high-quality randomized controlled trials describing the long-term clinical success or the cost–benefit ratio of the SMART technique. However, when good clinical judgment is exercised while performing this technique, it can be a plausible treatment option in cases, where pulpal

Table 5.2 Commercially available protective varnishes for Glass Ionomer restorations

	Product	Manufacturer	Mode of cure
1	G Coat Plus™	GC	Light cure
2	Equia Forte® Coat	GC	Light cure
3	GC Fuji Varnish™	GC	Self-cure
4	Vitremer™ Finishing Gloss	3 M™	Light cure
5	Easy Glaze	Voco	Light cure
6	Final Varnish LC	Voco	Light cure
7	COAT IT	Shofu	Light cure
8	Riva Coat	SDI	Light cure

preservation is the objective, and the extent of the cavity is such that a conventional restoration would succeed.

5.7.4 Resin Infiltration (RI)

The possibility of penetrating caries with resins was first described in the 1970s. The porous enamel lesion provided diffusion pathways for the acids and dissolved minerals that allowed the lesion to progress. Based on this principle, caries or Resin Infiltration technology was developed by Charite Berlin and the University of Kiel in 2012. It is currently marketed as Icon® (Infiltration CONcept) by DMG (Dental Material-Gesellschaft, Hamburg, Germany). This concept is a microinvasive approach that uses the same diffusion pathways to infiltrate the pores with a low-viscosity resin that reinforces, fills, and stabilizes demineralized enamel without sacrificing the healthy tooth structure [59]. While its early clinical application was aimed at treating initial-stage lesions on proximal and smooth surfaces, it was soon observed that treated lesions looked similar to sound enamel, when infiltrated with the resin. The esthetic value of Resin Infiltration technology was not only effective in treating post-orthodontic white spot lesions but also successfully masked the appearance of hypomineralized patches, particularly in the permanent anterior dentition [60, 61].

5.7.4.1 What Is the Rationale for Resin Infiltration? [62–64]

When the demineralization process starts to dominate at the enamel–plaque interface, there is a loss of ions making the enamel porous and leading to the formation of initial-stage lesions. Since the refractive index of water (1.33) or air (1.0) is less than that of sound enamel (1.62), these lesions appear whitish opaque, more so on-air drying. Resin is used to infiltrate these microporosities as it has a refractive index of 1.43, closer to that of sound enamel. The infiltrate blocks the channels serving the dual purpose of halting the progression of the lesion and restoring the esthetics of the tooth.

5.7.4.2 When Should Resin Infiltration Be Performed?

RI is indicated in proximal and smooth surface initial-stage lesions that do not exhibit microcavities or pitting. In case of proximal lesions, radiographically, the extent of the lesion should be limited to the outer half of enamel [65, 66]. Resin infiltration is an esthetic approach for the treatment of white spot lesions seen on smooth surfaces in the permanent dentition post-orthodontic debonding. RI can be used to treat mild cases of fluorosis, characterized by symmetrical lesions having a parchment or cloudy appearance and affecting homologous teeth. It can be successfully used in certain cases of traumatic hypomineralization limited to the superficial layers of the enamel [67].

5.7.4.3 In Which Cases Will RI Not Work?

It is difficult to mask discolored or brown spot initial-stage lesions in anterior teeth as the diffusion channels in these lesions are contaminated by chromophores and pigments. RI will not work in cases of severe Molar Incisor Hypomineralization (MIH), traumatic hypomineralization, or fluorosis as the defect originates at the DEJ and the diffusion channels seen in an initial-stage lesion may be lacking. For these lesions, a deep infiltration technique can be used, i.e., combination of micro-abrasion and Resin Infiltration (discussed later) or one can adopt a protocol of tooth whitening followed by resin infiltration. However, the desired esthetics may still not be achieved [68, 69].

RI must be used cautiously in posterior proximal lesions extending to the outer one third of dentin on a bitewing radiograph. Almost half of these lesions are likely to have microcavities that will deem RI ineffective. Therefore, it is advised to separate the teeth at a prior appointment to visualize the lesion clinically before planning infiltration. For proximal brown spot non-cavitated lesions in posterior teeth, rather than performing RI, regular monitoring and use of preventive measures are advised, as the brown appearance is a sign of arrest or slowing down of the caries process.

It must also be used judiciously in poorly compliant patients at high caries risk and children with special needs as the success of RI is bolstered with good professional and home care oral hygiene measures, including flossing for interproximal lesions.

5.7.4.4 Resin Infiltration Technique

The commercially available RI is the Icon by DMG which contains the following:

Proximal Kit [70]

- Disposable proximal tips that can rotate 360°. The green side of the tip should be aligned with the side to be treated. This side contains the perforated membrane that will express the etchant only on the treatment surface. The adjacent tooth is protected from the etchant with the non-perforated side of the membrane.
- Icon etchant (15% HCL) in a syringe that is dispensed using the proximal tip mentioned above.
- Icon dry (55–99% ethanol) in a syringe and needle that can be inserted interproximally.
- Icon infiltrant (Triethylene Glycol Dimethacrylate-70-95%, Camphoroquinone is less than 2.5%) is dispensed like the etchant with a new but similar proximal tip.
- A plastic wedge with a handle is used to create separation interproximally, which will allow the placement of the perforated membrane. Alternatively, elastic separators can be placed a day before the appointment.

Smooth Surface Kit [71]

The etchant and infiltrant are dispensed using disposable micro applicator brush tips attached to the syringes. All other components in the kit remain the same. Isolation with a rubber dam is a requisite for treating lesions involving the cervical third of the teeth. Lesions limited to the incisal half can be isolated with cotton rolls and suction tips. In addition, a liquid dam must be applied for both isolation methods to protect the soft tissues from the HCL etchant as it can erode the gingival margins on contact.

Role of ICON Dry

After applying the etchant for two minutes, the tooth is rinsed for 30 seconds and air dried. Icon Dry is applied for 30 seconds to desiccate the lesion by displacing water from enamel porosities, leaving the lesion completely dry. Additionally, it determines if the infiltrant will successfully mask the lesion, as the refractive index of Icon Dry (ethanol: 1.36) is closer to that of the resin infiltrant (1.43). If the defect is still visible after applying ICON Dry, then the resin infiltrant will not mask the lesion. The etching can be repeated 2–3 times, till the lesion is esthetically acceptable after application of Icon Dry [72]. If the lesion continues to appear the same after Icon Dry, a combination of microabrasion and resin infiltration should be used. If the lesion is masked by the Icon Dry, the Icon infiltrant is applied for three minutes and light cured for 40 seconds (Figs. 5.27 and 5.28).

5.7.4.5 Remineralization and Resin Infiltration in White Spot Lesions

On active chalky white spot lesions, three monthly applications of fluoride varnish along with remineralizing technology, Casein Phosphopeptide-Amorphous Calcium Phosphate (CPP-ACP), Amorphous Calcium Phosphate (ACP), Tri-calcium Phosphate (TCP) and regular home use of optimally fluoridated toothpaste (1000-1450 ppm fluoride) should be the first line of treatment. On the three monthly recall, only when the lesions are not covered with plaque and appear less chalky, RI may be performed to both treat and improve esthetics of the initial-stage lesion. If RI is done on active chalky lesions, the HCL component of Icon etch may cause microcavitation or crater-like defects.

In the permanent dentition, RI will afford better cosmetic outcomes than topical fluorides, as it penetrates and encapsulates the lesion from within, altering optical properties [67, 73–75]. As RI does not prevent the occurrence of new lesions, daily use of fluoridated toothpaste, remineralizing pastes such as TCP, ACP, or CPP–ACP, and professional topical fluoride applications must be continued following the caries risk-based recommendations.

5.7.4.6 Evaluating the Success of the Resin Infiltration Treatment

- *The esthetic appearance of the tooth and color stability*

The color stability of Resin Infiltrated anterior permanent teeth have shown that post-orthodontic white spot lesions and white defects (mild cases of MIH and fluorosis) show an immediate improvement in appearance after RI. The teeth treated with RI may discolor over two to four years due to water sorption by the hydrophilic TEGDMA component of the infiltrant. During follow-up visits, surface discoloration can often be managed through polishing or, in more severe cases, bleaching [76, 77].

- *Caries Arrest of the Lesion*

Systematic reviews conducted on the efficacy of resin infiltration in non-cavitated proximal lesions on permanent teeth have shown it has a better success rate than fluoride varnish applications, alone. The success rate is better in patients who floss

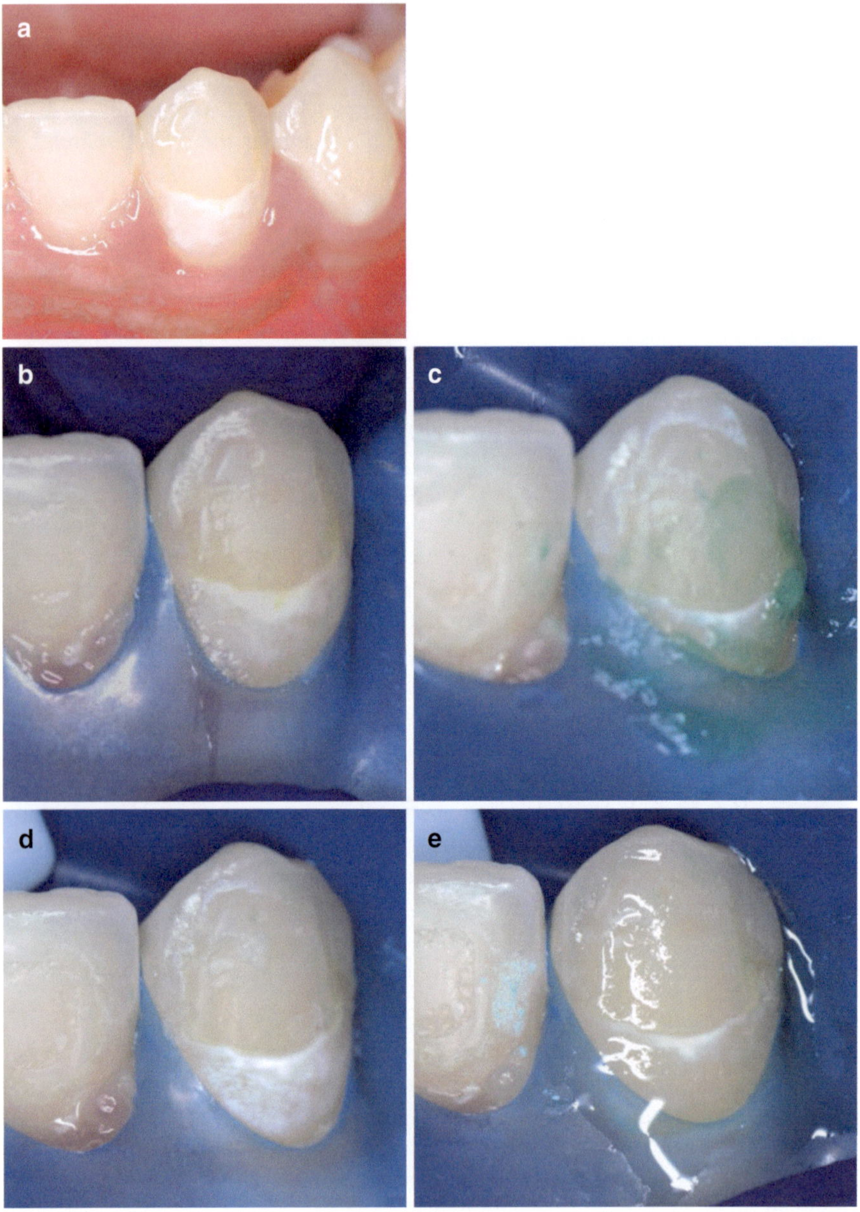

Fig. 5.27 Post-orthodontic white spot lesion on mandibular permanent left canine (**a**). The tooth is cleaned and isolated under rubber dam (**b**). Icon etch is applied on the lesion for two minutes (**c**). The etchant is left for 30 s and washed and airdried (**d**). Icon Dry is applied for 30 seconds to completely dessicate the lesion and determine if the infiltrant will successfully mask the lesion (**e**). Icon infiltrant is applied for three minutes and light cured for 40 seconds (**f**). Two-week follow-up (**g**)

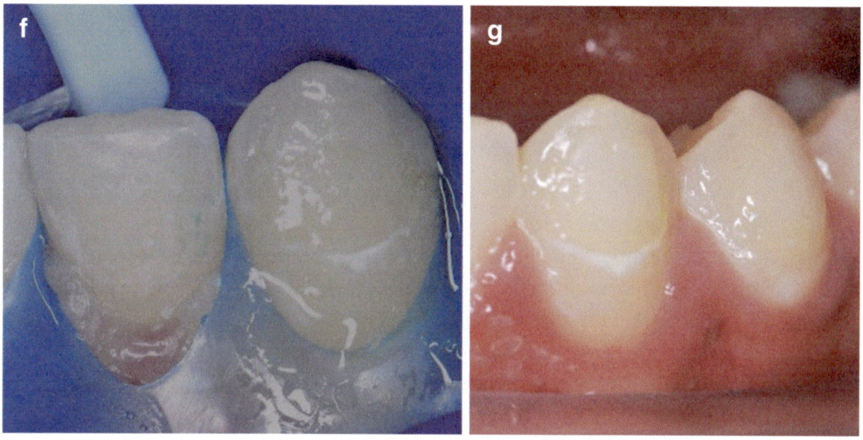

Fig. 5.27 (continued)

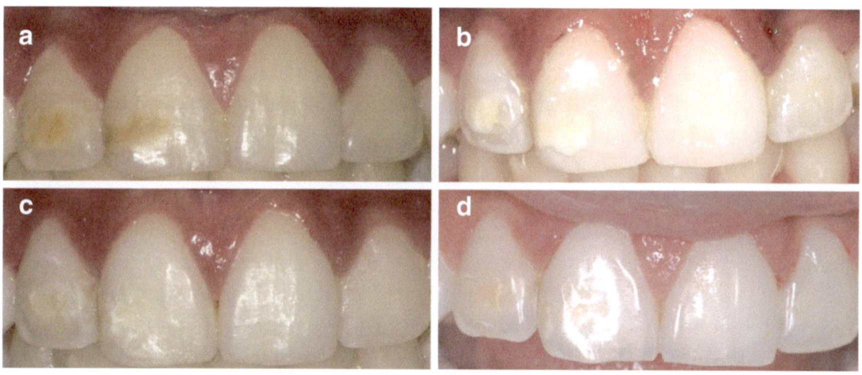

Fig. 5.28 Patient was concerned with the appearance of hypomineralized maxillary permanent right central and lateral incisors (**a**). The teeth were bleached to reduce the brown discoloration of the hypomineralized areas. Resin infiltration was done after one week (**b**). Follow-up after two years showed the infiltrant had not discolored (**c**). The teeth at five-year follow-up continued to appear esthetic (**d**)

regularly following RI than those who do not [78, 79]. However, Resin Infiltration's technique sensitivity and longer treatment time may limit its use in the primary dentition.

5.7.5 Management of Intrinsic Superficial and Deep White Defects

As discussed in the previous section, RI is less likely to be successful in teeth with intrinsic stains or defects such as

- Discoloration or texture alteration due to enamel hypoplasia, amelogenesis imperfecta, or mild to moderate fluorosis.
- Hypomineralized white spot lesions/brown spot lesions.

Microabrasion or tooth bleaching, alone or coupled with RI, can be the treatment of choice.

5.7.5.1 Microabrasion

It aims to remove intrinsic discoloration and textured defects that are superficial and do not require masking with an esthetic restorative material. 38% phosphoric acid or 6.6% HCL and silica containing gel (Opalustre™, Ultradent™, USA) is applied using a rubber cup attached to a slow-speed handpiece to remove the enamel stain or defect. The microabraded surface must be polished with felt discs followed by the application of sodium fluoride gel/varnish to promote the remineralization process (Fig. 5.29).

For lesions in the esthetic zone, microabrasion can be followed by RI. Tooth whitening is often necessary as microabraded teeth can acquire a darker or yellowish coloration after treatment, and the remaining enamel is thinner and more clearly reveals the dentin. Bleaching reduces the contrast between the remaining white spot lesions and the tooth surface. In-office or at home bleaching can be done after microabrasion and to further improve the esthetics, RI infiltration technique can be performed on the teeth [80].

5.7.5.2 Macroabrasion

It is a controlled method for removing enamel to improve discolorations or surface stains limited to the outer enamel layer and localized superficial white spots. In this technique, the area of concern is smoothened using high-speed handpieces with fine-grit diamond finishing burs or carbide burs. The natural contour and anatomy of the tooth surface should be maintained, and the enamel removed should be restricted to 0.5 mm. After this step, the tooth surface is further polished with commercially available flexible discs. Water should be used throughout as a lubricant, to provide cooling and prevent desiccation of the tooth surface. After performing macroabrasion, if there is loss of tooth structure, a Resin Composite restoration must be placed [81, 82].

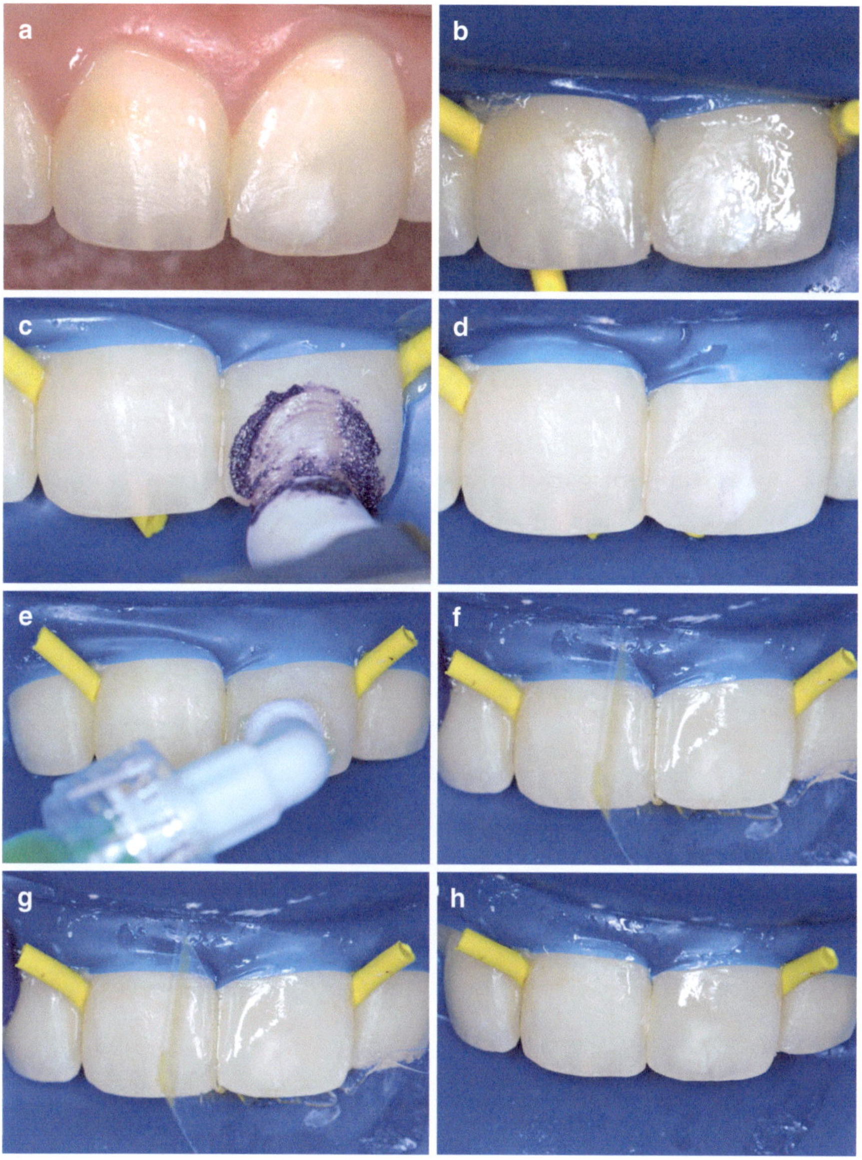

Fig. 5.29 Hypomineralized patch on maxillary permanent left central incisor (**a**). Teeth isolated with rubber dam. Cleaning and polishing done with prophy paste (**b**). The tooth is etched with 6.6% Hydrochloric acid slurry for 60 seconds. The slurry is applied to a rubber cup mounted on a slow-speed (500 RPM) micromotor handpiece (**c**). After washing and air drying, the tooth gives a frosted appearance (**d**). The lesion is etched with Icon etch for two minutes (**e**). The tooth is dried with Icon Dry and a mylar strip is placed to prevent the infiltrant from flowing interproximally (**f**). The infiltrant is applied for three minutes and cured for 40 seconds (**g**). Immediate post-operative photo (**h**). Follow-up after one month (**i**)

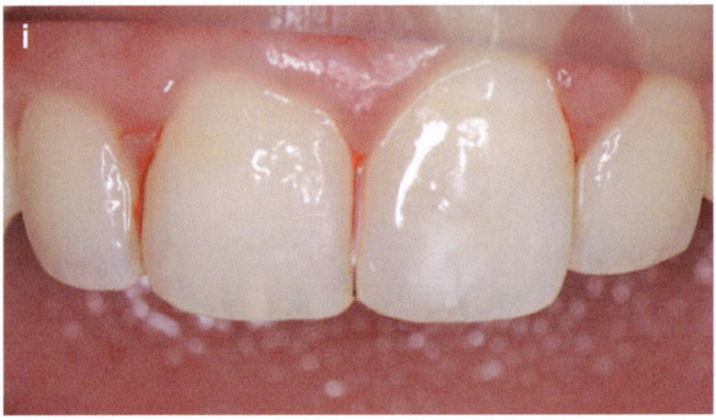

Fig. 5.29 (continued)

5.8 Correlation Between Staging of Carious Lesions and the Suggested Interventions (Table 5.3)

Table 5.3 In this table, the clinical and radiographic features of initial-, moderate-, and extensive-stage lesions are summarized (ICCMS™), along with the specific preventive and therapeutic measures, for each stage

Caries stages	Clinical appearance	Radiographic Appearance (RA)	Suggested intervention		
			Occlusal lesions	Proximal lesions	Smooth
Sound tooth	On cleaning and air-drying, the tooth surface appears sound with no evidence of caries.	No radiographic changes seen	Standardized home care and professional preventive measures		
Initial stage (ICDAS 1 and 2)	White or brown spot lesions seen without enamel breakdown and no underlying dentinal shadow seen.	Radiolucency seen in outer half of enamel and may extend to, but not beyond outer third of dentin. RA1 (limited to outer half of enamel) RA2 (limited to inner half of enamel) RA3 (limited to outer third of dentine)	Pit and fissure sealants	Topical fluoride gels and varnish Silver Diamine Fluoride Resin Infiltration	Extent of lesion and its relation with pulp space cannot be evaluated on a radiograph. Therefore, treatment decisions should be taken based on clinical signs and symptoms that will include the following: Topical fluoride gels and varnish Icon-Resin Infiltration (anterior)

(continued)

Table 5.3 (continued)

Caries stages	Clinical appearance	Radiographic Appearance (RA)	Suggested intervention		
			Occlusal lesions	Proximal lesions	Smooth
Moderate stage (ICDAS 3 and 4)	The lesion appears white or brown/black with localized enamel breakdown without dentinal exposure. An underlying dentin shadow may be seen in some cases.	Radiolucency extending to middle third of dentine	Conventional restoration Hall technique SMART	NRCC-fluoride varnish/SDF (anterior and posterior) SMART Conventional restoration Hall technique (posterior)	
Extensive stage (ICDAS 5 and 6)	Extensive-stage lesions reveal underlying dentin and are close to the pulp. To intervene with minimal operative procedure, there should be no clinical signs and symptoms of irreversible pulpitis.	Extending to the inner third of dentin or involve the pulp.	Restoration with Selective Caries Removal Hall technique SMART	NRCC-fluoride varnish/SDF (anterior) Restoration with selective caries removal Hall technique (posterior)	
			Endodontic treatment—If pulp exposure is seen.		

5.9 Concluding Remarks

Earlier, caries diagnosis was focused on identification of cavitated lesions and their treatment by traditional restorative or endodontic techniques. With the ICCMS, the focus has now shifted to identification of initial-stage lesions and their management by noninvasive or minimally invasive methods such as fluoride varnish application, SDF, NRCC, and Resin Infiltration. In extensive-stage lesions, Selective Caries Removal must be performed to preserve pulp vitality and avoid unnecessary pulp therapy. To ensure the success of these minimally invasive techniques, it is critical that the clinician reinforces home care measures to both the parent and the child.

References

1. Black GV. A work on operative dentistry; the technical procedures in filling teeth. Chicago: Medico-dental Publishing Co; 1917.
2. Beltran ED, Burt BA. The pre-and posteruptive effects of fluoride in the caries decline. J Public Health Dent. 1988;48(4):233–40.
3. Groeneveld A, Van Eck AA, Backer Dirks O. Fluoride in caries prevention: is the effect pre- or post-eruptive? J Dent Res. 1990;69 Spec No:751–5; discussion 820–3.
4. Fusayama T. Two layers of carious dentin; diagnosis and treatment. Oper Dent. 1979;4(2):63–70.
5. Massler M. Changing concepts in the treatment of carious lesions. Br Dent J. 1967;123:547–8.
6. Shovelton DS. A study of deep carious dentine. Int Dent J. 1968;18:392–405.
7. MacGregor AB, Marsland EA, Batty I. Experimental studies of dental caries. The relation of bacterial invasion to softening of the dentine. Br Dent J. 1956;101:230–5.
8. Ayna B, Çelenk S, Atakul F, Sezgin B, Özekinci T. Evaluation of clinical and microbiological features of deep carious lesions in primary molars. J Dent Childr. 2003;70(1):15–8.
9. Marsh PD. Microbial ecology of dental plaque and its significance in health and disease. Adv Dent Res. 1994;8(2):263–71.
10. Tjäderhane L, Tezvergil-Mutluay A. Performance of adhesives and restorative materials after selective removal of carious lesions: restorative materials with anticaries properties. Dental Clinics. 2019;63(4):715–29.
11. Horst JA, Ellenikiotis H, Milgrom PM. UCSF silver caries arrest committee. UCSF protocol for caries arrest using silver diamine fluoride: rationale, indications, and consent. JCDA. 2016;44(1):16.
12. Zaeneldin A, Ollie YY, Chu CH. Effect of silver diamine fluoride on vital dental pulp: a systematic review. J Dent. 2022;119:104066.
13. Frencken JE, Peters MC, Manton DJ, Leal SC, Gordan VV, Eden E. Minimal intervention dentistry for managing dental caries – a review: report of a FDI task group. Int Dent J. 2012;62(5):223–43.
14. Featherstone JD. The caries balance: contributing factors and early detection. CDA. 2003;31(2):129–34.
15. Pitts NB, Ekstrand KR, ICDAS Foundation. International Caries Detection and Assessment System (ICDAS) and its international Caries Classification and Management System (ICCMS) – methods for staging of the caries process and enabling dentists to manage caries. Community Dent Oral Epidemiol. 2013;41(1):e41–52.
16. Machiulskiene V, Campus G, Carvalho JC, Dige I, Ekstrand KR, Jablonski-Momeni A, Maltz M, Manton DJ, Martignon S, Martinez-Mier EA, Pitts NB, Schulte AG, Splieth CH, Tenuta LMA, Ferreira Zandona A, Nyvad B. Terminology of dental caries and dental caries management: consensus report of a workshop organized by ORCA and Cariology Research Group of IADR. Caries Res. 2020;54(1):7–14.
17. Ismail AI, Pitts NB, Tellez M. The International Caries Classification and Management System (ICCMS™) an example of a caries management pathway. BMC Oral Health. 2015;15(1):1–13.
18. IAPD Foundational articles and consensus recommendations: caries risk assessment and care pathways, 2022.
19. American Academy of Pediatric Dentistry. Prescribing dental radiographs for infants, children, adolescents, and individuals with special health care needs. In: The reference manual of pediatric dentistry. Chicago: American Academy of Pediatric Dentistry; 2024. p. 313–7.
20. Kühnisch J, Anttonen V, Duggal MS, Spyridonos ML, Rajasekharan S, Sobczak M, Stratigaki E, Van Acker JW, Aps JK, Horner K, Tsiklakis K. Best clinical practice guidance for prescribing dental radiographs in children and adolescents: an EAPD policy document. Eur Arc Paediatr Dent. 2020;21(4):375–86.

21. Scottish Dental Clinical Effectiveness Programme. Prevention and management of dental caries in children: dental clinical guidance. Scottish Dental Clinical Effectiveness Programme Dundee 2018.
22. Nyvad B, Baelum V. Nyvad criteria for caries lesion activity and severity assessment: a validated approach for clinical management and research. Caries Res. 2018;52(5):397–405.
23. Lussi A, Hibst R, Paulus R. DIAGNOdent: an optical method for caries detection. J Dent Res. 2004;83(1_suppl):80–3.
24. Innes N, Schwendicke F, Frencken J. An agreed terminology for carious tissue removal. Monogr Oral Sci. 2018;27:155–61.
25. Dhar V, Pilcher L, Fontana M, González-Cabezas C, Keels MA, Mascarenhas AK, Nascimento M, Platt JA, Sabino GJ, Slayton R, Tinanoff N. Evidence-based clinical practice guideline on restorative treatments for caries lesions: a report from the American Dental Association. J Am Dent Assoc. 2023;154(7):551–66.
26. Kidd EAM. How 'clean' must a cavity be before restoration? Caries Res. 2004;38:305–13.
27. Bjørndal L. Stepwise excavation. Monogr Oral Sci. 2018;27(1):68–81.
28. Schwendicke F, Frencken J, Innes N, editors. Caries excavation: evolution of treating cavitated carious lesions. Karger Medical and Scientific Publishers; 2018.
29. Schwendicke F, Frencken JE, Bjørndal L, Maltz M, Manton DJ, Ricketts D, Van Landuyt K, Banerjee A, Campus G, Doméjean S, Fontana M. Managing carious lesions: consensus recommendations on carious tissue removal. Adv Dent Res. 2016;28(2):58–67.
30. Bjørndal L, Larsen T, Thylstrup A. A clinical and microbiological study of deep carious lesions during stepwise excavation using long treatment intervals. Caries Res. 1997;31(6):411–7.
31. Bjørndal L, Larsen T. Changes in the cultivable flora in deep carious lesions following a stepwise excavation procedure. Caries Res. 2000;34(6):502–8.
32. Craig RG, Curro FA, Green WS, Ship JA. Treatment of deep carious lesions by complete excavation or partial removal: a critical review. JADA. 2008;139(6):705–12.
33. IAPD. Foundational articles and consensus recommendations: pulp therapy for primary and Young permanent teeth, 2022. http://www.iapdworld.org/2022_12_pulp-therapy-for-primary-and-young-permanent-teeth
34. Maltz M, Garcia R, Jardim JJ, De Paula LM, Yamaguti PM, Moura MS, Garcia F, Nascimento C, Oliveira A, Mestrinho HD. Randomized trial of partial vs. stepwise caries removal: 3-year follow-up. J Dent Res. 2012;91(11):1026–31.
35. Maltz M, Alves LS. Incomplete caries removal significantly reduces the risk of pulp exposure and post-operative pulpal symptoms. J Evid Based Dent Pract. 2013;13(3):120–2.
36. Hamouda M, Deery C. What is the best caries removal strategy for primary molars? Evid Based Dent. 2021;22(1):20–1. https://doi.org/10.1038/s41432-021-0150-x.
37. Santamaría RM, Abudrya MH, Gül G, Mourad MS, Gomez GF, Zandona AGF. How to intervene in the caries process: dentin caries in primary teeth. Caries Res. 2020;54(4):306–23. https://doi.org/10.1159/000508899. Epub 2020 Aug 27
38. Aïem E, Joseph C, Garcia A, Smaïl-Faugeron V, Muller-Bolla M. Caries removal strategies for deep carious lesions in primary teeth: systematic review. Int J Paediatr Dent. 2020;30(4):392–404.
39. Black GV. A work on operative dentistry vol 1. Management of children's teeth. Chicago: Medico Dental Publishing Company; 1908. p. 235–57.
40. van Strijp G, van Loveren C. No removal and inactivation of carious tissue: non-restorative cavity control. In: Caries excavation: evolution of treating Cavitated carious lesions, vol. 27. Karger Publishers; 2018. p. 124–36.
41. Gruythuysen RJ. Non-restorative cavity treatment Managing rather than masking caries activity. Nederlands tijdschrift voor tandheelkunde. 2010;117(3):173–80.
42. Gruythuysen RJ. Non-restorative cavity treatment: should this be the treatment of choice? Reflections of a teacher in paediatric dentistry. Dent Update. 2019;46(3):220–8.
43. Duangthip D, Jiang M, Chu CH, Lo E. Non-surgical treatment of dentin caries in preschool children–systematic review. BMC Oral Health. 2015;15(1):1.

44. Urquhart O, Tampi MP, Pilcher L, Slayton RL, Araujo MWB, Fontana M, Guzmán-Armstrong S, Nascimento MM, Nový BB, Tinanoff N, Weyant RJ, Wolff MS, Young DA, Zero DT, Brignardello-Petersen R, Banfield L, Parikh A, Joshi G, Carrasco-Labra A. Nonrestorative treatments for caries: systematic review and network meta-analysis. J Dent Res. 2019;98(1):14–26.
45. Innes NP, Evans DJ, Bonifacio CC, Geneser M, Hesse D, Heimer M, Kanellis M, Machiulskiene V, Narbutaité J, Olegário IC, Owais A. The Hall technique 10 years on: questions and answers. Bri Dent J. 2017;222(6):478–83.
46. Kaya MS, Kınay Taran P, Bakkal M. Temporomandibular dysfunction assessment in children treated with the Hall technique: a pilot study. Int J Paediatr Dent. 2020;30(4):429–35.
47. Joseph RM, Rao AP, Srikant N, Karuna YM, Nayak AP. Evaluation of changes in the occlusion and occlusal vertical dimension in children following the placement of preformed metal crowns using the hall technique. J Clin Pediatr Dent. 2020;44(2):130–4.
48. Welbury RR. The Hall technique 10 years on: its effect and influence. Br Dent J. 2017;222(6):421–2.
49. Badar SB, Tabassum S, Khan FR, Ghafoor R. Effectiveness of hall technique for primary carious molars: a systematic review and meta-analysis. Int J Clin Pediatr Dent. 2019;12(5):445.
50. Hu S, BaniHani A, Nevitt S, Maden M, Santamaria RM, Albadri S. Hall technique for primary teeth: a systematic review and meta-analysis. Jpn Dent Sci Rev. 2022;(58):286–97.
51. Innes NP, Evans DJ, et al. Sealing caries in primary molars: randomized control trial, 5-year results. J Dent Res. 2011;90:1405–10.
52. Santamaria RM, Innes NPT, et al. Alternative caries management options for primary molars: 2.5-year outcomes of a randomised clinical trial. Caries Res. 2017;51:605–14.
53. Boyd DH, Page LF, et al. The Hall technique and conventional restorative treatment in New Zealand children's primary oral health care – clinical outcomes at two years. Int J Paediatr Dent. 2018;28:180–8.
54. Innes NP, Stirrups DR, et al. A novel technique using preformed metal crowns for managing carious primary molars in general practice – a retrospective analysis. Br Dent J. 2006;200:451–4.
55. Ludwig KH, Fontana M, et al. The success of stainless steel crowns placed with the Hall technique: a retrospective study. J Am Dent Assoc. 2014;145:1248–53.
56. Natarajan D. Silver modified atraumatic restorative technique: a way towards "SMART" pediatric dentistry during the COVID-19 pandemic. Front Dent. 2022;19:12.
57. Aly AAM, Aziz AMA, Elghazawy RK, El Fadl RKA. Survival analysis and cost effectiveness of Silver Modified Atraumatic Restorative Treatment (SMART) and ART occlusal restorations in primary molars: a randomized controlled trial. J Dent. 2023 Jan;128:104379.
58. Fröhlich TT, Botton G, Rocha RO. Bonding of glass-ionomer cement and adhesives to silver diamine fluoride-treated dentin: an updated systematic review and meta-analysis. J Adhes Dent. 2022;24(1):29–38.
59. Paris S, Meyer-Lueckel H, Kielbassa AM. Resin infiltration of natural caries lesions. J Dent Res. 2007;86(7):662–6.
60. Kugel G, Arsenault P, Papas A. Treatment modalities for caries management, including a new resin infiltration system. Compend Contin Educ Dent (Jamesburg, NJ: 1995). 2009;30:1.
61. Son JH, Hur B, Kim HC, Park JK. Management of white spots: resin infiltration technique and microabrasion. J Korean Acad Conservat Dent. 2011;36(1):66–71.
62. Paris S, Meyer-Lueckel H. Masking of labial enamel white spot lesions by resin infiltration – a clinical report. Quintessence Int. 2009;40(9):713–8.
63. Meyer-Lueckel H, Paris S. Improved resin infiltration of natural caries lesions. J Dent Res. 2008;87(12):1112–6.
64. Paris S, Meyer-Lueckel H, Cölfen H, Kielbassa AM. Resin infiltration of artificial enamel caries lesions with experimental light curing resins. Dent Mater J. 2007;26(4):582–8.
65. Allen DN, Fine CM, Newton MN, Kabani F, Muzzin KB, Reed KM. Resin infiltration therapy: a micro-invasive treatment approach for white spot lesions. J Dent Hyg. 2021;95(6):31–5.
66. Phark JH, Duarte S, Meyer-Lueckel H, Paris S. Caries infiltration with resins: a novel treatment option for interproximal caries. Compend Contin Educ Dent. 2009;30 Spec No 3:13–7.
67. Borges AB, Caneppele TM, Masterson D, Maia LC. Is resin infiltration an effective esthetic treatment for enamel development defects and white spot lesions? A systematic review. J Dent. 2017;56:11–8.

68. Alwafi A. Resin infiltration may be considered as a color-masking treatment option for enamel development defects and white spot lesions. J Evid Based Dent Pract. 2017;17(2):113–5.
69. Casaña-Ruiz MD, Marqués Martínez L, García Miralles E. Management of Hypoplastic or Hypomineralized defects with resin infiltration at pediatric ages: systematic review. Int J Environ Res Public Health. 2023;20(6):5201.
70. https://www.dmg-dental.com/en/solutions/prevention-and-early-intervention/infiltration/icon-proximal#c7351
71. https://www.dmgamerica.com/fileadmin/DMG_America/IFU/IFU_Icon_Smooth_Surface.pdf
72. Atlan A, Denis M, Tirlet G, Attal JP. Orthodontics and enamel spots. Benefits of a minimally invasive approach, guidelines for the orthodontist. J Dent Anomal Orthodont. 2017;20(3):302.
73. Pliska BT, Warner GA, Tantbirojn D, Larson BE. Treatment of white spot lesions with ACP paste and microabrasion. Angle Orthod. 2012;82(5):765–9.
74. Aref NS, Alrasheed MK. Casein phosphopeptide amorphous calcium phosphate and universal adhesive resin as a complementary approach for management of white spot lesions: an in-vitro study. Prog Orthod. 2022;23(1):10.
75. Brignardello-Petersen R. Resin infiltration improves the appearance of enamel discolorations. J Am Dent Assoc. 2017;148(4):e34.
76. Saccucci M, Corridore D, Di Carlo G, Bonucci E, Cicciù M, Vozza I. Assessment of enamel color stability of resins infiltration treatment in human teeth: a systematic review. Int J Environ Health Res. 2022;19(18):11269.
77. Zhao X, Ren YF. Surface properties and color stability of resin-infiltrated enamel lesions. Oper Dent. 2016;41(6):617–26.
78. Puleio F, Fiorillo L, Gorassini F, Iandolo A, Meto A, D'Amico C, Cervino G, Pinizzotto M, Bruno G, Portelli M, Amato A, Lo Giudice R. Systematic review on white spot lesions treatments. Eur J Dent. 2022;16(1):41–8.
79. Doméjean S, Ducamp R, Léger S, Holmgren C. Resin infiltration of non-cavitated caries lesions: a systematic review. Med Princ Pract. 2015;24(3):216–21.
80. Pini NI, Sundfeld-Neto D, Aguiar FH, Sundfeld RH, Martins LR, Lovadino JR, Lima DA. Enamel microabrasion: an overview of clinical and scientific considerations. World J Clin Cases. 2015;3(1):34–41.
81. Amarlal D, Rayen R, Muthu MS. Macroabrasion in pediatric dentistry. J Clin Pediatr Dent. 2006;31(1):9.
82. Shenoi P, Kandhari A, Gunwal M. Esthetic enhancement of discolored teeth by macroabrasion microabrasion and its psychological impact on patients-a case series. Indian J Multidiscip Dent. 2011;2(1)

Direct Restorations

6

6.1 Introduction

Restorative dentistry has formed the mainstay of contemporary dental practices across the world. Over the years, the concepts and principles of restorative dentistry have undergone a significant transformation. Earlier, dental caries was considered a disease that was treated by complete elimination of decayed tooth structure. Further, it was believed that to prevent its recurrence; an "Extension for prevention" approach must be adopted wherein all susceptible pits and fissures were incorporated into the tooth preparation [1]. As the understanding of dental caries and tooth anatomy gradually improved, operators came to realize that aggressive tooth cutting not only reduced the strength of the tooth but often resulted in pulpal treatment that could have been avoided. With this realization, dentistry gradually shifted to performing conservative restorations in teeth with the added objective of pulpal preservation. The shift in the restorative approach towards "prevention of extension" and growing demand for esthetic restorations led to amalgam slowly becoming obsolete, despite it being an excellent restorative material. Concomitantly, there was development of newer biomaterials and improvement of materials like Glass Ionomer Cement (GIC) and Resin Composite, whose adhesive properties supported conservative preparations and provided esthetic advantages [2]. As restorative dentistry continues to advance, the focus of every new development is on replicating the appearance, form, and function of the natural tooth, while remaining respectful of healthy tooth structure and the dentino-pulpal complex.

H. Vyas et al., *Dental Caries and Traumatic Injuries in Pediatric Dentistry*,
https://doi.org/10.1007/978-3-031-98929-2_6

6.2 Tooth Preparation for Direct Restorations: Recommendations and Technique

6.2.1 What Are the Current Concepts in Tooth Preparation?

- *Design Extension*

G.V. Black's tooth preparation designs identified the position of a lesion and prescribed a cavity design that included all the fissures whether it was involved with caries or not. This resulted in cavity preparations often larger than it needed to be [3, 4]. *Contemporary cavity preparation designs* are conservative and dictated by the extent of the lesion. The adhesive properties of Resin Composites and GICs, which are the most widely used restorative materials, allow for such an approach [5]. Extension through the entire fissure system on the occlusal surface is undesirable because areas that are not involved in the carious lesion can be sealed. Additionally, retentive features like dove tails and undercuts need not be incorporated in the cavity design.

- *Depth of Restoration*

G.V. Black recommended a standard depth of 1.5-2 mm throughout the cavity preparation, to ensure sufficient bulk of amalgam to withstand the masticatory forces [4]. The "flat floor design" used for most silver amalgam restorations is no longer a requirement for the adhesive restorations [6, 7]. The *depth of contemporary cavity preparation* is dictated by the extent of the lesion and its proximity to the pulp [5]. In moderate-stage lesions, complete caries removal may be performed to allow for adequate bulk of the restoration. Selective caries excavation must be performed on the pulpal floor to soft or firm dentin in areas where deeper carious involvement is seen, thus, protecting the pulpo-dentinal complex [8, 9].

The *cavosurface margin* of the tooth preparation is determined by the type of restorative material used and the kind of bond it forms with the remaining tooth structure. Since amalgam forms a mechanical bond with the tooth and has a low edge strength, Black recommended a cavosurface angle of 90 degrees (butt joint) to give maximal strength to the restoration [4]. As Glass Ionomers form an ionic chemical bond with the tooth structure, a cavosurface butt joint is recommended as the material is brittle and has low edge strength. GIC will chip if placed on a bevel or feather edge margin as it requires a certain thickness to withstand occlusal forces [10]. On the other hand, Resin Composite exhibits micromechanical adhesion to the tooth, and hence, it is recommended to bevel the cavosurface margins of preparations to expose the enamel rods and increase the surface area on which the material can bond, improving both esthetics and the physical properties of the restoration [11].

The OXIS classification has described four types of proximal contacts in primary molars, i.e., O, X, I, S (Fig. 6.1). The authors have further shown that among the four groups, I and S contacts are more susceptible to dental caries due to their

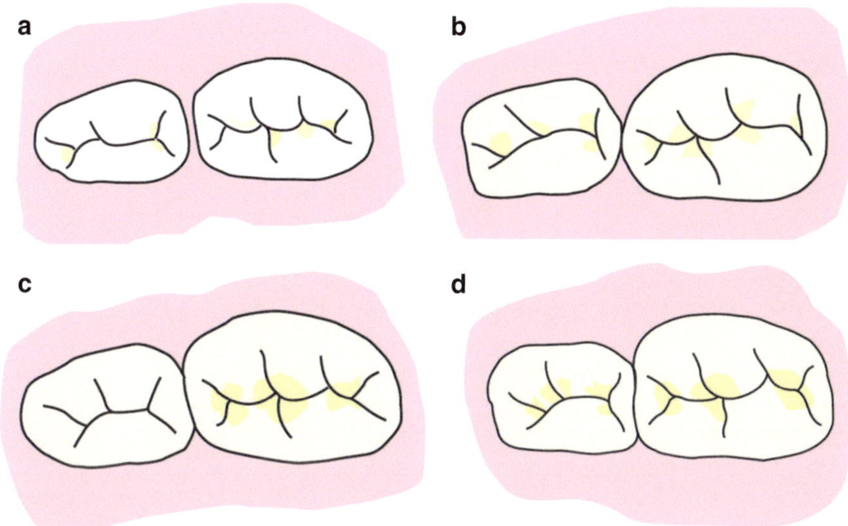

Fig. 6.1 The four interproximal contact types, O (**a**), X (**b**), I (**c**), and S (**d**)

Table 6.1 Correlating types of contact with caries susceptibility

	Type of contacts	Caries susceptibility
1	O	Low
2	X	Low
3	I	High
4	S	High

complex morphology which facilitates plaque accumulation and does not allow for effective cleansing with only tooth brushing (Table 6.1) [12]. In these contacts, any initial carious lesion requires active surveillance and preventive measures like fluoride varnish or 38% SDF application.

The tooth preparation designs for proximal lesions involve only the box preparation and need not have an occlusal extension unless the occlusal pits and fissures are involved with caries. Caries must be removed to healthy enamel and dentin on walls of interproximal box and the gingival seat. The axial wall may be excavated to sound or firm dentin [13]. The buccal and lingual walls of the proximal box must be in areas accessible for cleansing irrespective of the type of contact (OXIS) (Fig. 6.2).

The proximal box should not be beveled. In case of occlusal and proximal carious lesions on the same tooth, the preparations must be kept separate unless the intervening enamel is thin or undermined. In primary molars, if the gingival seat is lost or embrasures extend beyond the line angles and the proximal box is wide, then a full-coverage restoration must be placed (Figs. 6.3 and 6.4) [14–16]. Similarly in anterior teeth, if the incisal edge is involved or the proximal lesion is large, a full-coverage restoration is recommended.

While preparing a tooth to treat a proximal cavity, one must take care to avoid iatrogenic damage to the adjacent tooth. This can be achieved using products such

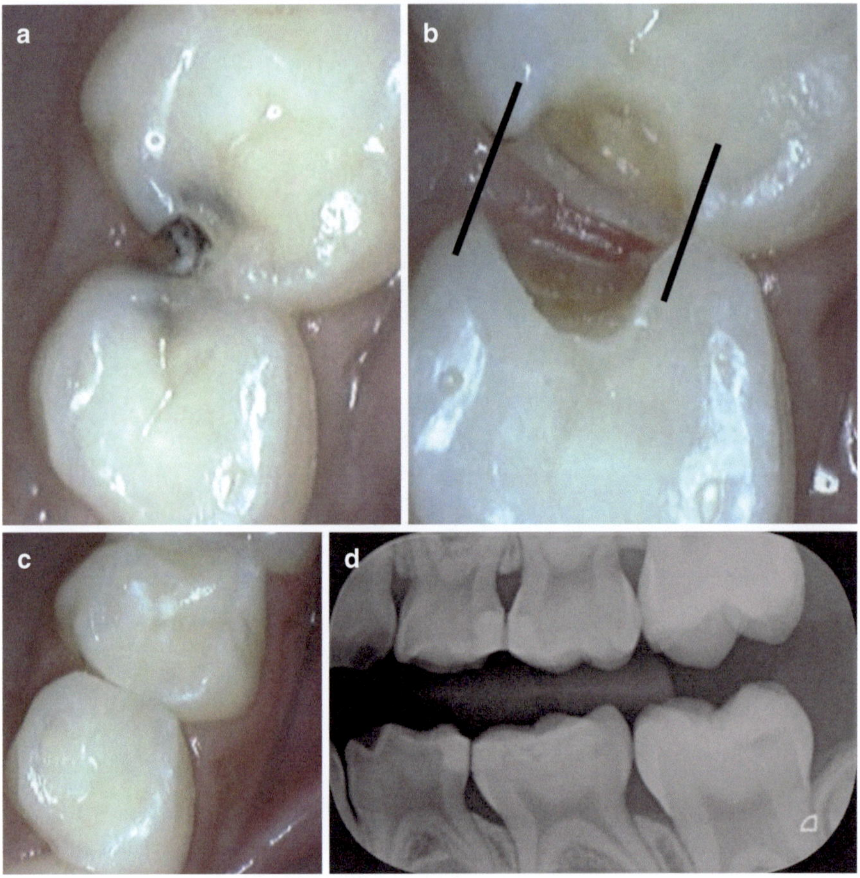

Fig. 6.2 Carious lesions in maxillary primary first and second molars (**a**). Complete Caries Removal is done to provide bulk to the Resin-Modified Glass Ionomer Cement. A box-type cavity is prepared without occlusal extension. The proximal box and gingival seat must not be beveled. The proximal walls of prepared cavity must be within line angles to receive a direct restoration (**b**). The restoration must not have overhangs or ledges, as seen clinically (**c**) and on the radiograph (**d**)

as InterGuard™ by Ultradent which is a straight metal band of a 4- or 5-mm thickness with stable curls at each end. Alternatively, a stainless-steel matrix band can also be placed between teeth during proximal tooth preparation to protect the adjacent tooth surface [17]. The etiological factors responsible for a proximal lesion in any tooth are likely to cause demineralization in the adjacent teeth. Preventive therapy such as fluoride varnish or 38% SDF should be applied on the adjacent tooth surface.

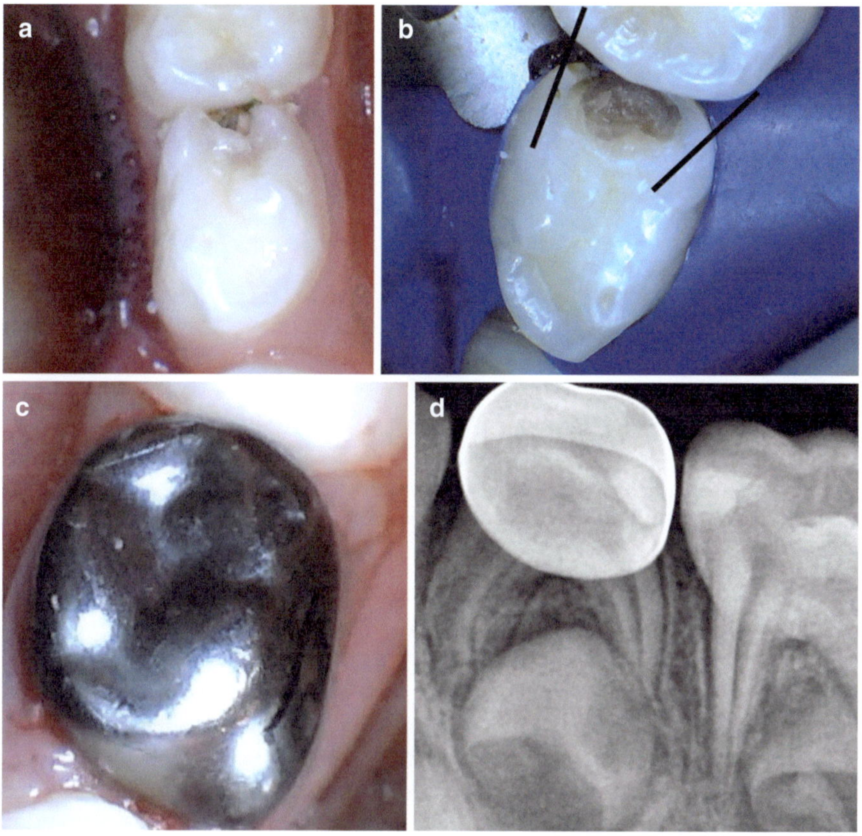

Fig. 6.3 Mandibular primary first molar showing proximal extensive-stage lesion (**a**). The cavity walls had extended beyond the interproximal embrasure (**b**) and a Stainless-Steel Crown was placed (**c**). Post-operative radiograph (**d**)

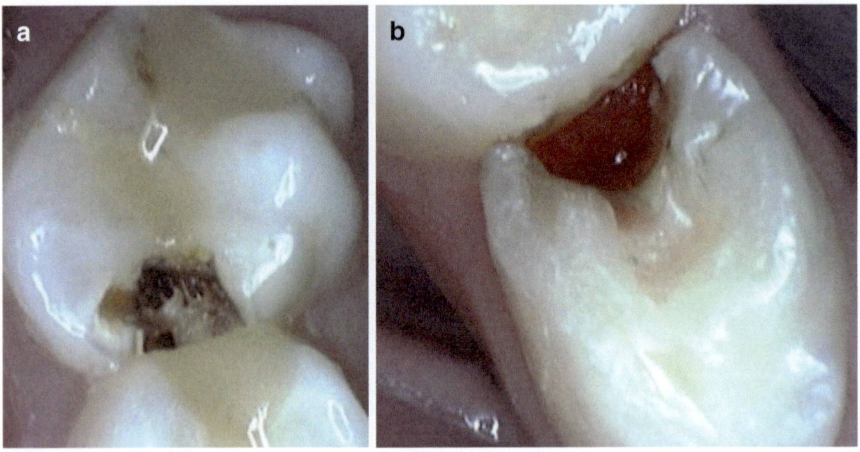

Fig. 6.4 Multisurface carious lesions or new carious lesions on a previously restored tooth (**a**) or a carious gingival seat (**b**) that does not support a direct restoration, are indications for a full-coverage restoration

6.3 Matrix Systems in Restorative Dentistry

When restoring proximal lesions, the goal is to provide tight contacts, good contours, and proper anatomy. A matrix system restores contour by simulating natural tooth structure and restores form and function [18, 19]. Incorrect replication of contact and contour will cause restoration overhangs leading to food lodgment and secondary caries, thus compromising the quality and longevity of a restoration [20, 21].

The dental matrix system comprises of the following three components:

1. The matrix is a metal or plastic band that compensates for the missing wall and contains the restorative material.
2. The retainer holds the matrix band in place and causes temporary separation of adjacent teeth.
3. The wedge adapts the matrix band gingivally and causes separation of the teeth.

Commercially available matrix systems are broadly classified as cervical matrices, sectional matrix systems (with a retainer), and circumferential (without a retainer) matrix system as given below [22, 23]:

6.3.1 Cervical Matrices

These are preformed matrices available in different sizes that correspond to the cervical contour of anterior and posterior teeth. It has a clear transparent tag on the outer surface that fits to a transparent holder. The matrix is flexible and adapts to the

Table 6.2 Commercially available cervical matrices

Matrix	Company	Country	Sizes
Cervical matrix	TDV	Brazil	5 sizes
Blue view™ Cervical Matrix Kit	Garrison® Dental solutions LLC	Germany	6 sizes
Hawe™ Transparent Cervical Matrices	Kerr™ corporation	USA	7 sizes
Cure-Thru® Clear Cervical Matrices	Premier®	USA	7 sizes
LM Cervical Matrices	LM-Dental™	Finland	4 sizes
SeptoMatrix Cervical	Septodont	France	3 sizes
Unica anterior matrix	Polydentia	Switzerland	1 size

These commercial products have been listed after visiting the manufacturers' website on 7th May 2025. The availability of these products may vary across different regions

cervical third of the tooth. The selected matrix must have a more pronounced curvature than the tooth being restored (Table 6.2). The adhesive restoration is placed on the tooth surface or the matrix itself and is compressed cervically or subgingivally as required. Placing a matrix before curing the final increment avoids formation of the oxygen inhibition layer and gives a smooth finish to the restoration. The edges of the matrix are thin and do not leave excess composite. Any excess material is removed before light curing. The material is cured for 10 seconds after which the matrix is removed, and the material is cured further as per manufacturer's instructions.

6.3.2 Mylar Strips

Mylar strips are used to contain the material while restoring anterior interproximal lesions. At the same time, the strip prevents the material from adhering to adjacent teeth. It may also be used to achieve favorable contour and provide a finish to the labial or proximal restoration. These are available as clear, plastic strips having a thickness of around 0.002 gauge (60 microns) and a length of 10 cm depending on the manufacturer. They are further categorized and color coded with a band of green, yellow, red, and blue, based on their width (Tables 6.3 and 6.4).

6.3.3 Circumferential and Sectional Matrices

While the anterior restorations can be contoured with a mylar strip, proximal restorations of canines and primary molars can be a challenge in a child's mouth. In a primary tooth, it is a common occurrence for adjacent teeth to require proximal restorations. Any system that allows for simultaneous placement of adjacent restorations must be preferred. Retainerless matrices not only allow for simultaneous adjacent proximal restorations but are also less likely to be dislodged by the child [24]. Primary teeth have shorter clinical height; hence, the use of a circumferential

Table 6.3 Color coding and sizes of mylar strips

	Color	Length	Width
1.	Yellow	100 mm	6 mm
2.	Red	100 mm	8 mm
3.	Blue	100 mm	10 mm
4.	Green	100 mm	12 mm

Table 6.4 Commercially available mylar strips

Matrix strips	Samit®
Tor VM transparent strips	Russia
Hawe™ Transparent strips	Kerr™ corporation
Prehma Mylar	Keystone industries

These commercial products have been listed after visiting the manufacturers' website on 7th May 2025. The availability of these products may vary across different regions

matrix that envelopes the tooth gives better stability and retention as compared to a sectional matrix. Most matrix systems, whether circumferential or sectional, are contoured such that cervical length is shorter than occlusal length that allow for better adaptation near the gingival seat.

The operator must be aware that based on individual manufacturing properties, matrices can also be categorized as conformed and laminated (memory-free matrices). Conformed matrices cannot be modified according to the shape and location of the contact areas of the tooth, as they have their own elastic memory. Silver amalgam on condensation pushes these matrices to the adjacent tooth, developing appropriate contours and contacts. Adhesive restorative materials cannot offer resistance to condensation forces and it is difficult for the operator to contour them, against the conformed matrix band. On the other hand, laminated matrices, that are memory free can be contoured by the operator using condensing instruments to establish contact with the adjacent teeth prior to restoration placement (Fig. 6.5).

While many of the available systems fulfill the criteria of a desired matrix system, the evidence is limited on their performance and comparison. Therefore, the choice of a matrix system is based on operator preference and patient comfort (Table 6.5).

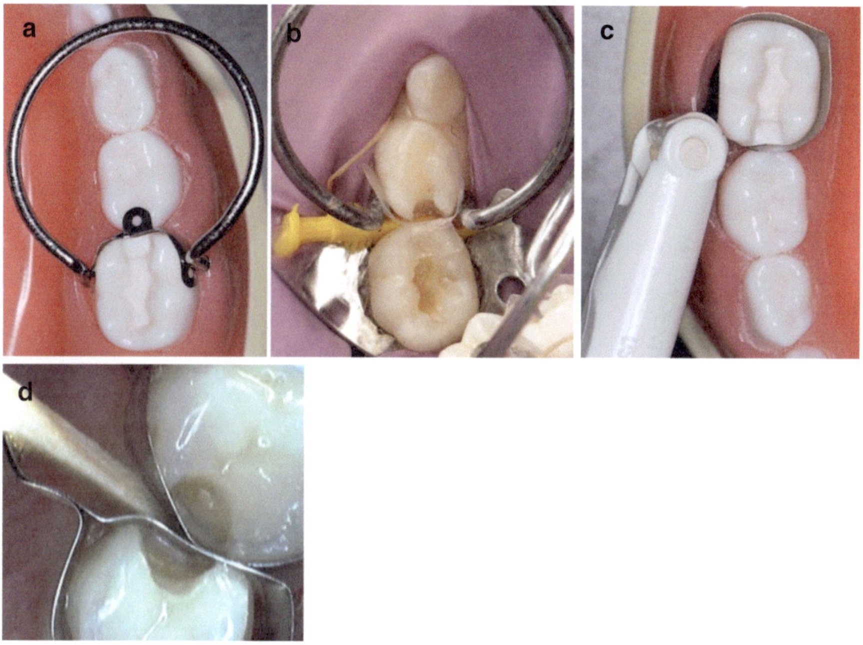

Fig. 6.5 A sectional matrix system with metal matrix band (**a**) and clear matrix (**b**), circumferential matrix system (**c**) or a circumferential matrix band (**d**) and wedge can be used to restore proximal cavities in primary molars. (Image 'b' courtesy: Dr Abhishek Soni, India)

6.4 Glass Ionomer Cement: Materials Science and Clinical Application

From the time they were first developed, GIC have gradually come to be recognized as one of the most versatile materials in dentistry. In recent years, their use has received an even greater impetus, as their properties align with the current practice of Minimal Intervention Dentistry. The conventional GIC devised by Wilson and Kent in 1969 was composed of a powder–liquid system containing an aqueous polyalkaenoic acid and a fluoroaluminosilicate glass. This material is characterized by chemical bonding, self-curing nature, and the ability to facilitate sustained fluoride release [25, 26].

6.4.1 What Are the Properties of Conventional GIC?

GIC is known to adhere chemically to the tooth structure. On placement into a cavity, GIC facilitates an ionic exchange at the cement–tooth interface leading to the development of an ion-enriched layer that is firmly attached to the tooth [27]. It allows for conservative cavity preparations and preserves healthy tooth structure. In

Table 6.5 Commercially available sectional and circumferential matrix systems

Type	Commercial name	Manufacturer
Sectional matrix system	Palodent BiTine	Dentsply Sirona, USA
	Palodent® V3	Dentsply Sirona, USA
	Palodent® Plus	Dentsply Sirona, USA
	NiTin™ Sectional Matrix System	Garrison Dental Solutions, USA
	Composi-Tight® Sectional Matrix System	
	Composi-Tight® Gold Sectional Matrix system	
	Composi-Tight® 3D XR Matrix System	
	Composi-Tight® 3D Fusion™ System	
	Strata-G Sectional Matrix System	
	myQuickmat Forte	Polydentia, Switzerland
	Bioclear Evolve	Bioclear, USA
	Biofit Blue series	
	Fendermate®	Directadental, Sweden
	Halo™ Sectional Matrix System	Ultradent, USA
	Contoured Metal Matrices	TOR VM, Russia
	Walser® Matrices	Walser, Germany
	X5 Sectional Matrix System™	Premier®, USA
	iMatrix™ Sectional Matrix System	PacDent, USA
	Unimatrix R	TDV, Septodont, Brazil
	Hawe Adapt™ Sectional Matrix System	Kerr™, USA
	LumiContrast Sectional Matrices	Polydentia, Switzerland
Circumferential matrix system	Denovo Dental Preformed Matrix System	Denovo dental, USA
	AutoMatrix® retainerless matrix system	Dentsply Sirona, USA
	Pro matrix®	Young innovations, Germany
	T bands	Pulpdent®, USA
	Palodent® 360	Dentsply Sirona, USA
	Adapt™ SuperCap™ Steel Matrix	Kerr™, Switzerland
	Lucifix™ Matrix System	
	SuperMat™ Retainerless Matrix System	
	MetaFix™	
	Omni-Matrix™	Ultradent, USA
	ReelMatrix™ Matrices	Garrison Dental Solutions, USA

These commercial products have been listed after visiting the manufacturers' website on 7th May 2025. The availability of these products may vary across different regions

case of fracture of the GIC restoration, the fractures are most often seen within the restoration and not at the tooth-restoration interface. This allows for repair of the restoration without the need to prepare the cavity again.

The coefficient of thermal expansion of conventional GIC is close to that of dentinal tissue. This factor has been shown to allow for better marginal adaptation and lesser leakage in Glass Ionomer restorations. The cement can be used as a liner in deep cavities prior to placing Resin Composite as it mimics the properties of dentin and helps in avoiding post-operative sensitivity. When GIC is placed close to the pulp, it shows an initial inflammatory response leading to the formation of reparative dentine [28, 29]. GIC bonds to caries-affected dentin and this property is useful when selective caries excavation is done or in the Silver-Modified Atraumatic Restorative Techique [30–34].

Additionally, GIC confers cariostatic benefits to the tooth due to its fluoride-releasing abilities [35]. Fluoride ions are released from the glass powder at the time of mixing and "burst release" in the oral environment during the first 24 hours. While the release of fluoride ions gradually tapers over 3 months, fluoride recharge of the cement takes place during every topical fluoride treatment [36–38].

6.4.2 What Are the Limitations of Conventional GIC?

GIC has poor flexural strength and resistance to abrasion and wear [39]. It may fracture if used as a restorative material in areas subjected to high occlusal forces or in cavities which are not well supported by healthy tooth structure. Also, conventional glass ionomer restorations are sensitive to moisture imbibition and desiccation during the early setting reaction causing cracks to appear on its surface and consequently leading to an increased micro-leakage or fracture of the restoration [40]. Therefore, a surface protection varnish must be applied once gross finishing of the restoration is done [41–43]. GICs are tooth colored and are available in different shades. However, they are not considered as a highly esthetic treatment option as they appear opaque after setting and do not closely replicate the translucent nature of enamel. To overcome these limitations of the conventional GIC, different modifications in the formulation were introduced in the market. The modifications follow a similar composition but differ from each other with the additives present.

- *Resin-Modified GIC (RMGIC)*

They were developed to override the problems attributed to conventional GIC associated with moisture sensitivity and low physical properties [44]. They have similar formulation to the traditional GIC, but with the addition of a small quantity (4.5% to 6%) of resin components, such as hydroxyethyl methacrylate (HEMA) or Bis-GMA (Bisphenol Glycidyl Methacrylate) in the powder. The water component of the conventional GIC is also replaced by a water/HEMA mixture [44, 45]. This ensures that two different polymerization reactions control the setting of the RMGIC namely, the fundamental acid–base curing reaction followed by a light polymerization reaction. RMGICs have received widespread acceptance from the dental community and have even replaced the conventional GICs in many areas of clinical application. Their primary advantages include greater working time and ability to "command set" on application of the relevant light source. Their esthetics are closer to resin-based materials. They also show better fracture strength and resistance to wear [46].

- *High-Viscosity Glass Ionomer Cement (HVGIC)*

A drawback of conventional GIC is its inferior physical properties, such as surface hardness and abrasion resistance, which are largely attributed to the material's low viscosity. HVGICs have a finer grain size distribution and incorporates polyacrylic acid into the powder, enhancing the compressive strength and wear resistance of the material. They are also referred to as condensable glass–ionomer cements because of the amalgam-like properties seen when longer mixing times were used [47–49]. This type of GIC was initially developed in response to the demand for a material that can be used with hand instrumentation in rural communities, as part of the Atraumatic Restorative Technique [50].

For example, 3 M™ Ketac™ Universal Aplicap, Fuji IX GIC by GC

- *Hybrid GIC*

Hybrid GICs are a modification of conventional GIC which been reinforced by incorporating reactive ultrafine glass particles and a high-molecular-weight polyacrylic acid [51–54]. This feature affects physical and mechanical properties of the material. Furthermore, the manufacturer provides a nano-protective coating to be applied over the restoration (micro-laminated technique) to improve the properties of the material.

For example, Equia Forte®, Equia Forte® HT, Equia Fil®, GC Gold label Hybrid

- *Metal-Reinforced GIC*

These were developed to improve the flexural strength of conventional GIC and consisted of a silver alloy and GIC admixture. They were manufactured by sintering fine metal particles onto the glass to form ceramic–metal materials or "Cermets." However, these metal-reinforced GICs are not superior in strength to other posterior restorative materials or even the conventional GIC. Their poor esthetic appearance and reduced fluoride-releasing ability have led to them being phased out from dental practices.

6.4.3 Types of GICs Based on Mode of Dispensation

The conventional GIC, RMGIC, and HVGIC are available as hand-mixed powder: liquid materials, capsulated versions, or paste systems. Hand-mixed materials require dispensing of the correct powder–liquid ratio as specified by the manufacturer, as an altered ratio can adversely affect the physical properties of the material. For example, use of increased quantity of powder may confer improved strength to the GIC mix but may decrease its bonding capabilities. The operator variability in method of manipulation and the time taken can affect the longevity of hand-mixed GIC restorations.

The use of capsulated materials reduces the possibility of errors in the powder: liquid ratio, as the capsule contains pre-measured amounts of powder and liquid wherein the liquid is separately encased in a "pillow." The capsule is activated to release the liquid, and it is then mixed in the capsule mixer for 4 to 5 seconds. The capsule is then attached to the applicator and the mixed glass ionomer is delivered directly into the cavity. This ensures consistency and standardization in the mixing process.

Another method of dispensing GIC is a paste–paste system. It uses a specially designed cartridge and material dispenser or double barreled "clicker" that delivers defined portions of two pastes to be mixed by spatulation or mixing syringes (Tables 6.6 and 6.7).

6.4.4 How is Dentin Conditioned Prior to Placing a GIC Restoration?

Following cavity preparation, the tooth is isolated, and a dentin conditioner (GC dentin conditioner, GC; Riva Conditioner, SDI) is applied to the bonding surfaces using a microbrush. After 20 seconds, the conditioner is washed with water from a three-way syringe. The cavity is blot dried so that the dentinal surfaces are moist and not overdried or desiccated as this may affect the retentiveness of the restoration (Fig. 6.6) [55].

Table 6.6 Commercially available conventional Glass Ionomer Cements

Product	Method of dispensation	Manufacturer
GC Fuji II	Powder–liquid system or capsules	GC
GC Gold Label II GC Gold Label IX GC Gold Label HS Posterior Extra	Powder–liquid system	
GC Fuji IX GP® Extra GC Fuji IX GP® Fast	Capsule	
3 M™ Ketac™ Universal Glass Ionomer Filling Material 3 M™ Vitremer™	Powder–liquid system	3 M
Ketac™ Molar Quick Aplicap™	Capsule	
Ionofil Molar Ionofil Plus IonoStar Molar Aqua Ionofil Plus	Powder liquid	Voco
IonoStar Plus Ionofil Molar AC Quick	Capsule	
ChemFil Rock	Capsule	Dentsply Sirona
Glass Ionomer Cement Type II Glass Ionomer FX ULTRA Glass Ionomer FX II	Powder Liquid	Shofu
Riva Self Cure Riva Self Cure HV	Capsule	SDI

These commercial products have been listed after visiting the manufacturers' website on 7th May 2025. The availability of these products may vary across different regions

Table 6.7 Commercially available Resin-Modified Glass Ionomer Cements

Product	Method of dispensation	Manufacturer
GC Fuji® Automix LC	Comes with an ergonomic dispenser	GC, Japan
GC Fuji Filling LC	Powder–liquid system	GC, Japan
GC Fuji II LC	Powder–liquid system or capsules	GC, Japan
GC Fuji II LC CORE Material	Powder–liquid system	GC, Japan
GC Fuji LINING LC Paste Pak	Paste–paste system	GC, Japan
Ketac™ Nano Light-Curing Glass Ionomer Restorative	Paste–paste system	3 M, USA
Equia forte	Capsules	GC, Japan
Ionolux	Powder–liquid capsules	Voco
Riva Light Cure Riva Light cure HV	Capsule	SDI

These commercial products have been listed after visiting the manufacturers' website on 7th May 2025. The availability of these products may vary across different regions

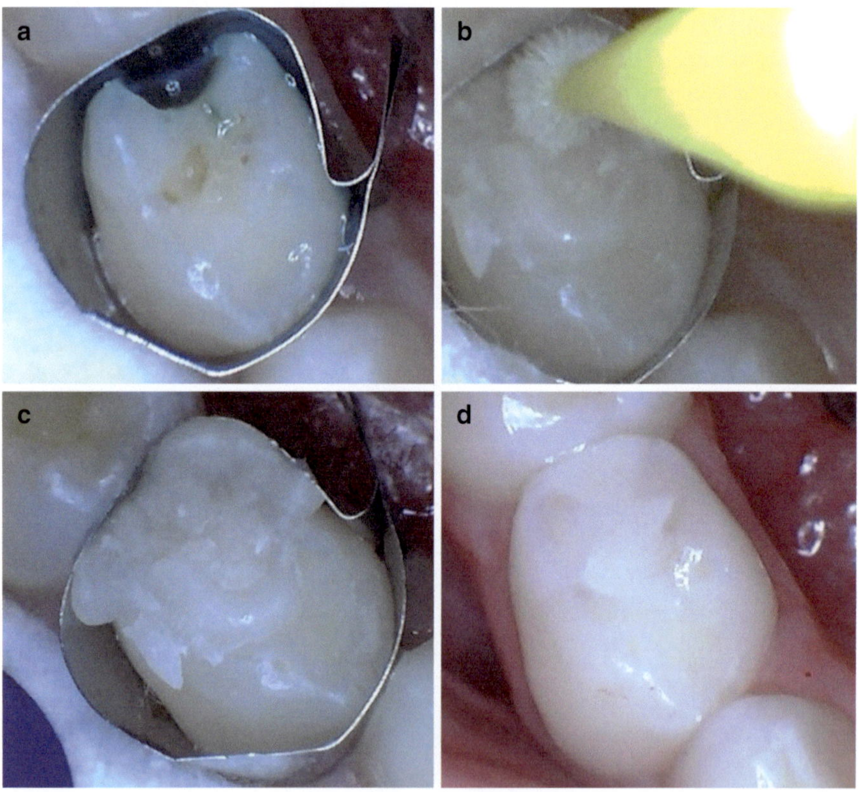

Fig. 6.6 Prepared proximal cavity conditioned with a commercial cavity conditioner for 10 seconds (**a**). Resin-Modified Glass Ionomer Cement in capsule form mixed and dispensed into the cavity with a capsule applier. The material is adapted with an applicator tip or microbrush (**b**). The cavity is overfilled (**c**). The restoration is finished and polished (**d**)

6.4.5 Why Is Dentin Conditioning Important?

Due to the lesser inorganic content (calcium and phosphate ions) of dentin, the ionic bond strength of GIC to dentin is lower as compared to enamel. Hence, the dentinal surface is conditioned with polyacrylic acid, which exposes the calcium and phosphate ions from hydroxyapatite crystals that are attached to the collagen fibrils of dentin, making them available to bond to the GIC. Dentin conditioning with 10% polyacrylic acid modifies the smear layer and improves the bond of both, GIC and RMGIC restorations, making it a necessary step before placing a restoration [55–57].

6.4.6 Can 37% Phosphoric Acid Be Used for Conditioning?

37% phosphoric acid is an enamel etchant and an aggressive dentin conditioner that can cause deep dentin hybridization and demineralization removing significant amounts of calcium and phosphate ions necessary for the bond to form between the GIC and the dentin [56, 57]. Hence, it should not be used as a dentin conditioner prior to GIC placement.

6.4.7 How Does One Place GIC Into the Prepared Cavity?

Following cavity conditioning and blot drying, the GIC is placed with a plastic instrument or delivered from a capsule into the prepared cavity. The glass ionomer must always be overfilled, and a micro brush can be used to adapt the material to the cavity walls (Fig. 6.7). A well-mixed GIC (capsule or hand mixed) that is sticky and adherent to the plastic instrument will have greater bond strength to the enamel and dentin as compared to a GIC that can be easily condensed (Figs. 6.8, 6.9, 6.10). After adequate placement and adaptation of the GIC, removal of excessive cement must be avoided as it may disturb the formation of the ionic bond.

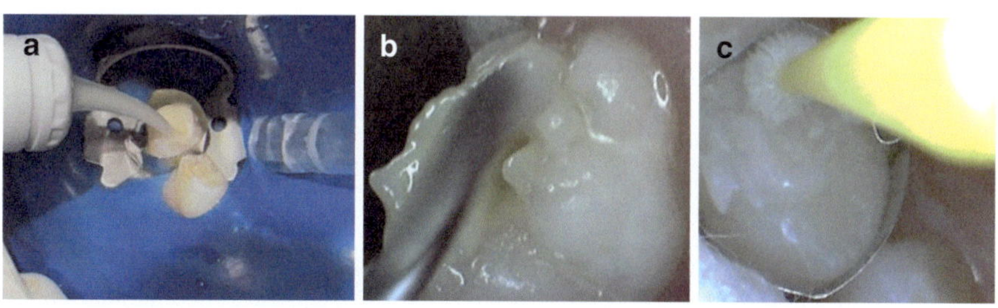

Fig. 6.7 Capsule mix Resin-Modified Glass Ionomer Cement is dispensed into the cavity with a capsule applier (**a**). The material is adapted with the flat end of a cement carrier (**b**) or an applicator tip (**c**)

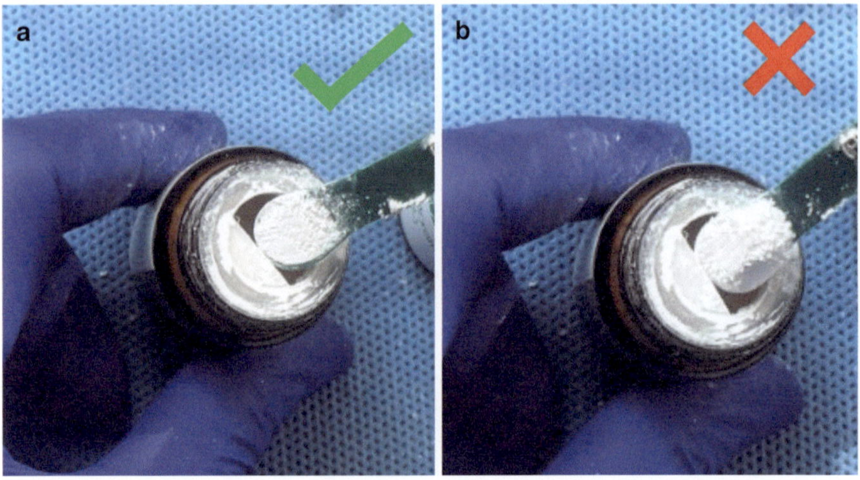

Fig. 6.8 The powder must always be dispensed with the scoop provided by the manufacturer. The powder: liquid ratio is usually mentioned on the cap of the bottle. The scoop is loaded with powder and leveled against the partition secured to the rim of the bottle (**a**). Excess powder will result in incorrect powder: liquid ratio affecting the final mix (**b**)

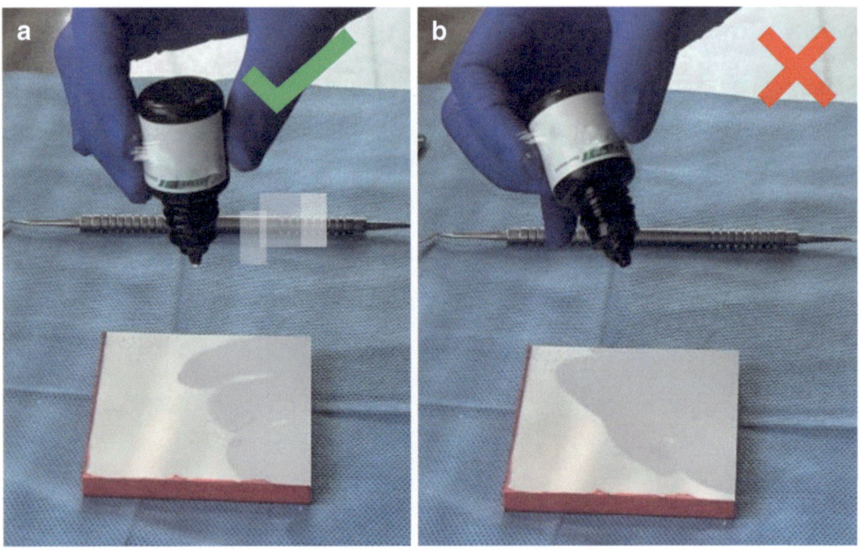

Fig. 6.9 While dispensing, the bottle must be held vertical to dispense exactly one drop of liquid (**a**). The bottle if held at an angle will dispense incorrect amount of liquid and affect the final mix (**b**)

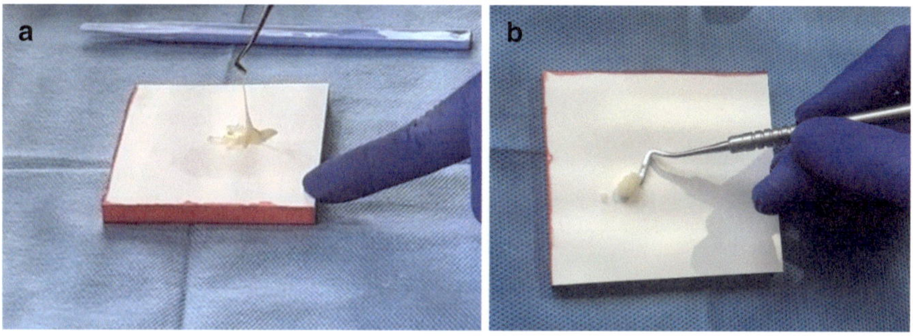

Fig. 6.10 The correct consistency of the final mix must be glossy and sticky, difficult to take off the instrument (**a**). A mix that can be molded to a shape and that does not stick to an instrument is said to be dry and shows poor bonding ability with the prepared cavity (**b**)

6.4.8 Is It Necessary to Apply a Protective Surface Coat Over the GIC Restoration?

Modern GICs, both RMGIC and the high-viscosity materials can be finished with dura white stones (Shofu, Japan). They are aluminum oxide impregnated stones with or without a friction grip attachment meant to be used at a recommended speed of 5000 to 20,000 rpm. They can also be used with an airotor under water coolant once the cement has set completely. The surface of a newly placed glass-ionomer must be protected from water exchange as this increases their vulnerability to dissolution and deterioration of physical properties [40]. Applying a coat fills surface voids and defects reducing the uptake of stains from food and drinks. There has been some debate in the past on whether the use of a waterproof coating like light-cured resin can hamper the fluoride release by a GIC system. In vitro studies have shown that these protective coatings do not remain on the surface long enough to prevent sustained fluoride release [58]. Various materials such as copal varnish, petroleum jelly, cocoa butter, and light-cured bonding adhesives have been used earlier. The nano-filled light-cured, self-adhesive surface coatings have been specifically developed for glass ionomer restorations (Table 6.8).

6.4.9 Why Has the Use of GIC Gained Importance in Pediatric Restorative Dentistry?

To preserve vitality of the tooth and maintain a healthy tooth structure, contemporary pediatric restorative dentistry recommends Selective Caries Removal. When a tooth requiring an intracoronal restoration is excavated to firm or soft dentin, the bonding capabilities of the restorative material to caries-affected dentin must be considered. Of all the restorative materials, GIC not only shows a better bond strength to carious dentin, but also supports the ability of the carious dentin to undergo physiological remineralization. In addition, GICs' fluoride-releasing and

Table 6.8 Commercially available protective surface coating

	Product	Manufacturer	Mode of cure
1	G Coat Plus™	GC	Light cure
2	Equia Forte® Coat	GC	Light cure
3	GC Fuji Varnish™	GC	Self-cure
4	Vitremer™ Finishing Gloss	3 M™	Light cure
5	Easy Glaze	Voco	Light cure
6	Final Varnish LC	Voco	Light cure
7	Coat it	Shofu	Light cure
8	Riva Coat	SDI	Light cure

These commercial products have been listed after visiting the manufacturers' website on 7th May 2025. The availability of these products may vary across different regions

recharging abilities also contribute to preventing secondary caries in adjacent teeth and help in maintaining a cario-protective environment in the oral cavity. Thus, it is recommended as a primary restorative material or as a liner below composites in teeth which have been selectively excavated to carious dentin.

The success rate of RMGIC is comparable to Resin Composite for restoring small-to-moderate-sized occlusal and proximal cavities in primary teeth. The American Academy of Pediatric Dentistry also gives strong recommendations for use of Resin Composite and RMGIC in Class I and Class II cavity preparations [59]. There is strong evidence to recommend the use of conventional GIC in occlusal cavity preparations, but the success rate is lesser for proximal preparations [59–61]. There is insufficient evidence to support the use of conventional or RMGIC as a long-term restorative material in permanent teeth.

HVGIC is recommended as a single surface temporary restoration, for both primary and permanent teeth in Atraumatic Restorative Technique (ART) [50].

Hybrid GICs such as Equia Forte are a recent addition to the range of commercially marketed GICs. While one would expect hybrid GICs to demonstrate superior physical properties; due to insufficient literature it is difficult to ascertain whether they would replace the highly viscous GICs such as Ketac molar or Fuji IX. Thus, in primary molars, RMGICs are preferred in moderate-sized occlusal and proximal cavities, whereas for larger sized occlusal cavities, one can opt for Hybrid or Highly viscous GICs [50, 59] (Figs. 6.11, 6.12, and 6.13).

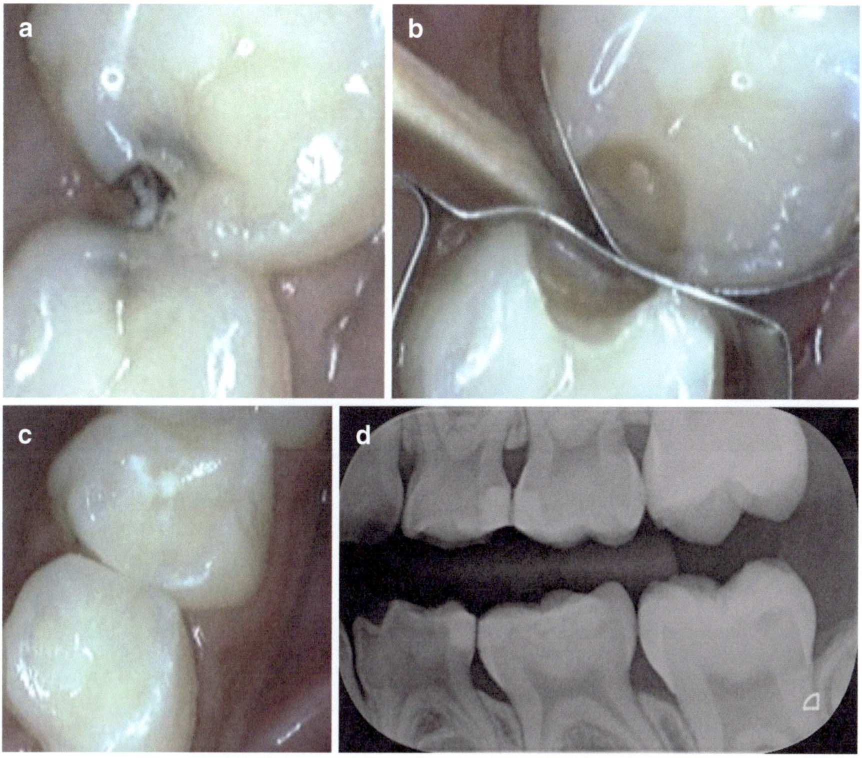

Fig. 6.11 Proximal carious lesion in maxillary primary left first and second molars (**a**). Complete Caries Excavation done, keeping a conservative box-type cavity preparation limited to the carious lesion. Circumferential matrices placed on both molars. A wooden wedge is used to minimally separate the teeth and help adapt the matrices to the close to the gingival wall of the prepared cavity (**b**). Restoration done with capsulated RMGIC. Finishing and polishing done (**c**). The proximal restoration should not have overhangs or gaps between the restoration and the gingival seat, as verified on the radiograph (**d**)

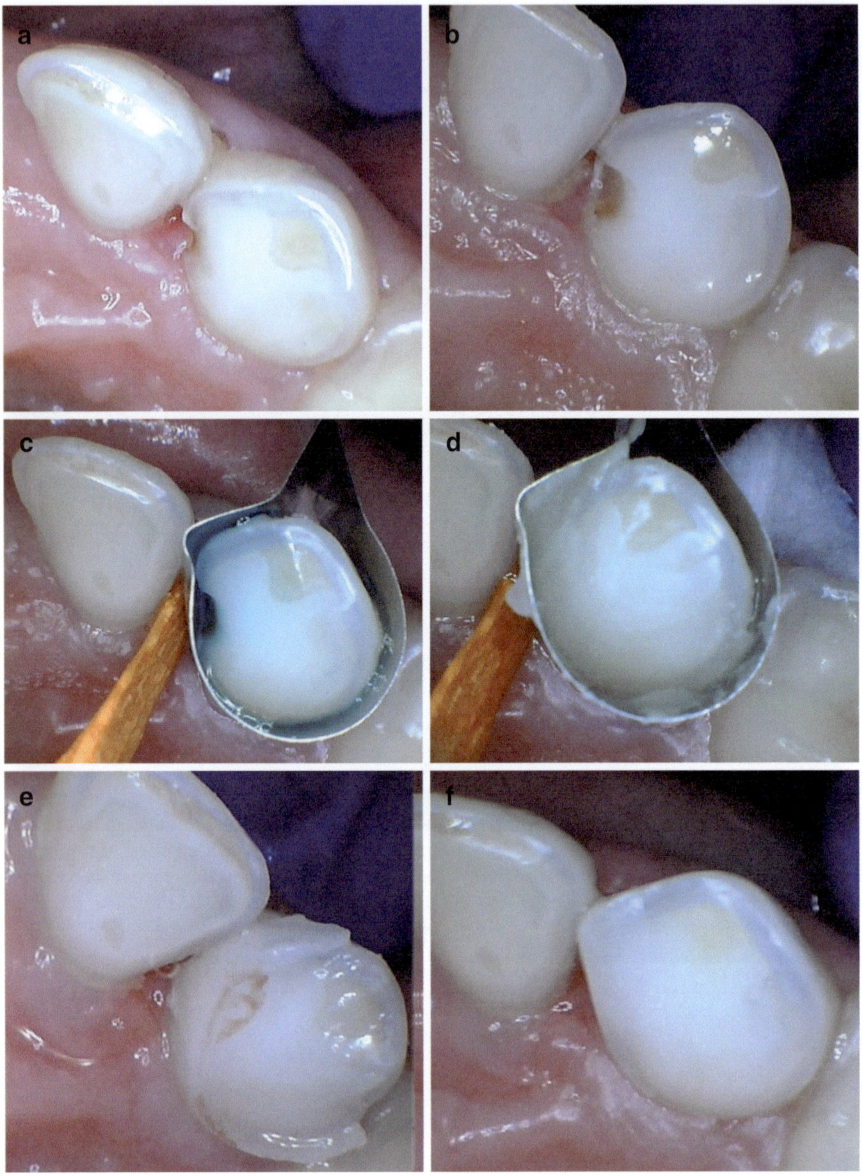

Fig. 6.12 Proximal carious lesion seen in maxillary primary left canine (**a**). Complete Caries Removal done (**b**). A circumferential matrix band is placed and adapted with a wooden wedge. Dentin conditioner is applied for 10 seconds (**c**). The conditioner is washed and blot dried after which the tooth is restored with capsulated RMGIC (**d**). The matrix band is removed (**e**). Finishing and polishing done and a surface protective agent applied (**f**)

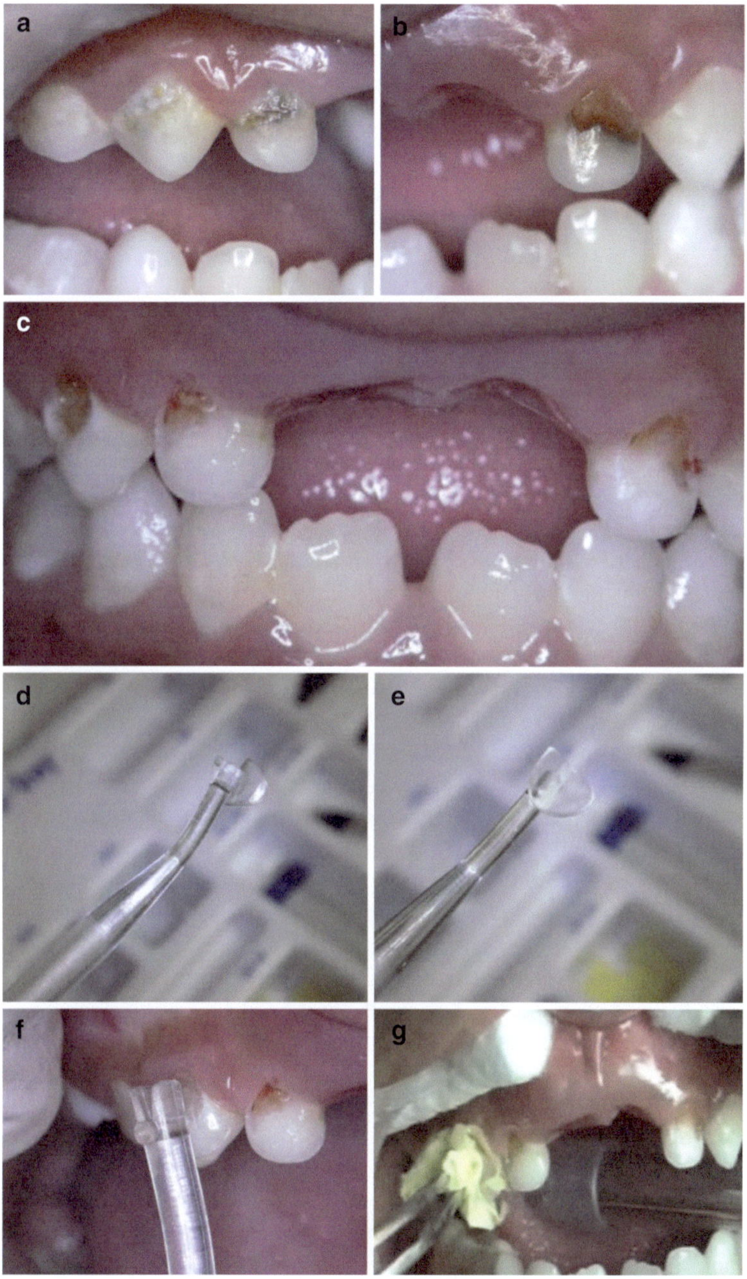

Fig. 6.13 Carious lesions on labial surfaces of maxillary primary lateral incisors and right canine (**a** and **b**). Complete caries excavation done (**c**). Side (**d**) and front view (**e**)of cervical matrix attached to the handle. The cervical matrix is checked for size and fit (**f**). Teeth are isolated with cotton rolls and saliva ejector. The tooth is etched, dried, and adhesive bond applied (**g**). Resin composite placed in prepared cavities and adapted with the cervical matrix (**h**). Finishing and polishing done (**i**)

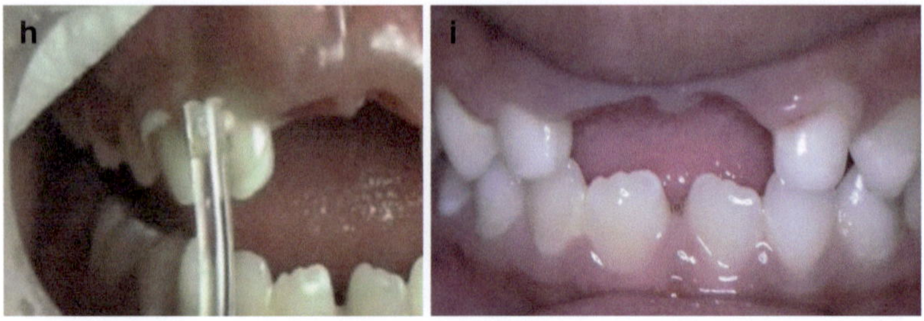

Fig. 6.13 (continued)

6.5 Resin Composite Restorations: Materials Science and Clinical Applications

Over the last few decades, the placement of tooth-like esthetic restorations in primary and permanent teeth has gained momentum due to the parental and patient demand for esthetic restorations. The two most widely used esthetic, direct restorative materials in pediatric practice that conform to the principles of Minimal Intervention Dentistry are GICs and Resin Composite. Certain physical properties of composites outrun Glass Ionomers such as flexural strength, surface hardness, and more importantly the esthetic characteristics such as shade matching, better color stability, and easier replication of dental anatomy. Resin composites were first introduced by Bowen in 1965 in a bid to improve the physical and esthetic properties of acrylic resins, and gradually they became the premier restorative materials to be used in dental practices. Though contemporary resin composites have performed excellently as a restorative material, research continues to focus on improving their physical properties and more importantly, their bond strengths to enamel and dentin [62]. The adhesive technology involving composite resin restorations is greatly influenced by the histological characteristics of the primary and permanent enamel and dentin. To deliver successful composite restorations in pediatric practice, it is important to keep in mind the key concepts related to these structures and the advances in the field of adhesive dentistry [63].

6.5.1 Bonding Protocol

The primary requisite for placing a successful composite restoration is to ensure optimal bonding of the resin to enamel and dentin. Buonocore (1956) introduced a time-controlled 30-second treatment of enamel with 85% phosphoric acid which resulted in the formation of microscopically roughened porous surfaces in which the resin could penetrate to form tags. This process is known as "etching" and is today considered to be essential to achieve enamel adhesion [64–66]. Currently, it is recommended that enamel should be etched with 37% phosphoric acid for

15 seconds only. This process must be done under adequate isolation as elimination of surface contaminants like saliva and surface pellicle is important for the hydrophobic resin to adhere to enamel. The etched enamel clinically appears white frosty after airdrying which increases the enamel surface energy making it receptive to bonding [66, 67].

- *Is There a Difference in Etching Times for Primary and Permanent Teeth?*

Earlier, it was believed that a longer etching time may be needed for primary enamel due to the presence of a thicker aprismatic layer and higher enamel rod density. However, most studies have not found any difference between the retention of resin restorations placed after longer etching times and have concluded that 15-second enamel etching is sufficient for optimal bonding to primary teeth. Similarly, the enamel of permanent teeth must be etched for 15 seconds only [68–70]. Etching beyond 15 seconds for both, primary and permanent teeth, can form precipitates of calcium phosphates that do not wash away easily and can lower the bond strength between the adhesive and the tooth structure [71].

- *How Does the Etching of Dentin Differ from That of Enamel?*

Unlike enamel, which is 95% mineralized and contains 5% organic tissue, dentin has 45% organic tissue making the adhesion of resin to dentin more complex and less predictable. The lower inorganic content of dentin results in a poor etching pattern as compared to enamel [72]. The outward flow of the dentinal fluid contaminates the surface, thereby reducing the adhesion of the hydrophobic resin to the dentin [73]. Additionally, mechanical tooth preparation of dentin leads to the formation of a layer of debris, *the smear layer* which creates *smear plugs* that prevents the penetration of the adhesive [74]. To ensure good adhesion at dentinal level, the smear layer must be removed or modified such that the adhesive can interlock into the dentin collagen matrix. This is achieved with the use of an acidic etchant (37% phosphoric acid or self-etch primer).

It is recommended that the dentin must be etched for a shorter time (10 seconds) than enamel (15 seconds) as it contains lesser inorganic tissue. The exposure of dentin to an etchant for longer than 10 seconds causes desiccation and collapse of the collagen fibrils compromising the bond between the tooth and the adhesive [65, 75, 76]. This etching of enamel and dentin with 37% phosphoric acid constitutes the total-etch concept.

- *Bonding Concepts*

The Resin Composite being hydrophobic needs an intermediate agent to bond to the moist dentin. This intermediate adhesive system or the bonding agent has low viscosity that improves the wettability of the etched enamel and dentin allowing better adhesion of the Resin Composite to the tooth. It has the following components:

Primer, a solvent (acetone, ethanol, or water)-based intermediate agent composed of hydrophilic monomers that penetrates to the depth of the etched dentin. This helps to carry the hydrophobic adhesive into the moist dentin.

Adhesive, a solvent-free hydrophobic resin applied to the primed dentin interlocks with the collagen matrix, that on polymerization forms a *hybrid layer* to which the Resin Composite bonds.

The hybrid layer is a collagen-resin phase wherein the adhesive has interlocked with the collagen fibers and penetrated the dentinal tubules [67, 77, 78].

- *Generations of Adhesive Systems*

The adhesive system has evolved over eight generations. Currently, the fourth to eighth generation bonding systems are in use, having different compositions and application protocols [67]. The adhesive systems presently available can be broadly categorized as *etch and rinse systems or the self-etch systems.*

Etch and rinse systems are based on the total etch concept which involves etching both enamel and dentin with 37% phosphoric acid. Etching creates porosities in enamel and ensures *complete removal of the smear layer,* thereby opening the dentinal tubules and intertubular space. This allows the primer and adhesive to penetrate the collagen network and form a hybrid layer that is analogous to the resin tag formation in the enamel. The *fourth-generation adhesive* is a 2-bottle bonding system wherein the primer is applied first followed by the dentin adhesive. The *fifth-generation adhesive* is a single bottle bonding system containing both the primer and the adhesive, which eliminates the extra step of application, reducing operator time and error. While the fifth-generation bonding system is considered an improvement and is used more commonly, the fourth-generation system is seen to have a higher bond strength.

- *What is Wet Bonding?*

Prolonged air-drying after rinsing of the 37% phosphoric acid can cause desiccation and collapse of the collagen matrix affecting the formation the of hybrid layer resulting in lowered bond strength and dentinal hypersensitivity. To prevent the collagen network from completely collapsing, a certain amount of moisture is needed, commonly referred to as *wet bonding* [78–80]. Wet bonding does not mean allowing salivary contamination or a visibly clear film of water on the conditioned dentinal surface. Clinically, a moist dentin surface can best be achieved by removing excess water by blot drying with a dry tissue pellet so that the surface looks glossy. After blot drying, the primer is immediately applied allowing it to penetrate to the depth of the etchant. A delay in application of primer will lead to outward flow of the dentinal tubular fluids causing the formation of a poor hybrid layer [78–82].

- *Etch and Rinse Technique*

The prepared cavity must be isolated preferably with a rubber dam or with cotton rolls and saliva ejector. 37% phosphoric acid is applied on the enamel first and then flowed onto the dentin. Etching of dentin should not exceed 10 seconds and the total etching time of enamel and dentin is 15 seconds. Etchant is washed with water from a 3-way syringe for 30 seconds. The tooth is blot dried with tissue or blotting paper pellets which results in enamel appearing white frosty and the dentin moist. For the *4th-generation adhesive system*, the primer is applied for 5 seconds. After air drying, the adhesive is applied for 10 seconds. For the *5th-generation adhesive system*, the primer and adhesive available in one bottle are applied on the etched tooth for 10 seconds. Both, the 4th and 5th-generation adhesives, are air dried for 5 seconds followed by light curing. The duration of application of primer and adhesive can vary for different bonding systems, and it is recommended to follow manufacturer's instructions.

Resin Composite restoration is done with the incremental layering technique (Table 6.9).

- *Self-etch Adhesive System*

The self-etch system was developed by incorporating an acidic component to the primer so that the penetration of the primer and etching of the tooth structure occurred simultaneously [83]. The adhesive component applied separately (sixth

Table 6.9 Commercially available fourth- and fifth-generation bonding agents

Generation	Commercial names
Fourth generation (three-step etch and rinse) *37% phosphoric acid (step 1) + primer (step 2) + adhesive (step 3)*	All-Bond 3® (Bisco) OptiBond™ FL (Kerr™) PermaQuick (Ultradent) Adper Scotchbond™ Multi-Purpose (3 M™) Syntac (Ivoclar) ProBond® (Dentsply) LuxaBond Total Etch (DMG) Clearfil™ Photo Bond (Kuraray)
Fifth generation (two-step etch and rinse) *- 37% phosphoric acid (step 1) + primer and adhesive in a single bottle (step 2)*	ExciTE® (Ivoclar) Solobond M (Voco) Gluma® 2 Bond (Kulzer) Gluma® Bond 5 (Kulzer) iBond® Total Etch (-Kulzer) One-Step® (Bisco) One- Step® Plus (Bisco) OptiBond™ Solo Plus (Kerr™) Prime & Bond elect® (Dentsply Sirona) Prime & Bond active® (Dentsply Sirona) Prime & Bond® NT (Dentsply Sirona) Prime and Bond® XP (Dentsply Sirona) Adper™ Scotchbond 1 (3 M™) Adper™ Single Bond (3 M™) Adper™ Single Bond Plus (3 M™) TECO (DMG) One Coat Bond (Coltene) Stae (SDI) Bond-1™ (Pentron)

These commercial products have been listed after visiting the manufacturers' website on 7th May 2025. The availability of these products may vary across different regions

generation) or concomitantly (seventh generation) was able to infiltrate the interfibrillar space and form the hybrid layer.

The sixth-generation adhesive system consists of etchant and primer in one bottle and the adhesive in another bottle. These are applied separately in two steps as per the manufacturer's instructions. In some sixth-generation systems, the acidic primer and adhesive are available in separate wells, in the same product. Both are mixed and applied in a single step. *The seventh-generation adhesive systems* are single-component, one-step, self-etch adhesives. They are available as one-bottle or all-in-one adhesives combining etching, priming, and bonding without the need for mixing (Table 6.10).

The self-etch systems can be categorized according to their pH as [84].

Table 6.10 Commercially available sixth-, seventh-, and eighth-generation bonding agents

Generation	Commercial names
Sixth generation (two step)—*etchant and primer (step 1) + adhesive (step 2)*	AdheSE (Ivoclar-Vivadent) Clearfil™ SE Bond (Kuraray) Clearfil™ SE Protect (Kuraray) Clearfil™ Liner Bond F (Kuraray) Contax (DMG) FL-Bond II (Shofu) A.R.T Bond (Coltene®) OptiBond™ eXTRa Universal (Kerr™)
Sixth generation (one step, two component)—*acidic primer and adhesive in separate reservoirs in the same unit dose or bottles that need mixing before application*	Adper™ Prompt L-Pop (3 M) One-up Bond F (Tokuyama) Xeno III (Dentsply) All Bond SE (Bisco)
Seventh generation *All components in a single bottle for direct application without prior etching and mixing*	Adper™ Easy Bond (3 M™) Scotchbond™ Universal (3 M™) Single Bond™ Universal (3 M™) Bond Force (Tokuyama) Clearfil™ S^3 Bond Plus (Kuraray) Clearfil™ Universal Bond Quick 2 (Kuraray) G-Bond and G-aenial Bond (GC) iBond Universal (Kulzer) Xeno V (Dentsply) Brush and Bond® (Parkell®) Futurabond NR (Voco) Futura bond DC (Voco) Bond-1 SF (Pentron) One Coat 7.0 (Coltene) Xeno IV® (Dentsply Sirona) AdheSE® Universal (Ivolcar) OptiBond™ Universal 360 (Kerr)
Eighth generation All components in a single bottle used for direct and indirect restoration.	G-Premio Bond™ (GC) All Bond Universal® (Bisco) Single Bond™ Universal (3 M™) GLUMA® Bond Universal (Kulzer)

These commercial products have been listed after visiting the manufacturers' website on 7th May 2025. The availability of these products may vary across different regions

- Strong (pH < 1).
- Intermediately strong (pH ~1.5).
- Mild (pH ~2).
- Ultra-mild (pH > 2.5).

While the strong self-etch adhesives simultaneously etched and conditioned the dentin and were adequate to etch the enamel, it was found that the milder self-etch adhesives were not strong enough to create etch pits in enamel, resulting in compromised resin tags that affected bond strength [85, 86]. Therefore, the concept of *selective etching technique* was introduced wherein the enamel was selectively etched and rinsed with 37% phosphoric acid followed by the application of an ultra-mild to mild self-etch adhesive on enamel and dentin [87].

- *Self-etch Adhesive Technique*

The prepared cavity must be isolated preferably with a rubber dam or with cotton rolls and saliva ejector.

37% phosphoric acid is applied only on the prepared enamel for 15 seconds. Etchant is washed for 30 seconds and the tooth is blot dried with tissue or blotting paper, resulting in enamel appearing white frosty.

If strong acidic primers are used, the above steps of selective etch protocol are not required. In *sixth-generation system*, the acidic primer is applied on enamel and dentin and left for 20 seconds following which it is air dried for 5 seconds. The adhesive is applied with a micro brush and left for 10 seconds. In the *seventh-generation system*, the acidic primer and adhesive are in a single bottle or may need to be premixed prior to application on the tooth surface for 20 seconds. It is then spread uniformly with a gentle stream of oil-free air. The primer and adhesive are light cured together as per manufacturer's instructions. Composite restoration is done with the incremental layering technique.

- *Can an Adhesive Be Applied Over Carious Dentin?*

Carious dentin shows reduction in mineral content and loss of crystallinity of the mineral phase along with the changes in the structure of collagen. This affects the depth of primer and adhesive penetration leading to the formation of a poor hybrid layer and unfavorable bond strength. Consequently, this results in microleakage and compromises the longevity of the restoration. It is critical to excavate to healthy tooth structure, both peripherally and on the floor of the cavity to ensure optimal bonding and a successful restoration. In case of moderate- to extensive-stage lesions, if carious dentin is left on the floor of the cavity, it should be lined with a glass ionomer base prior to composite restoration [88, 89]. The bond strengths achieved with primary teeth are lower as compared to that in permanent teeth. The fourth- and fifth-generation adhesive systems are considered the gold standard as they have the maximum bond strength. Hence, they are the preferred adhesive systems for restoring primary teeth. In patients who have a gag reflex and are uncomfortable with the use of the etch and rinse, strong self-etch adhesives can be used that eliminate the rinse step.

6.6 Resin Composite—The Material

Resin Composites are presently the only direct restorative filling material that come close to replacing enamel or dentin in both appearance and function. They were first introduced in dentistry in the 1950s and 1960s by Bowen, who developed the monomer Bisphenol A-Glycidyl Methacrylate (Bis-GMA) and added inorganic filler particles to synthesize the first-ever dental composite [62, 76]. The first generation of composites presented with rough surfaces that abraded easily, showed high polymerization shrinkage, were difficult to polish and were available in only a few shades. Over the years, there has been considerable change in the formulation of Resin Composite with respect to both the monomers and fillers used to improve their physical and esthetic properties. Consequently, different types of composites such as hybrid and nano composites are now being commercially marketed. While the availability of a wide range of composites such as packable, bulk fill, and flowable provides the operator the best opportunity of placing a successful restoration, its long-term prognosis remains dependent on knowing which type of composite to use in each clinical situation and the technique of placement [90].

- *What is Composite Resin Made of?*

Composite resins are broadly composed of three distinct components:

Polymerizable monomers Bis-GMA, Hydroxyethyl Methacrylate (HEMA), Triethylene Diglycol Dimethacrylate (TEGDMA), Urethrane Dimethacrylate (UDMA) which convert from a liquid to a highly crosslinked polymer upon exposure to visible light.

Filler particles (silica, quartz, other glass powders, surface pre-reacted glass ionomer S-PRG fillers) provide hardness, wear resistance, radiopacity, and translucency to the composite and reduce the tendency of the polymer to undergo shrinkage.

Coupling agent containing organic silanes binds the polymer matrix with the inorganic filler particles.

Additionally, the composite contains a light initiator system, such as camphoroquinone (CQ), and catalysts to control the polymerization speed [91, 92].

- *What Are the Types of Resin Composites?*

Earlier, composites used to be broadly distinguished based on the distribution and average filler particle size such as *Macrofilled* (approximately 8 μm) and Microfilled (0.01–0.04 μm). However, due to the inherent limitations in the esthetic properties of macrofilled and physical properties of microfilled composites, they were gradually phased out of practice and a *hybrid composite* (0.04–0.1 mm), came to the forefront [93, 94]. In subsequent years, the addition of micro (0.01–0.04 μm) and nano fillers (0.005–0.01um) to hybrid composites has paved the way for *micro-hybrid* and *nanohybrid* composites. These materials have a high wear resistance, impart a smooth texture to the restoration, and are available in a variety of shades with tailored opacity and translucency. Today, the commercially available composites are microhyrid or nanohybrid which are suitable for high-quality restorations on both anterior and posterior teeth.

In terms of clinical applicability, composites can be classified as

Packable composites are the most used materials for anterior and posterior restorations. Most packable composites available today are nanohybrid while some

Table 6.11 Commercially packable Resin Composite material

Commercial name	Opacities	Shades
3 M™ Filtek Z350 XT Universal Restorative (Nanofilled) Syringe	3 M™	A1, A1B, A1D, A2, A2B, A2D, A2E, A3,A3.5, A3.5B, A3B, A3D, A3E, A4B, A4D, AT, B1, B1B, B2, B2B, B3, BT, C1, C2, C2B, C3B, CT, D2, WD, White, Extra white, Clear, Blue Gray, Amber
3 M™ Filtek™ Z250 XT Universal Restorative (Nano Hybrid) Capsule and syringe		A1, A2, A3, A3.5, A4, B1, B2, B3, C2, D3, OA2, OA3, O (opaque)
3 M™ Filtek™ P60 posterior restorative (Microhybrid) Syringe		A3, B2, C2
3 M™ Filtek™ Z250 Universal restorative (Microhybrid) Capsule and syringe		B1, A1, B2, C2, A2, B3, D3, A3, A3.5, A4, I, UD
3 M™ Filtek™ Easy Match Universal Restorative (Nano composite)		Bright, natural, warm
3 M™ Filtek™ Universal Restorative (Nano composite)		A1, B1, A2, B2, A3, D3, A3.5, A4, PO, XW
Tetric® Prime	Ivoclar	A1, A2, A3, A3.5, A4, B1, B2, C1, T A2 dentin A3.5 dentin L bleach
Mosaic by Ultradent (Anterior and posterior restorative)		A0.5, A1, A2, A3, A3.5, A4, A5 B0.5, B1, B2, C2, C3, D2 OW, EW, EN, EB, EG, EY, ET
G-ænial™ A'CHORD	GC	A1, A2A3, A3.5, A4
GRADIA® DIRECT GRADIA® DIRECT X (Nanofilled)		A1, A2A3, A3.5, A4, O2, O3, O4, B1, B2, B3, BW, C3, CT, CV, CVD, CVT, DT, GT, NT, P-A1, P-A2, P-A3, P-A3.5, P-NT, P-WT, WT, XBW
G-ænial Sculpt®		A1, A2A3, A3.5, A4, AE (Adult Enamel), AO1, AO2, AO3, B1, B2, B3, BW, C3, CV (Cervical), JE (Junior Enamel), XBW (Extra Bleach White)
KALORE™		A1, A2A3, A3.5, A4, AO2, AO3, AO4, B1, B2, B3, BW, C2, C3, CT, CV, CVD, CVT, D2, DT, GT, NT, OBW, OXBW, WT, XBW

(continued)

Table 6.11 (continued)

Commercial name	Opacities	Shades
BEAUTIFIL II (Nanohybrid dentin shades)	Shofu Inc	A1, A2, A3, A3.5, A4, B1, B2, B3, C2, C3, INC (Incisal), BW (Bleach White), A2O, A3O
BEAUTIFIL II pink and white (Nanohybrid enamel shades)		Gingival (pink)- G-DP (Dark Pink), G-LP (Light Pink), G-Or (Orange)0, G-Br (Brown), G-V (Violet) Enamel (white)- HVT (High Value Translucent), T (Translucent), LVT (Low Value Translucent), AM (Amber)
BEAUTIFIL II LS		A1, A2, A3, A3.5, A4, B1, B2, B3, C2, C3, INC (Incisal), BW (Bleach White), A2O, A3O
BRILLIANT EverGlow (Microhybrid)	Coltene	OBL (Opaque BL), OA1 (Opaque A1), OA3 (Opaque A3), Bleach, A1/B1, A2/B2, A3/D3, A3.5/B3, A4/C4, C2/C3
BRILLIANT NG (Nanofilled)		Enamel- A1/B1, A2/B2, A3/D3, A3.5/B3, A4/C4, C2/C3, Enamel Bleach, Transparent Dentin- A1/B1, A2/B2, A3/D3, A3.5/B3, A4/C4, C2/C3, Dentin Bleach
Synergy Nano Formula Duo Shade and Synergy Nano Formula Compact (Nanohybrid)		A1/D2, A2/B2, A3/D3, A3.5/B3
CLEARFIL™ AP-X ES-2 Universal	Kuraray	U (Universal), UW (Universal White), UL (Universal Light), UD (Universal Dark)
CLEARFIL™ AP-X ES-2 (Nanohybrid)		A1, A2, A3, A3.5, A1E, A2E, A3E, A3.5E, A1D, A2D, A3D, A3.5D, Clear, Amber, Blue, Gray
CLEARFIL™ AP-X Esthetics		A1, A2, A3, A3.5, B2, B3, C3, T, XL, OC, OA3, HO
CLEARFIL™ AP-X		A2, A3, A3.5, A4, B2, B3, B4, C2, C3, C4, XL
Nanohybrid restorative material GrandioSO Unlimited Admira® Fusion 5 Admira® Fusion GrandioSO Grandio	Voco	A1, A2, A3, A3.5, A4 A1, A2, A3, A3.5, A4 A1, A2, A3, A3.5, A4, B1, B2, B3, C2, C3, OA1, OA2, OA3, OA3.5, BL, BXL, Incisal, GA3.25, GA5 A1, A2, A3, A3.5, A4, B1, B2, B3, C2, D3, Incisal, OA1, OA2, OA3.5, BL, GA3.25, GA5 A1, A2, A3, A3.5, A4, B1, B2, B3, C2, C3, D2, D3, Incisal, OA2, OA3.5, BL

These commercial products have been listed after visiting the manufacturers' website on 7th May 2025. The availability of these products may vary across different regions

belong to the microhybrid type with a filler loading of 70 to 85% (Table 6.11) [93, 94].

Due to their decreased viscosity and increased flowability, *flowable composites* (Table 6.12) can penetrate the small crevices or corners of a cavity with an injection syringe, thus simplifying the handling operation and shortening the working time. Their reduced filler loading and higher resin component results in a lowered modulus of elasticity that withstands tooth flexure making it a suitable material for cervical restorations. This property also helps it to act as a stress absorber, when placed as a liner below packable composite. Certain flowable composites have higher filler loading that approaches that of packable composites (3 M Filtek, GC Genial flow). While their flowability is decreased, these materials can be used in stress-bearing

Table 6.12 Commercially available flowable resin composite material

Flowable composite	Manufacturer	Shades
ever X FLOW™ (Short, glass micofiber reinforced)	GC	Universal Dentin
G-aenial™ universal flo	GC	A1, A2, A3, A3.5, A4, B1, B2, B3, C3, CV, BW, AO2, AO3, JE, AE
G-aenial™ flow X	GC	A1, A2, A3, A3.5, A4, CV, AO2, AO3
GRADIA® Direct LoFlo (Microfilled hybrid)	GC	A1, A2, A3, A3.5, A4, CV, AO2, AO3
GRADIA® DIRECT flo (Microfilled hybrid)	GC	A1, A2, A3, A3.5, A03, BW, CV
3 M™ Filtek™ Supreme™ Flowable Restorative (Nanofilled)	3 M™	A1, A3.5, A3, A2
3 M™ Filtek™ Bulk Fill Flowable Restorative (Microhybrid)	3 M™	A1, A2, A3, Universal
Synergy D6/Brilliant Flow (Nanofilled)	Coltene	A1/B1, A2/B2, A3/D3, A3.5/B3
CLEARFIL MAJESTY™ flow	Kuraray	A1, A2, A3, A3.5, B1, B2, C3, D3, E2, CV, OA3, BL2
CLEARFIL MAJESTY™ ES flow	Kuraray	A1, A2, A3, A3.5, A4, KA6, B1, B2, XW, W
CLEARFIL MAJESTY™ ES Flow Universal	Kuraray	U, UD
CLEARFIL MAJESTY™ AP-X Esthetics Flow (Hybrid)	Kuraray	A1, A2, A3, A3.5, A4, KA6, B1, B2, XW, W
Revolution™ Formula 2 (Hybrid resin)	Kerr™	A1, A2, A3, A3.5, A4, B1, B2, B3, B3, C1, C2, C3, C4, D2, D3, D4, XL, G2, Light, Opaque, White
Herculite™ Ultra Flow (Nanohybrid)	Kerr™	A1, A2, A3, A3.5, A4, B1, B2, C2, D2, XL1, XL2, Universal Opaque
Premise™ flow (Nanofilled)	Kerr™	A1, A2, A3, B1
Vertise™ Flow	Kerr™	A1, A2, A3, A3.5, B1, B2, Universal Opaque, XL, Translucent
SimpliShade™ Self Adhesive flow	Kerr™	Light, Medium, Dark, Universal Opaque
BEAUTIFIL Flow (Giomer)	Shofu Inc	A1, A2, A3, A3.5, A4, A3OP, Gum (Low flow) A1, A2, A3, A3.5, A4, A3O, A3T (High flow)
BEAUTIFIL Flow Plus® (Hybrid) BEAUTIFIL Flow Plus® X (Bioactive nanohybrid)	Shofu Inc	A0.5, A1, A2, A3, A3.5, A4, B1, B2, C2, D2, A0.5O, A1O, A2O, INC, BW, MI, CV

(continued)

Table 6.12 (continued)

Flowable composite	Manufacturer	Shades
Tetric Evoflo® (Nano hybrid)	Ivoclar	A1, A2, A3, A3.5, A4, B1, B3, A2 dentin, A3.5 dentin, B2 dentin, Bleach XL, Bleach L, Bleach M
Tetric® plus flow (Micro hybrid)	Ivoclar	A2 plus, A3 plus, A3.5 plus, Bleach plus
Heliomolar® Flow (Reinforced Microfill)	Ivoclar	A1, A2, A3, D3, T
Wave, Wave MV, Wave HV	SDI	A1, A2, A3, A3.5, B1, B2, B3, C2, C3, D3, OA2, Gingival and Bleach.
Flow-It™ ALC™ (Hybrid)	Pentron	A1, A2, A3, A3.5, A4, B1, B2, B3, B4, C1, C2, C3, C4, D2, D3, D4, Clear, Universal Opaque. Pedo Lgt, Pedo XLgt, AO, BO, Incisal, White Opaque
AeliteFlo™ (Microhybrid)	Bisco	12 shades
AlignerFlow LC (Nanohybrid)	Voco	A1, A2, A3
Admira® Fusion Flow (Nanohybrid)	Voco	A1, A2, A3, A3.5, A4, B1, B2, C2, I, Opaque OA2, BL, WO
Admira® Flow	Voco	A1, A2, A3, A3.5
Grandio® flow Grandio® SO flow Grandio®SO Light flow Grandio®SO Heavy flow (Nanohybrid)	Voco	A1, A2, A3, A3.5, A4, B1, B2, C2, D2, OA2, BL, WO A1, A2, A3, A3.5, A4, B1, B2, C2, OA2, BL, WO, Incisal, GA5 A1, A2, A3, A3.5, B1, OA2, WO, Incisal A1, A2, A3, A3.5, A4, B1, B2, C2, OA2, BL, WO, Incisal, GA5

These commercial products have been listed after visiting the manufacturers' website on 7th May 2025. The availability of these products may vary across different regions
O opaque, *CV* cervical, *BW* bleach white, *JE* junior enamel, *AE* adult enamel, *BL* bleach, *WO* White opaque

areas such as on the surface of a preventive resin restoration, as they have greater wear resistance and can withstand masticatory forces [95, 96].

Bulk-fill composites were developed to improve the time-consuming incremental cavity-filling technique for core build ups and restorations in young children, where it may be difficult to achieve prolonged isolation. The newer bulk-fill composites allow incremental filling of up to 4 mm in thickness as compared to the 2 mm increments of packable and flowable composites. Due to high color translucency of these materials, the depth of cure is ensured, and innovative initiator system shortens the light-curing time (Table 6.13) [97, 98].

- *Types of Composites Based On Shade Matching*

Resin Composite stand out from all direct restorative materials, due to their availability in a variety of shades which allows them to merge with the remaining tooth structure and mimic the appearance of adjacent teeth [99]. Different shades of

Table 6.13 Commercially available bulk fill resin composite material

Bulk-fill composite	Manufacturer	Shades
Beautifil Bulk Flowable Beautifil Bulk Restorative (Giomer-based direct Resin Composite)	Shofu Inc	Universal Dentin Shade A Shade Universal
G-aenial™ BULK injectable	GC	A1, A2
Tetric EvoCeram® Bulk fill	Ivoclar	B2, B3, C1, C2, C3, A4 dentin, T, A3.5 dentin, Bleach L, D2, D3, Bleach I, Bleach M, B2 dentin
SimpliShade™ Bulk fill (Unidose and syringe)	Kerr™	One shade
SonicFill™ 3		A1, A2, A3, B1
Filtek™ One bulk fill (Unidose and syringe)	3 M™	A1, A2, A3, B1, C2
Aura (Unidose and syringe)	SDI	One shade
Fill-Up!™	Coltene	One shade
VisCalor Bulk Grandio® SO x-tra	Voco	A1, A2, A3, Universal
SDR® Plus	Dentsply Sirona	A1, A2, A3, Universal

These commercial products have been listed after visiting the manufacturers' website on 7th May 2025. The availability of these products may vary across different regions

composites were first developed by studying the natural tooth color and were modeled on the Vita shade guide, which is commonly used for shade selection of custom-made crowns. Most of the commercial formulations of composites currently available are broadly categorized into four distinct shades A, B, C, and D. These base shades represent parts of the visible color spectrum as follows [100]:

- A (orange-red).
- B (orange yellow).
- C (brown-gray).
- D (brown).

Shade A is most often used in children and young adults and on a few occasions, shade B may be selected as well. Shades C and D are generally reserved for older patients. These base shades are each further subdivided from 1 to 4, i.e., A1 to A4 *based on the intensity of the color* with A1 having the lowest intensity or lightest shades and A4 being the darkest [99, 100]. However, for ease of use, many companies have divided the shades into broad categories where enamel shades have more translucency and dentin shades show more opacity.

- *Clinical Considerations While Using Resin Composite*

While the use of newer resin materials containing HEMA and TEGDMA has reduced *polymerization shrinkage*, this inherent limitation of composites continues to persist even in the new generations. This can cause restorative failures such as

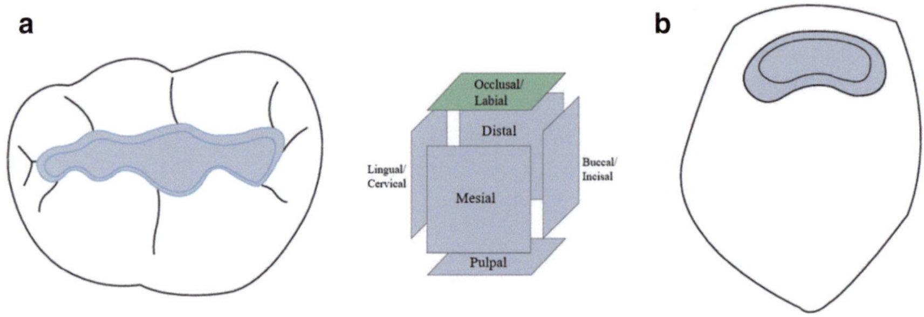

Fig. 6.14 The greatest polymerization shrinkage is seen in occlusal (Class I) (**a**) and cervical (Class V) (**b**) tooth preparations which have a C factor of 5, because the restoration is bonded to five walls of the cavity (buccal/incisal, lingual/cervical, mesial, distal, pulpal-blue) and only the occlusal/labial surface is free or unbonded (green)

interfacial gap formation, postoperative sensitivity, secondary caries, and crack formation [101].

Upon polymerization, the Resin Composite shrinks towards the center of the cavity creating stress at the resin–tooth interface. Hence, there is a chance of bond disruption, as the force of shrinkage is greater than the strength of the bond developed between the composite and the prepared tooth. The magnitude of this pull is dependent on the Configuration factor (C -factor) [101]. The C-factor is the ratio of bonded surfaces to unbonded or free surfaces of the prepared tooth. The higher the C-factor, greater is the chance of bond disruption [102, 103] (Figs. 6.14, 6.15, 6.16, and 6.17).

- *How Can Polymerization Shrinkage Be Reduced Keeping the C-Factor in Mind?*

Incremental filling of composites in layers of less than 2 mm decreases stress caused by polymerization shrinkage. While placing each increment, the composite material should not contact more than two walls of the cavity, especially in those preparations that have a high C-factor. The different incremental layering techniques that follow this principle are placing composites in horizontal layers, oblique layers, or by building each cusp individually. This method of curing ensures complete polymerization and helps to achieve better marginal seal. In anterior teeth, a multilayer buildup not only ensures adequate polymerization but also allows the operator to add esthetic value to the restoration [101–103].

The placement of a material with low modulus of elasticity as a base, acts as an intermediate stress-absorbing layer to compensate for the polymerization shrinkage of the Resin Composite restoration placed above. The use of flowable composite (*snow plough technique*) in 2 mm increments or a glass ionomer material (*sandwich technique*) will reduce the stress at the tooth resin interface preventing microleakage and secondary caries [104]. Many *light curing units* have soft or ramp curing mode to reduce the polymerization shrinkage associated with high-intensity light curing. The gradual intensity curing retards the polymerization process, which provides

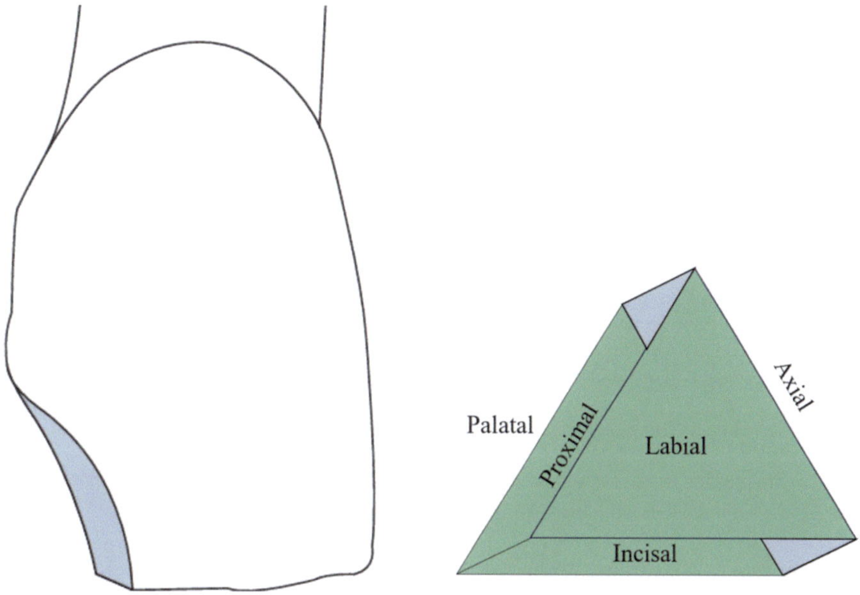

Fig. 6.15 The lowest polymerization shrinkage is seen in tooth preparations involving the incisal edge (Class IV), as it has a C-factor of 0.25; with only one bonded surface (pulpal-blue) and four surfaces free (labial, palatal/lingual, mesial, distal-green) providing stress relief

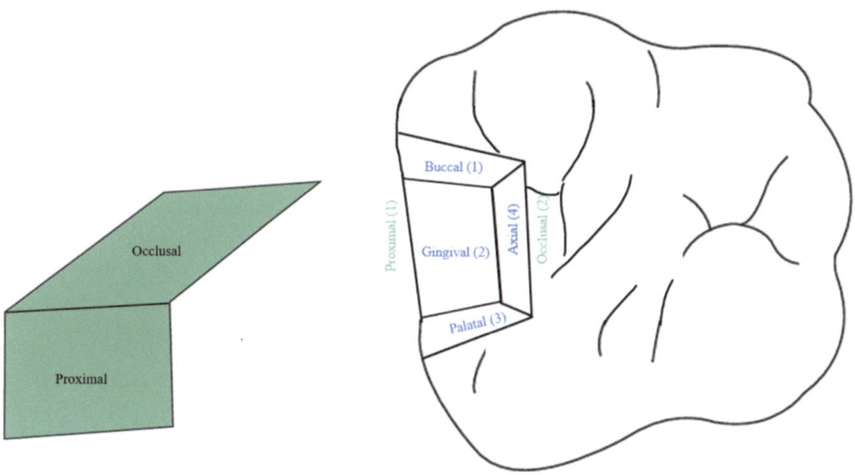

Fig. 6.16 Proximal box (Class II) preparations have an intermediate C factor of 2 (bonded: buccal, gingival, lingual/palatal, axial-blue; unbonded: occlusal and proximal-green)

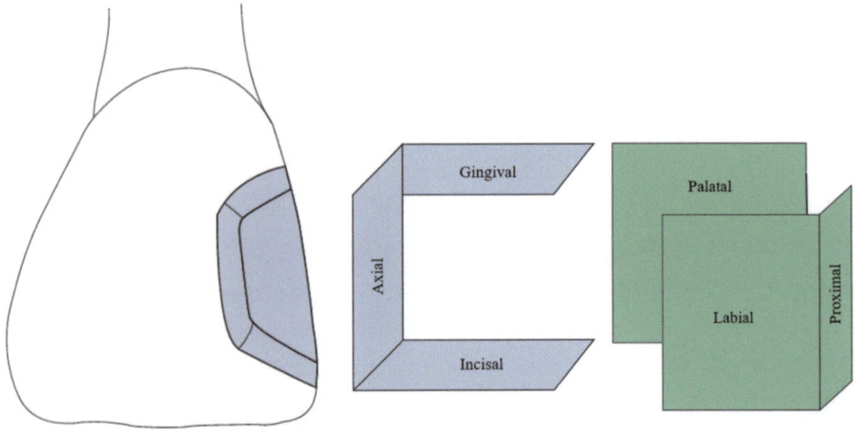

Fig. 6.17 Anterior proximal (Class III) preparations (bonded: pulpal, incisal, cervical-blue; unbonded: labial, palatal/lingual, proximal-green) have a C-factor of 1

time for stress relaxation. While the newer LED lights may have a high-intensity setting with a lesser curing time, it is always advisable that the increments are cured as per manufacturer's instructions [102, 103].

- *Application of Resin Composite in Pediatric Dentistry*

  1. *Preventive Resin Restoration (PRR)*

Preventive Resin Restoration, introduced by Simonsen, integrates the use of preventive agents like sealants indicated for caries-susceptible pits and fissures along with the restoration of lesions on the same occlusal surface, using Resin Composite [105, 106]. PRR is indicated after a thorough visual examination with air drying, to reveal an opaque, chalky appearance exhibiting loss of translucency along pits and fissures. Stained or carious pits and fissures or deep pits and fissures that could inhibit complete penetration of sealant material or could be carious at their bases, are also indicated for a PRR [106, 107]. Based on the extent and depth of the carious lesion as determined by tooth preparation, PRR is classified as follows [106].

Type A
This involves sealing of the susceptible pits and fissures limited to enamel.

Type B
This involves sealing susceptible areas and restoring carious lesions that extend substantially into enamel or even into dentin but are limited to pits and fissures.

Type C
More extensive carious lesions with dentinal involvement requiring removal of carious tissue using a carbide or stainless-steel bur, while the remaining pits and fissures

are then sealed [108]. Most Resin Composite restorations today fall into the category of Type C PRR.

- *Technique for Placing a PRR Restoration* [109–111]

Burs Used

The Fissurotomy® conservative preparation and exploration bur kit (SS White®) has three tungsten carbide burs, the Fissurotomy® Original, the Fissurotomy® Narrow Tapered Fissure (NTF), and the Fissurotomy® Shallow Tapered Fissure (STF) which have diameters of 1.1 mm, 0.7 mm, and 0.6 mm, respectively. The Fissurotomy® (STF) has a shorter head length of 1.5 mm as compared to 2.5 mm in the other variants. The other burs that can be used in a PRR are the SS White FG 330 S. It has a working head length of 1.6 mm and a diameter of 0.8 mm. The Nos ¼, ½, 1, and 2 round tungsten carbide have a diameter of 0.25, 0.5, 1, and 2 mm, respectively.

The Fissurotomy® burs (Original/NTF/STF) along with the tungsten carbide round burs (sizes ¼ or ½) can be used for initial fissure preparation to enable the operator to know the extent of the lesion. If caries is seen on the floor or along the walls after fissurotomy, excavation can be done with a ¼ or ½ stainless-steel round bur. If further preparation is needed, it must be done with a 330 pear-shaped carbide bur (SS White® FG 330 S) or a no. 2 stainless-steel round bur. The cavosurface margins for a Type A or Type B PRR that receives a sealant or flowable composite need not be beveled as the preparation is minimal and restricted to occlusal pits and fissures.

Apply the etchant (37% phosphoric acid) on enamel first and then flow to dentin for a total of 15 to 20 seconds only. Rinse and blot dry for a white frosty appearance. Scrub the bonding agent and air dry after 10 seconds. Air dry till the bonding agent stops rippling to ensure that there is no pooling of the material at the base of the fissure. Self-etch bonding systems may also be applied using the selective etch concept.

In a *Type A PRR*, a filled sealant is delivered into all the pits and fissures on the occlusal surface. A sharp explorer is used to ensure that the sealant penetrates completely. The material is allowed to rest for 10 seconds before curing.

Type B PRR, where the fissurotomy has resulted in a wider preparation, can be restored by placing a flowable resin at the base of the fissure. After curing, a sealant can be applied over the occlusal surface to seal the remaining narrow fissures.

In certain Type A and Type B PRRs which show narrow fissures after tooth preparation, a filled sealant or flowable Resin Composite may not penetrate to the base of the fissure. In these cases, an unfilled sealant can be placed after bonding and the remaining fissure which is wider towards the occlusal surface can be restored with a filled sealant or flowable resin.

Type C PRR

While deciding on the type of Resin Composite to restore a Type C PRR, it is the width of the preparation that is more critical than the depth. A flowable composite is placed first and allowed to penetrate before light curing. Wherever a 330 FG bur or a no. 2 stainless-steel bur is used for caries excavation, the cavity prepared will

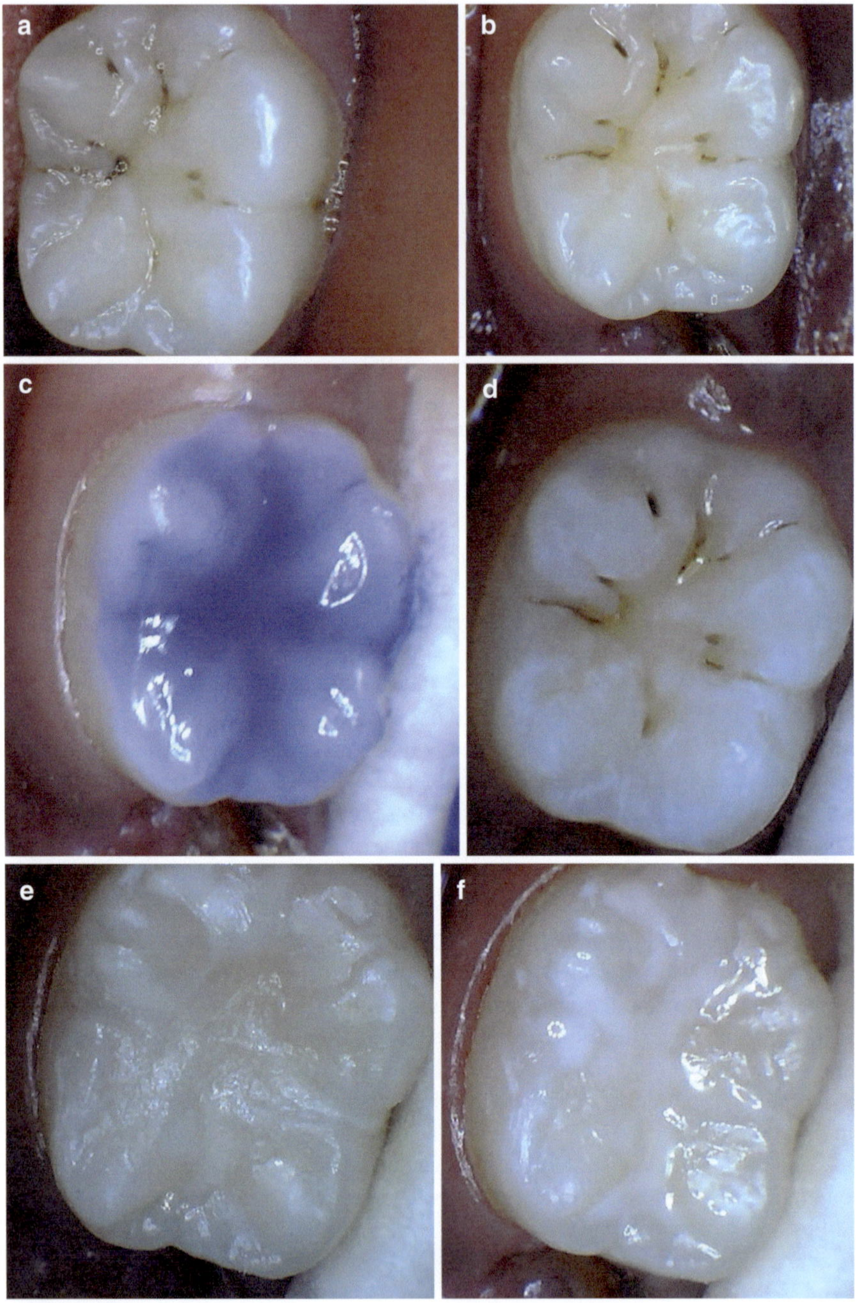

Fig. 6.18 Occlusal carious lesion in mandibular permanent left first molar (**a**). Fissures opened with a fissurotomy bur. The walls of the fissures are left caries free (**b**). Etching done with 37% phosphoric acid for 15 seconds (**c**). The tooth is washed and air dried to a white frosty appearance (**d**). The tooth is washed and air dried to a white frosty appearance (**d**). The remaining unprepared fissures were covered with sealants (**e**). Finishing and polishing done (**f**)

be wide enough and a packable Resin Composite should be placed over the flowable composite. If the preparation narrows along the remaining fissure, a flowable composite can be placed. A sealant is then applied over the entire occlusal surface to complete the preventive resin restoration.

Type A PRR generally does not require occlusal adjustment, while Type B and Type C PRR need to be checked for high points and occlusal adjustments (Fig. 6.18).

- *Success of Preventive Resin Restorations*

Several clinical studies have cited different criteria such as longevity of sealant, wear of sealant, need for re-restoration or occurrence of secondary caries to judge the success of a PRR [112–114]. The one-year success rate judged on the basis of the complete retention of PRR was 100% (Simonsen and Stallard), while the 7-year success rate (complete retention) was seen to be 90%. The most common failure was loss of sealant which can be repaired during follow-up visits [111].

6.7 Conventional Resin Composite Restorations for Occlusal and Proximal Surfaces

While restoring a cavity with Resin Composite, the walls must always be prepared to healthy tooth structure and the cavosurface margin beveled. In completely excavated moderate-stage lesions, a flowable composite placed on the floor acts as a stress-absorbing layer. If the floor of an extensive carious lesion is excavated to soft or firm dentin, using the selective caries removal approach, a Glass Ionomer base (sandwich technique) must be applied before placing the resin restoration.

In a proximal cavity, if glass ionomer is placed as a base, an open sandwich technique can be performed wherein the glass ionomer extends to the outer wall of the restoration or a closed sandwich technique done, where the Glass Ionomer is placed short of the cavosurface margin of the gingival seat. It is important to not leave remnants of a base or liner on the walls of the prepared tooth as this will compromise the seal between the resin and healthy tooth structure ensuing microleakage. Following this, packable Resin Composite is then placed using the incremental layering technique.

There are numerous layering techniques advocated in literature (Table 6.14). However, there is no consensus on which technique is better; the underlying principle is that the operator should place the composites such that each increment does not contact more than two surfaces of the cavity wall, when placing each layer. This ensures reduction in polymerization shrinkage due to the higher C-factor seen in occlusal and proximal restorations [115]. Resin Composite should always be overfilled slightly and flushed well onto and beyond the beveled cavosurface margin. Maintaining tooth anatomy by sculpting the Resin Composite during placement not only improves the final esthetics and function but also reduces the time taken to finish and polish the restoration. Any fissure not involved in the restoration must be sealed.

Table 6.14 Resin Composite layering techniques

Technique	Description	Diagram
Horizontal layering technique	The horizontal placement technique utilizes composite layers, each less than 2.0 mm thick placed one atop the other.	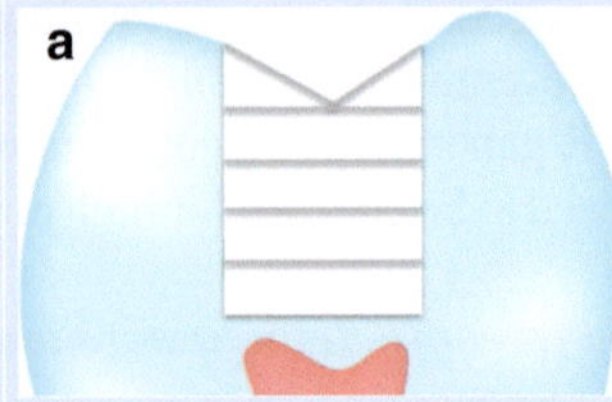
Oblique layering technique	The oblique technique is accomplished by placing a series of wedge-shaped composite increments.	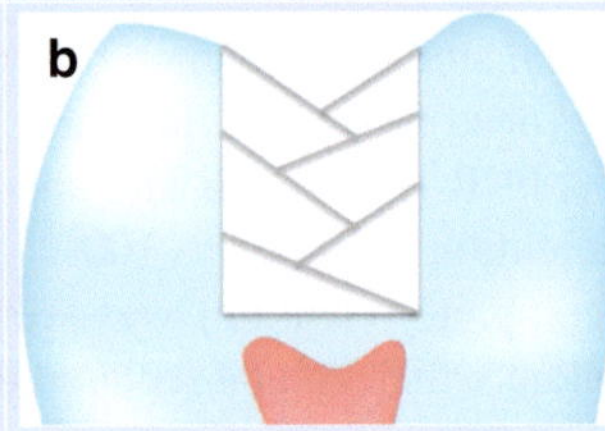
Vertical layering technique	Place small increments in vertical pattern starting from one wall, i.e., buccal or lingual and carried to another wall.	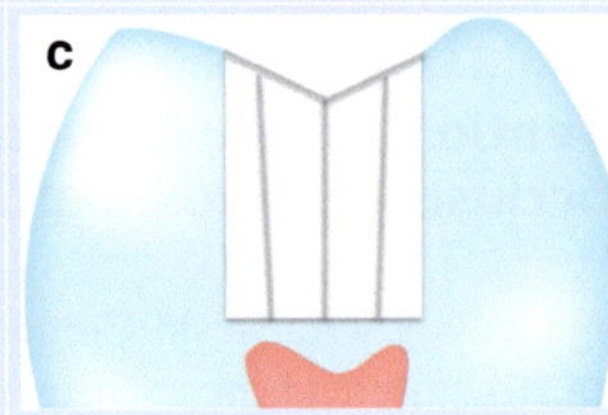
Split-increment horizontal layering technique	Each horizontal increment is split, before curing, into four triangle-shaped portions, with each portion placed against only one cavity wall.	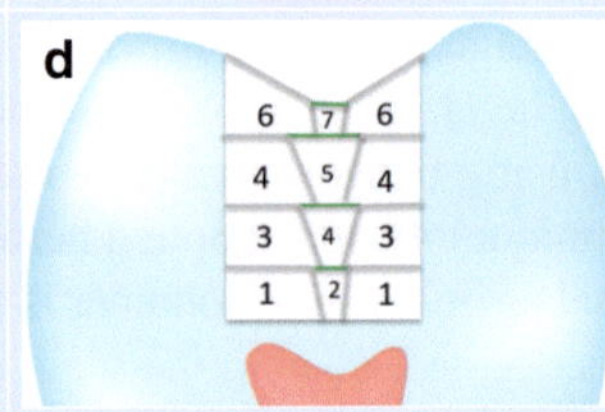
Stratified layering technique	It involves placing dentin shades of Resin Composite with a higher chroma in the middle of the preparation and placing a lower chroma resin close to the cusp walls.	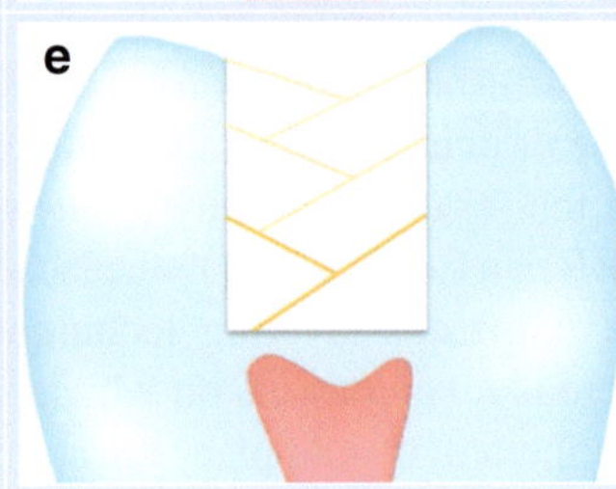

(continued)

Table 6.14 (continued)

Technique	Description	Diagram
Successive cusp buildup technique	Here, individual cusps are restored one at a time up to the level of the occlusal enamel. Small sloping increments are applied to each corner of the cavity in turn and manipulation is kept to a minimum, to avoid folding voids into the material.	f 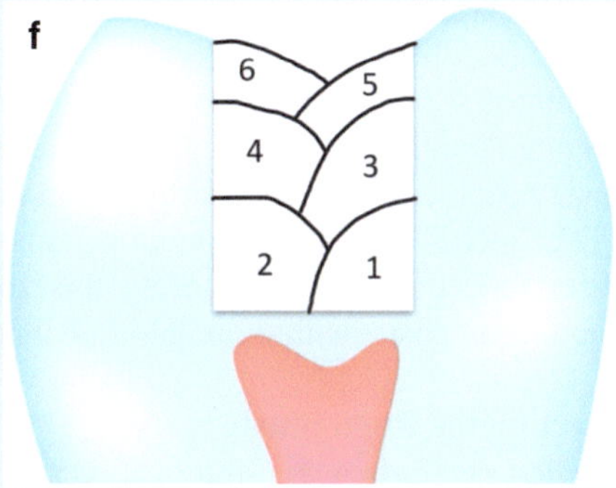

Success of Conventional Resin Composite Restoration

The overall success rate for Class I Resin Composite restorations in the primary dentition over a period of 4 years was 79.3%, and the annual fracture rate ranged from 1.7% to 12.9% [115]. Studies in primary teeth have shown the success rate of composites to be higher in occlusal than proximal posterior restorations. While the fracture toughness of composites is certainly superior as compared to both GICs, the lower success rates could be attributed to poor bond strength in primary enamel and dentin. Additionally, difficulty in isolation can not only contaminate the restoration but also prevent the operator from placing incremental layers. Resin Composite is considered the best restorative material for all types of direct restorations in permanent teeth. [61, 116, 117]

- *Anterior Composite Restorations*

Layering of Composite Based on Tooth Morphology [100, 114, 118, 119]

Composite restorations should emulate the optical characteristics of natural teeth, which can only be achieved by the critical first step of accurate shade selection. The process of shade selection and stratification becomes easier if one is familiar with the basic morphological characteristics of an anterior tooth. For the purpose of understanding, it is important for the operator to visualize the tooth in a cross-sectional view. The enamel is the thinnest at the gingival or cervical margin and the dentin is close to the surface. As we move towards the incisal edge, the dentin reduces as the enamel thickness increases.

To obtain a life-like buildup of the resin composite, stratification should always be done using a darker composite in the inner layers and moving to a lighter shade in the outer layer. The dentinal composite in the buildup should always be sandwiched between a layer of palatal and labial enamel.

In the cervical third, there is more reflection and virtually no passage of light. As there is greater color saturation due to the underlying dentin being seen, one should use dentin shades and a very thin or no enamel layer.

The middle third will have less dentinal color as compared to the cervical third. This can be achieved by layering the dentin composite to one shade lighter than seen on the cervical third or by placing a thicker layer of overlying enamel.

The middle third also shows more reflection and prevents passage of light so as to minimize the "see through effect" which will show the demarcation between the fractured tooth and the Resin Composite buildup. Dentin composites from higher to lower opacities are placed starting from the deeper layer.

The incisal aspect of the tooth is translucent and allows more light passage and lesser reflection. When restoring this zone, it is advisable to place translucent enamel composite with minimal or no inner dentinal layer.

Selecting the Right Shade

The first step during this stratification procedure is to select the base shade from the middle one-third of the tooth. Place a small amount of composite on the adjacent tooth and light cure (button dry technique). If after curing, the composite matches the adjacent enamel, then it is selected as the base shade. To give depth to the composite buildup, the underlying composites should be a shade darker than the outermost layer simulating the enamel. If the operator chooses to restore the tooth with Resin Composites having base color A2 (Vita Shade Guide™), the surface enamel on the palatal and labial surfaces should be built with A2 enamel shade and the deeper dentinal layers with darker dentin shades.

Step-by-Step Workflow of the Resin Composite Restoration of a Fractured Anterior Tooth

- At the first appointment, make a sectional impression of the fractured tooth and adjacent teeth with alginate.
- Apply a layer of bonding agent on the stone model and do a mock composite buildup of the fractured tooth. Replicate the palatal anatomy accurately and ensure the surface is polished well.
- Make a putty impression of the palatal surface to create a stent. The stent should extend onto the adjacent teeth on either side and up to the incisal edge taking care not to cover any portion of the labial surface.
- This allows building of the palatal shell or first layer of stratification on which the remaining layers can be placed.
- At the second appointment, clean and polish the tooth to remove debris and plaque.
- Select the base shade using the composite button dry technique. Let us consider that we are restoring a tooth with a base shade of A2. An example of the composite stratification would be as follows:
- Base shade A2 = A3 dentin shade (innermost layer) + A2 dentin shade (second layer) + A2 enamel shade (outermost layer)

- Isolate the segment with a rubber dam. Additional retraction can be achieved with floss ties or gingival retraction cord. The adjacent teeth can be covered with Teflon tape.
- A 3 to 4 mm bevel must be placed along the fracture line to ensure a seamless and well-blended final restoration.
- Etch with 37% phosphoric acid for 20 seconds. Rinse and blot dry.
- Apply one or two coats of bonding agent, air dry, and light cure. It is important to avoid pooling and curing of a thick layer of bonding agent, especially those containing HEMA, as this may not only compromise the bond strength but also degrade over time and lead to discoloration of the restoration.
- The silicone stent should be held against the fractured tooth and a 0.5 mm layer of A2 enamel shade should be constructed to replicate the palatal enamel.
- Once the palatal shell is built, the stent may be removed, and matrices can be used to build proximal contours.
- Proceeding to the stratification of dentin, the first dentin layer placed should have a higher chroma (A3 dentin shade) and must be opaque. This will prevent the see through effect. It should be placed such that it is thickest cervically and thins out as it approaches the incisal.
- This layer of composite should not extend into the incisal zone. It should be sculpted to create the three developmental lobes of the incisors.
- The next layer of composite should be of a lighter shade and less opaque than the previous layer (A2 dentin shade) and is placed in a similar manner. Should internal mamelons be recreated, they must be sculpted in this layer.
- The outermost layer of composite replaces labial enamel and it should be more translucent and have lesser chroma as compared to the dentinal shades used. A thin layer of A2 enamel shade is placed cervically, increasing in thickness as it extends incisally and proximally.
- The incisal edge can be built using only enamel shades to ensure translucency. Incisal shades having a bluish gray tinge may be used to replicate the incisal esthetics [40, 41].
- The restoration should be finished using final grit diamond points to remove gross irregularities. Polishing is done using polishing discs and interdental strips from the coarser to the finer grits.
- A surface sealant (Fortify™, Bisco, USA Permaseal™, Ultradent, USA) must be applied after polishing to seal microporosities.
- The final restoration should not only match the base shade chosen but mimic the natural tooth. This is achieved by using a combination of composites with different opacities and chromas as outlined above (Figs. 6.19, 6.20, and 6.21).

Cervical and Proximal Restorations of Anterior Teeth

- The technique of layering or stratification essentially remain the same as used above.
- For proximal anterior restorations, a mylar strip is used and lingually an enamel shade is placed on the mylar strip.

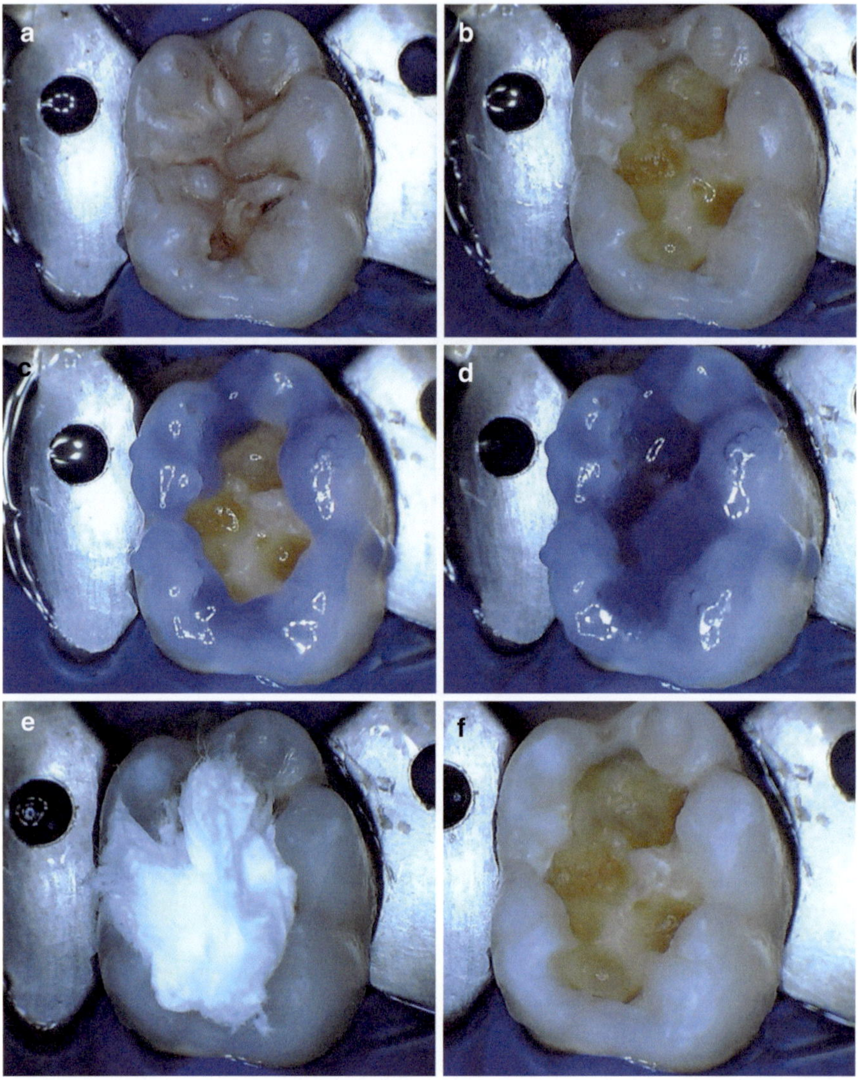

Fig. 6.19 Occlusal carious lesion in mandibular primary left second molar (**a**). Complete Caries Removal done from walls and floor of the lesion (**b**). Enamel etched with 37% phosphoric acid first (**c**), and then spread to dentin (**d**), for a total of 15 seconds. Etchant was washed and cavity blot dried (**e**). The enamel must appear frosty white and the dentin moist (**f**). Bonding agent applied and air dried to a thin uniform layer. The bonding agent was cured for 10 seconds (**g**). First increment was placed to build individual cusps without contacting each other. Each increment did not touch more than two walls at the time of curing (**h**). Second increment was placed in similar manner and the unprepared buccal and lingual fissures were sealed with pit and fissure sealant material (**i**). The third increment was placed in excess and cured (**j**). The restoration was finished and polished (**k**)

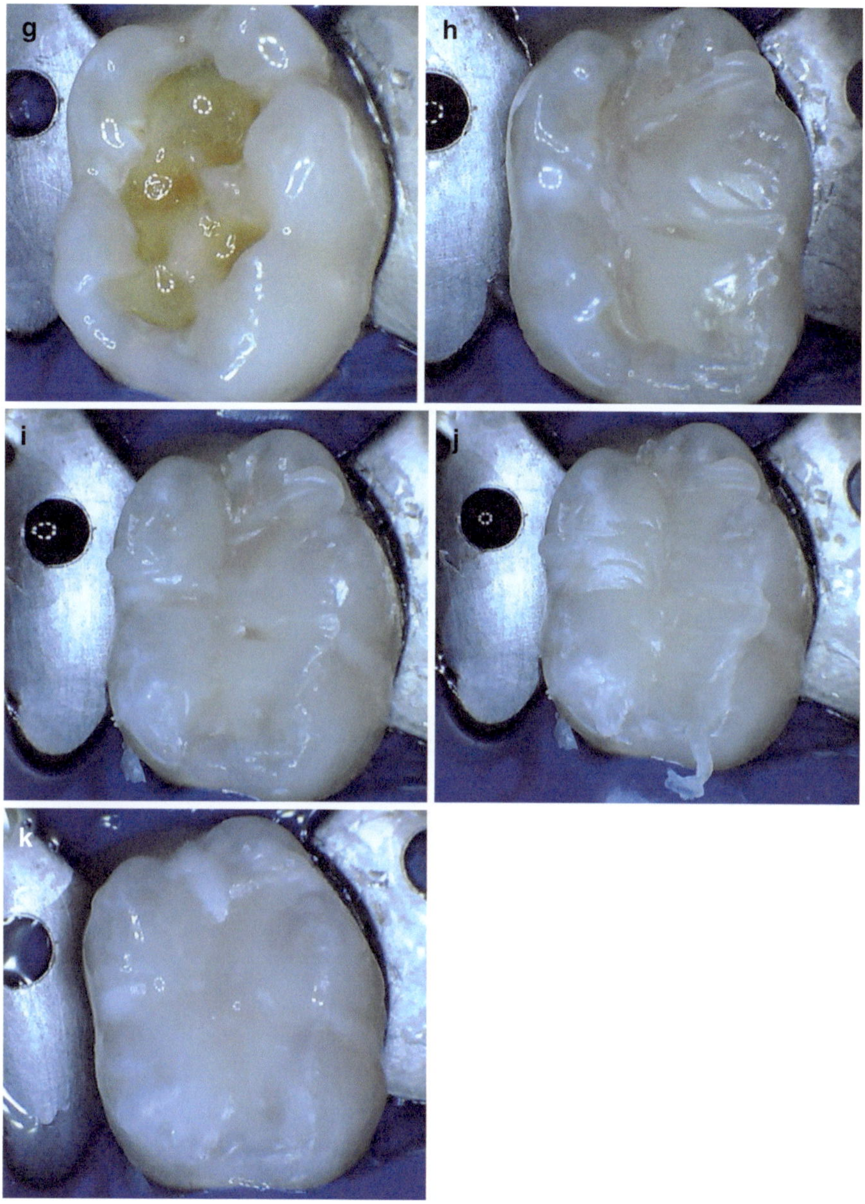

Fig. 6.19 (continued)

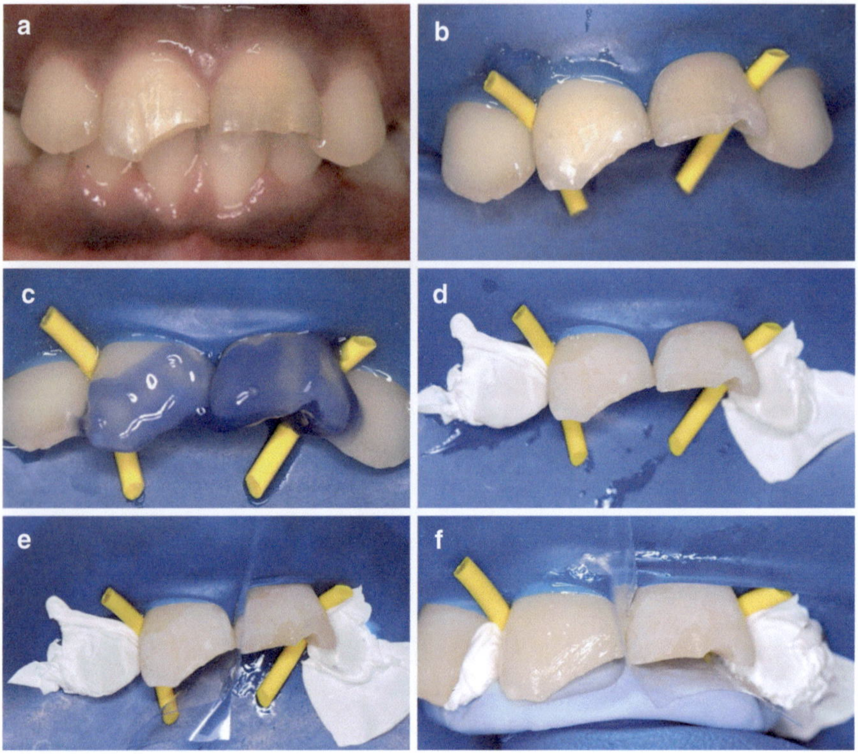

Fig. 6.20 Uncomplicated crown fracture of maxillary permanent central incisors (**a**). The teeth were isolated under rubber dam and the fractured edges were prepared with a short bevel to improve retention of the Resin Composite (**b**). Both incisors were etched with 37% phosphoric acid for 15 seconds (**c**). The etchant was washed and air dried such that the enamel appeared frosty (**d**). A mylar strip placed to prevent bonding agent from adhering to the adjacent tooth and to build proximal contacts. Adjacent teeth were covered with Teflon tape (**e**). Bonding agent applied on maxillary right central incisor and putty index held in place (**f**). The first increment of enamel shade built using a flat-bladed instrument, to replicate the palatal shell (**g**). The palatal shell was cured (**h**). The second increment, replicating dentin was layered on the palatal shell, such that it was thick in the middle and thinned down as it approached the incisal region. The material was extended to build contact mesially (**i**). Mammelons or developmental lobes, if required, should be sculpted in this layer (**j**). The third layer of a darker dentin shade built in the same manner. Internal mamelons were sculpted in this layer (**k**). The last layer of Resin Composite replicating enamel (same shade used to build palatal shell) placed. It should be thinnest at the cervical zone and thickest at the incisal zone, extending proximally to blend with the restoration (**l**). The left central incisor was built in a similar manner (**m**). Gross finishing of both teeth done to desired shape (**n**). Polishing done with discs and polishing paste (**o**). Teeth in palatal view showing identical contour, thickness and alignment to arch form (**p**)

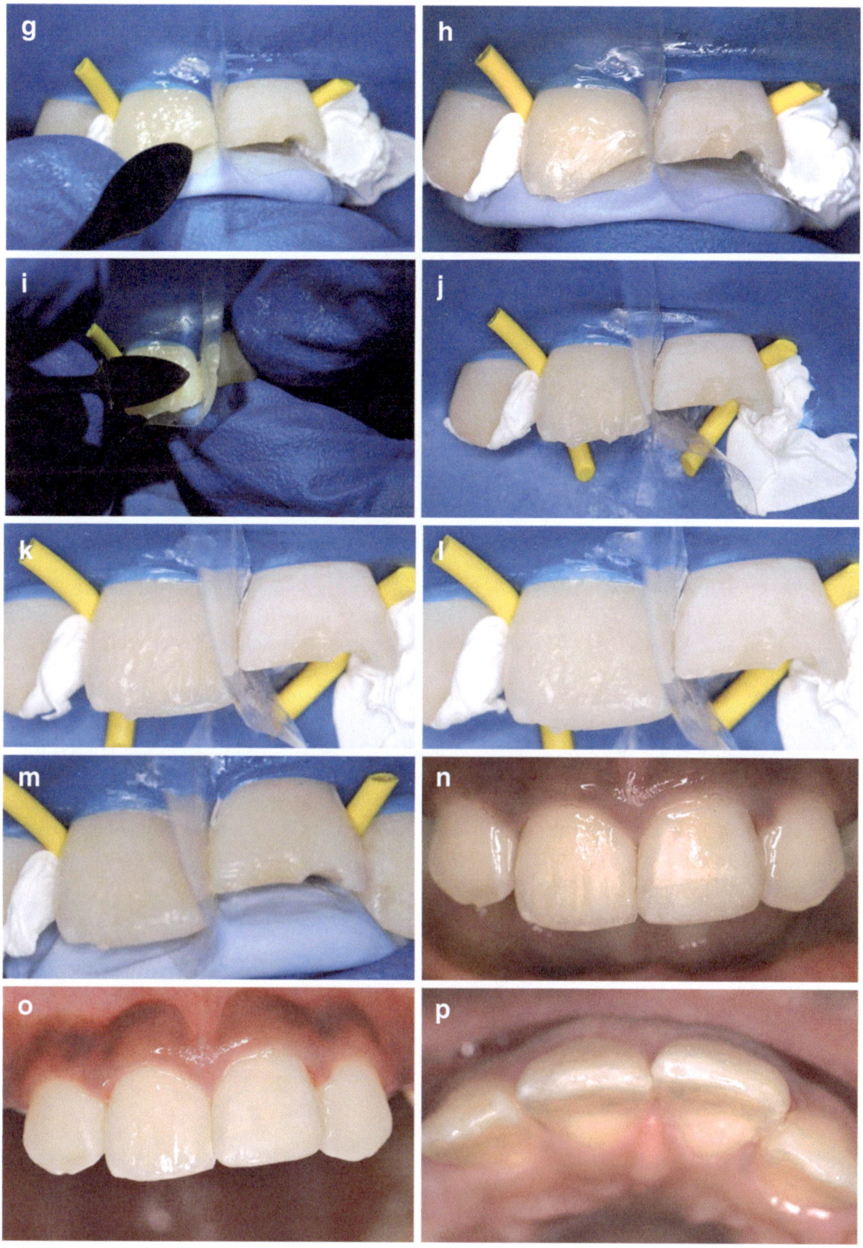

Fig. 6.20 (continued)

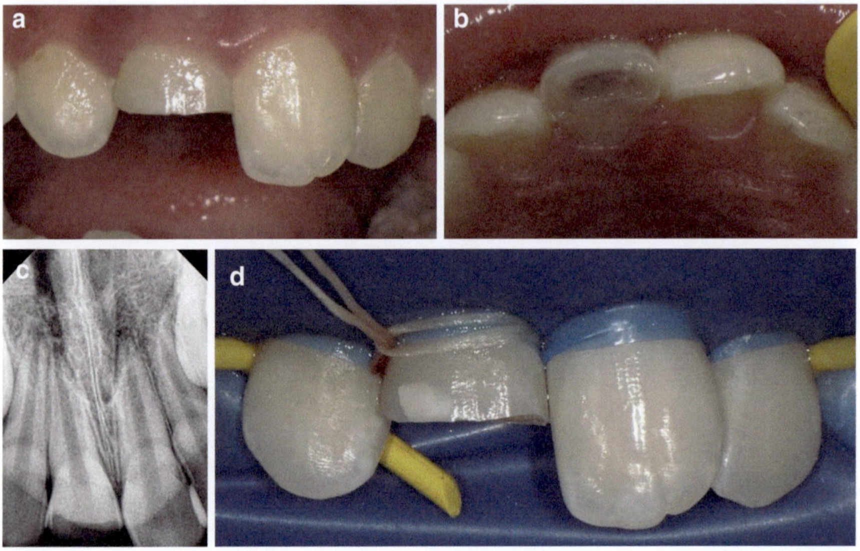

Fig. 6.21 Complicated crown fracture of maxillary permanent right central incisor (**a**). Patient presented with a larger pulp exposure few hours after trauma (**b**). The diagnostic radiograph revealed immature root apex (**c**). The tooth was anesthetized and isolated under rubber dam (**d**). Complete pulpotomy was done (**e**) and remaining pulp tissue capped with Calcium Silicate Cement (**f**). The access cavity was sealed with Resin-Modified Glass Ionomer Cement and flowable Resin Composite (**g**). A post-pulpotomy radiograph was taken (**h**). Alginate impression was made for fabricating a putty stent for Resin Composite buildup (**i**). A dental stone model is poured for a mock tooth buildup (**j**). The mock buildup done with Resin Composite in labial (**k**) and palatal view (**l**). The material should flush with the stone model. A putty impression of the buildup made (**m**). Putty stent in place (**n**). The tooth is built with stratified composite layering technique. Immediate post-operative image (**o**). Follow-up at 6 months (**p**). Radiograph shows continued root maturation and calcific bridge formation below the Calcium Silicate Cement (**q**)

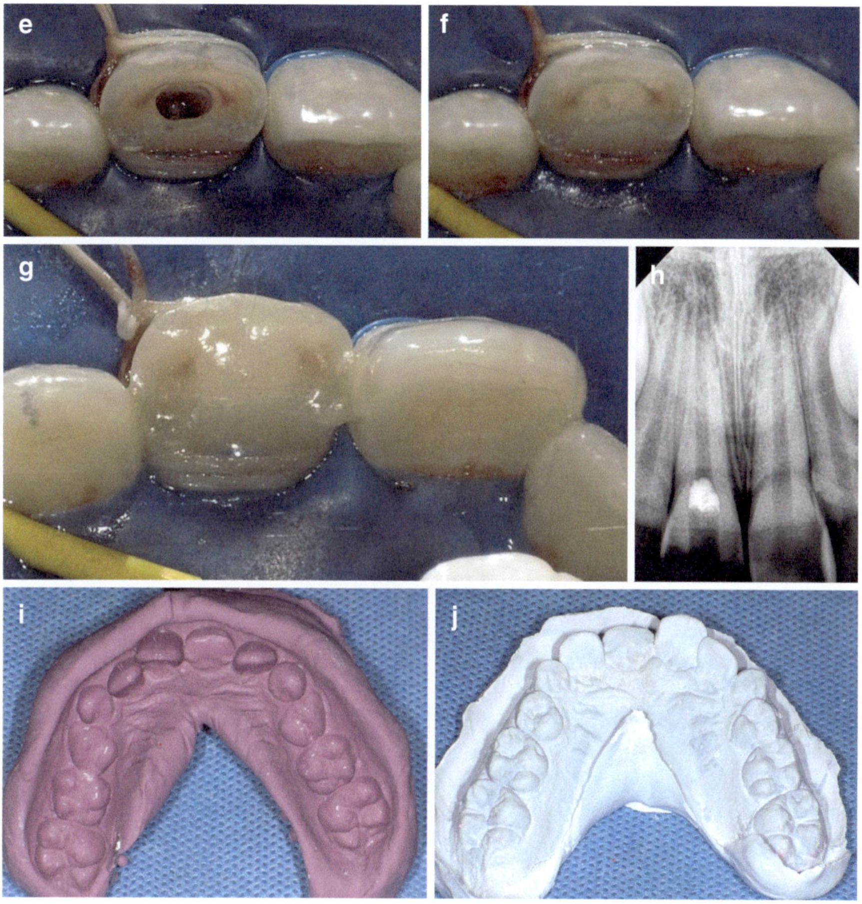

Fig. 6.21 (continued)

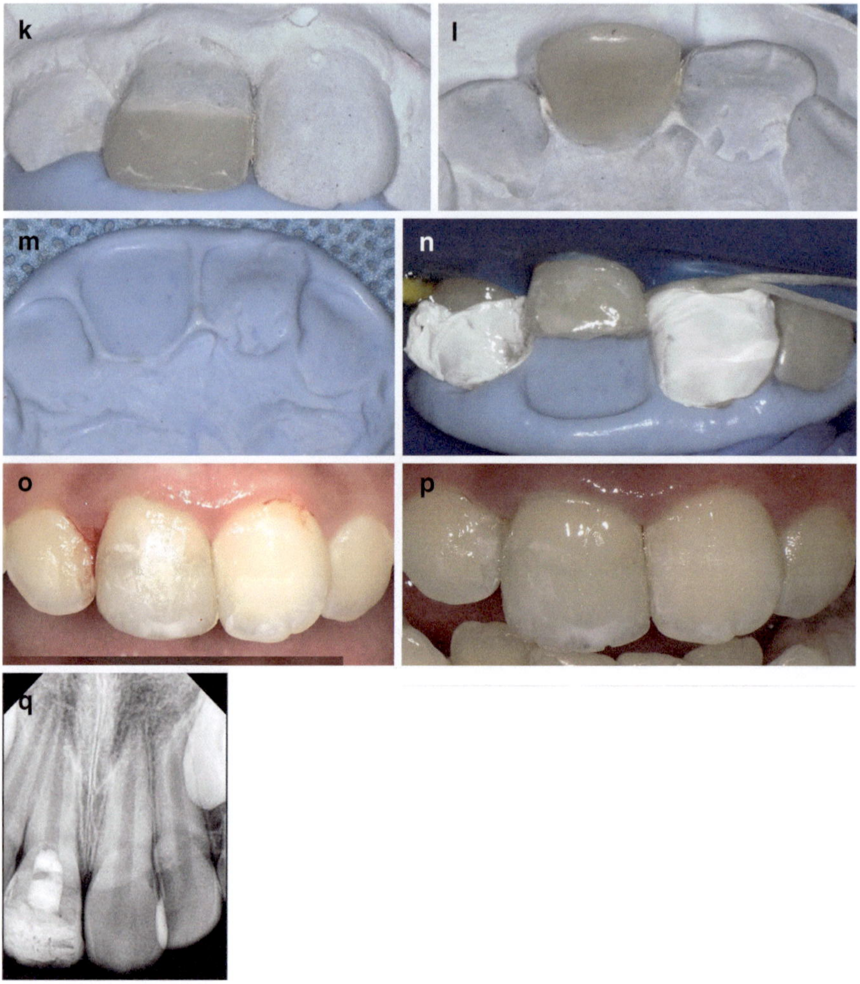

Fig. 6.21 (continued)

- Dentin composites from darker to lighter shades depending upon the size of the lesion are then layered onto the palatal wall of the enamel. This is essential as dentin shades provide the necessary opacity to avoid the restorations looking translucent and darker in appearance.
- A final layer of enamel composite is then placed on the labial surface that corresponds to the selected base shade of the tooth to be restored.
- Cervical lesions must be restored using a flowable composite of a darker dentinal shade followed by a second layer of dentinal composite to match the tooth.
- A thin layer of translucent enamel composite may be placed, if required (Figs. 6.22 and 6.23).

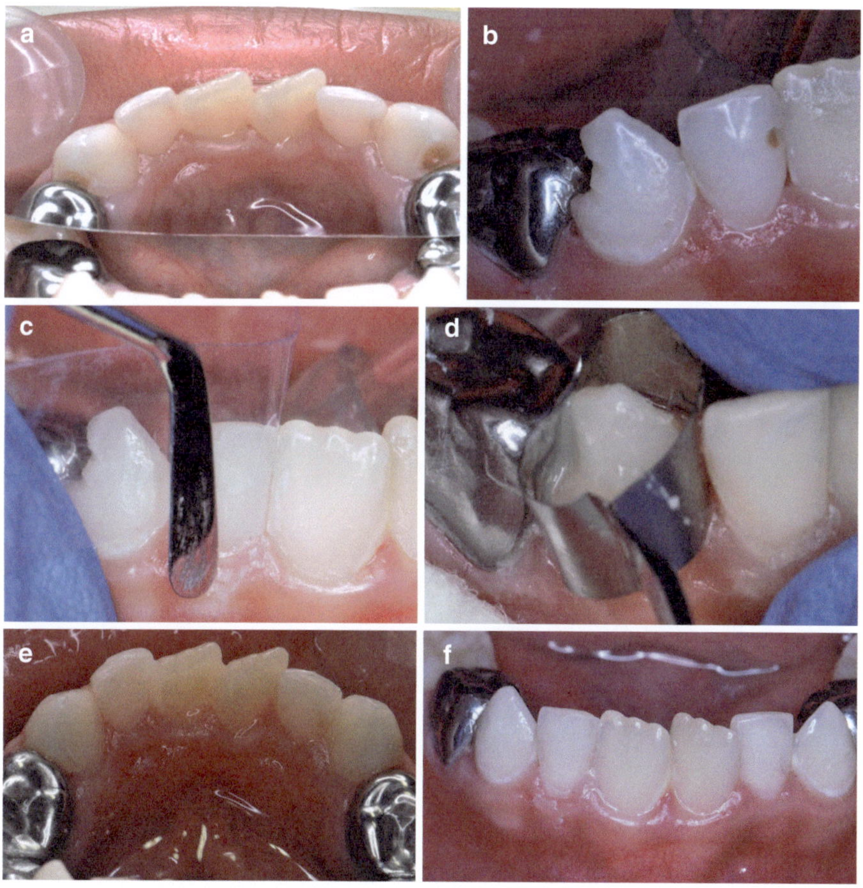

Fig. 6.22 Carious lesions in mandibular primary lateral incisors and canines (**a**). Complete Caries Removal done. Bevel and retention grooves given in the incisor and canine preparation, respectively. The teeth were etched, washed, and bonding agent applied (**b**). A mylar strip was placed interproximally before curing. Packable Resin Composite was placed in the cavity of lateral incisor and the mylar strip adapted to the restoration and cured (**c**). A circumferential matrix band was adapted around the canine to hold the restoration (**d**). The mandibular left lateral incisor and canine were restored in a similar manner (**e**). Finishing and polishing completed (**f**)

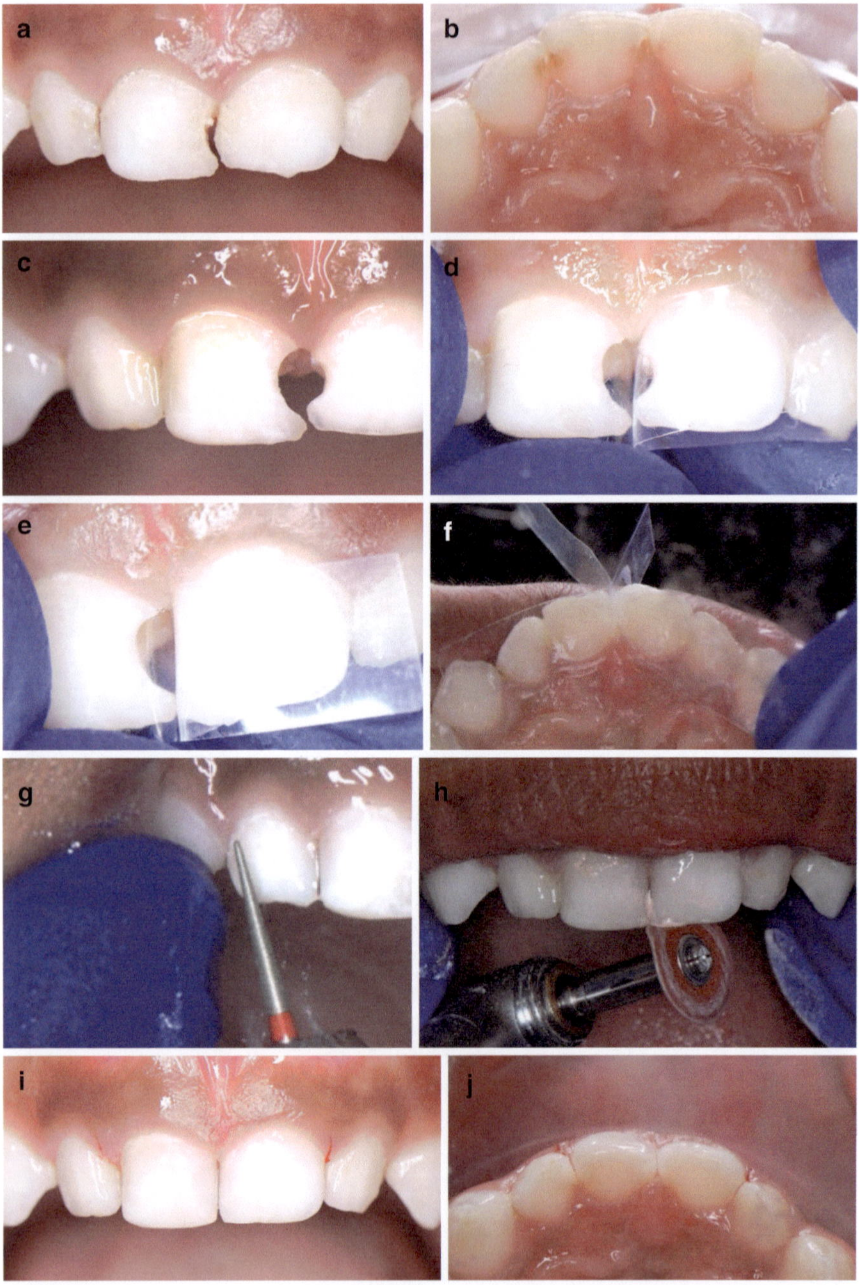

Fig. 6.23 Labial (**a**) and palatal view (**b**) of carious lesions in maxillary primary incisors. Caries was excavated from mesial lesions of central incisors. A short bevel was given at the cavosurface margin to improve Resin Composite retention (**c**). The mylar strip must be placed into the gingival sulcus of the tooth being restored so as to prevent restoration overhang. The mylar strip must be closely adapted to one tooth at a time, here it was adapted to the left central incisor (**d**) and the Resin Composite is cured (**e**). Two mylar strips can be placed simultaneously to restored adjacent proximal lesions, such that they are in gingival sulci of respective tooth (**f**). The restorations were finished (**g**) and polished (**h**). The restorations in labial (**i**) and palatal view (**j**)

6.8 Finishing and Polishing of Resin Composite Restorations [120, 121]

While placing a Resin Composite restoration, attention is often solely focused on shade selection and layering of the restoration. While these steps play an important role in restoring the esthetics of the treated tooth, equal time must be dedicated to finishing and polishing the restoration. Finishing is a procedure whereby an abrasive instrument is used to remove surface irregularities and contour the Resin Composite restoration; polishing involves the use of abrasives of progressively lesser roughness and hardness to create an optically and physically smooth surface texture. Inadequate finishing and polishing can lead to esthetic failure due to increased surface staining, roughness, and crack formation. This further results in excessive plaque accumulation and gingival irritation that gives rise to recurrent caries, periodontal problems, and failure of the restoration.

- *What Are the Esthetic Characterizations Required for Young Permanent Anterior Teeth?*

The *first step* is to perform a gross contouring and finishing of the restorative margins to determine the outline and the shape of the tooth. The shape of the tooth is determined by the mesiodistal width of the Resin Composite buildup and the sharpness or roundness given to the line angles. The tooth can be made to appear wider or narrower by increasing or decreasing the distance between the two line angles. To make the tooth appear wider, the area between the mesial and distal line angles must be flattened and these line angles pushed as far apart as possible, using either medium to fine diamond points or carbide burs or intermediate abrasive discs (Table 6.15). Conversely, to make the tooth appear narrow, the line angles are brought closer, thereby reducing the flattened area. The tooth can further be made to look narrow by interproximal reduction using finishing strips without creating diastemas. For central incisors, the distoincisal angle must be rounded, while the mesioincisal angle kept slightly sharp. In a narrow and rounded tooth like the maxillary lateral incisor, both angles must be rounded, with the distoincisal angle still being more rounded than the mesial to give a tapered, convex look.

The *second step* is to replicate the features on the labial surface of the incisors such as the developmental lobes and the mammelons. For these features to appear distinctly in the finished and polished Resin Composite restoration, they must be first replicated during Resin Composite buildup. The mammelons can be further emphasized during the gross contouring process using abrasive discs or diamond points. To accentuate the developmental lobes, these discs can be held perpendicular on the labial surface to create two inverted V-shaped depressions, wider incisally and tapering cervically. Further characterization can be done by creating a few horizontal grooves between the line angles.

After the above steps, *polishing* can be commenced, or it can be performed after every step of gross contouring and finishing to eliminate and identify the scratches seen on the Resin Composite surface due to the use of abrasives. Rubber discs,

Table 6.15 Commercially available polishing systems

Manufacturer	Gross finishing	Fine finishing	Polishing	Polishing paste
Shofu (For anterior and posterior teeth)	Diamond Point FG # SF104R: for finishing labial, interdental, cervical, and flat surfaces Diamond Point FG # 215: for finishing interdental and cervical areas Diamond Point FG # 219: for finishing palatal/lingual surfaces	Dura-Green Stones—for reduction of excess material Dura-White Stones—for finishing without damaging enamel	CompoSite Polishers, Knife, Wheel—for Pre-Polishing CompoSite Fine Polisher cup and disk—for Polishing without damaging enamel	CompoSite Polishing paste
Shofu super snap	Black	Violet	Green	Pink
3 M (Anterior)	Soflex finishing discs Black (coarse)- contouring	Dark blue (medium)-finishing	Blue (fine)-polishing	Light blue (Superfine)-super polishing
	Soflex Xt by 3 M Dark orange (coarse)-contouring	Orange(medium)-finishing	Light orange(fine)-polishing	Yellow (Superfine)-super polishing
3 M (Anterior and posterior)		3 M Soflex diamond polishing spirals (beige)—to be used after gross contouring		3 M Soflex diamond polishing spirals (pink)—to be used after fine finishing and polishing
Ultradent	Jiffy composite finishing burs 30 blade flame-shaped bur Flat cylinder bur Beveled cylinder bur Jiffy original composite system Green (cups, points, discs)	Yellow (cups, points, discs) Jiffly spiral wheels and twirls (yellow)	Jiffy polishing brushes Silicone carbide impregnated brushes White (cups, points, discs) Jiffly spiral wheels and twirls (white)	Diamond polish mint Blue (cups, points, discs)

These commercial products have been listed after visiting the manufacturers' website on 7th May 2025. The availability of these products may vary across different regions

Table 6.16 Commercially available plastic strips

Sr No.	Brand name	
1	Flexistrips (Cosmodent)	Available in two grits, one for finishing and one for polishing.
2	Sof-Lex Strips (3 M™)	They come in two widths and two pairs of grits, one for finishing and one for polishing.
3	Vivadent Strip	They come in two widths and two pairs of grits, one for finishing and one for polishing.

rubber spirals, abrasive strips along with diamond or aluminum oxide pastes in increasingly finer grits can be used for the polishing process (Table 6.16).

- *What Are the Instruments Used In Finishing and Polishing?*

Carbide burs are available in a variety of shapes (flame shaped, tapered, pear shaped) for gross contouring and smoothing of various restorative materials and tooth structures. Due to their less abrasive action, they are kinder to soft tissue at the gingival margin as compared with diamond bur or bonded abrasive contouring instruments.

Finishing *diamond points* are used to contour, adjust, and smoothen Resin Composite and come in different grits, ranging from 7 to 50 μm depending on the manufacturer.

Strips are available in metal and plastic, both. They are excellent for gross interproximal reduction, particularly as a first step in interproximal finishing. Presently, there are a wide variety of metal strips available in market with different grit sizes from 15 μm to 45 μm.

Flexible discs give an excellent finish. As heat and friction weaken the composite and enamel–resin interface, they should be used with water and be moved constantly to prevent heat and flat spots. The range of particle size distributions noted for coated abrasive discs vary from 55 to 100 μm for coarse-grade finishing discs, to 7 to 8 μm for the ultra- or superfine grade of finishing disc (Table 6.17).

Finally, to give the composite resin a natural appearance of enamel gloss, it is recommended to apply low-grade (less than 0.5 μm) *diamond pastes or aluminum oxide pastes* with a felt disc or a soft-bristle brush (Table 6.18). Circular movements should be made with low pressure and low speed rotation (maximum of 5000 rpm) must be used.

It is advised to pair a resin composite with a polishing system from the same manufacturer due to variations in filler particles and types of resin. However, the operator can choose to use one system from start to finish or combine different systems based on the preference and location of the restoration. During each stage of finishing and polishing, the operator should proceed in one direction only. Then, after the use of the next abrasive in the sequence, polishing should continue in a direction perpendicular to the previous one. This process ensures that scratches become more visible, and that the effectiveness of scratch removal can be assessed

Table 6.17 Commercially available flexible discs

	Contouring	Finishing	Polishing	Super polishing
Type/commercial name	Coarse	Medium	Fine	Superfine
Soflex discs by 3 M	Black	Dark blue	Blue	Light blue
Soflex Xt by 3 M	Dark orange	Orange	Light orange	Yellow
Shofu super snap	Black	Violet	Green	Pink
Flexi discs	Gray	Blue	Yellow	Red
Moore discs	White	Green	Blue	Tan

These commercial products have been listed after visiting the manufacturers' website on 7th May 2025. The availability of these products may vary across different regions

Table 6.18 Commercially available polishing pastes

Type of paste	Manufacturer	Abrasive
CompoSite Polishing paste	Shofu	Aluminum oxide particles
Platina Hi Gloss Composite Polishing Paste	Prevest Denpro	Aluminum oxide particles
DiaShine polish	DiaShine	Diamond particles
Prisma Gloss	DentsplySirona	Aluminum oxide particles
Diamond polish mint	Ultradent	Titanium dioxide particles

These commercial products have been listed after visiting the manufacturers' website on 7th May 2025. The availability of these products may vary across different regions

more rapidly. Dry finishing is harmful to most restorations, as the heat and friction generated can open tooth composite margins. Wet finishing reduces heat and friction, and thus, reduces surface damage to the body and margins of the restoration.

6.9 Concluding Remarks

Advancements in material science and an improved understanding of caries dynamics have redefined pediatric restorative dentistry. A contemporary approach emphasizes conservation of tooth structure, preservation of pulpal vitality, and adherence to minimally invasive techniques. Resin-Modified Glass Ionomer Cements and Resin Composites have been used successfully for restoring occlusal, proximal, and cervical carious lesions in primary teeth. While Resin Composites have superior esthetics and better wear resistance, GICs are preferred in children with high caries risk and where optimal isolation is not possible. The adherence to material protocols which includes conditioning and manipulation of GIC and beveling, bonding and incremental layering for Resin Composite improves overall success of restorations.

References

1. Black GV. Operative dentistry. Medico-Dental Publishing Company; 1955.
2. Mount GJ. A new paradigm for operative dentistry. Aust Dent J. 2007;52(4):264–70.
3. Welk DA, Laswell HR. Rationale for designing cavity preparations in light of current knowledge and technology. Dent Clin N Am. 1976;20(2):231–9.

4. Black GV. A work on operative dentistry; the technical procedures in filling teeth. Chicago: Medico-Dental Publishing Company; 1917.
5. Mount G. Minimal intervention in dentistry: how should a cavity be prepared? J Minim Interv Dent. 2012;5(1):7–10.
6. Full CA, Hollander WR. The composite resin restoration: a literature review. Part I. Proper cavity preparation and placement techniques. ASDC J Dent Child. 1993;60(1):48–51.
7. Lynch CD. Successful posterior resin composites. London: Quintessence Publishing Co.; 2008.
8. Ricketts D, Innes N, Schwendicke F. Selective removal of carious tissue. In: Caries excavation: evolution of treating cavitated carious lesions, vol. 27. Karger Publishers; 2018. p. 82–91.
9. Innes NP, Frencken JE, Bjørndal L, Maltz M, Manton DJ, Ricketts D, Van Landuyt K, Banerjee A, Campus G, Doméjean S, Fontana M. Managing carious lesions: consensus recommendations on terminology. Adv Dent Res. 2016;28(2):49–57.
10. Gudapati S. Cavosurface margins for various restorations.
11. Opdam NJ, Roeters JJ, Kuijs R, Burgersdijk RC. Necessity of bevels for box only Class II resin composite restorations. J Prosthet Dent. 1998;80:274–9.
12. Kirthiga M, Muthu MS, Kayalvizhi G, Krithika C. Proposed classification for interproximal contacts of primary molars using CBCT: a pilot study. Wellcome Open Res. 2018;3:98.
13. Schwendicke F, Frencken JE, Bjørndal L, Maltz M, Manton DJ, Ricketts D, Van Landuyt K, Banerjee A, Campus G, Doméjean S, Fontana M, Leal S, Lo E, Machiulskiene V, Schulte A, Splieth C, Zandona AF, Innes NP. Managing carious lesions: consensus recommendations on carious tissue removal. Adv Dent Res. 2016;28(2):58–67. https://doi.org/10.1177/0022034516639271. PMID: 27099358
14. Wu E, Yang YJ, Munz SM, Hsiao CC, Boynton JR. Restorations versus stainless steel crowns in primary molars: a retrospective split-mouth study. Pediatr Dent. 2021;43(4):290–5. PMID: 34467846
15. Chadwick BL, Evans DJP. Restoration of class II cavities in primary molar teeth with conventionaland resin modifed glass ionomer cements: a systematic review of the literature. Eur Arc Pediatr Dent. 2007;8(1):14–21.
16. American Academy of Paediatrics Dentistry (AAPD). Guidelines for Paediatric Restorative Dentistry. Revised 2016. https://www.aapd.org/research/oral-health-policies-recommendations/pediatric-restorative-dentistry/
17. Lenters M, van Amerongen WE, Mandari GJ. Iatrogenic damage to the adjacent surfaces of primary molars, in three different ways of cavity preparation. Eur Arch Paediatr Dent. 2006;7(1):6–10. https://doi.org/10.1007/BF03320808. PMID: 17140521
18. Loomans BAC. Proximal contact tightness of posterior composite resin restorations.
19. Nijmegen, the Netherlands: Radboud University; 2006. 3. Raghu R, Srinivasan R. Optimizing tooth form with direct posterior composite restorations. J Conserv Dent. 2011;14(4):330–336.
20. Hancock EB, Mayo CV, Schwab RR, Wirthlin MR. Influence of interdental contacts on periodontal status. J Periodonl. 1980;51:445–9.
21. Jernberg GR, Bakdash MB, Keenan KM. Relationship between proximal tooth open contacts and periodontal disease. J Periodontol. 1983;54:529–33.
22. Bauer JG, Crispin BJ. Evolution of the matrix for Class 2 restorations. Oper Dent. 1986;Suppl 4:1–37.
23. Owens BM, Phebus JG. An evidence-based review of dental matrix systems. Gen Dent. 2016;64(5):64–70.
24. Bailey O. Sectional matrix solutions: the distorted truth. Br Dent J. 2021;231(9):547–55.
25. Wilson AD, Kent BE. A new translucent cement for dentistry. The glass ionomer cement. Br Dent J. 1972;132:133–5.
26. Wilson AD, McLean JW. Glass ionomer cement. Chicago: Quintessence; 1988.
27. Ngo H, Mount GJ, Peters MC. A study of glassionomer cement and its interface with enamel and dentin using a low-temperature, high-resolution scanning electron microscopic technique. Quintessence Int. 1997;28:63–9.

28. Hatibovic-Kofman S, Suljak JP, Koch G. Remineralization of natural carious lesions with a glass ionomer cement. Swed Dent J. 1997;21(1–2):11–7.
29. Ngo HC, Mount G, McIntyre J, Do L. An in vitro model for the study of chemical exchange between glass ionomer restorations and partially demineralized dentin using a minimally invasive restorative technique. J Dent. 2011;39(Suppl 2):S20–6.
30. Chen CA, Chen YL, Huang JS, Huang GT, Chuang SF. Effects of restorative materials on dental pulp stem cell properties. J Endodont. 2019;45(4):420–6.
31. Council O. Policy on Interim Therapeutic Restorations (ITR). Pediatr Dent. 2008;30(7 Suppl):38–9.
32. Mertz-Fairhurst EJ, Curtis JW Jr, Ergle JW, Rueggeberg FA, Adair SM. Ultraconservative and cariostatic sealed restorations: results at year 10. J Am Dent Assoc. 1998;129:55–66.
33. Alleman DS, Magne P. A systematic approach to deep caries removal end points: the peripheral seal concept in adhesive dentistry. Quintessence Int. 2012;43:197–208.
34. Gruythuysen RJ, van Strijp AJ, Wu MK. Long-term survival of indirect pulp treatment performed in primary and permanent teeth with clinically diagnosed deep carious lesions. J Endodont. 2010;36:1490–3.
35. Mickenautsch S, Yengopal V. Absence of carious lesions at margins of glass-ionomer cement and amalgam restorations: an update of systematic review evidence. BMC Res Notes. 2011;4:58.
36. Gjorgievska E, Nicholson JW, Grcev AT. Ion migration from fluoride-releasing dental restorative materials into dental hard tissues. J Mater Sci Mater Med. 2012;23:1811–21.
37. Wiegand A, Buchalla W, Attin T. Review on fluoride releasing restorative materials-fluoride release and uptake characteristics, antibacterial activity and influence on caries formation. Dent Mater. 2007;23:343–62.
38. Cranfield M, Kuhn AT, Winter GB. Factors relating to the rate of fluoride-ion release from glass-ionomer cement. J Dent. 1982;10:333–41.
39. Lohbauer U. Dental glass ionomer cements as permanent filling materials?—properties, limitations future trends. Materials. 2009;3(1):76–96.
40. Roberts H, Berzins D, Nicholson J. Long-term water balance evaluation in glass ionomer restorative materials. Materials (Basel). 2022;15(3):807.
41. Bonifácio CC, Werner A, Kleverlaan CJ. Coating glass-ionomer cements with a nanofilled resin. Acta Odontol Scand. 2012;70(6):471–7.
42. Hotta M, Hirukawa H, Yamamoto K. Effect of coating materials on restorative glass-ionomer cement surface. Oper Dent. 1992;17(2):57–61.
43. VG S. To evaluate the effect of surface coating on three different types glass ionomer restorations. Biomed Pharmacol J 2015;8(October Spl Edition):445–449.
44. Mathis RL, Ferracane JL. Properties of a glass-ionomer/resin composite hybrid material. Dent Mater. 1989;5:355–8.
45. McCabe JF. Resin-modified glass-ionomers. Biomaterials. 1998;19(6):521–7.
46. Wilson AD. Resin-modified glass-ionomer cements. Int J Prosthet. 1990;5:425–9.
47. Frencken JE, van't Hof MA, van Amerongen WE, Holmgren CJ. Effectiveness of single-surface ART restorations in the permanent dentition: a meta-analysis. J Dent Res. 2004;83(2):120–3.
48. Mickenautsch S, Yengopal Y. Failure rate of high-viscosity GIC based ART compared with that of conventional amalgam restorations–evidence from an update of a systematic review. S A D J. 2012;67(7):329–31.
49. Schmalz G. ART–a method on its way into dentistry. Clin Oral Investig. 2012;16(5):1335–6.
50. Frencken JE. Atraumatic restorative treatment and minimal intervention dentistry. Br Dent J. 2017;223(3):183–9.
51. https://www.aegisdentalnetwork.com/news/2020/09/21/equia-restorative-system
52. Singh S, Goel D, Awasthi N, Khandelwal D, Sharma A, Patil S. Comparative evaluation of marginal integrity of three esthetic restorative materials – an *In-vitro* Study Contemp Clin. Dent. 2021;12(3):241–6.

53. Gurgan S, Kutuk ZB, Ergin E, Oztas SS, Cakir FY. Clinical performance of a glass ionomer restorative system: a 6-year evaluation. Clin Oral Investig. 2017;21:2335–43.
54. Šalinović I, Stunja M, Schauperl Z, Verzak Ž, Ivanišević Malčić A, Brzović Rajić V. Mechanical properties of high viscosity glass ionomer and glass hybrid restorative materials. Acta Stomatol Croat. 2019;53(2):125–31. https://doi.org/10.15644/asc53/2/4.
55. Lopes LE, Tedesco TK, Calvo AF, Imparato JC, Raggio DP, Mendes FM, Gimenez T. Is prior conditioning of dentin necessary in restoration with glass-ionomer cement? A systematic review and network meta-analysis. Int J Adhes Adhes. 2021 Jan;1(104):102748.
56. Avila WM, Hesse D, Bonifacio CC. Surface conditioning prior to the application of glass-ionomer cement: a systematic review and meta-analysis. J Adhes Dent. 2019;21(5):391–9. https://doi.org/10.3290/j.jad.a43183. PMID: 31624804
57. Sauro S, Watson T, Moscardó AP, Luzi A, Feitosa VP, Banerjee A. The effect of dentine pre-treatment using bioglass and/or polyacrylic acid on the interfacial characteristics of resin-modified glass ionomer cements. J Dent. 2018;73:32–9. https://doi.org/10.1016/j.jdent.2018.03.014. Epub 2018 Mar 30. PMID: 29609016
58. Kamatham R, Reddy SJ. Surface coatings on glass ionomer restorations in Pediatric dentistry-Worthy or not? J Indian Soc Pedod Prev Dent. 2013;31(4):229–33.
59. Dhar V, Hsu KL, Coll JA, Ginsberg E, Ball BM, Chhibber S, Johnson M, Kim M, Modaresi N, Tinanoff N. Evidence-based update of pediatric dental restorative procedures: dental materials. J Clin Pediatr Dent. 2015 Summer;39(4):303–10.
60. Chadwick BL, Evans DJ. Restoration of class II cavities in primary molar teeth with conventional and resin modified glass ionomer cements: a systematic review of the literature. Eur Arch Paediatr Dent. 2007;8(1):14–21.
61. Toh SL, Messer LB. Evidence-based assessment of tooth-colored restorations in proximal lesions of primary molars. Pediatr Dent. 2007;29(1):8–15.
62. Bowen RL, Marjenhoff WA. Development of an adhesive bonding system. Oper Dent. 1992;Suppl 5:75–80.
63. Rueggeberg FA. From vulcanite to vinyl, a history of resins in restorative dentistry. J Prosthet Dent. 2002;87(4):364–79.
64. Buonocore MG. A simple method of increasing the adhesion of acrylic filling materials to enamel surfaces. J Dent Res. 1955;34:849–53.
65. Buonocore MG. Principles of adhesive retention and adhesive restorative materials. JADA. 1963;67:382–91.
66. Buonocore MG, Matsui A, Gwinnett AJ. Penetration of resin dental materials into enamel surfaces with reference to bonding. Arch Oral Biol. 1968;13(1):61–70.
67. Kugel G, Ferrari M. The science of bonding: from first to sixth generation. J Am Dent Assoc. 2000 Jun;1(131):20S–5S.
68. Gindri LD, Fröhlich TT, Rosso CR, Rocha RD. Etching time and bonding of adhesive systems to dentin of primary teeth: a systematic review and meta-analysis. Int J Paediatr Dent. 2021 Jan;31(1):122–30.
69. Lenzi TL, Braga MM, Raggio DP. Shortening the etching time for etch-and-rinse adhesives increases the bond stability to simulated caries-affected primary dentin. J Adhes Dent. 2014;16(3):235–41. https://doi.org/10.3290/j.jad.a31103. PMID: 24669366
70. Redford DA, Clarkson BH, Jensen M. The effect of different etching times on the sealant bond strength, etch depth, and pattern in primary teeth. Pediatr Dent. 1986;8(1):11–5.
71. Gwinnett AJ. Histologic changes in human enamel following treatment with acidic adhesive conditioning agents. Arch Oral Biol. 1971;16(7):731–8. https://doi.org/10.1016/0003-9969(71)90118-x. PMID: 5283531
72. Duke ES, Lindemuth J. Variability of clinical dentin substrates. Am J Dent. 1991;4:241–6.
73. Nakabayashi N, Kojima K, Masuhara E. The promotion of adhesion by the infiltration of monomers into tooth states. J Biomed Mater Res. 1982;16:265–73.
74. Pashley DH, Michelich V, Kehl T. Dentin permeability: effects of smear layer removal. J Prosthet Dent. 1981;46:531–7.

75. Fusayama T, Nakamura M, Kurosaki N, Iwaku M. Non-pressure adhesion of a new adhesive restorative resin. J Dent Res. 1979;58:1364–72.
76. Bowen RL. Investigations of the surface of hard tooth tissues by a surface cavity test. In: Adhesive restorative dental materials. Phillips RW, Ryge G, eds. Spencer, Ind.: Owen Litho Service; 1961:177.
77. Nakabayashi N, Pashley DH. Hybridization of dental hard tissues. Tokyo: Quintessence; 1998.
78. Titley K, Chercnecky R, Chan A, Smith DC. The composition and ultrastructure of resin tags in etched dentin. Am J Dent. 1995;8:224–30.
79. Tay FR, Gwinnett AJ, Wei SHY. Structural evidence of a sealed tissue interface with total etch wet bonding technique, in vivo. J Dent Res. 1994;73:629–36.
80. Kanca J. Wet bonding: effect of drying time and distance. Am J Dent. 1996;9:273–6.
81. Gwinnett AJ, Tay FR, Wei SHY. Bridging the gap between overly dry and overwet bonding phenomenon of dentin hybridization and tubular seal. In: Shimono M, Maeda T, Suda H, Takayashi K, editors. Dentin/pulp complex. Tokyo: Quintessence; 1996. p. 359–63. 23.
82. Tay FR, Gwinnett AJ, Wei SH. The over wet phenomenon: an optical, micromorphological study of surface moisture in acid-conditioned, resin-dentin interface. Am J Dent. 1996;9(1):43–8.
83. Giannini M, Makishi P, Ayres AP, Vermelho PM, Fronza BM, Nikaido T, Tagami J. Self-etch adhesive systems: a literature review. Braz Dent J. 2015;26:3–10.
84. Moszner N, Salz U, Zimmermann J. Chemical aspects of self etching enamel-dentin adhesives: a systematic review. Dent Mater. 2005;21:895–910.
85. Toida K, Watanabe A, Nakabayashi N. Effect of smear layer on bonding to dentin prepared with bur. J Jpn Dent Mater. 1995;14:109–16.
86. Van Landuyt KL, Kanumilli P, De Munck J, Peumans M, Lambrechts P, Van Meerbeek B. Bond strength of a mild self-etch adhesive with and without prior acid-etching. J Dent. 2006;34(77–85):24.
87. Nazari A, Shimada Y, Sadr A, Tagami J. Pre-etching vs. grinding in promotion of adhesion to intact enamel using self-etch adhesives. Dent Mater J. 2012;31:394–400.
88. Nakajima M, Kunawarote S, Prasansuttiporn T, Tagami J. Bonding to caries-affected dentin. Jpn Dent Sci Rev. 2011;47(2):102–14.
89. Yoshiyama M, Urayama A, Kimochi T, Matsuo T, Pashley DH. Comparison of conventional vs self-etching adhesive bonds to caries-affected dentin. Oper Dent. 2000;25(3):163–9.
90. Moraes RR, Cenci MS, Moura JR, Demarco FF, Loomans B, Opdam N. Clinical performance of resin composite restorations. Curr Oral Health Rep. 2022;9(2):22–31.
91. Riva YR, Rahman SF. Dental composite resin: a review. In AIP conference proceedings. 2019, vol. 2193, No. 1. AIP Publishing.
92. Hervás García A, Lozano M, Cabanes Vila J, Barjau Escribano A, Fos GP. Composite resins: a review of the materials and clinical indications. Med Oral Patol Oral Cir Bucal. 2006;11(2):E215–20.
93. Sakaguchi RL, Powers JM. Craig's restorative dental materials-e-book. Elsevier Health Sciences; 2011.
94. Anusavice KJ, Shen C, Rawls HR, editors. Phillips' science of dental materials. Elsevier Health Sciences; 2012.
95. Baroudi K, Rodrigues JC. Flowable resin composites: a systematic review and clinical considerations. J Clin Diagn Res. 2015;9(6):ZE18.
96. Unterbrink GL, Liebenberg WH. Flowable resin composites as "filled adhesives": literature review and clinical recommendations. Quintessence Int. 1999;30(4):249.
97. Gupta R, Tomer AK, Kumari A, Perle N, Chauhan P, Rana S. Recent advances in bulkfill flowable composite resins: a review. Int J App Dent Sci. 2017;3(3):79–81.
98. Eweis AH, Yap AU, Yahya NA. Comparison of flexural properties of bulk-fill restorative/flowable composites and their conventional counterparts. Oper Dent. 2020;45(1):41–51.
99. Stevenson B. Current methods of shade matching in dentistry: a review of the supporting literature. Dent Update. 2009;36(5):270–6.
100. Manuata J, Salat A. Layers: an atlas of composite resin stratification. Milan: Style Italiano. 2012.

101. Schricker SR. Composite resin polymerization and relevant parameters. Orthodontic Applications of Biomaterials 2017:153–170.
102. Mondelli RF, Velo MM, Gonçalves RS, Tostes BO, Ishikiriama SK, Bombonatti JF. Influence of composite resin volume and C-factor on the polymerization shrinkage stress. Braz Dent Sci. 2016;19(2):72–81.
103. Braga RR, Ballester RY, Ferracane JL. Factors involved in the development of polymerization shrinkage stress in resincomposites: a systematic review. Dent Mater. 2005;21(10):962–70.
104. Borouziniat A, Khaki H, Majidinia S. Retrospective evaluation of the clinical performance of direct composite restorations using the snow-plow technique: up to 4 years follow-up. J Clin Exp Dent. 2019;11(11):e964–8.
105. Simonsen, R.J. Preventive resin restorations. Quintessence Int. 1978;9(l):69–76.
106. Simonsen RJ. Preventive resin restorations: three-year results. JADA. 1980;100(4):535–9.
107. Mackenzie LM, Banerjee A. The minimally invasive management of early occlusal caries: a practical guide. Prim Dent J. 2014;3:42–9.
108. Swift EJ Jr. Preventive resin restorations. J Am Dent Assoc. 1987;114(6):819–21.
109. Hassall DC, Mellor AC. The sealant restoration: indications, success and clinical technique. Br Dent J. 2001;191(7):358–62.
110. Simonsen RJ. Preventive resin restorations and sealants in light of current evidence. Dent Clin. 2005;49(4):815–23.
111. Houpt M, Fuks A, Eidelman E. The preventive resin (composite resin/sealant) restoration: nine-year results. Quintessence Int-English Edition. 1994;25:155.
112. Granath L, Schroder U, Sundin B. Clinical evaluation of preventive and class-I composite resin restorations. Acta Odontol Scand. 1992;50(6):359–64.
113. King NM, Yung LK, Holmgren CJ. Clinical performance of preventive resin restorations placed in a hospital environment. Quintessence Int. 1996;27(9):627.
114. Chandrasekhar V, Rudrapati L, Badami V, Tummala M. Incremental techniques in direct composite restoration. J Conserv Dent. 2017;20(6):386–91. https://doi.org/10.4103/JCD.JCD_157_16. PMID: 29430088; PMCID: PMC5799982
115. Chisini LA, Collares K, Cademartori MG, de Oliveira LJC, Conde MCM, Demarco FF, Corrêa MB. Restorations in primary teeth: a systematic review on survival and reasons for failures. Int J Pediatr Dent. 2018;28(2):123–39.
116. Ortiz-Ruiz AJ, Pérez-Guzmán N, Rubio-Aparicio M, et al. Success rate of proximal tooth-coloured direct restorations in primary teeth at 24 months: a meta-analysis. Sci Rep. 2020;10:6409.
117. Dietschi D, Fahl N. Shading concepts and layering techniques to master direct anterior composite restorations: an update. Br Dent J. 2016;221:765–71.
118. Leven A. Layers: an atlas of composite resin stratification. Br Dent J. 2013;214:319.
119. https://www.styleitaliano.org/the-step-by-step-in-finishing-and-polishing-part-i/
120. https://www.styleitaliano.org/polishing-lifelike-composite/
121. Peyton JH. Finishing and polishing techniques: direct composite resin restorations. Pract Proc Aesth Dent. 2004;16(4):293–8.

7 Preformed Crowns in Pediatric Dentistry: Clinical Considerations and Techniques

7.1 Introduction

Extracoronal restorations in Pediatric Dentistry evolved from the need to place durable and retentive restorations on teeth with multi-surface caries. For a long time, amalgam was used to restore badly decayed teeth; however, the longevity of these restorations was short-lived. Later, dentists began placing orthodontic bands around teeth with multi-surface caries and filled them with amalgam. While this restorative technique afforded limited success, it did provide inspiration for the discovery of the first preformed crowns [1, 2]. With the manufacturing of the first Stainless-Steel Crown in the 1960s and more recently the zirconia crowns in 2008, prefabricated crowns for primary teeth are the most successful and versatile restorative options in pediatric dental practice (Fig. 7.1).

H. Vyas et al., *Dental Caries and Traumatic Injuries in Pediatric Dentistry*,
https://doi.org/10.1007/978-3-031-98929-2_7

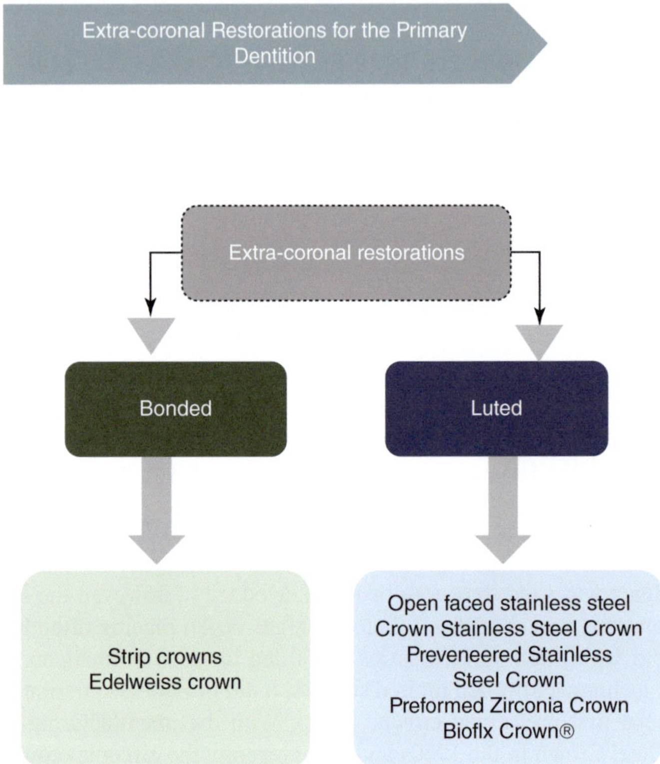

Fig. 7.1 Extra-coronal restorations for the primary dentition

7.2 When Should the Clinician Place an Extracoronal Restoration?

For most clinicians, it is an established practice to place an extracoronal restoration on teeth that have multi-surface caries, teeth that have undergone endodontic treatment, and hypoplastic teeth [3–6]. Current trends in caries management necessitate the use of full-coverage restorations in extensive-stage lesions that have been selectively excavated or as part of the Hall technique. Extracoronal restorations may be preferred in teeth showing initial or moderate-stage lesions that would otherwise receive conventional restorations in children with high caries risk or those undergoing treatment under general anesthesia.

7.3 Stainless-Steel Crowns

> Gold has its cost, amalgam its controversy, and plastic its limits. Maybe the success of the stainless steel crown has been that it never claimed to be more than it is, yet when called upon to do more, responded so well [7].
>
> -Paul Casamassimo

Table 7.1 Commercially available stainless-steel crowns

	Brand name	Country
1.	3M™	USA
2.	Hu Friedy	USA
3.	NuSmile®	USA
4.	Denovo dental	USA
5.	SML® (Space Maintainer Laboratory)	USA
6.	Kids crown	South Korea
7.	Prime Pedo	India
8.	Rainbow crown®	India
9.	Oro® Little crown	India

Stainless steel crowns are the oldest, most evidence-based extracoronal restorative option available in the primary dentition. They are manufactured from austenitic or 18-8 stainless steel and are composed of iron (76%), nickel (10%–13%), chromium (17%–19%), and other minor elements. They are a final restoration in primary teeth and a semipermanent restoration in the adult dentition [8] (Table 7.1).

7.3.1 Stainless-Steel Crown Placement Technique

The *tooth preparation* for placement of a posterior primary Stainless-Steel Crown involves [6, 8–11]

- Occlusal reduction of 1.5–2 mm using a flame-shaped or pear-shaped bur.
- Proximal preparation with a thin tapered cone diamond point is done such that the proximal contacts are broken.
- Alternatively, elastics can be placed at an earlier appointment to create separation between the adjacent teeth. This not only reduces the amount of proximal reduction required but also prevents damage to the adjacent teeth.
- The tooth preparation should be rounded at the corners and tapered to the occlusal.
- Reduction of the buccal cervical bulge should be done only if the crown is unable to flex over the surface.
- While the presence of undercuts is desirable for improving crown retention, the tooth must be prepared to a feather edge margin for better crown adaptation.

Selection of crown may be completed prior to tooth preparation by correlating the mesiodistal diameter of the tooth with the sizes provided by manufacturers or by trial and error after preparation is complete.

Crown Adaptation

- During trial, the crown must be rotated from lingual or palatal to buccal to achieve a snap fit.
- While it is desirable to restore the original occlusion, a 1.5–2 mm discrepancy is acceptable as the occlusion of the primary dentition is dynamic. This is the reasoning behind placing a crown using the Hall technique.

- The newer SSCs are pre-crimped, pre-contoured and hence cause minimal gingival blanching. It is not recommended to trim the SSC unless gingival blanching is excessive and causes discomfort to the child.
- If the crown is removed easily with finger pressure or rotates, a smaller crown must be used.
- If the selected smaller size does not flex over the cervical contours, the operator should prepare the tooth to allow for complete placement of the smaller crown. Alternately, the crown can be squeezed mesiodistally with the Johnson's 114 plier to increase the buccolingual dimension. If the buccolingual dimension of the prepared tooth is still larger and the crown cannot be squeezed further mesiodistally to match the tooth preparation, the cervical crimp of the crown should be trimmed by using a crown cutting scissor or a metal cutting carbide bur. This will allow the crown to flex over the cervical contours and seat subgingivally. The cut margins of the crown must be polished and re-crimped.
- In case of space loss due to proximal caries, a Howe's plier is used to flatten the proximal surfaces of the crown to replicate the reduced mesiodistal dimension of the tooth receiving the crown. Alternatively, a maxillary crown of the contralateral side can be placed on the corresponding mandibular molar.
- If the smallest crown is oversized and needs to be adapted, a cut is made on the buccal surface using crown scissors. The cut edges are then approximated, and the overlapping margins are spot welded together following which the crown is finished and polished.
- Conversely, if the largest crown size is too small, the crown can be cut buccally or lingually, and an additional piece of 0.004-inch orthodontic stainless-steel band can be spot welded over the gap that is then contoured to the desired form.

7.3.2 Permanent Stainless-Steel Crown

The choice of extracoronal restoration for a permanent molar till the age of 18 years continues to be the Stainless-Steel Crown. The rationale behind their use is that minimal tooth preparation is required allowing for preservation of original coronal tooth structure and vitality of the dentino-pulpal complex. Most importantly, these crowns can be placed in permanent molars that are newly erupted and have not achieved full clinical height. It is recommended that the original occlusion is maintained as far as possible, to allow for continued eruption of other permanent molars. The permanent stainless-steel crowns are pre-crimped, pre-contoured and have an increased occluso-cervical height corresponding to that of the permanent molars. As they need to be placed on molars in varying stages of eruption, the height of the crown may be reduced by trimming the margins for better seating and to achieve a proper occlusion. This also results in closer adaptation of the crown thereby minimizing the thickness of the cement interface. After try in, the crown margins need to be polished and re-crimped if necessary, so that crown is flushed with the feather edge margins. The crown should be extended subgingivally to cover as much of the crown as possible, as the margins may become supragingival due to continued passive eruption [10].

7.3.3 Is It Necessary to Administer Local Anesthesia Before Tooth Preparation for SSC?

The preparation for the SSC will cause some injury to the gingival tissues leading to patient discomfort. The discomfort may be particularly heightened in cases, where the molar is yet to completely erupt to its full occlusal height and the crown needs to slip beneath the distal bulge. As the inferior margin of the crown extends subgingivally, even trial placement and removal of the crown can cause discomfort. Therefore, topical anesthesia should be applied to the gingival margins prior to crown placement. If the teeth are vital, hypomineralized or require extensive tooth preparation, local anesthesia will ensure comfort and ease of placement. In teeth undergoing pulpal therapy under local anesthesia, the post-endodontic restoration should be placed at the same appointment [11].

7.3.4 What Are the Consequences of Placing an Oversized Stainless-Steel Crown?

If an oversized SSC is placed and the crown margins are not adapted to the tooth, the resultant overhang can impede the eruption of the adjacent permanent teeth. In such a situation, either a smaller sized crown should be selected, or the crown margins should be contoured with a Johnson's 114 plier and crimped to achieve a better fit. The above discussion is relevant in contemporary Pediatric Dentistry where the placement of an oversized crown using the Hall technique is the practice. It is important for clinicians to ensure the crown fitting be as precise as possible with minimal overhang and if needed, the marginal adaptation confirmed with radiographs.

7.4 Open-Faced Stainless-Steel Crowns

These are stainless steel crowns for anterior teeth which have been made esthetically acceptable by removing the labial surface of the crown and bonding composite resin onto the open facing. While the preveneered stainless steel crowns, the adhesive resin strip crowns, and the preformed zirconia crowns are far more esthetic, these open-faced stainless-steel crowns are the "go to" restorations for primary anterior teeth that have short clinical height or at least one-third of remaining healthy tooth structure after endodontic treatment.

The preparation required for these teeth with less crown structure is restricted to minimal circumferential reduction extending subgingivally. The smallest SSC that fits must be selected. A band pusher is used to seat a tightly fitting crown over the cervical contours of the tooth. The ability to crimp these crowns circumferentially or even squeeze the crown buccolingually results in active retention.

To further improve bonding between the metal and glass ionomer luting cement, an alloy primer (Shofu AZ primer, Japan; Kuraray, Japan) is applied on the inner surface of the crown and is allowed to dry prior to luting. Alternatively, the crown can be sandblasted with aluminum oxide particles.

A rubber dam is placed to isolate the oral cavity from the metal shavings generated while creating the open-faced stainless-steel crown. The labial window is prepared using a Great White #2 (GW2) carbide bur (SS White, USA) and is then extended cervically, incisally, and to the proximal line angles so that minimal metal margins are seen. The underlying tooth is made visible by removing the surface-luting cement. The tooth is etched using 37% phosphoric acid for 15 s and then washed and dried. The metal margins are primed again with an alloy primer for 10 s and allowed to dry. The bonding agent is applied on the tooth and the metal margins, air dried and cured after 20 s.

Resin composite is then placed incrementally starting with an opaque shade to mask the metallic margins. A dentin shade (more opaque, less translucent) can be used for the later increments. An enamel shade that is more translucent can be used as a final layer. The labial surface is then finished and polished (Fig. 7.2) [12].

The limitations of these crowns include:

- Increased operating time
- Technique sensitive to create an esthetic labial veneer
- Exposure of metallic border of the SSC at the gingival margin if the biological width is not preserved and due to continued passive eruption over time (Fig. 7.3).

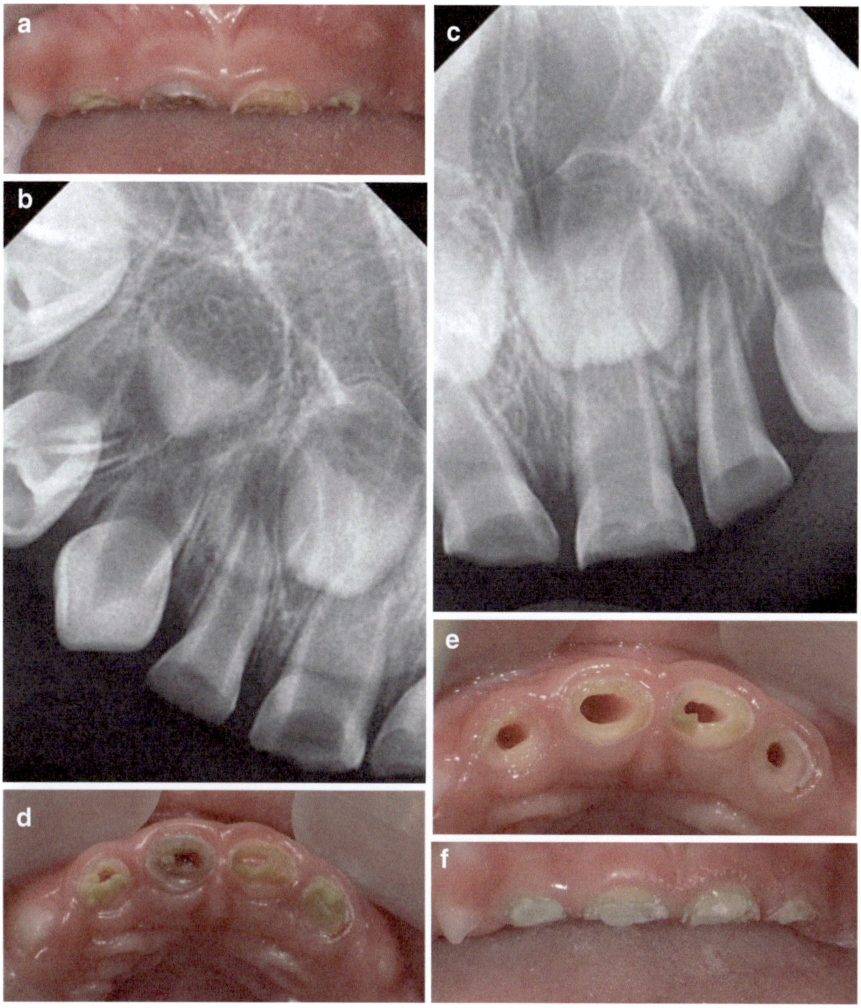

Fig. 7.2 Maxillary primary incisors showing extensive stage lesion (**a**). Radiographs showing pulpal involvement and sufficient root length (**b**, **c**). Occlusal view showing soft dentin and pulp exposure (**d**). The teeth were nonvital and endodontic treatment was done for all the maxillary incisors (**e**). The post-endodontic restoration was done with Resin-Modified Glass Ionomer Cement (**f**). Radiographs taken post-endodontic treatment to verify the obturation (**g**, **h**). Minimal tooth preparation was done circumferentially and subgingivally with a tapered diamond point (**i**). Occlusal view (**j**). Trial placement of anterior stainless-steel crown (**k**). Rubber dam isolation before preparing labial window with Stainless Steel Carbide Bur (GW2- Great White® Gold Series, SS White, USA) (**l**). The labial window preparation is extended cervically, incisally, and proximally leaving thin metal margins (**m**). Resin Composite restoration of labial surface done followed by finishing and polishing (**n**). Two-year follow-up (**o**). Radiograph at 2 years showing physiologic root resorption (**p**)

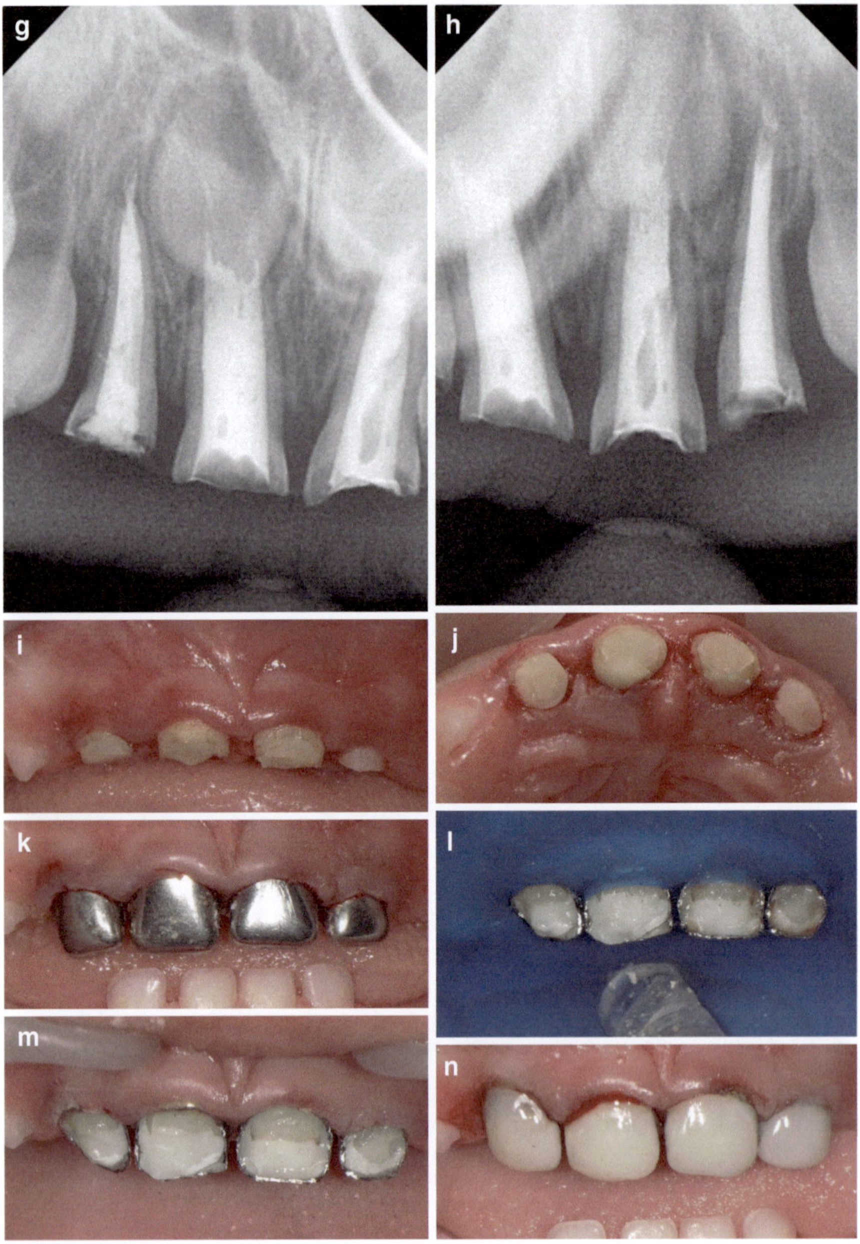

Fig. 7.2 (continued)

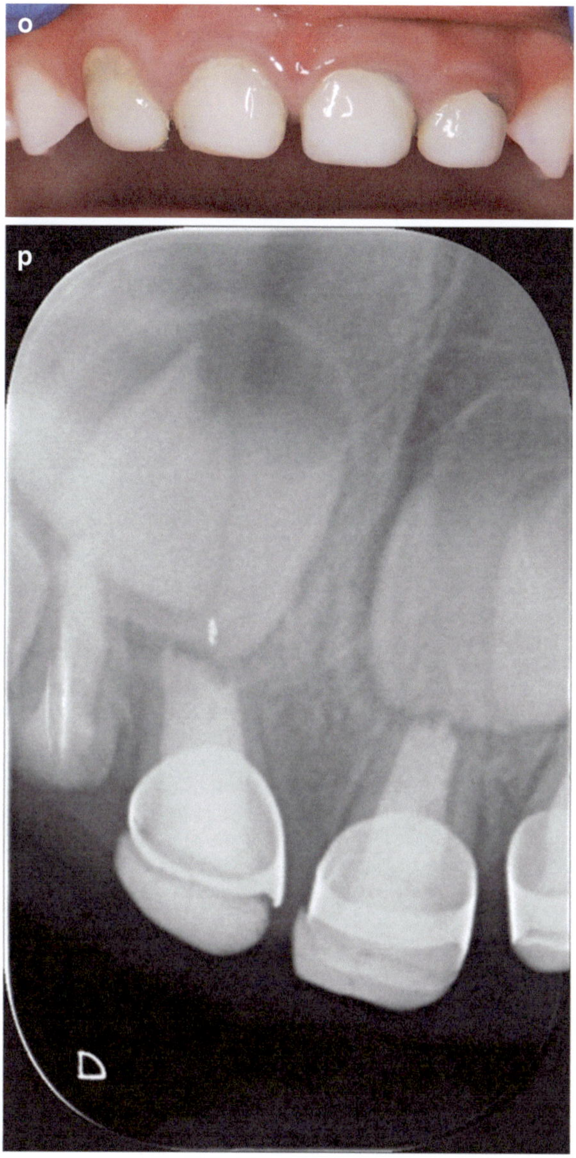

Fig. 7.2 (continued)

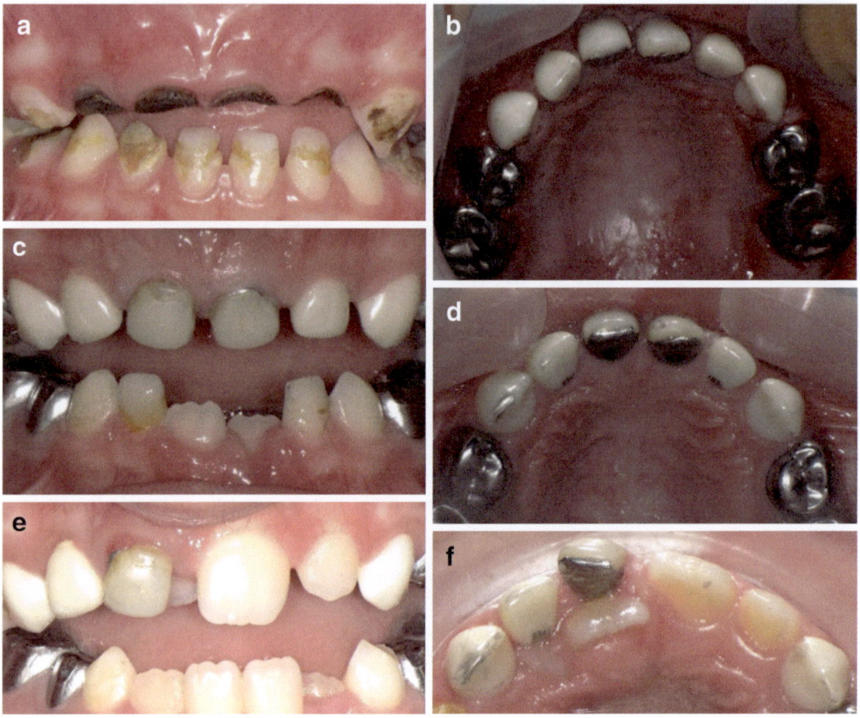

Fig. 7.3 Extensive stage lesions of maxillary primary anterior teeth (**a**). Immediate post operative photograph of anterior veneered stainless-steel crown on maxillary central incisors and preformed zirconia crowns on lateral incisors and canines (**b**). Front view (**c**) and occlusal view at 2-year follow-up (**d**). Four-year follow-up showing exfoliated maxillary primary left central and lateral incisor (**e**). The maxillary primary right central and lateral incisors were mobile and allowed to exfoliate. The permanent right incisors were erupting palatally but were not in crossbite (**f**)

7.5 Preveneered Stainless-Steel Crowns

Preveneered stainless-steel crowns were developed to overcome the poor esthetics of the conventional SSC. While these crowns had superior esthetics as compared to the open-faced crowns, the inability to crimp these crowns labially limits their retentiveness in teeth having short clinical height. Also, the high fracture rate of the veneer due to mastication was a limitation to their replacing the full stainless-steel crown for posterior teeth [13, 14]. The success of zirconia in terms of esthetics and retention has further limited the use of the preveneered stainless steel crown in clinical practice (Table 7.2).

Table 7.2 Commercially available preveneered stainless steel crowns

	Brand name	Country
1	NuSmile® Signature Crowns	USA
2	Cheng Crowns	USA
3	Kinder krowns	USA
4	Dura Crowns	USA

7.5.1 Technique of Placement

The technique of placement of a preveneered SSC is similar to that of a conventional SSC. The modifications in the process are as follows:

- The labial reduction is more than that of a conventional SSC to accommodate for the esthetic veneer.
- Vertical striations must be cut onto the labial surface of the tooth to ensure increased surface area and optimal retention of the crown to the tooth.

After desired tooth preparation, the tooth should be isolated with cotton rolls and the crown should be filled 2/3rd with the glass ionomer luting cement. The crown is then slid over the tooth and stabilized by finger pressure, until the cement sets. Excess cement should be removed with an explorer and a dental floss should be passed between the proximal contacts of the crown.

7.6 Strip Crowns

Strip crowns are celluloid crown forms that are meant to contain a Resin or Glass ionomer-based material and bonded to anterior teeth. These are an ideal restorative option in anterior teeth having proximal lesion(s) with an intact incisal edge. It should be placed on teeth in which more than 2/3rd of healthy tooth structure and particularly, *enamel is present*. This is because the bond of enamel with composite is stronger and more predictable, as compared to dentin (Table 7.3).

7.6.1 Clinical Technique [15, 16] (Fig. 7.5)

- Place the incisal edge of the strip crown against the tooth to select the size.
- Using a fine tapering cone diamond point, circumferential reduction of 0.5–1 mm should be done. The incisal edge is reduced by 2 mm and retention grooves are placed on the labial and lingual surface.
- Trim the neck of the strip crown, if required with crown cutting scissors.
- Check the fit of the crown and make sure that it is passive especially on the lingual surface and around the cervical margins (Fig. 7.4). This ensures for sufficient thickness of the composite resin. If it is active, further tooth preparation must be performed or a larger crown size must be selected.

Table 7.3 Commercially available strip crowns

Product	Manufacturer
3M™ strip crowns	USA
SML®Space maintainer laboratory strip crowns	USA
TDV strip crowns	Brazil
Nowak strip crowns	USA
Kids Strip Crown	South Korea
Tor VM	Russia

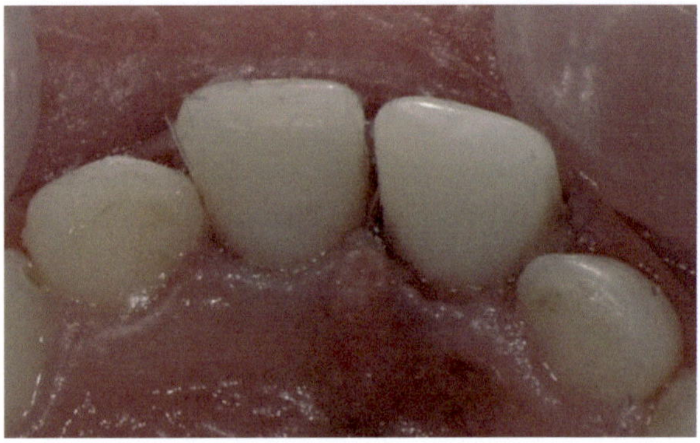

Fig. 7.4 Palatal view of strip crowns. The crowns should flush with the tooth subgingivally without leaving flash of excessive material or ledge

- Make a vent hole on the palatal surface of the strip crown with a diamond point or sharp explorer to allow excess resin to escape.
- The crown must be filled with the composite resin leaving space at the core to accommodate the prepared tooth. Ensure that there are no air bubbles in the filled composite resin.
- Isolate the tooth with rubber dam or cotton rolls and saliva ejector.
- Etch and bond the prepared tooth surface.
- Seat the filled strip crown and remove excess cervically and from the palatal vent. Cure the crown from both the labial and lingual surfaces.
- Adjacent strip crowns can be placed simultaneously and then cured.
- Peel the crown form with a sharp instrument while stabilizing the tooth with digital pressure.
- Finishing of the strip crown must be done to remove excess cervical flash if present with tapered composite finishing burs. The vent must be smoothened with polishing discs. The surface of the resin crown should be untouched as the finish provided by the strip crown form is excellent (Figs. 7.5 and 7.6).

7.6.2 What Are the Limitations of Strip Crowns?

- Technique sensitive requiring adequate moisture control and hemostasis
- Stains over time (Figs. 7.7 and 7.8)
- Low fracture resistance

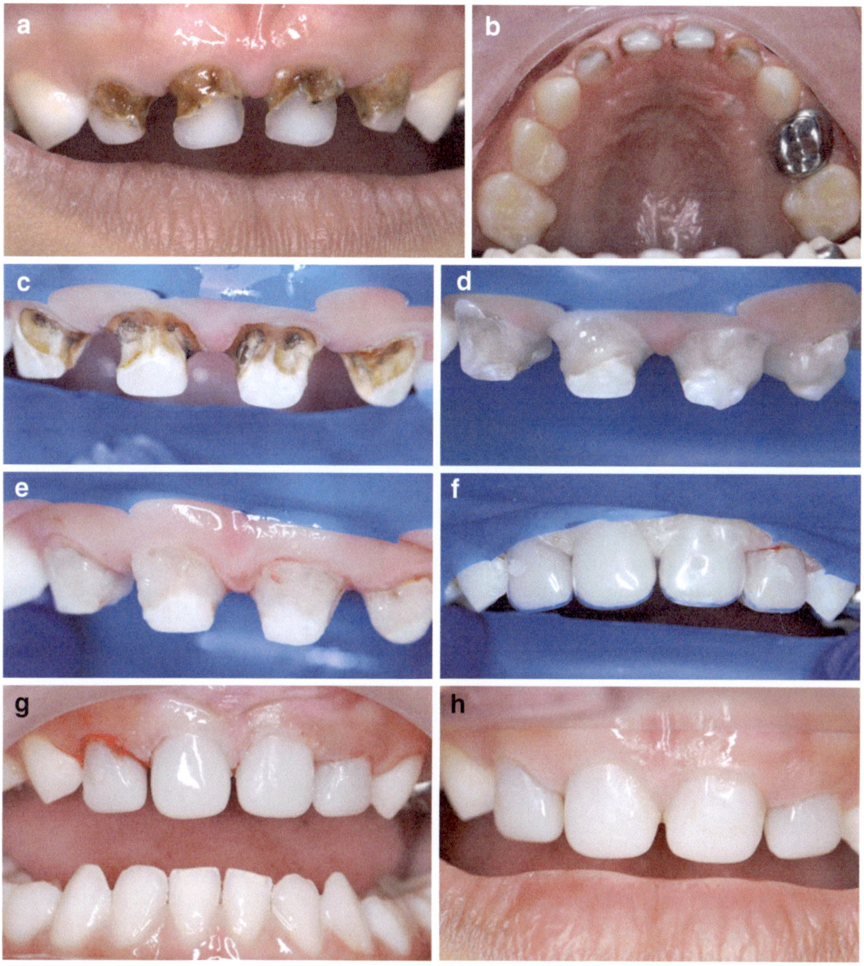

Fig. 7.5 Carious lesions in maxillary incisors, labial (**a**) and palatal view (**b**). The teeth were isolated under rubber dam and selective caries excavation was done (**c**). The lesions were conditioned with commercially available dentin conditioner and restored with Resin Modified Glass Ionomer Cement (**d**). Circumferential tooth preparation was done and extended to feather-edge margin subgingivally (**e**). Strip crowns were loaded with Resin Composite and bonded to the teeth. Vent holes were made on the labial surface of the crown to allow excess material to escape (**f**). The crowns were peeled after curing (**g**). Recall in 1 week (**h**)

Adequate cervical preparation of the tooth should be performed so that the strip crown form fits passively during try in. This ensures sufficient thickness of resin near the crown margins, thereby preventing chipping at the edges. Ensure excellent hemostasis and if required, a gingival retraction cord (size 0-0) may be placed. While hemostasis is essential, care must also be taken to avoid contamination with sulcular fluids, as this too will lead to marginal discoloration and breakdown over time.

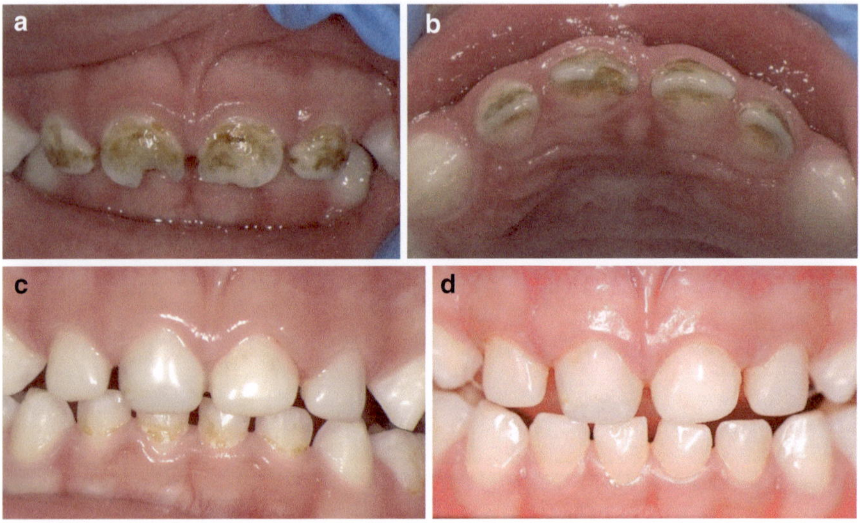

Fig. 7.6 Carious lesions on maxillary incisors, in labial (**a**) and palatal view (**b**). Immediate postoperative photograph of maxillary incisors restored with strip crowns (**c**). Follow-up at 5 years. The mandibular incisors were restored with Resin Composite at a previous visit (**d**)

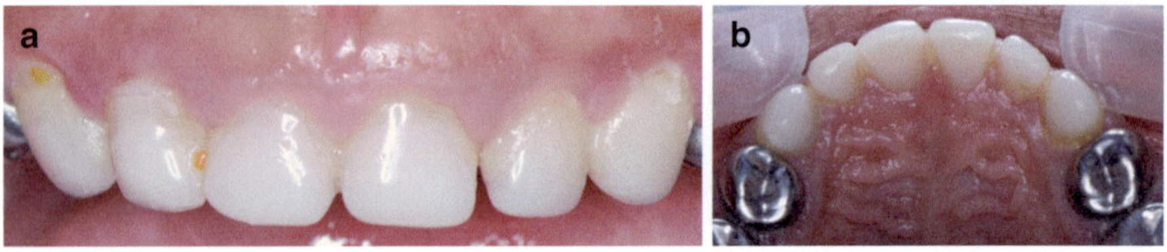

Fig. 7.7 Staining of restorations along the gingival margin of anterior teeth, labial (**a**) and palatal view (**b**)

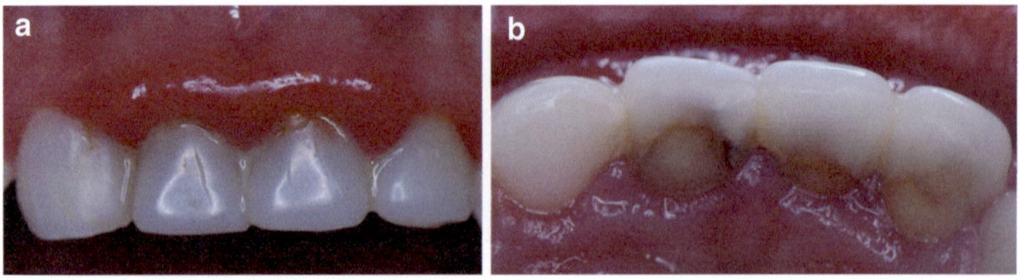

Fig. 7.8 Note the gingival puffiness (**a**) and inadequate cervical third preparation causing the restorations to chip and stain (**b**)

7.6.3 What Is the Success Rate of Strip Crowns?

The retention rate of composite resin strip crowns was 88% and 80% at the end of 18 and 24 months, respectively. The success of strip crowns primarily depends on case selection and technique of placement. Under adequate isolation, the strip crowns are more likely to retain longer if the tooth structure preoperatively has only proximal involvement and more of a healthy enamel surface to allow bonding of the material. In case of chips or cracks during follow-up visits, the restored tooth form can be repaired conventionally with the same material [17–19].

7.7 Preformed Zirconia Crowns

For many years, dentistry remained in search of a material that could match the esthetics of the natural tooth, yet possess the strength and longevity of metal. The introduction of a restorative material like zirconia in the 1990s sparked an esthetic revolution, which was later expanded to Pediatric Dentistry by the marketing of prefabricated zirconia crowns for the primary dentition and permanent molars. While as a metal, zirconia is available in nature in three main forms—monoclinic, tetragonal, and cubic; Yttrium-stabilized tetragonal zirconia (Y-TZP) is the most stable form. The preformed zirconia crowns used in Pediatric Dentistry are primarily monolithic-milled from a single block of Y-TZP. They are broadly composed of zirconium oxide (>85%), yttrium oxide (5%–6%), along with organic binders and pigments. The crowns are tooth colored, anatomically shaped, and have highly polished surfaces enabling them to mimic the natural appearance of the primary tooth [20].

7.7.1 What Are the Indications of Zirconia Crowns?

Zirconia crowns are indicated in cases where 2/3rd or at least half of the healthy tooth is intact, and the remaining tooth structure is predominantly dentine. As of today, zirconia crowns are the best esthetic options for primary teeth showing excellent color stability and retention (Table 7.4).

Table 7.4 Commercially available preformed zirconia crowns

Product	Country
EZ Pedo	USA
Cheng crowns	USA
Nusmile® ZR	USA
KinderKrowns	USA
Kids-e-Dental®	India
Kids Zirconia Crown	India
Signature crowns	India

7.7.2 Technique of Placement for Anterior and Posterior Zirconia Crowns (Fig. 7.4)

- Incisal or occlusal reduction of 1.5–2 mm is performed using a coarse diamond bur.
- Labial (anterior) or buccal and lingual or palatal (posterior teeth) depth cuts of 0.5–1.25 mm are made and merged using a straight fissure bur.
- An equigingival shoulder of approximately 1–1.25 mm thickness is created.
- The preparation is extended proximally and lingually, thereby creating a circumferential shoulder.
- The proximal walls are maintained near parallel by contouring the middle to cervical third with a slight taper towards the incisal.
- A fine tapering cone diamond point is now used to flush the shoulder to a feather edge margin subgingivally.
- Run a probe or explorer circumferentially to identify ledges or shoulders subgingivally.

Earlier, it was believed that due to the thickness of the zirconia crown, aggressive occlusal and proximal reduction was needed. The *occlusal thickness* of the first and second primary molar zirconia crowns (NuSmile ZR, USA) is only 0.75 mm to 0.85 mm, respectively. Hence, the occlusal preparation for a zirconia crown should be 1.5–2 mm similar to that of a stainless-steel crown. Unlike a SSC where the cervical bulge is preserved; the key to zirconia preparations is to *perform reduction of the middle to cervical one-third*, thereby reducing the crest of contour to allow for passive seating of the crown. The above method ensures good crown height with nearly parallel walls and minimal taper and preserves the vitality of the pulp. The *cervical margin* of a zirconia crown is 0.2 mm in thickness allowing it to flush with the prepared feather edge margins.

7.7.3 Crown Trial

- The crown must be tried to check the fit. It should seat passively without the use of digital pressure or a band seater.
- If the selected crown does not slide easily over the prepared tooth surface, avoid forcibly fitting the crown or asking the child to bite down as it will lead to fracture of the crown. Instead, check the fit of a larger sized crown. If the larger sized crown rotates or is loose on manipulation, the tooth must be prepared further, especially in the region of the cervical bulge.
- During trial placement, one must check that the labial surface of the crown is in alignment with the rest of the arch. If the crown appears more labially rotated than the remaining dentition, it indicates that the labial reduction is insufficient.
- Due to space loss, the regular crown may not fit in the mesiodistal space available. The following options may be considered:

(a) Use a narrow crown if provided by the manufacturer.
(b) Use a contralateral crown for lower primary molar.
(c) Further tooth reduction to select a smaller crown size.
(d) Lastly, do minimal proximal wall reduction of the final crown with a diamond point under water spray to ensure that it seats passively.

- Similarly, if zirconia crowns are to be placed on adjacent teeth, the crowns at try-in must be placed simultaneously to ensure they seat passively side by side. If the crowns do not seat passively,

  (a) Follow steps a to d, as mentioned above.
  (b) A combination of stainless steel and zirconia crowns may be placed.

- In children having anterior deep bite or crossbite, the anterior zirconia crowns may get dislodged due to occlusal interference. The bite may be raised bilaterally by placing Glass Ionomer Cement, Resin Composite on the occlusal surfaces posteriorly. Teeth needing posterior extracoronal restorations can be placed high in occlusion, thereby creating more clearance and allowing for anterior zirconia crown placement.
- In case of high points during try-in or post cementation, adjustments can be made with the opposing tooth instead of reducing the crown height of the tooth being prepared.
- Once the crown trial is complete, fine tapering cone diamond bur is used to place retentive grooves on the labial/buccal surfaces to improve retention (Figs. 7.9, 7.10, 7.11, 7.12, 7.13, and 7.14).

7.7.4 Hemostatic Control

The clinical technique for placement of zirconia crowns involves circumferential and subgingival preparation of the tooth. This causes bleeding from the gingival tissues, which can contaminate the zirconia crown affecting its retentive abilities. Thus, it is important to achieve hemostatic control prior to crown cementation. This can be achieved by applying pressure to the gingival margins with a damp cotton or by the application of a hemostatic agent like ferric sulphate or aluminum chloride [21].

7.7.5 Relative Contraindications to Placement of Zirconia Crowns

- In cases where retention of the crown may be compromised due to extensive loss of tooth structure.
- Presence of crossbite and deep bite causes aberrant masticatory forces that may dislodge the zirconia crown.
- In children with bruxism.

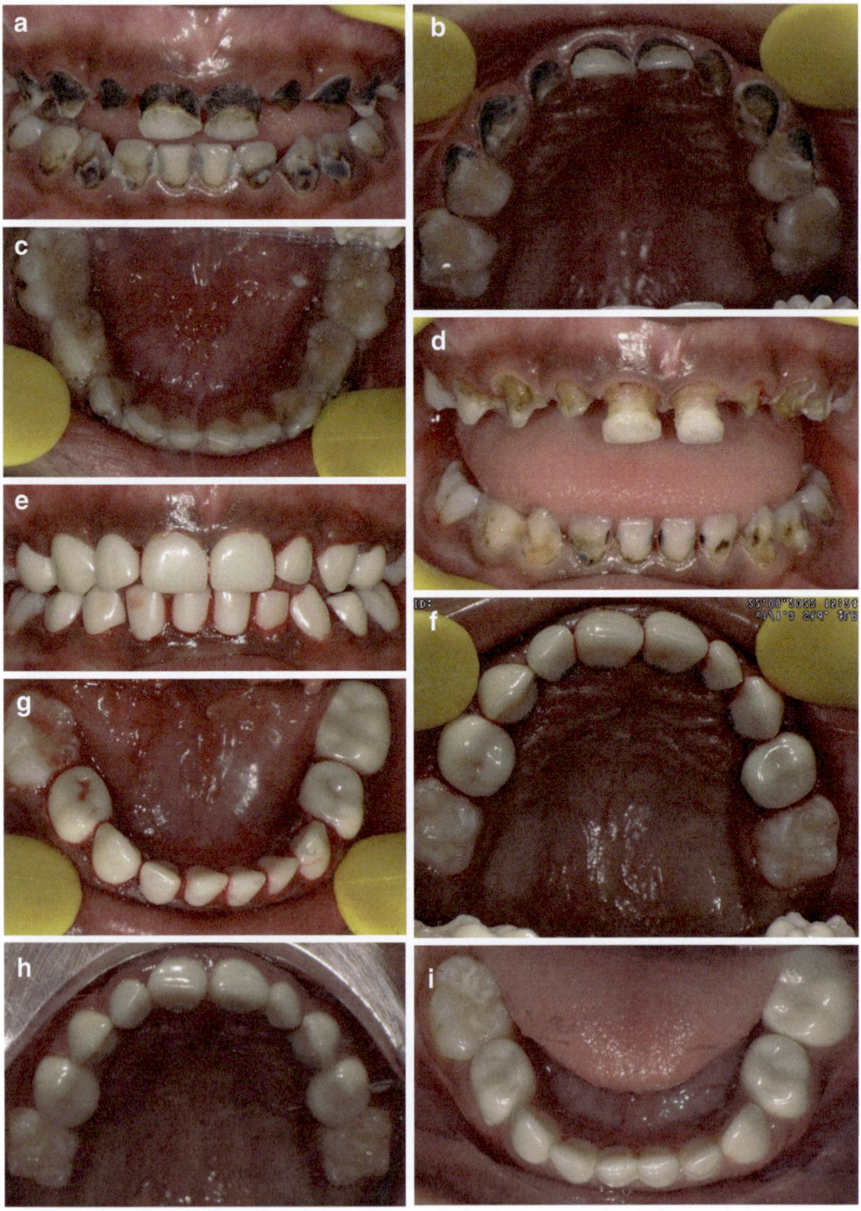

Fig. 7.9 Full mouth 38% Silver Diamine Fluoride application was done as an interim procedure to arrest the lesions (**a**). Preoperative maxillary and mandibular occlusal photographs (**b**, **c**). Full mouth rehabilitation was planned under General Anesthesia. Complete caries removal was done on all carious lesions (**d**). Immediate post-operative photograph of preformed zirconia crowns placed on all teeth except maxillary second molars and mandibular right second molar as these teeth received pit and fissure sealants (**e–g**). Follow-up at 1 year showed excellent gingival health and oral hygiene maintenance (**h**, **i**). Child reported with avulsion injury of maxillary right central incisor after 2 years (**j**). Three-year follow-up showed exfoliation of mandibular central incisors (**k**). Maxillary and mandibular occlusal view at 3-year follow-up (**l**, **m**). 3.5-year follow-up showing exfoliating mandibular lateral incisors (**n**)

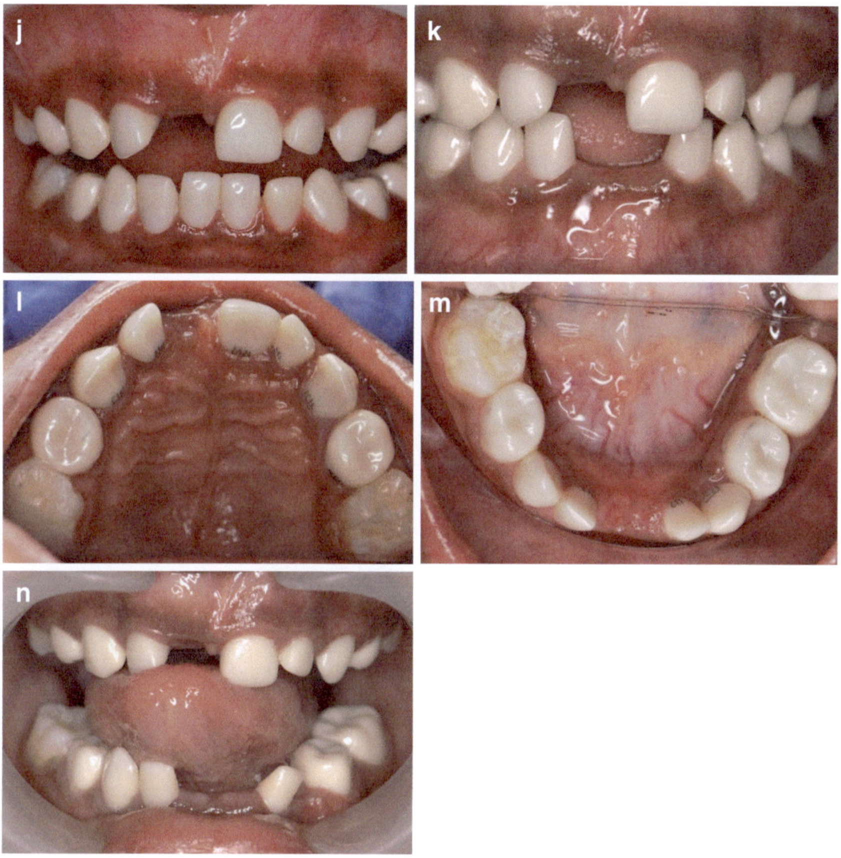

Fig. 7.9 (continued)

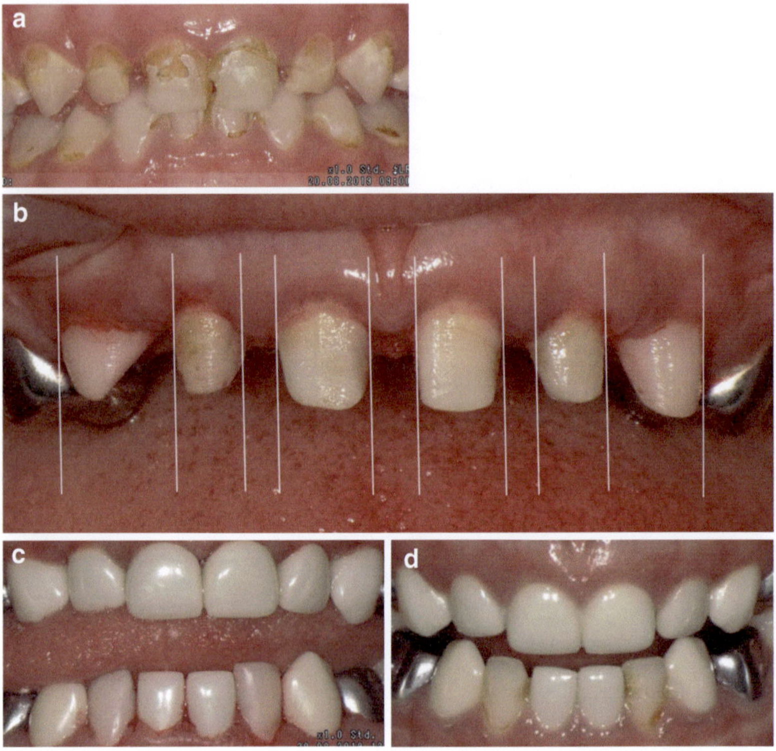

Fig. 7.10 Extensive stage lesions on maxillary anterior teeth (**a**). Complete caries removal was done, and the maxillary anterior teeth were restored with Resin Modified Glass Ionomer Cement. The teeth were prepared to receive zirconia crowns. The preparation is maintained near parallel by contouring the middle to cervical third with a slight taper towards the incisal (**b**). Immediate post-operative photograph. The mandibular central incisors and canines were restored with preformed zirconia crowns and lateral incisors with strip crowns (**c**). At 3-year follow-up (**d**)

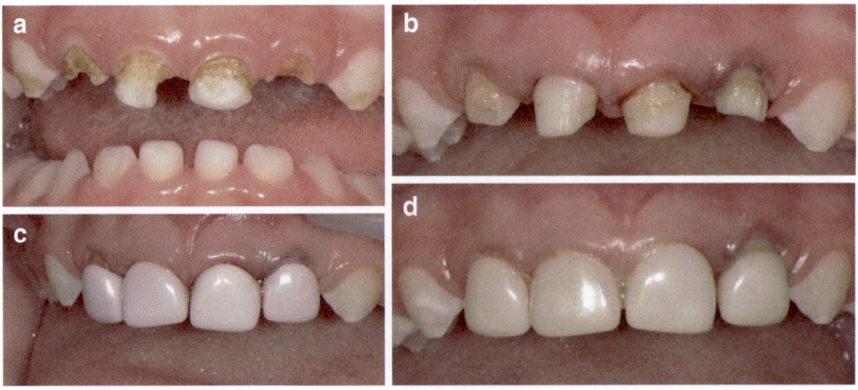

Fig. 7.11 Extensive stage lesions in maxillary anterior teeth (**a**). Post-endodontic restoration was done with Resin Modified Glass Ionomer Cement (**b**). All try in crowns must be placed at the same time (**c**). Preformed zirconia crowns cemented with Resin Modified Glass Ionomer Cement (**d**)

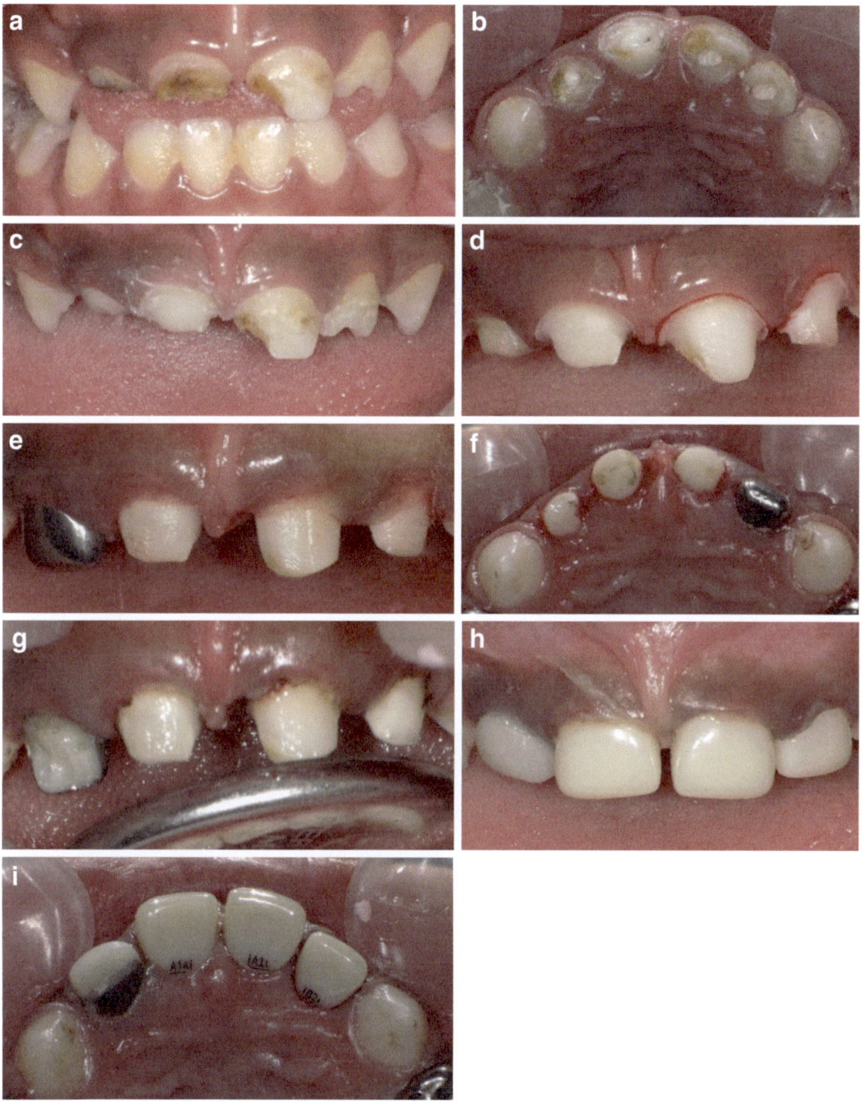

Fig. 7.12 Extensive stage lesions in maxillary incisors (**a**), treated with pulpectomy (**b**). Post-endodontic restoration done with Resin Modified Glass Ionomer Cement (**c**). Maxillary right lateral incisor was prepared to receive an open-faced stainless-steel crown due to less than one-third remaining tooth structure. The central incisors and left lateral incisor were prepared to receive preformed zirconia crowns. An equigingival shoulder of approximately 1–1.25 mm thickness was created circumferentially, while maintaining parallelism between teeth. The right lateral incisor was prepared circumferentially and subgingivally to a feather edge margin (**d**). Stainless Steel Crown was placed to check for fit. The crown was adapted in place with a band pusher. The other incisors were prepared subgingivally and circumferentially to a feather edge margin, with a tapered diamond point (**e**). Occlusal view of the preparation (**f**). A labial window was prepared on the Stainless Steel Crown (**g**). Resin Composite build-up done on the open-faced Stainless-Steel Crown. Preformed zirconia crowns placed on other incisors (**h**). Occlusal view of the restorations (**i**)

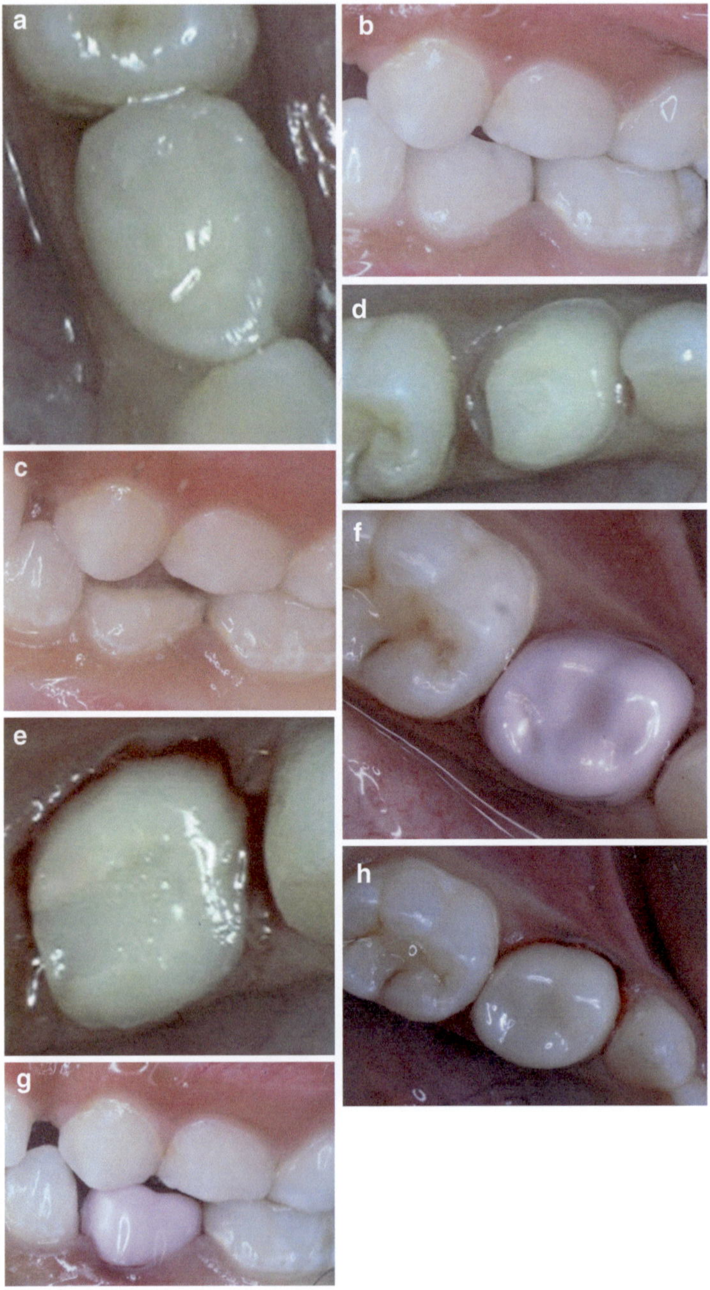

Fig. 7.13 Mandibular primary left first molar treated for pulpectomy and post-endodontic restoration with Resin Modified Glass Ionomer Cement (**a**). Occlusion checked before preparing the tooth for preformed zirconia crown (**b**). Occlusal reduction of 1.5–2 mm done (**c**). Equigingival circumferential reduction was done to a shoulder of 1–1.5 mm (**d**). Subgingival tooth preparation to a feather edge margin with a tapered diamond point (**e**). Try in crown in place. The trial crown should have a passive fit and remain in arch alignment (**f**). The occlusion is checked. Slight opening of bite is expected (**g**). Preformed zirconia crown cemented (**h**)

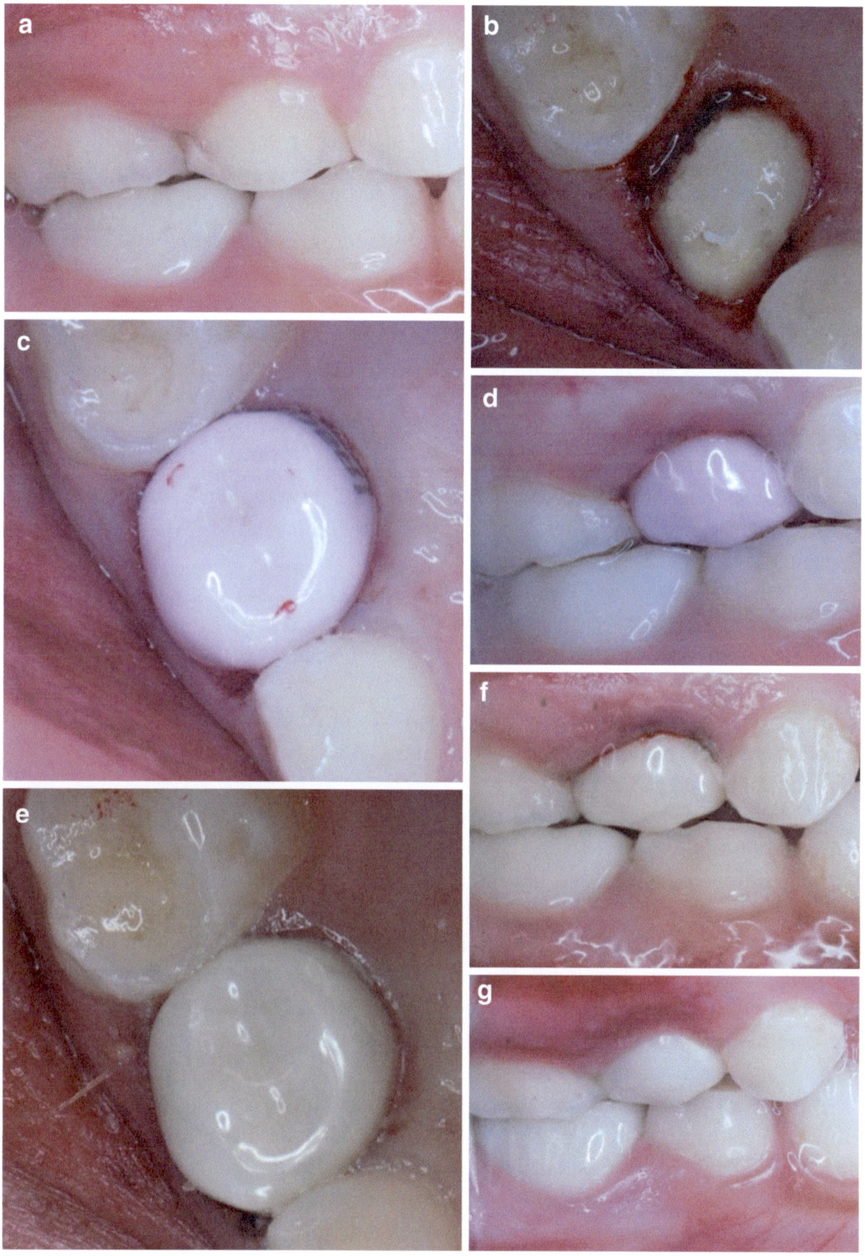

Fig. 7.14 Maxillary primary first molar was treated for pulpotomy and a post-endodontic restoration with Resin Modified Glass Ionomer Cement done (**a**). Tooth preparation completed (**b**). Occlusal view of try in crown in place (**c**) and in occlusion (**d**). Immediate post-operative photograph of crown cemented (**e**) and in occlusion (**f**). Follow-up at 1 year showing excellent gingival health and oral hygiene (**g**)

- Placement of zirconia crowns may be difficult in a crowded dentition, as one may not achieve sufficient proximal clearance even after substantial tooth preparation.
- Young children between 2 and 4 years of age, wherein passive eruption of the primary molars is still occurring. In these cases, stainless-steel crowns will offer better retention and ensure the cervical margins of the tooth are not exposed, when the clinical height of the tooth increases after completion of the eruption process.
- It is difficult to restore a single anterior tooth in the esthetic zone with a zirconia crown as it is a challenge to match the shade and merge the crown with the remaining dentition.
- Placing a zirconia crown in occlusion with a stainless-steel crown will lead to grayish marks on the zirconia crown which may or may not be removed with polishing.
- The placement of zirconia crowns is a technique-sensitive process requiring a longer operating time and more effective pain control, i.e., administration of an injectable local anesthetic as compared to SSC crowns. Thus, in children with limited cooperative abilities, a SSC crown may be preferred.

7.7.6 Which Is an Appropriate Cement for Luting Zirconia Crowns?

Zirconia crowns must be luted with a Resin-Modified Glass Ionomer Cement as it bonds to the tooth as well as the crown unlike a conventional Glass Ionomer Cement that does not bond to zirconia.

While using a glass ionomer luting cement, the tooth should be conditioned with a dentin conditioner prior to crown cementation. Two-thirds of the crown is filling with the luting cement and seated on the prepared tooth in the appropriate position. The seated crown should be stabilized with finger pressure for 20 s. Following this, it can be tack cured for 5 s if a dual cure cement has been used or continued to be held in position for 2 min till the initial set has occurred. The excess cement surrounding the crown margins can be removed with a sharp instrument, while taking care to maintain the crown stability. A floss can be passed interproximally to remove any excess cement that may be present (Table 7.5).

Bioactive cements that have been recently introduced for luting Zr crowns are BioCem® (Nusmile, USA) and Ceramir® (Doxa Dental). Both cements show evidence of hydroxyapatite formation at the tooth–cement interface. According to the manufacturers, Ceramir, a calcium aluminate cement sets to a basic pH making it a strong antibacterial. BioCem®, a hydrophilic dual cure cement, after bonding to the tooth, remains flexible because of a rubberized urethane component that is able to absorb masticatory forces.

Table 7.5 Commercially available Resin-Modified Glass Ionomer luting cement are as follows

Product	Manufacturer	Country
FujiCEM® 2	GC	USA
RelyX™ U200	3M™	USA
Fusion Ultra D/C™	Prevest DenPro®	India
TheraCem®	Bisco	USA
Wizdent Wonder lute	Pidilite	India
Speedcem Plus®	Ivoclar	USA
Calibra® Universal	Dentsply Sirona	USA
ClearFil™ SA	Kuraray	Japan
Dual Force	Maquira	Brazil
Fylla Connect dual cure	Mothers dental®	Australia
Bifix SE	Voco	Germany
Riva CEM Automix	SDI	Australia

7.7.7 What Is the Role of Try-In Crowns?

Certain manufacturers (Nusmile ZR, USA; Kids ZR crowns, India) offer try-in crowns in their kits that are identical in size and shape to the actual zirconia crowns. These crowns allow for tooth preparation refinement and prevent contamination of the actual ZR crown. The inner surface of zirconia crowns has an inherent affinity towards phospholipids in saliva and blood or phosphoric acid from the etchant. This depletes the sites available for bonding of resin cement to the interior surface, thus reducing bond strength and compromising retention. Therefore, an alkaline solution is necessary to neutralize the phosphate contamination [21].

For kits that do not have try-in crowns, the inner surface can be cleaned with the following (Table 7.6).

Alternate methods like sodium hypochlorite, hydrogen peroxide, and additional sandblasting can also be done. Rinsing of the crown with water must precede the process of decontamination. During recementation of dislodged preformed zirconia crowns, the remanants of the luting cement is first removed with an ultrasonic scaler or a diamond point under water spray. Then, the inner surface of the crown is sandblasted and cleaned with the decontaminants mentioned above to ensure a good bond between the tooth and the crown.

7.7.8 Do Zirconia Crowns Cause Temporomandibular Joint Dysfunction or Attrition of Opposing Teeth in Children?

At present there is no positive evidence correlating temporomandibular joint dysfunction after rehabilitation of posterior teeth with zirconia crowns. Attrition of opposing teeth due to the zirconia crown is within acceptable limits. However, zirconia crowns may be avoided in children with bruxism.

Table 7.6 Commercially available surface cleaning agents

Product	Manufacturer
ZirClean® (potassium hydroxide)	Bisco, USA
Ivoclean (sodium hydroxide)	Ivoclar, USA

7.7.9 Can the Tooth Be Treated for Pulp Therapy After Cementation of Zirconia Crown?

The clinician can gain access to the pulpal space through the crown in a way similar to conventional endodontic preparation using a diamond point at high speed with water as a coolant. After completion of the procedure, the access opening can be sealed with a Resin Composite restoration.

7.7.10 Can the Zirconia Crown Receive a Stainless-Steel Band and Loop Space Maintainer?

In such a situation, the surface of the zirconia crown can be polished with pumice and the stainless-steel space maintainer be cemented with a resin-modified glass ionomer luting cement. If this situation is anticipated at the time of treatment planning, the parents must be informed of the questionable retention of the stainless-steel space maintainer.

7.7.11 Can Zirconia Crowns Be Trimmed?

It is not recommended to trim zirconia crowns routinely as it will cause microcrack propagation within the material that may weaken the crown and leave rough margins leading to plaque accumulation. However, for crown adjustments, zirconia crowns can be trimmed minimally on the proximal surfaces or cervical margins if required.

7.7.12 What Is the Success Rate of Preformed Zirconia Crown?

While comparing the performance of preformed zirconia crowns with other extracoronal restorations, it was seen that the former outperformed in terms of periodontal health, parental satisfaction, color stability, crown retention, contour, fracture resistance, marginal integrity, surface roughness, and recurrent caries. It was found that the primary posterior teeth rehabilitated with preformed zirconia crowns may have lesser risk of experiencing clinical failure and probably better gingival health after 12 months than SSCs [22–24]. Despite certain challenges like cost and technique of placement that can be time-consuming and daunting to the child, preformed zirconia crowns make a promising esthetic option for extracoronal restoration in children.

7.8 Bioflx Crowns

Recently, a new range of metal-free, monochromatic tooth-colored crowns called the Bioflx crowns made of a hybrid resin polymer have been introduced to the market. These crowns require minimal tooth preparation prior to placement like an SSC, while providing a more esthetic appearance. Unlike zirconia crowns, Bioflx crowns can be trimmed with scissors and the proximal surfaces, contoured, or flattened with Howe's pliers. Crimping is not recommended, and they are not indicated for use with the Hall technique. These crowns flatten or show "dimple" in areas of high occlusion, and must not be used with the Hall technique (Fig. 7.15).

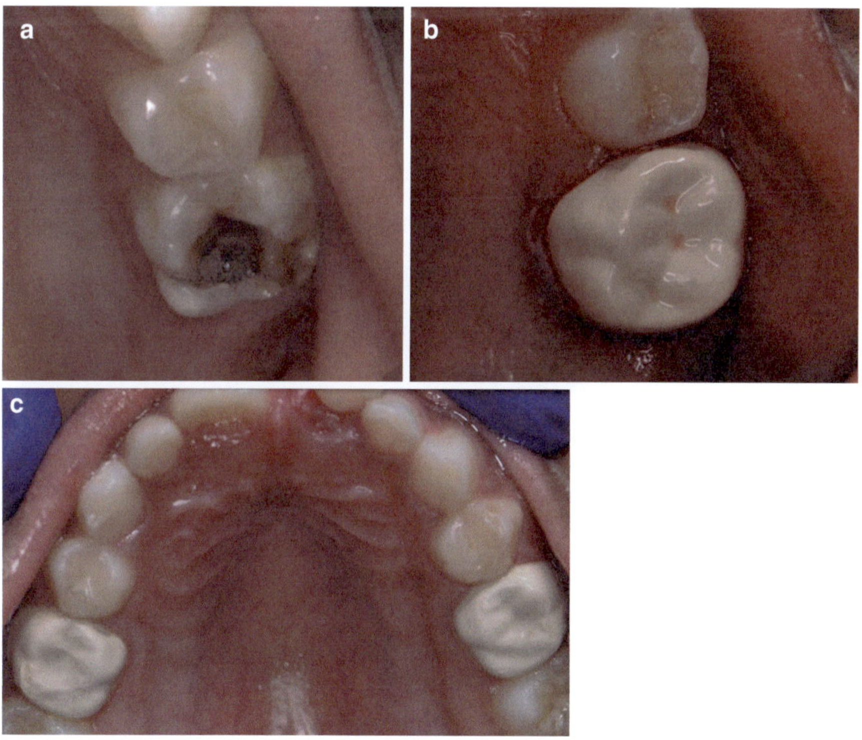

Fig. 7.15 Extensive stage lesion in maxillary primary left second molar (**a**). Immediate post-cementation photograph of Bioflx® crown (Kids-e-dental®, India) (**b**). Both maxillary primary second molars restored with Bioflx® crowns. Six-month follow-up photograph showing facets or dimpling of the crown (**c**)

7.9 Concluding Remarks

Preformed zirconia crowns are an ideal restoratitive option in anterior teeth owing to their superior esthetics, color stability, and strength. When a single tooth in the anterior segment is to be restored and in cases where there is crowding, a strip crown may be preferred over a zirconia crown. In situations wherein less than one-third of the tooth structure is present, an open-faced stainless-steel crown must be the restoration of choice as long as there is a ferrule of sound tooth structure. The mechanical retention due to crimping of the SSC provides additional retention for better longevity. There is little evidence to support the use of one type of crown over another for primary molars, particularly for preformed zirconia crowns that were introduced much later than SSC to Pediatric Dentistry. The gold standard for restoring decayed primary molars is still the preformed Stainless-Steel Crown. Ultimately, the choice of extracoronal restoration should depend on the clinical situation, patient, and clinician preference for successful primary teeth rehabilitation.

References

1. Randall RC. Preformed metal crowns for primary and permanent molar teeth: review of the literature. Pediatr Dent. 2002;24(5):489–500.
2. Seale NS, Randall R. The use of stainless steel crowns: a systematic literature review. Pediatr Dent. 2015;37(2):145–60.
3. Croll T, Resienberger R. Primary molar stainless steel crown restoration. Quintessence Int. 1986;17(4):221–6.
4. Patel RV, Thikkurissy S, Schwartz SB, Gosnell ES, Sun Q, Cully JL. Preferential use of stainless steel crowns as a strategy to minimize retreatment of primary molars under general anesthesia. Pediatr Dent. 2021;43(1):24–7.
5. Badar SB, Tabassum S, Khan FR, Ghafoor R. Effectiveness of hall technique for primary carious molars: a systematic review and meta-analysis. Int J Clin Pediatr Dent. 2019;12(5):445–52.
6. Mathewson RJ, Primosch RE. Fundamentals of pediatric dentistry. In: Stainless steel crown procedures for primary molars. 3rd ed. Chicago, USA: Quintessence Books;1995. p. 257–84.
7. Casamassimo PS. The venerable stainless steel crown. Pediatr Dent. 1994;16(2):83.
8. Stewart RE, Barber TK, Troutman KC, Wei SH. Pediatric dentistry: scientific foundation and clinical practice. London: The C.V. Mosby Company; 1982.
9. Croll TP, Castaldi CR. The preformed stainless steel crown for restoration of permanent posterior teeth in special cases. J Am Dent Assoc. 1978;97(4):644–9.
10. Padminee K, Hemalatha R, Shankar P, Senthil D, Trophimus GJ. Topical anesthesia for stainless steel crown tooth preparation in primary molars: a pilot study. J Dent Anesth Pain Med. 2020;20(4):241–50.
11. Doykos JD 3rd, Valachovic RW. Precementation radiographic assessment for permanent posterior stainless steel crowns. J Pedod. 1979;3(3):216–20.
12. Hartmann C. The open-face stainless steel crown: an esthetic technique. ASDC J Dent Child. 1983;50(1):31–3.
13. Shah PV, Lee JY, Wright JT. Clinical success and parental satisfaction with anterior preveneered primary stainless steel crowns. Pediatr Dent. 2004;26(5):391–5.
14. O'Connell AC, Kratunova E, Leith R. Posterior preveneered stainless steel crowns: clinical performance after three years. Pediatr Dent. 2014;36(3):254–8.
15. Webber D, Epstein N, Tsamtsouris A. A method of restoring primary anterior teeth with the aid of a celluloid crown form and composite resins. Pediatr Dent. 1979;1:244–6.

16. Kupietzky A. Bonded resin composite strip crowns for primary incisors: clinical tips for a successful outcome. Pediatr Dent. 2002;24(2):145–8.
17. Kupietzky A, Waggoner WF, Galea J. The clinical and radiographic success of bonded resin composite strip crowns for primary incisors. Pediatr Dent. 2003;25(6):577–81.
18. Grewal N, Jha S, Kaur N. Clinical and radiographic success of resin-bonded strip crowns in primary incisors with varying extents of sound tooth structure available for bonding. Int J Clin Pediatr Dent. 2021;14(4):454–61.
19. Radu F, Leon A, Luca R. Clinical performance of strip crowns in restoring primary incisors: preliminary study. P Romanian Acad A. 2015; Vol 1, No.B :190–3.
20. Larsson C. Zirconium dioxide based dental restorations. Studies on clinical performance and fracture behaviour. Swed Dent J. 2011;(213):9–84.
21. Tian F, Londono J, Villalobos V, Pan Y, Ho HX, Eshera R, Sidow SJ, Bergeron BE, Wang X, Tay FR. Effectiveness of different cleaning measures on the bonding of resin cement to saliva-contaminated or blood-contaminated zirconia. J Dent. 2022;120:104084.
22. Alzanbaqi SD, Alogaiel RM, Alasmari MA, Al Essa AM, Khogeer LN, Alanazi BS, Hawsah ES, Shaikh AM, Ibrahim MS. Zirconia crowns for primary teeth: a systematic review and meta-analyses. Int J Environ Res Public Health. 2022;19(5):2838.
23. Alrashdi M, Ardoin J, Liu JA. Zirconia crowns for children: a systematic review. Int J Paediatr Dent. 2022;32(1):66–81.
24. Patnana AK, Chugh VK, Chugh A, Vanga NRV, Kumar P. Effectiveness of zirconia crowns compared with stainless steel crowns in primary posterior teeth rehabilitation: a systematic review and meta-analysis. J Am Dent Assoc. 2022;153(2):158–66.

Pediatric Endodontics in Primary Teeth: Vital Pulp Therapy

8

8.1 Introduction

Pulpotomy was considered the treatment of choice for managing vital primary teeth with extensive-stage lesions based on the type of carious dentin and its proximity to the pulp. A better understanding of the layers of carious dentin suggests that the innermost layer (affected dentin), overlying the pulp, was capable of remineralization, even if the outer infected layer was not removed completely and the tooth restored to prevent reactivation of the caries process. In the last few decades, the concept of Minimal Intervention Dentistry has changed the complexion of pediatric endodontics and once again laid emphasis on the dental pulp's ability to heal from reversible injuries bringing Indirect Pulp Treatment (IPT) back to the forefront. The emergence of Calcium Silicate Cements (CSCs) with regenerative properties has improved the success of Direct Pulp Capping (DPC) and pulpotomy. Today, a successful practice of pediatric endodontics depends on the clinician's acumen in accurately diagnosing the extent of pulpal inflammation and adopting a conservative approach to its management.

8.2 Vital Pulp Therapy

Vital Pulp Therapy (VPT) is based on the premise that reversible pulpal injuries in both primary and permanent teeth have the capacity to heal [1]. The basic principles of vital pulp treatment are:

- Removing diseased and bacterially contaminated tissue.
- Establishing an environment that will prevent any further bacterial contamination [2, 3].

Currently, VPT options for the treatment of teeth with extensive carious lesions presenting with reversible pulpitis are Indirect Pulp Treatment (IPT), Direct Pulp Capping (DPC), and Pulpotomy. These procedures also form the basis of

H. Vyas et al., *Dental Caries and Traumatic Injuries in Pediatric Dentistry*,
https://doi.org/10.1007/978-3-031-98929-2_8

apexogenesis, performed in an immature permanent tooth with the primary objective of maintaining pulp vitality and promoting continued root development [4–7].

VPT is indicated in teeth with extensive carious lesions that are asymptomatic or exhibit a history of provoked pain that subsides on the removal of stimulus, indicative of reversible pulpitis. The chief complaint, specifically, the description of pain, is crucial to the initial diagnosis of the pulp status. It must not be performed if the child has a history of spontaneous and nocturnal pain [1, 4, 5, 7–9]. The tooth should not have a carious exposure or be associated with a dentoalveolar abscess or facial swelling.

Radiographic assessment of teeth deemed to undergo VPT procedures must be correlated with clinical findings. The extensive-stage lesions show radiolucency approaching the pulp with or without a layer of dentin capping the pulp. The bone surrounding the tooth must appear normal, with no pathologic root resorption or periapical radiolucency [4, 5, 10].

8.3 Indirect Pulp Treatment (IPT)

Indirect Pulp Treatment is a procedure that leaves the deepest caries adjacent to the pulp undisturbed, to avoid pulp exposure. The remaining dentin is covered with a biocompatible material to stimulate healing and repair [4, 5, 10].

8.3.1 What Is the Rationale for Indirect Pulp Treatment?

Earlier, it was believed that the outer layer of *infected dentin* was contaminated with bacteria and needed to be removed while the inner *affected dentin* overlying the pulp was capable of remineralization and could be left behind. The few bacteria present in the *affected dentin* did not survive once the cavity was restored and their nutrition supply cut off. Further, this "*affected dentin*" had an intact collagen matrix and could be remineralized by placing an appropriate pulp capping agent [11–13]. The dentinopulpal complex under favorable conditions induced the formation of tertiary dentin, thereby maintaining pulp vitality [14, 15]. Clinicians tried to distinguish between affected and infected dentin based on broad generic criteria such as color and texture [11, 12, 15].

Presently, carious dentin can be categorized into four separate layers, namely, soft, leathery, firm, and hard; with soft dentin lying as the outermost layer and hard or sound dentin at the base of the lesion towards the pulp. The modern technique of IPT takes cognizance of these separate layers and recommends a clinically decipherable method of caries excavation based on the tactile hardness [16–19].

To help clinicians with the same, the International Caries Consensus Collaboration (ICCC) has developed the following terminology for layers of carious dentin [16, 17].

Hard dentin is the part that requires a pushing force "with a hard instrument to engage the dentin, and only a sharp cutting edge or a bur will lift it. A scratchy sound or 'cri dentinaire' can be heard when a straight probe is taken across the dentine (Fig. 8.1a)" [16, 17].

Firm dentine is physically resistant to hand excavation, and "some pressure needs to be exerted through an instrument to lift it (Fig. 8.1b)" [16, 17].

Leathery dentine "does not deform when an instrument is pressed onto it but can still be easily lifted without much force being required (Fig. 8.1c)" [16, 17].

Soft dentine will deform when a hard instrument is "pressed onto it and can be easily scooped up (e.g., with a sharp hand excavator) with little force being required (Fig. 8.1d)" [16, 17].

There may be little difference between leathery and soft dentine, with leathery being a transition on the spectrum between soft and firm dentine. A distinguishing feature between the two layers is that firm dentin appears dry and soft or leathery dentin appears moist.

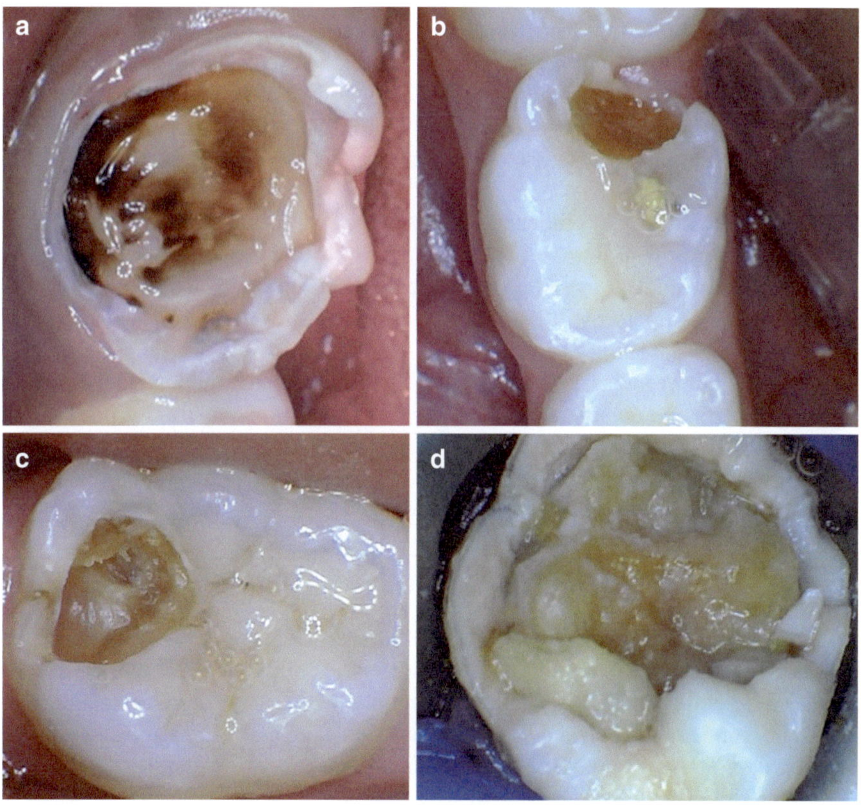

Fig. 8.1 Hard dentin (**a**). Firm dentin (**b**). Leathery dentin (**c**). Soft dentin (**d**)

8.3.2 What Are the Indications of Indirect Pulp Treatment?

IPT is recommended in teeth with carious lesions that have penetrated into the inner third of the dentin, with or without a band of dentin capping the pulp on the radiograph. If there is no evident band of dentin between the advancing carious lesion and the pulp, the clinician may still opt to perform an IPT, provided the **tooth is asymptomatic or exhibits clinical signs and symptoms of reversible pulpitis** [4, 5, 10, 20].

8.3.3 What Must Be the Threshold of Caries Excavation in Indirect Pulp Treatment?

While complete caries removal has been the standard practice, the approach of Selective Caries Removal (SCR) is now the established norm while treating extensive-stage lesions that are adjacent to the pulp [4, 5, 10, 20].

In this method, the periphery or walls of the carious lesion must be excavated to hard dentin or healthy tooth structure. This is ascertained when a scratchy sound or "cri dentinaire" is heard upon reaching this layer. The excavation on the floor of the lesion should not extend to hard dentin and a layer of firm or soft dentin is left overlying the pulp. This prevents pulp exposure and allows for a successful IPT, provided the tooth is asymptomatic or shows signs and symptoms of reversible pulpitis only [10, 16, 17].

One of the concerns of clinicians in leaving behind soft dentin is that it is teeming with bacteria, resulting in the underlying pulp being inflamed and possibly infected. As a result, these teeth are subjected to the more invasive forms of pulp therapy such as pulpotomy, if the pulp is deemed vital or pulpectomy/extraction if the pulp is non-vital [21].

It is now understood that the inner layer has minimal bacterial load and *diagnosing pulp vitality and completely sealing in the caries* forms the crux of performing a successful IPT, no matter what layer of carious dentin is left overlying the pulp [22, 23].

8.3.4 Pulp Diagnosis

While the absence of spontaneous or nocturnal pain is one of the best indicators of a vital pulp [24], at times the symptoms given by the child may be varied and unreliable. Often a child presents with pain while eating, which may continue for a slightly longer duration after removal of the stimulus. This pain due to food impaction in the gingival papilla maybe mistaken for tenderness, indicating irreversible pulpitis. It is important to corroborate the pain history with the radiographic picture wherein there should be no periapical or significant furcal radiolucency in addition to pathological root resorption. Clinically, after removing the food debris, the carious lesion must be inspected under magnification to rule out pulp exposure. There should be no abscess or swelling associated with the tooth.

At times, despite a thorough assessment, the pulp status cannot be ascertained. An Interim Therapeutic Restoration (ITR) can be used as an additional tool to determine pulp vitality in asymptomatic teeth where the clinician is unsure of the pulp status. In this technique, the periphery of the lesion is excavated to hard dentin with minimal or no excavation on the floor. The tooth is restored with a Glass Ionomer Cement. The patient is recalled after 4–6 weeks to determine the pulp response, if any. If the tooth is asymptomatic, IPT can be done. On the other hand, if the patient returns with symptoms of irreversible pulpitis, a pulpectomy or extraction must be performed (Fig. 8.2) [25–27].

ITR should be done only if the patient is sure to return in 4–6 weeks for a definitive restoration [27]. In situations where the patient is unable to return and the clinician is still unsure of the pulp status, the best indicator of pulp vitality is direct inspection of the pulp tissue. The clinician can completely excavate the lesion and expose the pulp. A bleeding pulp with the absence of necrotic tissue or yellow exudate in the pulp chamber ascertains pulp vitality, allowing the clinician to complete a VPT procedure, such as pulpotomy [19].

Most times, the pulp status can be assessed fairly accurately by correlating the pain history and clinical and radiographic findings. IPT as a technique using SCR has shown great success in pulp preservation [4, 20, 28, 29].

8.3.5 Technique of IPT for Primary Teeth (Figs. 8.3 and 8.4)

- Rubber dam isolation is preferred over a combination of saliva ejector and cotton rolls.
- Clean the walls of the carious lesion with an airotor and/or sharp spoon excavator. Remove all enamel overhangs and excavate to hard or sound dentin.
- Excavate the floor of the carious lesion to firm or soft dentin using a sharp spoon excavator [29].
- In primary teeth, Glass Ionomer Cement is placed on the floor of the lesion either as a direct restoration or as a liner below resin composite or as a luting cement with a preformed crown [30, 31].
- The coronal seal after pulp capping is more critical to the success of IPT than the capping material itself [22, 32].

Under the umbrella of Minimal Intervention Dentistry (MID), one can also opt for no removal of caries and restore the tooth with the Hall or the Silver-Modified Atraumatic Restorative Technique.

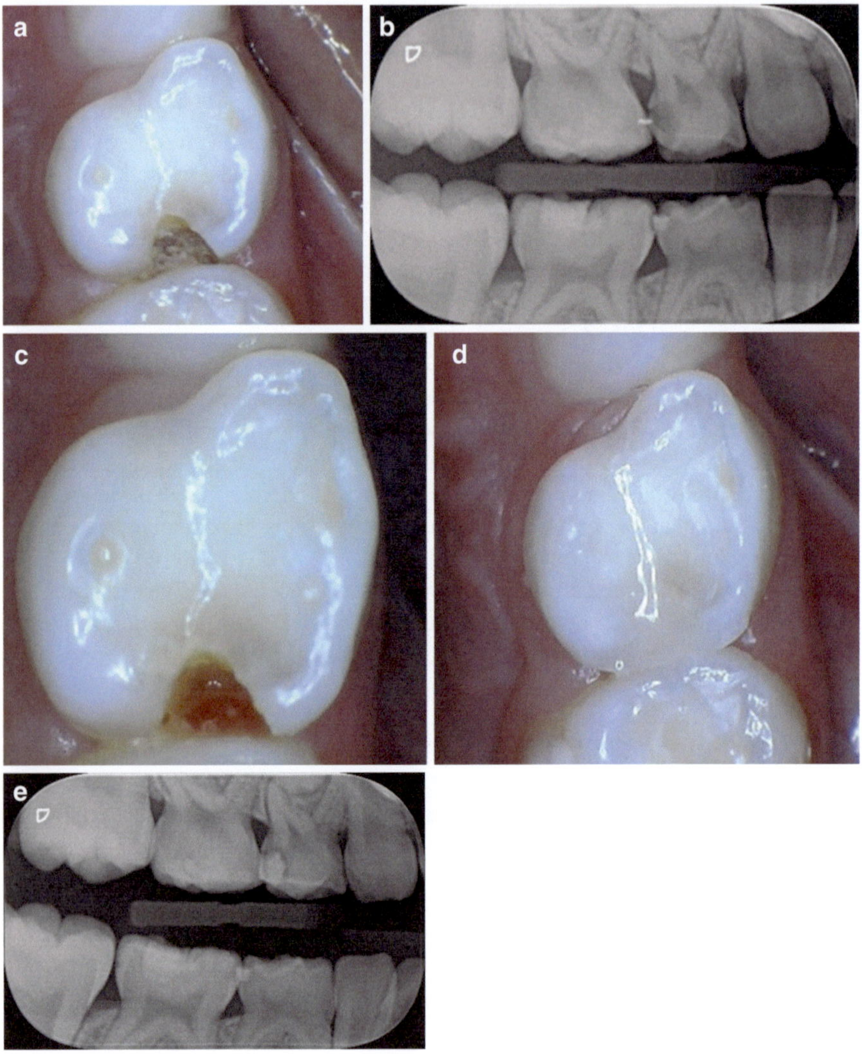

Fig. 8.2 Extensive stage lesion on the maxillary primary right first molar (**a**). Radiolucency was seen approaching the pulp. As pulpal diagnosis was uncertain, an Interim Therapeutic Restoration was planned (**b**). The walls of the lesion were excavated to sound tooth structure, and minimal excavation was performed on the floor of the lesion (**c**). A Resin Modified Glass Ionomer restoration was done (**d**). At the one-month follow-up, the child complained of spontaneous pain and PDL widening was seen (**e**). The tooth was extracted

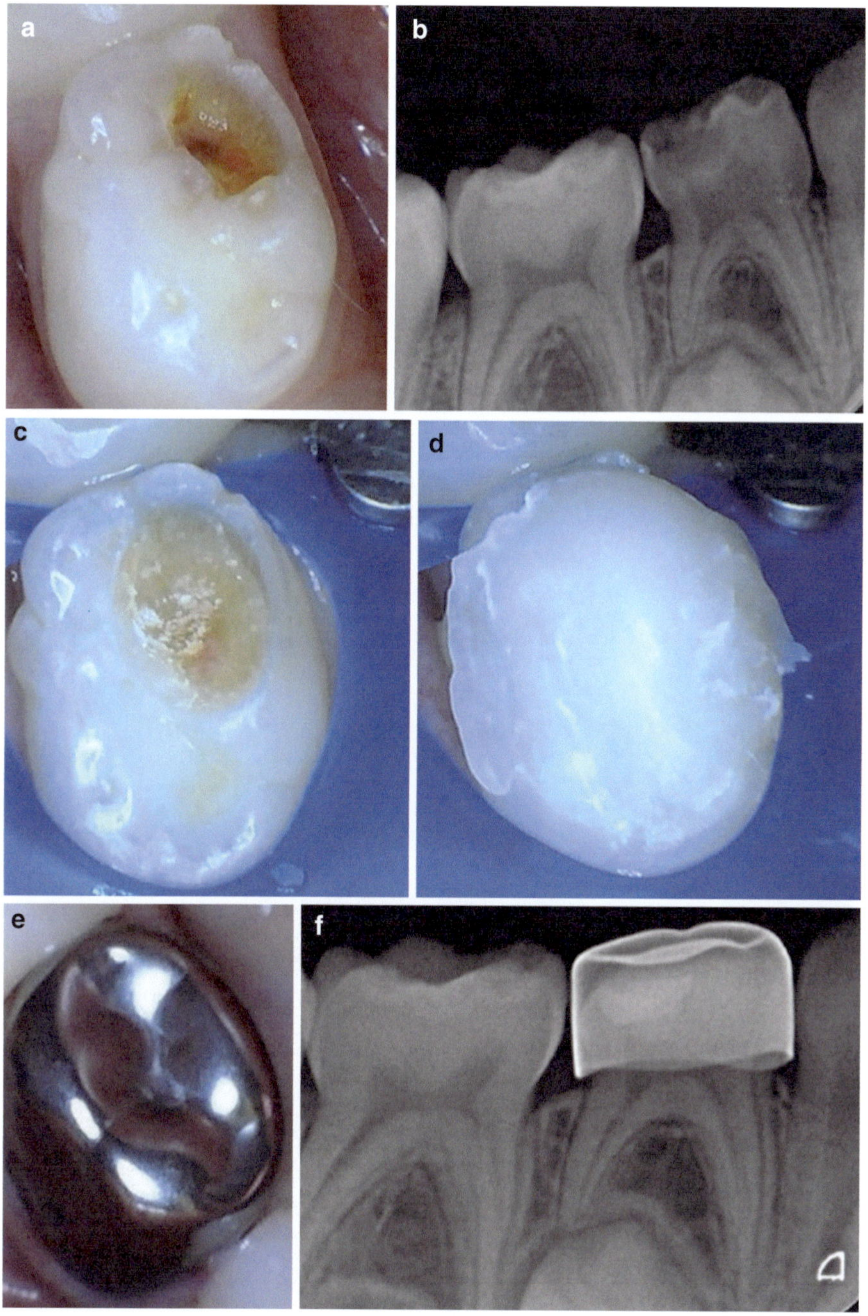

Fig. 8.3 Extensive stage lesion on mandibular primary right first molar. The tooth was asymptomatic and did not show clinical (**a**) and radiographic signs (**b**) of periapical pathology. Peripheral walls excavated to sound dentin and Selective Caries Removal performed on the floor of the lesion (**c**). Tooth was restored with a glass ionomer restoration (**d**) followed by a Stainless Steel Crown to ensure coronal seal (**e**). Radiograph taken at three-month follow-up (**f**)

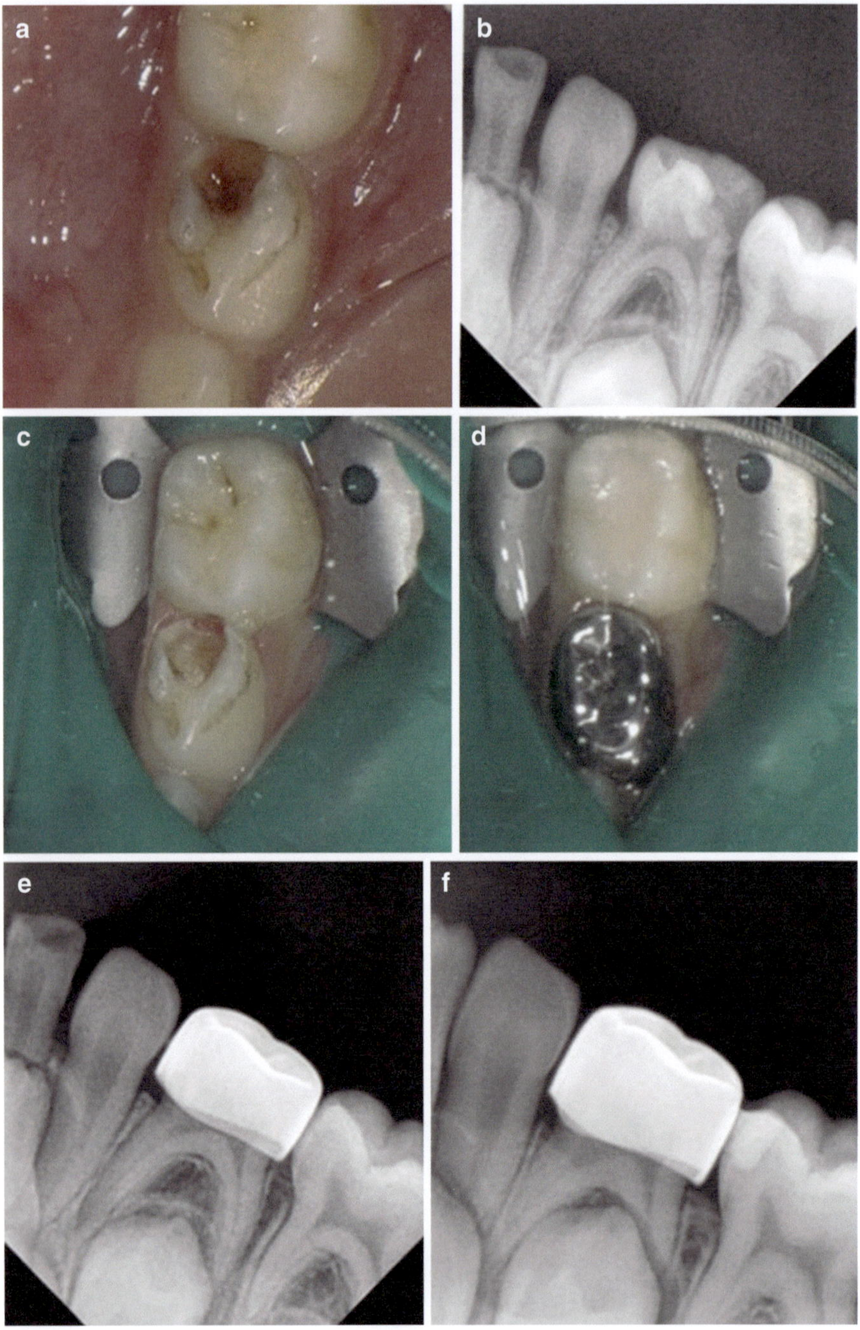

Fig. 8.4 Extensive stage lesion seen on mandibular primary left first molar (**a**). The tooth was asymptomatic and did not show clinical and radiographic signs of pulpal pathology (**b**). Selective Caries Removal performed on the floor of the lesion (**c**). The tooth was restored with a Stainless Steel Crown to ensure coronal seal (**d**). Radiograph taken at 1-year (**e**) and three-year follow-up (**f**)

8.3.6 Do Liners Have a Role in IPT?

CSCs used as liners in SCR have not improved the success rate of IPT in primary teeth. Placement of GIC in contact with the carious dentin either as a restoration or as a luting cement for a crown has been shown to be as successful. The coronal seal after pulp capping is more critical to the success of IPT than the capping material itself [33–35].

8.4 Direct Pulp Capping (DPC)

Direct Pulp Capping (DPC) is performed when a pinpoint exposure (one millimeter or less) of the pulp is encountered during cavity preparation or following a traumatic injury; a biocompatible material is placed in contact with the exposed pulp tissue and the tooth is restored [5, 36, 37].

8.4.1 What Are the Indications of DPC?

Mechanical exposure is one that occurs during cavity preparation after Complete Caries Removal (CCR) and there is sound dentin surrounding the exposure site [5]. Earlier, these exposures occurred more frequently during complete caries excavation or while flattening the pulpal floor as a part of cavity preparation to receive an amalgam restoration. The contemporary practice of caries management recommends Selective Caries Removal (SCR) in primary molars with extensive-stage lesions and has considerably reduced the chances of mechanical exposure [5, 10, 20].

During SCR, the clinician may still accidentally expose the pulp due to the subjective nature of the layers of carious dentin. This should be considered a carious exposure and not a mechanical one. An attempt to do DPC in such instances is associated with questionable prognosis due to preexisting pulpal inflammation, possible bacterial contamination, and areas of focal necrosis seen in carious lesions, the extent of which cannot be judged clinically [38, 39]. While carious exposures capped with Calcium Silicate Cements (CSCs) have shown improved success rates, DPC in mechanical exposures continue to show better results in primary teeth [38].

8.4.2 What Are the Different Direct Pulp Capping Agents?

Earlier, Calcium Hydroxide (CH) was the most widely used DPC agent. In recent years, CSCs have become the preferred DPC agents. Histological studies have shown that the highly alkaline CH induces chronic inflammation and liquefaction necrosis when placed in direct contact with pulp tissue. The resultant dentinal bridge formed is irregular with multiple tunnel defects. Additionally, CH is highly soluble and provides poor seal. In carious exposures in primary teeth, CH can often stimulate the undifferentiated mesenchymal cells to form odontoclasts leading to an elevated risk of internal resorption or obliteration of root canals. Hence, it should not be used in primary teeth [40–42].

When placed as DPC agents, CSCs release calcium oxide that react with the pulpal tissue to form calcium hydroxide. This reaction induces only mild inflammation in the dentinopulpal complex stimulating the formation of a much thicker and consistent hard tissue dentin bridge. They have low solubility and establish a better seal than CH [41]. The success rate of DPC declines over time for Calcium Hydroxide, while Calcium Silicate Cements perform better [43–45].

8.4.3 Direct Pulp Capping Technique

- If a pinpoint exposure occurs, place a moist cotton pellet on the exposure site.
- Examine the area around the exposure to determine if it is a mechanical or carious exposure.
- A layer of Calcium Silicate Cement (Mineral Trioxide Aggregrate/Biodentine™) is placed covering the exposure site and allowed to set.
- The final restoration must be placed at the same appointment [5]. (Figs. 8.5 and 8.6).

Following a Direct Pulp Capping procedure, bacterial leakage through the final restoration is considered more detrimental to the outcome than bacterial contamination at the treatment time. This finding underlines the need for the placement of a full coronal restoration to ensure an excellent coronal seal after completion of the procedure [2, 40].

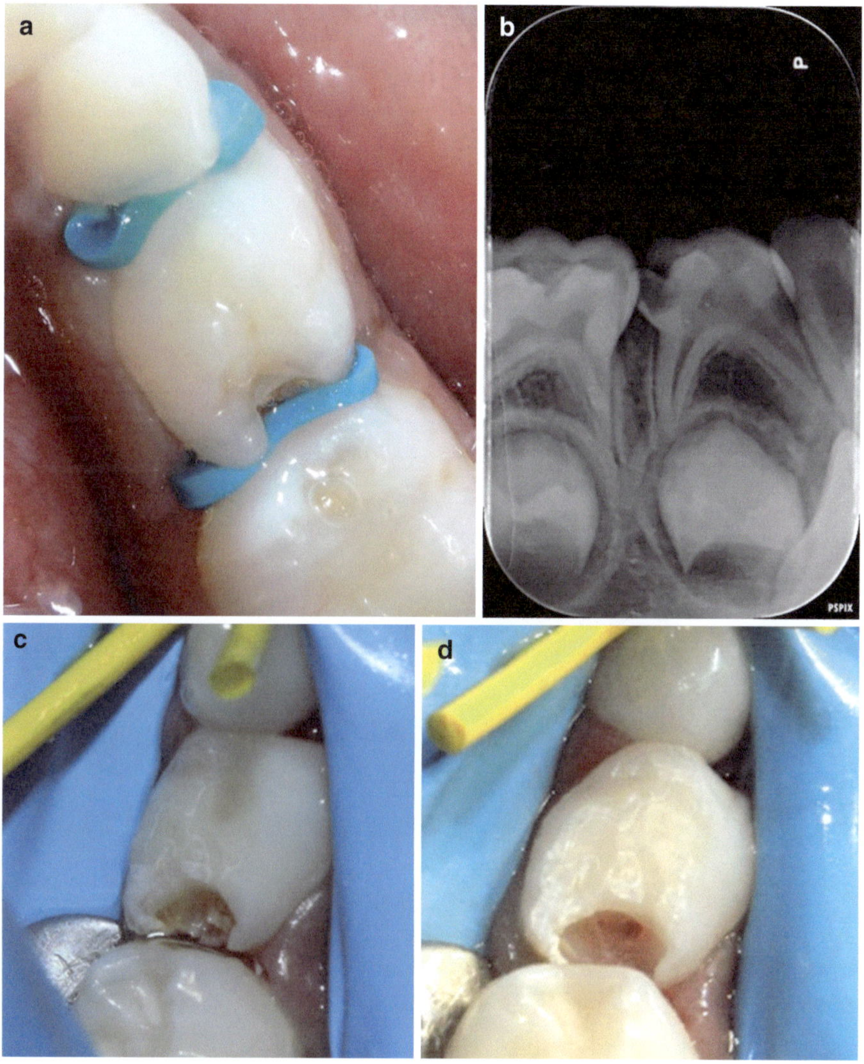

Fig. 8.5 Extensive stage lesion seen on the mandibular primary right first molar (**a**). Radiograph shows a radiolucency almost involving the distal pulp horn. (**b**). The cavity was widened to access the lesion for carious tissue removal (**c**). Mechanical carious exposure seen surrounded by sound dentin (**d**). Calcium Silicate Cement as capping agent placed on the exposure (**e**). The tooth was restored with a Stainless Steel Crown to ensure coronal seal (**f**). The 5-year follow-up shows uneventful physiological exfoliation of the treated tooth (**g**). (Image Courtesy: Dr Abhishek Soni, India)

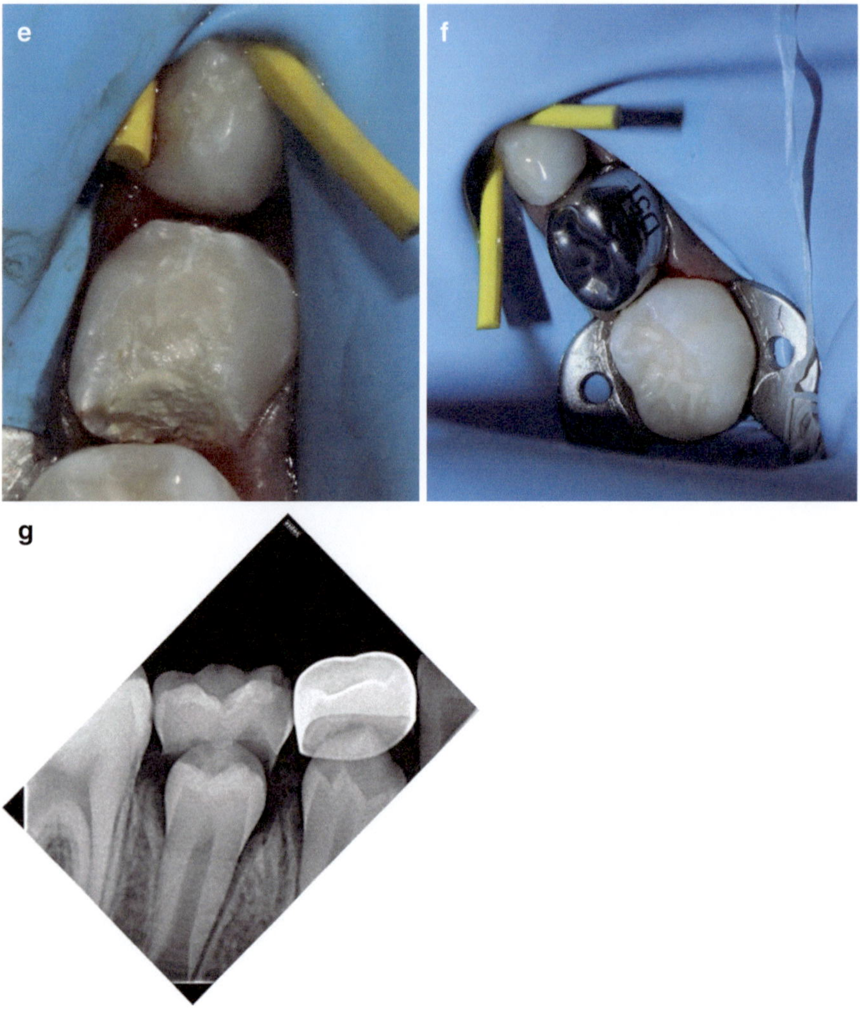

Fig. 8.5 (continued)

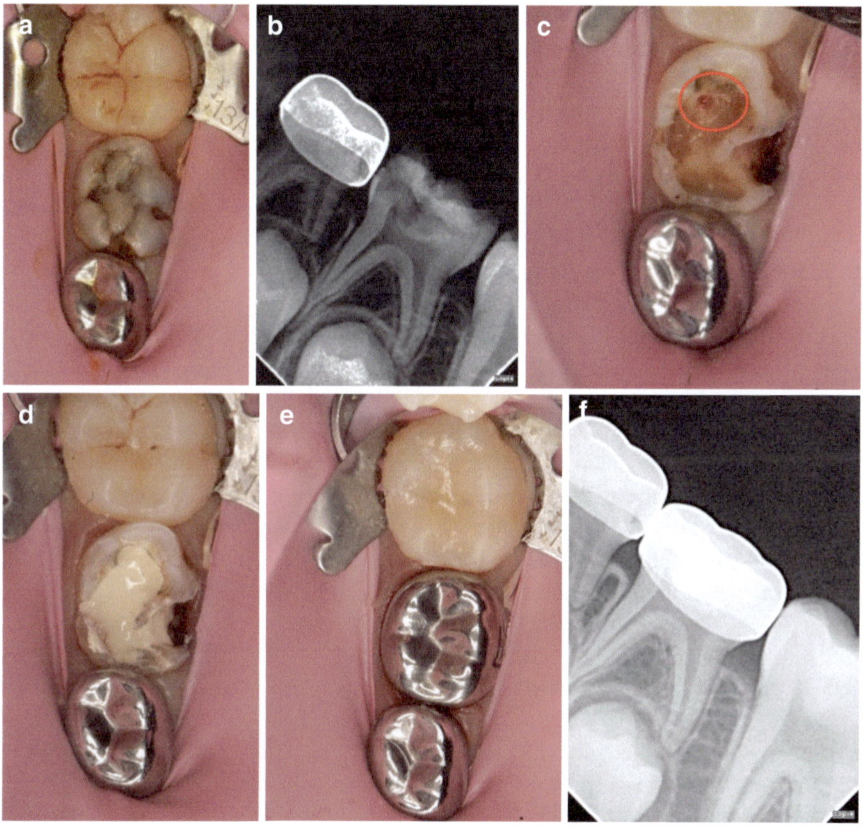

Fig. 8.6 Secondary carious lesion in mandibular primary left second molar. The tooth was asymptomatic (**a**). Radiolucency seen approaching the pulp with absence of periapical pathology (**b**). Mechanical exposure seen surrounded by sound dentin (**c**). Calcium Silicate Cement was placed on the exposure (**d**), and tooth was restored with a Stainless Steel Crown to ensure coronal seal (**e**). Immediate post-operative radiograph (**f**). (Courtesy: Dr Abhishek Soni, India)

8.5 Pulpotomy

A pulpotomy involves the complete removal of the coronal portion of the dental pulp, followed by the placement of a suitable dressing or medicament that will promote healing and preserve vitality of the tooth [5].

8.5.1 What Are the Indications of Pulpotomy?

Pulpotomy is indicated in mechanical exposures larger than pinpoint (>1 mm) or carious exposures in extensive-stage lesions in primary teeth that are asymptomatic or show signs and symptoms limited to reversible pulpitis (Figs. 8.7 and 8.8) [4, 5, 10, 19, 28]. While the indications appear similar to the Direct Pulp Capping (DPC) procedure, the size of the exposure and the presence of carious dentin around the exposed vital pulp decide the treatment choice between DPC and pulpotomy. If the operator is unsure of the pulpal status in extensive-stage lesions, a prophylactic pulpotomy can be performed to ascertain if the pulp is vital.

8.5.2 Pulpotomy Medicaments

Historically, formocresol was considered the gold standard for single-visit pulpotomies. Concerns with its toxicity profile have led to the emergence of newer agents like Ferric Sulfate that caused minimal insult to the pulp [46]. The introduction of Calcium Silicate Cements revolutionized healthy radicular pulp. The current guidelines recommend using Mineral Trioxide Aggregate (MTA) as the material of choice for pulpotomy in primary teeth, as it has a higher success rate and excellent clinical performance compared to other agents [5, 47–49]. The other material with a similar success rate is Biodentine™ [50]. Calcium hydroxide is not recommended as a pulpotomy agent in primary teeth [5].

8.5.3 Pulpotomy Technique

- The tooth is anesthetized and a rubber dam placed before performing the procedure to ensure the pulp chamber and radicular pulp remain free from salivary contamination.
- The walls of the lesion must be completely excavated to avoid bacterial infiltration before gaining access to the pulp chamber.
- A no.5 sterile round bur is used to access the pulp from the exposure site and the chamber is deroofed.
- The coronal pulp must be inspected under magnification to rule out the presence of necrotic tissue or exudate which make the tooth unsuitable for pulpotomy.
- A bleeding pulp irrespective of the color and the time taken to achieve hemostasis is a vital pulp.
- A sterile sharp spoon excavator or a round bur is used to remove the remaining coronal pulp tissue including all tissue tags, to avoid leaving behind pulp that may hemorrhage.
- Hemostasis is achieved with placement of a cotton pellet soaked in saline.
- Place MTA or Biodentine™ in a thickness of 1.5 to 2 mm covering the floor of the chamber.
- If MTA is used, a moist sterile cotton pellet is placed with minimal pressure and the material is allowed to set.
- Place a Glass Ionomer Cement or Intermediate Restorative Material followed by a full coronal restoration. (Figs. 8.7 and 8.8).

The long-term success of a pulpotomy is dependent on the placement of an extracoronal restoration on the tooth, as this ensures that marginal leakage is avoided [2, 32].

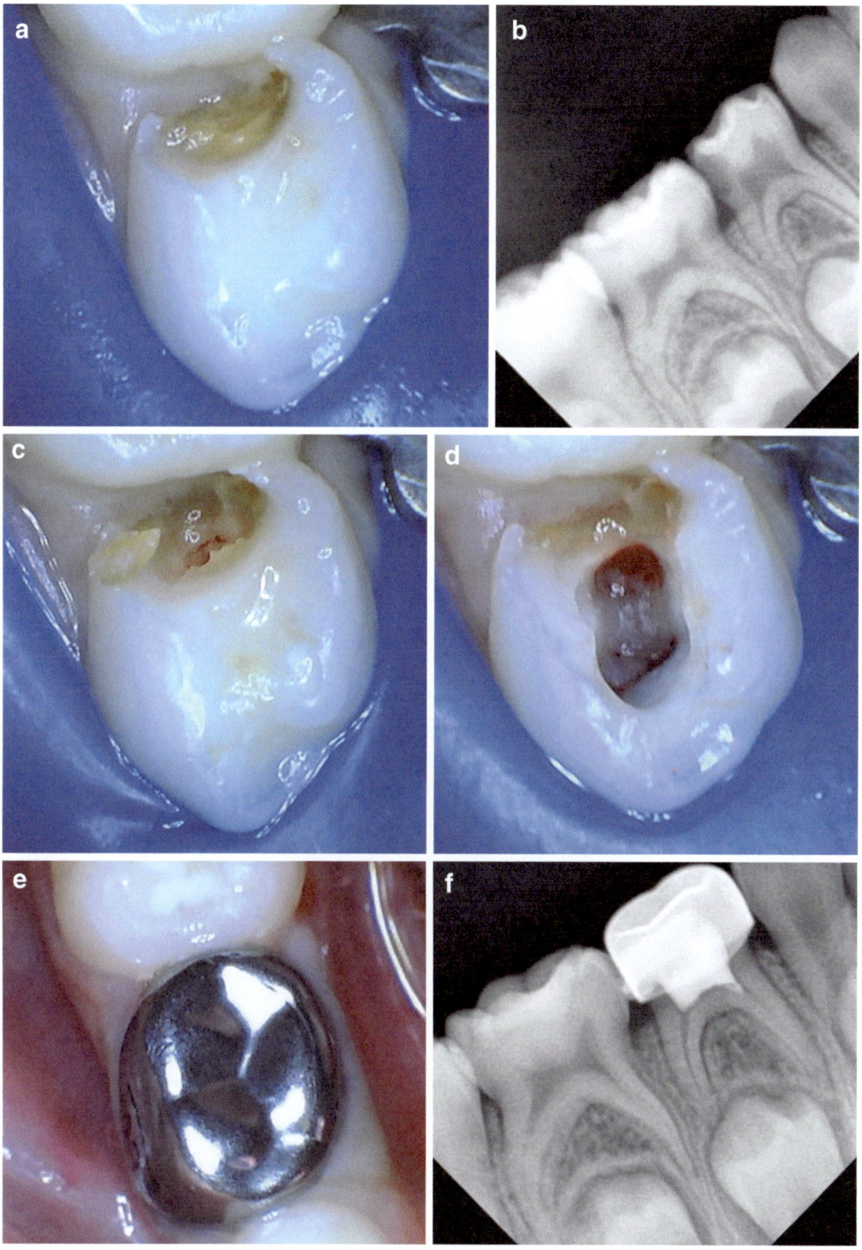

Fig. 8.7 Extensive stage lesion in mandibular primary right first molar (**a**). Radiograph shows a radiolucency approaching the pulp and the absence of periapical pathology (**b**). Carious exposure occurred during Selective Caries Removal (**c**). Access opening performed for pulpotomy and haemostasis achieved at the canal orifices (**d**). MTA placed on the canal orifices and the tooth restored with Glass Ionomer Cement and Stainless Steel Crown (**e**). Post-operative radiograph taken (**f**)

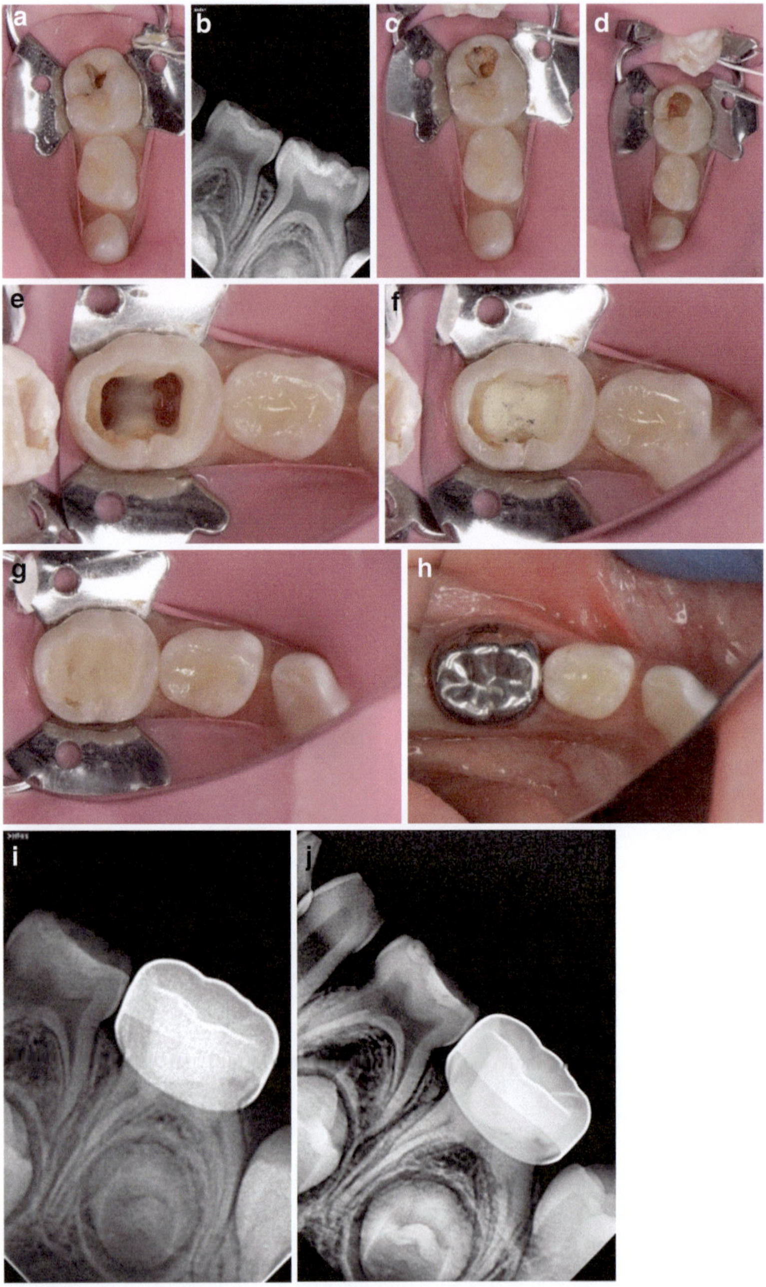

Fig. 8.8 Extensive stage lesion in mandibular primary left second molar (**a**). Radiolucency approaching the pulp and the absence of periapical pathology (**b**). Carious exposure seen during Selective Caries Removal (**c**, **d**). Pulpotomy performed, Calcium Silicate Cement placed on the canal orifices and the tooth restored with Glass Ionomer Cement followed by a Stainless Steel Crown (**e**–**h**). Post-operative radiograph (**i**). Two-year follow-up (**j**). (Image courtesy: Dr Abhishek Soni, India)

8.6 Concluding Remarks

In teeth with extensive-stage lesions that are asymptomatic or show symptoms of reversible pulpitis only, IPT can be performed even if there is soft caries overlying the pulp. If a carious exposure occurs during Selective Caries Removal, pulpotomy using Calcium Silicate Cements can be performed if the pulp appears vital under magnification. While DPC is indicated in mechanical exposures, it must be performed with caution in small carious exposures. Vital Pulp Therapy procedures should not be performed in teeth with a history of spontaneous or nocturnal pain, history of dentoalveolar abscess or facial swelling and presence of root resorption or periapical radiolucency (Fig. 8.9).

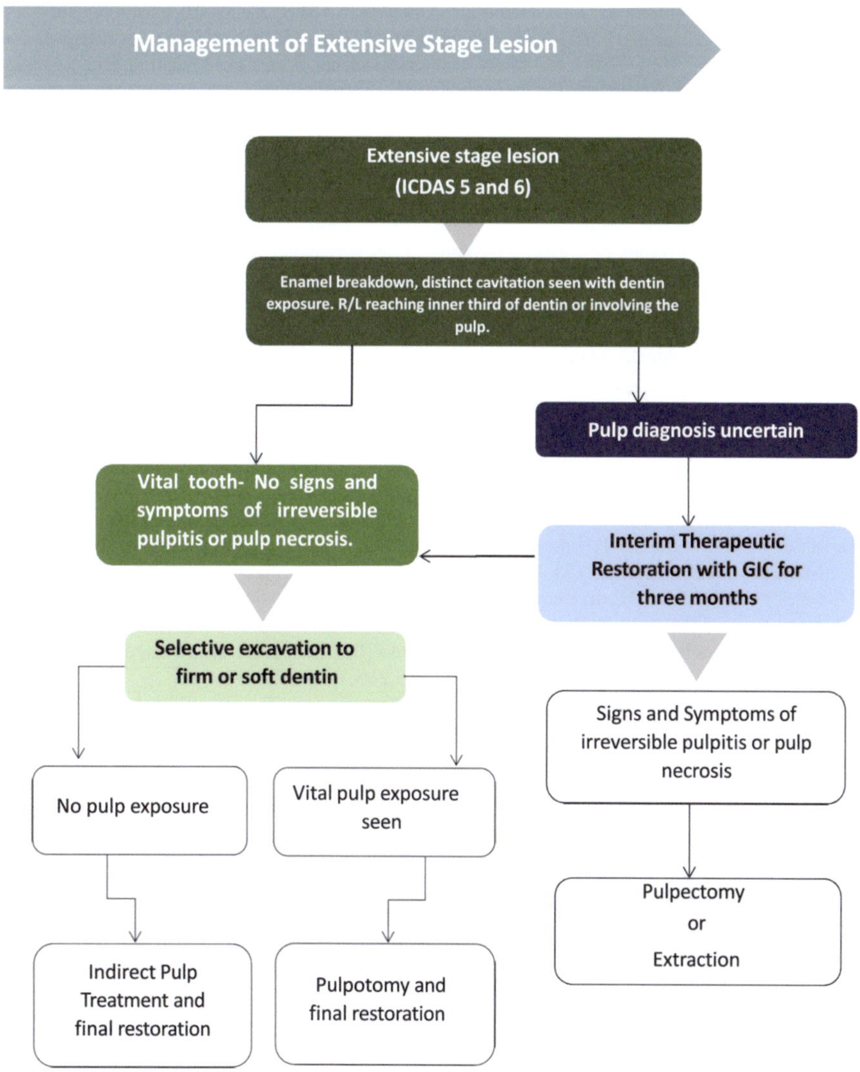

Fig. 8.9 Management of extensive stage lesions

References

1. Baume LJ. The biology of pulp and dentine. Monogr Oral Sci. 1980;8:1–246.
2. Vij R, Coll JA, Shelton P, Farooq NS. Caries control and other variables associated with success of primary molar vital pulp therapy. Pediatr Dent. 2004;26(3):214–20.
3. Ricucci D, Siqueira JF Jr, Li Y, Tay FR. Vital pulp therapy: histopathology and histobacteriology-based guidelines to treat teeth with deep caries and pulp exposure. J Dent. 2019;86:41–52.
4. Coll JA, Dhar V, Chen CY, et al. Use of vital pulp therapies in primary teeth 2024. Pediatr Dent. 2024;46(1):13–26.
5. American Academy of Pediatric Dentistry. Pulp therapy for primary and immature permanent teeth. The reference manual of pediatric dentistry. Chicago: American Academy of Pediatric Dentistry; 2024. p. 466–74.
6. Kratunova E, Silva D. Pulp therapy for primary and immature permanent teeth: an overview. Gen Dent. 2018;66(6):30–8.
7. Alsadat FA, El-Housseiny AA, Alamoudi, Alnowaiser AM. Conservative treatment for deep carious lesions in primary and young permanent teeth. Niger J Clin Pract. 2018;21(12):1549–56.
8. Ismail AI, Pitts NB, Tellez M, et al. The international caries classification and management system (ICCMS™) an example of a caries management pathway. BMC Oral Health. 2015;15(Suppl 1):S9.
9. Martignon S, Pitts NB, Goffin G, et al. CariesCare practice guide: consensus on evidence into practice. BDJ. 2019;227(5):353–62.
10. IAPD. Foundational articles and consensus recommendations: pulp therapy for primary and young permanent teeth; 2022. http://www.iapdworld.org/2022_12_pulp-therapy-for-primary-and-young-permanent-teeth.
11. Fusayama T. Two layers of caries dentine-diagnosis and treatment. Oper Dent. 1979;4:63–70.
12. Fusayama T. New concepts in operative dentistry: differentiating two layers of carious denitin and using an adhesive resin. Quintessence Pub. Co; 1980. p. 61–156.
13. Ogawa K, Yamashita Y, Ichijo T, Fusayama T. The ultrastructure and hardness of the transparent layer of human carious dentin. J Dent Res. 1983;62(1):7–10.
14. Smith AJ, Murray PE, Sloan AJ, Matthews JB, Zhao S. Trans-dentinal stimulation of tertiary dentinogenesis. Adv Dent Res. 2001;15(1):51–4.
15. Wambier DS, dos Santos FA, Guedes-Pinto AC, Jaeger RG, Simionato MR. Ultrastructural and microbiological analysis of the dentin layers affected by caries lesions in primary molars treated by minimal intervention. Pediatr Dent. 2007;29(3):228–34.
16. Innes N, Schwendicke F, Frencken J. An agreed terminology for carious tissue removal. Monogr Oral Sci. 2018;27:155–61.
17. Innes NPT, Frencken JE, Bjørndal L, et al. Managing carious lesions: consensus recommendations on terminology. Adv Dent Res. 2016;28(2):49–57.
18. Ricketts D, Lamont T, Innes NP, Kidd E, Clarkson JE. Operative caries management in adults and children. Cochrane Database Syst Rev. 2013;28:CD003808.
19. AAE position statement on vital pulp therapy. J Endodont. 2021;47(9):1340–4.
20. Duggal M, Gizani S, Albadri S, Krämer N, Stratigaki E, Tong HJ, Seremidi K, Kloukos D, BaniHani A, Santamaría RM, Hu S. Best clinical practice guidance for treating deep carious lesions in primary teeth: an EAPD policy document. Eur Arch Paediatr Dent. 2022;23(5):659–66.
21. Besic F. The fate of bacteria sealed in dental cavities. J Dent Res. 1943;22:349–54.
22. Maltz M, de Oliveira E, Fontanella V, Bianchi R. A clinical, microbiologic, and radiographic study of deep caries lesions after incomplete caries removal. Quintessence Int. 2002;33:151–15.
23. Lula EC, Monteiro-Neto V, Alves CM, Ribeiro CC. Microbiological analysis after complete or partial removal of carious dentin in primary teeth: a randomized clinical trial. Caries Res. 2009;43(5):354–8.

24. Dhillon IK, Hong CH, Hu S, Sim YF, Goh BKC, Duggal MS, Sriram G. Accuracy of the American Association of Endodontists diagnostic criteria for assessing pulp health in primary teeth. Clin Oral Investig. 2023;27(10):6043–53.
25. Soxman JA. Handbook of clinical techniques in pediatric dentistry. 1st ed. Wiley Blackwell; 2015. p. 47–50.
26. Coll JA, Campbell A, Chalmers NI. Effects of glass ionomer temporary restorations on pulpal diagnosis and treatment outcomes in primary molars. Pediatr Dent. 2013;35(5):416–21.
27. American Academy of Pediatric Dentistry. Policy on interim therapeutic restorations (ITR). The reference manual of pediatric dentistry. Chicago: American Academy of Pediatric Dentistry; 2024. p. 107–8.
28. Coll JA, Dhar V, Chen CY, Crystal YO, Guelmann M, Marghalani AA, AlShamali S, Xu Z, Glickman GN, Wedeward R. Use of vital pulp therapies in primary teeth 2024. Pediatr Dent. 2024;46(1):13–26.
29. Dhar V, et al. Evidence-based clinical practice guideline on restorative treatments for caries lesions: a report from the American dental association. JADA. 2023;154(7):551–66.
30. Alves FB, Hesse D, Lenzi TL, Guglielmi CD, Reis A, Loguercio AD, Carvalho TS, Raggio DP. The bonding of glass ionomer cements to caries-affected primary tooth dentin. Pediatr Dent. 2013;35(4):320–4.
31. Mickenautsch S, Yengopal V, Banerjee A. Pulp response to resin-modified glass ionomer and calcium hydroxide cements in deep cavities: a quantitative systematic review. Dent Mater. 2010;26(8):761–70.
32. Hilton TJ. Keys to clinical success with pulp capping: a review of the literature. Oper Dent. 2009;34(5):615–25. https://doi.org/10.2341/09-132-0.
33. Miotti LL, Vissotto C, De Nardin L, de Andrades MB, Tuchtenhagen S, Münchow EA, Emmanuelli B. Does the liner material influence pulpal vitality in deep carious cavities submitted to selective caries removal? A network meta-analysis review. Clin Oral Investig. 2023;27(12):7143–56.
34. Lourenço N, Jorge PK, Ambrosio EC, Vitor LL, Rios D, Cruvinel T, Machado MA, Oliveira TM. Is cavity lining really necessary after selective caries removal in primary teeth? Pesquisa Brasileira em Odontopediatria e Clínica Integrada. 2024;24:e23012.
35. Santos PS, Pedrotti D, Braga MM, Rocha RD, Lenzi TL. Materials used for indirect pulp treatment in primary teeth: a mixed treatment comparisons meta-analysis. Braz Oral Res. 2017;18:31.
36. Çalışkan MK, Güneri P. Prognostic factors in direct pulp capping with mineral trioxide aggregate or calcium hydroxide: 2- to 6-year follow-up. Clin Oral Investig. 2017;21(1):357–67.
37. Matoug-Elwerfelli M, ElSheshtawy AS, Duggal M, Tong HJ, Nazzal H. Vital pulp treatment for traumatized permanent teeth: a systematic review. Int Endod J. 2022;55(6):613–29.
38. Garrocho-Rangel A, Esparza-Villalpando V, Pozos-Guillen A. Outcomes of direct pulp capping in vital primary teeth with cariously and non-cariously exposed pulp: a systematic review. Int J Paediatr Dent. 2020;30(5):536–46.
39. Ouni M, Kallel I, Douki N. Direct pulp capping of carious immature tooth using bioactive material: a case report. SAGE Open Med Case Rep. 2022;10:2050313X221087565.
40. Sujlana A, Pannu PK. Direct pulp capping: a treatment option in primary teeth?? Pediatr Dent J. 2017;27(1):1–7.
41. Witherspoon DE. Vital pulp therapy with new materials: new directions and treatment perspectives–permanent teeth. Pediatr Dent. 2008;30(3):220–4.
42. Modena KC, Casas-Apayco LC, Atta MT, Costa CA, Hebling J, Sipert CR, Navarro MF, Santos CF. Cytotoxicity and biocompatibility of direct and indirect pulp treatment materials. J Appl Oral Sci. 2009;17:544–54.
43. Canoğlu E, Güngör HC, Uysal S. Direct pulp capping of primary molars with calcium hydroxide or MTA following hemorrhage control with different medicaments: randomized clinical trial. Pediatr Dent. 2022;44(3):167–73.

44. Jha S, Namdev R, Singhal R, Goel N, Singhal P, Rani R. Comparative evaluation of effectiveness of TheraCal LC, MTA, and calcium hydroxide in direct pulp capping in primary molars: randomized clinical study. Int J Clin Pediatr Dent. 2023;16(Suppl 2):213–9.
45. Mente J, Hufnagel S, Leo M, Michel A, Gehrig H, Panagidis D, Saure D, Pfefferle T. Treatment outcome of mineral trioxide aggregate or calcium hydroxide direct pulp capping: long-term results. J Endodont. 2014;40(11):1.
46. Ranly DM. Pulpotomy therapy in primary teeth: new modalities for old rationales. Pediatr Dent. 1994;16:403.
47. Lin PY, Chen HS, Wang YH, Tu YK. Primary molar pulpotomy: a systematic review and network meta-analysis. J Dent. 2014;42(9):1060–77.
48. Tewari N, Goel S, Mathur VP, O'Connell AC, Johnson RM, Rahul M, Sultan F, Goswami M, Srivastav S, Ritwik P. Success of medicaments and techniques for pulpotomy of primary teeth: an overview of systematic reviews. Int J Paediatr Dent. 2022;32(6):828–42.
49. Taneja S, Singh A. Evaluation of effectiveness of calcium hydroxide and MTA as pulpotomy agents in permanent teeth: a meta-analysis. Pediatr Dent J. 2019;29(2):90–6.
50. Stringhini Junior E, Dos Santos MG, Oliveira LB, Mercadé M. MTA and biodentine for primary teeth pulpotomy: a systematic review and meta-analysis of clinical trials. Clin Oral Investig. 2019;23:1967–76.

9 Non-Vital Pulp Therapy Clinical Considerations, Chemicomechanical Preparation Including Rotary File Systems and Obturation Techniques

9.1 Introduction

Initially, pulpectomies in primary teeth only referred to the removal of the pulp. Earlier, clinicians were apprehensive of performing pulpectomies due to the difficulties encountered in adequately navigating and cleaning the tortuous root canal system in primary teeth, and causing damage to the developing permanent tooth bud [1–3]. Moreover, these procedures were performed over multiple visits testing the cooperative ability of the pediatric patient. A better understanding of treatment outcomes and technological advancements have helped substantially decrease the operating time and allow clinicians to deliver predictable results in a single visit. Pulpectomy now encompasses the removal of inflamed or necrotic pulp, cleaning and shaping the root canals, and obturation of the root with a resorbable filling material [4, 5].

9.2 How Does a Pulpectomy Differ from the Root Canal Treatment Performed in Permanent Teeth?

The clinical considerations and techniques of pulpectomy and root canal treatment vary due to certain anatomical, morphological, and histological differences between the primary and permanent teeth [3–5]. The dentinal walls of the primary roots are thinner and show a greater curvature that originates from the cervical constriction of the crown. While accessory canals are common to both dentitions, those leading to the furcation are seen more commonly in primary teeth [6, 7].

The cleaning and shaping of canals for both primary and permanent dentition involves mechanical preparation using hand or rotary files and chemical disinfection with irrigants. In primary teeth, the focus is more on chemical debridement, which along with mechanical preparation ensures adequate cleaning of the complex

H. Vyas et al., *Dental Caries and Traumatic Injuries in Pediatric Dentistry*,
https://doi.org/10.1007/978-3-031-98929-2_9

canal systems [6]. The continuous change in position of the apical foramen makes accurate working length estimation difficult. The nature of the primary tooth to undergo physiological or pathological root resorption necessitates the use of resorbable obturating materials [8, 9].

9.3 What Are the Clinical Situations in Which a Pulpectomy Is Indicated?

(i) A pulpectomy must be performed in primary teeth showing clinical signs and symptoms of irreversible pulpitis [1, 10–13] (Fig. 9.1).
  - Presence of spontaneous pain.
  - Pain that lingers after removal of stimulus
  - Nocturnal pain or pain that aggravates on posture change.
  - Acute dentoalveolar abscess.

(ii) While performing a pulpotomy, if the clinician finds necrotic tissue or exudate in the pulp chamber, a pulpectomy should be performed.

(iii) A pulpectomy is also indicated in longstanding traumatic exposures showing necrotic pulp.

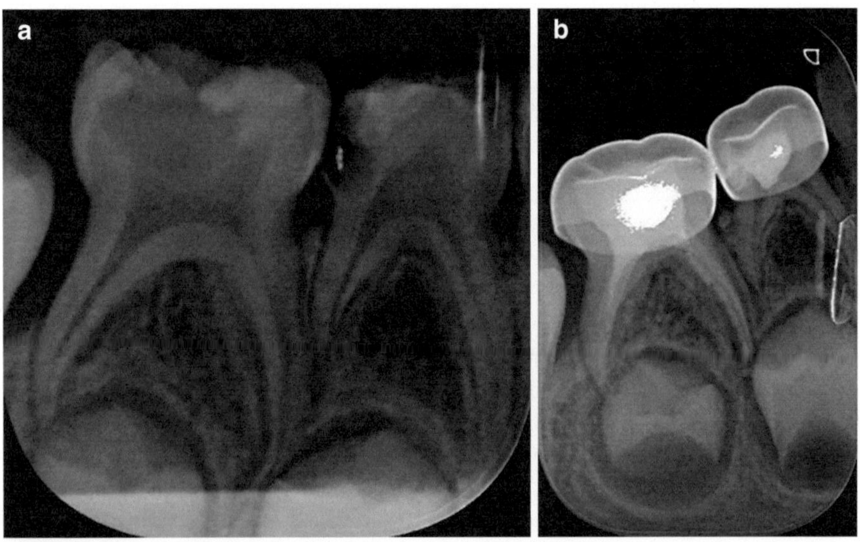

Fig. 9.1 Radiolucency involving the pulp seen in the mandibular primary right second molar. The patient history was indicative of irreversible pulpitis. The mandibular primary first molar was asymptomatic, and the radiograph showed a radiolucency approaching the pulp. No periapical changes or root resorption noted with either tooth (**a**). Pulpectomy performed with the mandibular primary second molar and a pulpotomy performed with the mandibular primary first molar. Stainless Steel Crown cemented on both teeth (**b**)

9.4 In Which Situations Should Pulpectomy Be Avoided?

Pulpectomy is contraindicated in primary teeth that are non-restorable due to inadequate crown structure or presence of subgingival caries, as the operator may not achieve a good coronal and cervical seal. Teeth showing more than 1/3rd of physiological or any pathological internal or external root resorption and extensive furcal or periapical radiolucency are not suitable candidates for pulpectomy (Fig. 9.2). It is not advised in teeth with recurrent episodes of dentoalveolar abscesses, presence of sinus tracts, or intraoral or extraoral swellings, even if complete root morphology is seen. Extraction would ensure a more predictable elimination of the source of infection allowing the periapical area to heal faster and preventing further damage to the succedaneous tooth bud. It should also be avoided in patients undergoing immunosuppressive treatment such as chemotherapy, organ transplants, or corticosteroid therapy [1, 10–13].

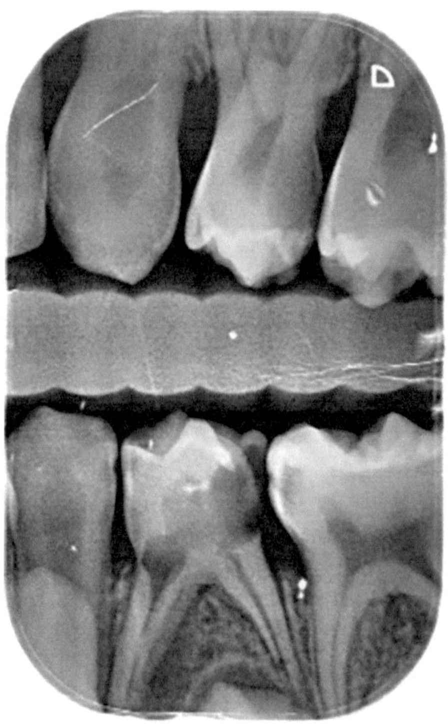

Fig. 9.2 Radiolucency involving the pulp with mandibular primary first molar. The tooth shows signs of severe internal root resorption on the radiograph and is not indicated for a pulpectomy

9.5 Pulpectomy Technique

9.5.1 Access Opening

9.5.1.1 Clinical Considerations [14–19]

Primary teeth have a thin pulpal floor, due to which furcal perforation during access opening is a possible mishap. The teeth are constricted in the cervical region at the Cementoenamel Junction (CEJ) increasing the chance of crown perforation while extending the access opening.

9.5.1.2 Procedure [5, 13–18]

- After complete excavation of caries, the access opening should always be initiated from the lingual surface of anterior teeth or occlusal surface of posterior teeth, regardless of the site of the carious lesion.
- A straight diamond point must first drill through the enamel and dentin and “drop” into the pulp chamber.
- The pulp chamber is unroofed such that the diamond point does not extend more than half into the coronal pulp space. Alternatively, a safe end bur can be used to avoid perforating the pulpal floor. It should remain parallel to the walls of the tooth to avoid perforating the crown.
- The number or anatomy of the canals dictates the cavity preparation (Fig. 9.3).

Maxillary and mandibular anterior teeth have single roots and single canals. In less than 10% of cases, mandibular incisors may be present with two canals. The access opening for maxillary incisors is triangular, with the base oriented towards the incisal edge. The mandibular incisors, as well as maxillary and mandibular canines, have an ovoid access opening.

Maxillary molars generally have three roots and three canals (mesiobuccal, distobuccal, and palatal). The most common accessory canal in maxillary second molar

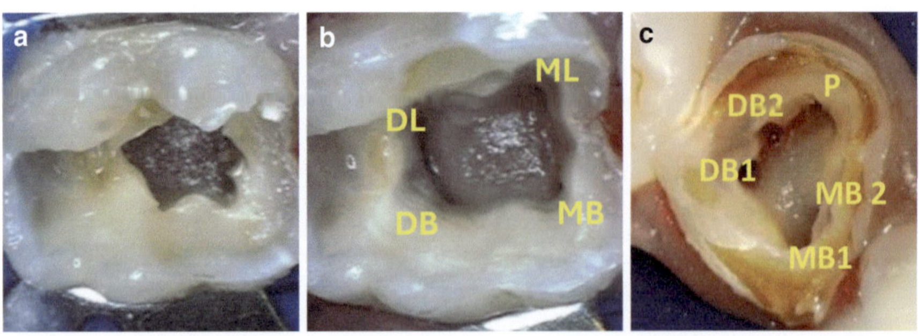

Fig. 9.3 Incomplete access cavity preparation for mandibular primary second molar with undercuts still present (**a**). Completed access cavity preparation for mandibular primary second molar showing four canal orifices (mesiobuccal, mesiolingual, distobuccal, and distolingual). (**b**). Access cavity preparation for maxillary first molar showing five canals (mesiobuccal, mesiobuccal 2, distobuccal, distolingual, and palatal canals (**c**) (Image ‘c’ courtesy: Dr Mayur Bhattad, India)

is the MB2 that is just adjacent to the mesiobuccal canal. In some cases, variations may occur, such as two roots, where the distobuccal and palatal roots are fused. Another variation is the presence of four roots, commonly seen in maxillary second primary molars with bifurcated palatal roots. The access opening for maxillary first primary molars is triangular with rounded corners, with the base towards the buccal aspect (Fig. 9.4d). For second primary molars, the access opening is rhomboid (Fig. 9.4e).

Mandibular molars have two roots but may occasionally show three. They usually have three root canals (mesiobuccal, mesiolingual, and one distal canal). Often, there could be two distal canals (distobuccal and distolingual). Rarely a middle mesial canal maybe present between the mesiobuccal and mesiolingual orifices of mandibular primary second molars. The access opening for mandibular primary first molar is ovoid, while for primary second molar, it is trapezoidal with rounded corners, with the longest side facing the buccal surface (Figs. 9.4a, b, c) [14–19].

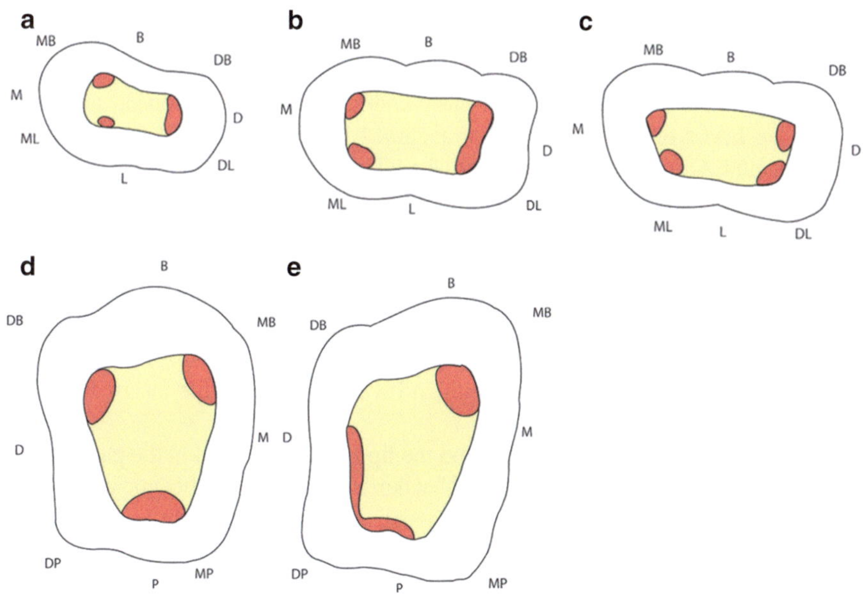

Fig. 9.4 Access opening of mandibular primary first molar showing three canal orifices, mesiobuccal, mesiolingual, and joined distobuccal and distolingual canals (**a**). Access opening of mandibular primary second molar showing three canal orifices, mesiobuccal, mesiolingual, and a large distal canal (**b**). Access opening of mandibular primary second molar showing four canal orifices, mesiobuccal, mesiolingual, distobuccal, and distolingual (**c**). Access opening of maxillary primary first molar showing three canal orifices, mesiobuccal, distobuccal, and palatal (**d**). Access opening of maxillary primary second molar showing two canal orifices, mesiobuccal and a joined distal and palatal canal (**e**)

9.5.2 Canal Scouting [14]

Following access opening, canal scouting is performed to identify and know the orientation and number of canals. It is done with ISO (International Organization of Standardization) No 8 or 10 K file. These stainless-steel files are pre-curved and are introduced up to the middle third without binding inside the canals.

9.5.3 Working Length Determination

9.5.3.1 Clinical Consideration

Establishing an accurate working length is crucial, as primary teeth have shorter root lengths and show a continuous change in the position of the apical opening. This helps in preventing over-instrumentation and reducing the risk of damage to the developing succedaneous tooth bud [20].

9.5.3.2 Electronic Apex Locators (EALs)

EALs are the gold standard for working length estimation in permanent teeth, and their use has also extended to the primary dentition [21], as the fourth- and fifth-generation EALs offer a high level of accuracy in primary teeth. In vitro studies show that an EAL can give a false-positive reading which is 0.5 mm shorter than the actual working length [21–23]. The primary tooth does not have a definite apical constriction, as seen in a permanent tooth. Instead, an apical opening is seen due to the resorptive process, and therefore a 0.5 mm short reading is beneficial, so that the instrumentation and obturation remains within the canal.

9.5.3.3 Procedure

- The working length is measured with an ISO No 8 or 10 K file inserted into the canal till a stop is felt.
- The file clip is attached to the file, and the lip hook is engaged in the patient's lip vestibule. The monitor will output "0" when the file touches the apical opening.

While the EALs are part of routine practice, at times there is no reading, or the output keeps fluctuating or shows over-instrumentation even when the file is in the coronal third of the canal. These readings may indicate resorption, excessive hemorrhaging, or infection. If the history and radiographic picture are indicative of pulpectomy with a good prognosis and the EAL readings seem incorrect, then the clinician should use the radiographic method for working length determination.

9.5.4 Radiographic Method for Working Length

9.5.4.1 Procedure

- The original diagnostic radiograph is used to estimate the working length of the tooth from a stable reference point to the root apex.

- A diagnostic file (usually no. 10–15 K file) that fits into the root canal is gently teased till it reaches the estimated working length or a definite apical stop (Fig. 9.5).
- A radiograph is taken to compare the exact position of the instrument in the root canal.
- If the file is 1 mm longer or shorter of the radiographic foramen, one should subtract or add the necessary length to obtain the root canal measurement.
- If the difference is greater than 1 mm, one should make necessary adjustments on the file and take another radiograph.

Compared to the radiographic method, it is easier to determine the working length with the EAL. It also reduces chairside time and radiation exposure while providing accurate and precise readings [21–23].

9.5.5 Cleaning and Shaping the Canals with Rotary Files

Earlier root canals in primary teeth were prepared with ISO 2% taper stainless-steel hand files (H or K files) [22, 23]. The rotary file systems were developed by Barr et al. in 2002. Rotary files made of Nickel Titanium (NiTi) are memory free and flexible enough to conform to the canal shape as compared to the stainless-steel hand files that require to be pre-curved to the canal orientation [24, 25]. Rotary files reduce working time and operator fatigue, have good cutting efficiency, prepare funnel-shaped canals that allow predictable obturation. They also reduce chances of ledging and perforation, especially in the apical third of the root canal [25, 26]. In recent years, pediatric rotary file systems have been developed having a shorter length (17 mm) ideal for the primary teeth.

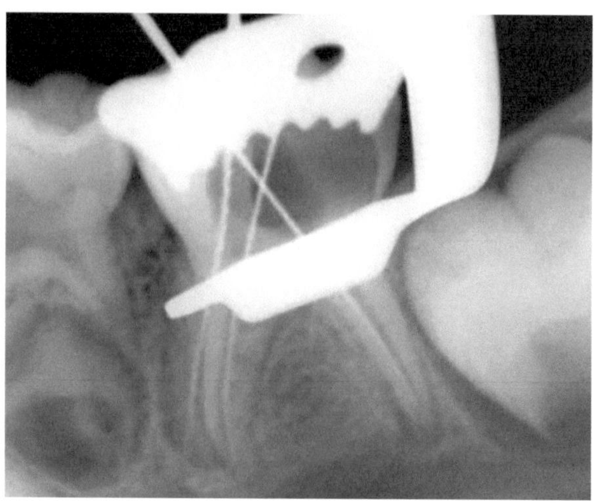

Fig. 9.5 Radiographic method for working length determination

9.5.5.1 Clinical Considerations

- *Roots* of primary teeth are predictably *curved* to cradle the succedaneous tooth.
- The *dentin near the furcation* is thin.
- Canals are *flatter, ribbon-shaped, and tortuous.*

When the roots are curved, it is important to have a straight-line access that provides a straight or outwardly flared unimpeded path from the occlusal surface to the apex. It is difficult to achieve a straight-line access in primary teeth due to significant constriction present at the cervical region along with predictable flaring of the roots (Fig. 9.6). This is pronounced in the mesial canals of mandibular molars and palatal canals of maxillary molars [23–25]. *Coronal flaring* is performed to achieve a straight-line access by using files in a brush stroke motion directed towards the wall that shows the least curvature, which in the primary tooth is away from the furcation. This not only improves straight-line access but also prevents stripping of the thin radicular areas near the furcation. Additionally, the coronal preparation prevents the apical extrusion of debris besides allowing irrigants and the obturating material to reach the apical third of the root canal. The above technique forms the basis for *the Crown Down preparation* [27].

Fig. 9.6 Curvature of roots in the maxillary and mandibular primary molars

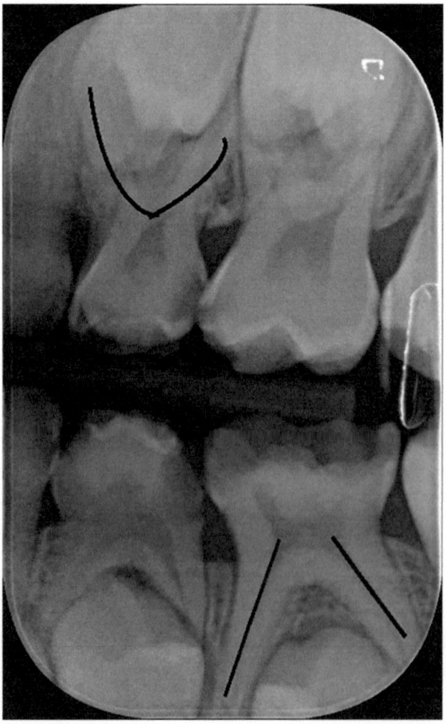

9.5.5.2 Coronal and Middle Third Preparation (Crown Down Technique)

- Rotary files having a greater taper are used to prepare the coronal and middle third of the canal. The size and taper of the file is based on the width of the canal.
- To determine the canal width, a no. 10 K or 15 K file is introduced in watch winding motion (approximately quarter turn anti-clockwise, then clockwise). A no. 10 or 15 size is selected depending on which file passes through the coronal third without binding and at the same time is not too loose in the canal.
- If it remains short of the working length, then the canal is considered *narrow*.
- If the file can be teased to the entire working length, the canal is considered *intermediate*.
- If the file is loose throughout the working length, then the canal is considered *large*.
- Various rotary file systems have devised their own protocol based on the file size and taper (4%, 6%, 8%) that are meant to be used in narrow, intermediate, and wide canals [27–30]. While most file systems have a standard taper, some systems have a variable or progressive taper within each file.
- For most rotary systems, files with 6–8% taper are the first to be introduced in the canal for *coronal and middle third preparation*. The selected file is eased into the canal with Ethylene Diamine Tetracetic Acid (EDTA) up to middle third (Table 9.1).
- The file is withdrawn using brush strokes in a direction away from the furcation.
- For further canal preparation, the rotary file systems recommend either a similar taper file with a smaller size or a file with lesser taper and larger size than that used earlier (Table 9.1).

Table 9.1 Protocol for coronal and middle third root canal preparation based on commercially available file systems

File system For coronal and middle third preparation	Narrow (File no/taper)	Intermediate (File no/taper)	Large (File no/taper)
ProTaper®	Sx—Orifice enlargement S1and S2—Coronal and middle 1/3rd		
HERO 642®	20/0.06 20/0.04	25/0.06 25/0.04	30/0.06 30/0.04
Flexmaster®	20/0.06 30/0.04	25/0.06 20/0.06	30/0.0625/0.06
Profile® ISO	25/0.06 20/0.06 25/0.04 20/0.04	30/0.06 25/0.06 30/0.04 25/0.04	35/0.06 30/0.06 35/0.04 30/0.04

The protocol for using these commercial products has been listed after visiting the manufacturers' websites on 7th May 2025. The availability of these products may vary across different regions

This systematic decrease or increase in taper or size prepares the canal in a funnel shape while preserving the dentinal wall thickness. It mitigates any adverse events like zipping, ledging, or stripping of the canal walls.

9.5.5.3 Apical Preparation [31]

The extent of apical preparation in a primary tooth is performed keeping in mind the continuous change in the position of the apical opening. Rotary file systems are available having varied tapers and sizes for canal preparation. The systems developed for permanent teeth are adapted in the primary teeth keeping the root morphology in mind. Zoremchingi et al. [32] showed the mean apical diameter of the distobuccal canal and mesiolingual canal in the maxillary and mandibular first molars were the narrowest at 0.30 and 0.38 mm, respectively. Applying this information, no. 20, 25, or 30 size files can be used for apical preparation. While 4% taper seems to be the norm, a system like the Protaper that has variable tapers of 7% (0.20 mm), 8% (0.25 mm), and 9% (0.30 mm) for their F1, F2, and F3 finishing files can also be used as the primary canal morphology does permit the use of more aggressive tapers.

9.5.5.4 Procedure

- The file chosen for apical preparation should have the same taper or one taper lesser than the file used for the middle third preparation (4% or 2% taper). (Table 9.2).
- Using rotary files with the above selected taper, apical preparation is done to a size 20. If Protaper® is being used, the preparation is done till F1(size 20).
- An ISO no. 20 file is now tapped to length, to see if it binds in the apical 1/3rd. If it binds, apical preparation is complete. This is known as apical gauging.
- If it is loose, then the canal is prepared to length with a no. 25 (2% or 4%) rotary file or a F2 Protaper® finishing file (size 25).

Table 9.2 Apical preparation protocol for different commercially available adult file systems used in pulpectomy

File system	Narrow	Intermediate	Large	Manufacturer	Country
ProFile®	20/0.04 25/0.04	25/0.04 30/0.04	30/0.04 35/0.04	Dentsply Sirona	USA
Flexmaster®	20/0.02 25/0.02 30/0.02 35/0.02	25/0.02 30/0.02 35/0.02	30/0.02 35/0.02	VDW dental	Germany
HERO 642®	20/0.02	25/0.02	30/0.02	Micromega	France
ProTaper®	F1 (20/07), F2(25/08), F3(30/09)—Finishing canal preparation to full working length			Dentsply Maillefer	Asia

The protocol for using these commercial products has been listed after visiting the manufacturers' websites on 7th May 2025. The availability of these products may vary across different regions

- An ISO file no. 25 is now tapped to length, to see if it binds to the apical one third. If it binds, the apical preparation is considered complete.
- If it is loose, the same procedure is repeated till the file size binds in the apical one third.
- In anterior teeth, file sizes can be increased to no. 35 or 40 depending on the diameter of the canal, as ascertained by apical gauging (Fig. 9.7).

At present, the choice of a rotary file system for primary teeth is based on the operator's clinical judgement and ease of use (Table 9.3).

9.5.5.5 Cleaning and Shaping the Canals with Hand Files—Is Hand Instrumentation No Longer Practiced?

Even though the use of rotary systems in pediatric endodontics is gaining more popularity, the use of hand files continues to deliver good results. ISO H or K hand files made of stainless steel or nickel titanium with increasing taper can be used for cleaning and shaping the canals. While rotary systems use the crown down technique, mechanical preparation with hand files *may be better suited* to the step back technique (Table 9.4).

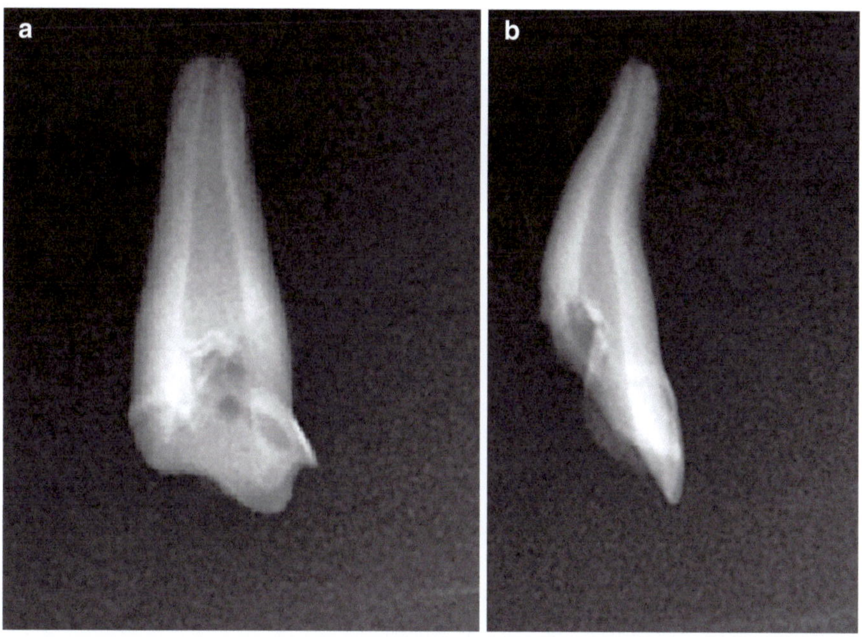

Fig. 9.7 Buccolingual view of maxillary incisor showing round tapered canals (**a**). Mesiodistal view of maxillary incisor showing ovoid, elliptical canals (**b**)

Table 9.3 Commercially available pediatric rotary file systems

File system	File no	Taper	Manufacturer	Country
Pro AF baby	Orifice enlarger (B0) —Up to middle third The canal is prepared to full length with the following files: Yellow (B1)—No 20 Red (B2) —No 25 Blue (B4) —No 30 Black (B5) —No 40	Single ring—4% Double ring—6%	Kids-e-dental	India
Prime Pedo	Starter 16 mm (orifice shaper) up to middle third 18 mm P1-white-no 15 (narrow canals) P2-white-no 25 (standard/wide canals) Endosonic file—Apical third preparation	8% 6% 6% 2%	Prime pedo	India
DXL Pro Niti files	16 mm Yellow—No 20 Red—No 25 Blue—No 30	4%	Dexel™	India
Kedo SG Kedo SG blue Kedo SG square	16 mm D1—No 25 (narrow canals) E1—No 30 (standard or wide canals) U1- no 40 (primary anterior teeth)	Variable taper	Reeganz Dental Care Pvt Ltd	India

The protocol for using these commercial products has been listed after visiting the manufacturers' websites on 7th May 2025. The availability of these products may vary across different regions

Table 9.4 Commercially available NiTi hand files

File	Manufacturer
Niti flex®	Dentsply
ProTaper® Universal	Dentsply
Endostar™	Kerr
Hero shaper®	MicroMega
NeoBlue NiTi®	Orikam

These commercial products have been listed after visiting the manufacturers' website on 7th May 2025. The availability of these products may vary across different regions

9.5.5.6 Step Back Technique

In the *step back preparation*, coronal flaring is performed after the apical instrumentation is completed. This can be performed using H or K hand files, to provide a funnel shape that ensures good obturation (Fig. 9.8).

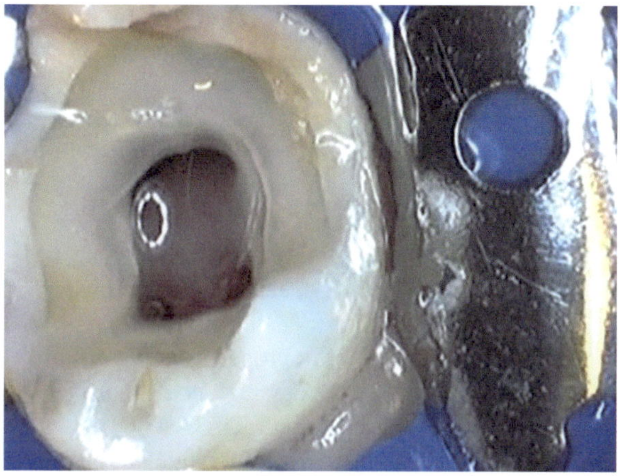

Fig. 9.8 Orifices enlarged with a greater taper file or an orifice opener to facilitate flow of the irrigant and obturating material

9.5.5.7 Procedure

- After canal scouting, the initial files (ISO nos. 10–15 K files) are slowly advanced to the full working length.
- Depending upon the width of the canal, the file size that first binds snugly at working length is selected.
- The apical preparation is done to three sizes larger than the selected file.
- The middle and coronal one third of the canals are prepared by using progressively larger files in a step back manner.
- If stainless steel files are used, the files should be pre-curved according to the root curvature.
- Instrumentation should be performed towards the lesser curvature of the tooth in a direction away from the furcation.
- After step back with every file, the canal is recapitulated with the file used for apical preparation to full working length, to ensure canal patency [33].

As the step back procedure prepares the apical one third first, there is a chance that the root canal debris may be pushed apically. Whereas the crown down technique prepares the coronal and middle third removing the infected debris from two thirds of the canal, before beginning apical preparation.

9.6 Irrigants in Pulpectomy

9.6.1 Clinical Consideration

Mechanical instrumentation does not ensure complete debridement, especially in primary molars that have thin canals with several channels and accessory recesses. Commercially available irrigants include sodium hypochlorite (NaOCL), chlorhexidine gluconate, ethyleneiaminetetraacetic acid (EDTA), citric acid, mixture of tetracycline, citric acid and detergent (Tween 80) (mixture commercially available as BioPure® MTAD® root canal cleanser, Dentsply, Tulsa, USA), and hydrogen peroxide.

The functions of an irrigant are as follows:

- Soft tissue dissolution.
- Broad antimicrobial activity.
- Lubrication and smear layer removal.
- Flushing out debris and necrotic pulpal remnants.

Each irrigant has specific properties and current literature does not support the use of one irrigant over the other. Hence, a combination of irrigants suitable to the clinical situation must be used. The AAPD recommends the use of 1% sodium hypochlorite and chlorhexidine gluconate [12].

Sodium Hypochlorite is known for its strong antibacterial activity, as it kills gram-positive and gram-negative bacteria and highly resistant yeast within the root canal system even at 1%. Unlike most irrigants, it can dissolve pulpal tissue remnants [34]. Warm NaOCl demonstrates better dissolving and disinfecting properties in permanent teeth. Warming of NaOCl can be done by either preheating the solution in a water bath or heating it inside the canal with a heat carrier (System B™, Kerr™). The tip of the carrier must be heated and placed in the canal to warm the sodium hypochlorite irrigant. The irrigant is heated for 3 to 5 s twice at an interval of 5 s to allow sufficient cooling time as continuous activation is likely to overheat the irrigant and irritate the periapical tissue [35]. The limitations of sodium hypochlorite are its inability to remove the smear layer, its unpleasant odor and taste, and it is a potential irritant, if it contacts the surrounding soft tissue [3].

Ethylenediaminetetraacetic acid (EDTA) is mostly used as a 17% neutralized solution, either as a gel or liquid. It dissolves the inorganic component and removes the smear layer within the root canal [36]. Removing the smear layer allows penetration of the irrigants into the irregularities of the root-canal system [35, 36]. During mechanical preparation, it is recommended that every file should be coated with EDTA gel prior to insertion into the canal. Besides smear layer removal, it also acts as a lubricant which reduces stress on the instruments and improves hard-tissue debridement. However, EDTA does not possess any antimicrobial activity and has little or no effect on organic tissue [36–38].

Chlorhexidene Gluconate (CHX) in 2% concentration is effective against Gram-positive and -negative bacteria, spores of bacteria, lipophilic viruses, yeast, and fungi [38]. Its primary advantages include relatively low toxicity and substantivity wherein the antimicrobial action lingers even after the irrigant is flushed from the canal [38]. Its effectivity is reduced in the presence of organic matter and it is incapable of removing biofilms and other organic debris [39, 40].

The primary function of *Normal Saline (NS)* is to lubricate the canals and flush out pulpal remnants and debris. As it has no antimicrobial activity, it must be used in conjunction with other irrigants. Normal saline must be used in between two different irrigants and as a last rinse to flush out leftover irrigant.

A preheated solution of 1% sodium hypochlorite has been found to be as effective as the 5.2% solution. This lower concentration is less irritant to the soft tissues and does not have a strong odor, which is unpleasant to children. In combination with normal saline or chlorhexidine gluconate, 1% sodium hypochlorite along with mechanical instrumentation using EDTA as a lubricant, ensures optimal cleaning and shaping of the primary root canals [41–44].

The most common *irrigation technique* is with a 24-gauge, 1.5′ beveled disposable needle bent at a 45-degree angle. While copious irrigation is advised, flushing the solution under positive pressure causes extrusion of the debris periapically. Therefore, it is recommended to place 1 or 2 drops of the irrigant in the canal with the needle inserted passively to the middle third. The plunger of the syringe is withdrawn to aspirate the irrigant and this causes movement of solution within the canal. The action of alternately expressing and aspirating the irrigant is carried out multiple times to flush out the debris [45].

There are few commercially available *irrigation systems* to assist irrigation between instrumentation. The EndoVac™ system (Kerr Dental) uses negative pressure to pull the irrigant down the root canal, and then up and away with the help of a Hi-Vac suction unit [46].

The 30G Side vent needle (Neoendo, Orikam) has a non-cutting tip with a diameter of 0.3 mm. It has single or double openings on the side to allow for irrigation. It prevents extrusion of the solution beyond the apex as this can be damaging to the periapical tissues and the succedaneous tooth.

Irrigant activation [47, 48] done with a U blade file or the Endoactivator® (Dentsply) with polyethylene tips creates ultrasonic waves that activates the irrigant and causes its movement within the complex canal system. A U blade file (Mani, INC.) can be fixed onto a special carrier attached to the ultrasonic handpiece. Alternatively, the Endoactivator® (Dentsply) is available as a separate handpiece to which a non-cutting polyethylene tip is attached. The U blade file or the polyethylene tip is inserted passively into the canal that has the desired irrigant and is activated for 10 s. The file or tip causes oscillation of the irrigants and flushes out debris. On completion of chemo-mechanical preparation, if bleeding or oozing is encountered, the canals should be re-instrumented and irrigated to remove any remnant pulpal tissue.

All the methods of irrigation described above effectively debride the root canals of primary teeth. Following every change of instrument, irrigation is performed till all debris is flushed out and no bleeding or oozing from the canal is seen. The canals are then dried using paper points and are ready for obturation.

9.7 Obturation of the Primary Tooth

9.7.1 Clinical Considerations

- As roots of the primary tooth undergo physiological resorption, the material used for obturation must also have resorptive property.
- The clinical goal of endodontic obturation is to fill the empty root canal spaces, promote sealing, and prevent microbial leakage from the apical third.

Zinc Oxide Eugenol (ZOE) was the first material recommended by Sweet in 1930 for obturating primary teeth and it continues to remain the gold standard. Studies have shown that the eugenol released in the periapical zone immediately after placement of ZOE has antimicrobial, anti-inflammatory, and analgesic properties that are useful after a pulpectomy procedure (Fig. 9.9). Also, ZOE does not dissolve easily from within the canals, thereby improving the apical seal of the obturation. A thicker consistency of ZOE may demonstrate a slower resorption rate than the primary root structure. Extrusion of a thick mix of ZOE may take months to resorb and possibly cause deflection of the succedaneous tooth [49–51].

Initially, *Calcium Hydroxide and Iodoform* were used separately as standalone root canal filling materials for primary teeth. However, it was seen that obturation with Calcium Hydroxide frequently resulted in the development of internal root resorption. On the other hand, iodoform can discolor the tooth and cause periapical irritation when extruded beyond the apex. Later, both agents were combined in commercial formulations available (Vitapex®, Neo Dental International Inc, Japan and Metapex Plus®, Meta Biomed, Korea) in a premixed syringe with similar compositions, except in slightly different percentages. The advantages of combining the two agents showed a higher success rate, slower resorption, and better handling properties. The calcium hydroxide–iodoform-based pastes resorb at a much faster rate than the primary roots. When this material extrudes into the furcal or apical areas, they either diffuse away or are resorbed in part by macrophages within 3 months. Their primary disadvantage is that they tend to resorb within the canals much prior to the exfoliation of the tooth, leaving the canals empty and causing a "hollow tube effect" (Fig. 9.10). This can cause the canals to be permeated with tissue fluid, possibly leading to reinfection [49–54].

Endoflas FS (Sanlor Laboratories S.A.S, Columbia) is available as a powder and liquid system composed primarily of ZOE and calcium hydroxide–iodoform. Due to the presence of both iodoform and eugenol, Endoflas has a broad spectrum of antibacterial efficacy and the ability to disinfect dentinal tubules and hard-to-reach accessory canals. The resorption of Endoflas® is limited to the extruded material and does not occur within the canal. This does not result in the hollow tube effect. However, if Endoflas® is mixed to a thin consistency, its eugenol content has been reported to cause periapical irritation. It also has been linked to tooth discoloration due to the presence of iodoform [49–52, 55].

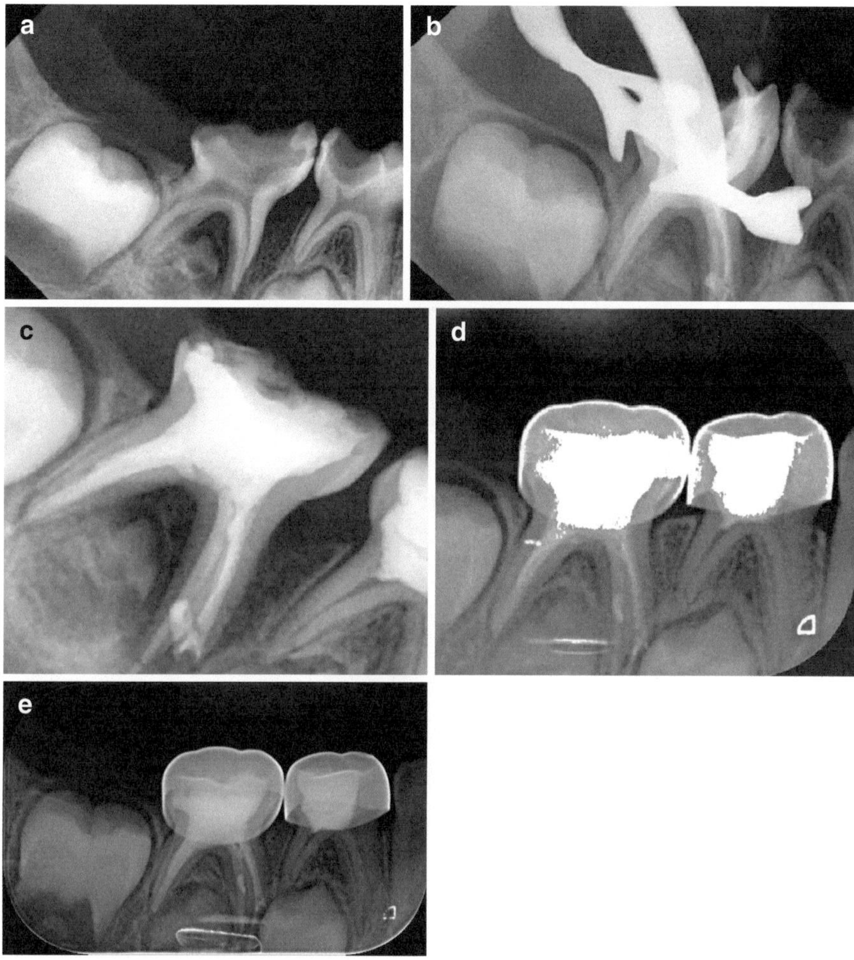

Fig. 9.9 Mandibular primary second molar showing furcal radiolucency. No signs of root resorption seen (**a**). Chemo-mechanical preparation was done and the tooth was obturated with Zinc Oxide Eugenol (**b**). Immediate postoperative follow-up (**c**). Six monthly follow-up shows complete resolution of the radiolucency (**d**). One-year follow-up (**e**)

A systematic review by Coll et al. in 2020 showed that Endoflas® and ZOE demonstrated a 90% success rate compared to the 71% success rate shown by iodoform formulations at 18 months [56]. Another systematic review by Fidaglo et al. in 2020 concluded that there was no convincing evidence to support the superiority of any material over ZOE, and both ZOE and Calcium hydroxide–iodoform formulation appear to be suitable as root canal fillings for deciduous teeth [57]. The antibacterial efficacy of ZOE was the best followed by Endoflas®, Vitapex®, and Metapex® in decreasing order [58, 59]. The AAPD guidelines recommend the use of zinc oxide

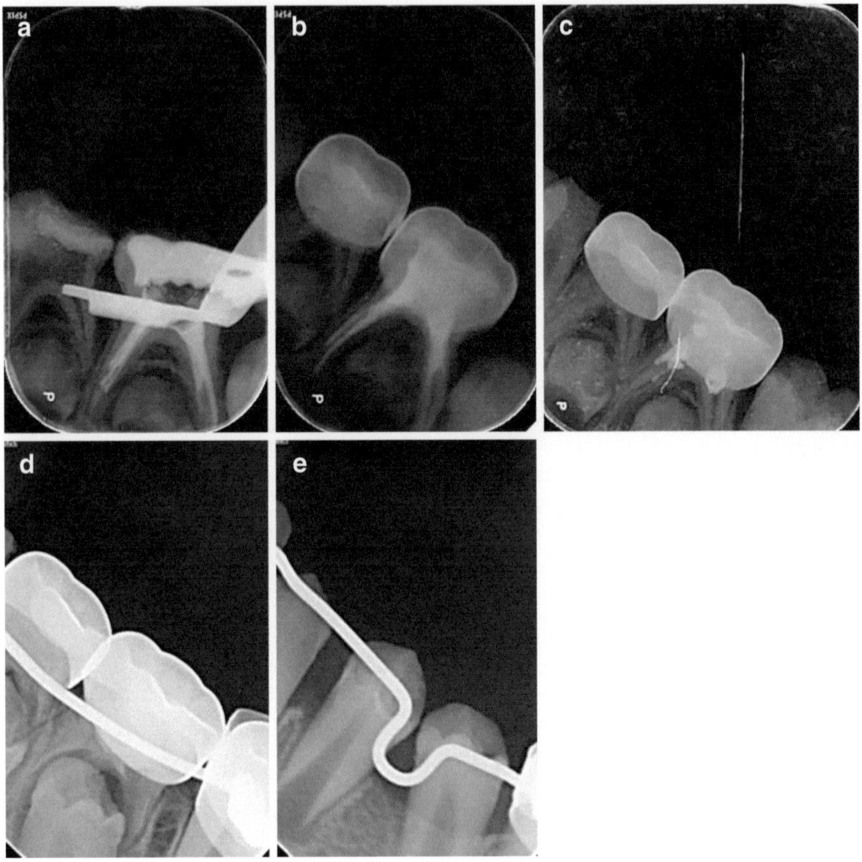

Fig. 9.10 Pulpectomized mandibular primary molar obturated with calcium hydroxide-iodoform mixture (**a**). Twelve months follow-up showing resorption of the obturating material from distal root creating a hollow tube effect (**b**). Twenty-four months follow-up showing resorption of obturating material from both mesial and distal canals (**c**). Thirty-six months follow-up (**d**). Four-year follow-up showing eruption of premolar (**e**). (Courtesy: Dr. Abhishek Soni, India)

eugenol (ZOE) and Endoflas® as obturating materials for primary teeth, that are to be retained for more than 18 months [12, 13]. The IAPD recommends Endoflas®, non-reinforced ZOE and calcium hydroxide–iodoform paste (Vitapex®, Metapex®) for pulpectomies [10].

9.8 Procedure—The Obturating Technique [60, 61]

The obturation technique depends on the choice of the root canal filling material (Table 9.5). The tooth must be isolated and residual moisture must be withdrawn from all the canals using an aspirating needle and syringe and paper points must be placed inside all the canals for drying. They should be placed 2–3 mm short of the working length and allowed to absorb the moisture in the canals.

9.8.1 Obturation with ZOE and Endoflas®

A premeasured scoop for the powder and a dropper for the liquid must be used to standardize the amount dispensed to achieve a thin or thick consistency.

9.8.2 Thin Consistency

- The thin mix should have as much powder incorporated as possible, yet thin enough to flow with a lentulospiral.

Table 9.5 Commercial formulations of calcium hydroxide and iodoform obturating materials

Commercial name	Composition	Manufacturer	Country
Vitapex®	40.4% Iodoform, 30.3% Calcium Hydroxide, and 22.4% Silicon oil	Neo Dental International Inc.	Japan
Metapex Plus®	<40% Iodoform, <40% Calcium Hydroxide, <30% Polydimethylsiloxane (Silicon oil)	Meta Biomed CO., LTD.	Korea
Endoflas	Powder Tri-iodomethane. Zinc oxide. Calcium hydroxide. Barium sulphate. Iodine dibutilorthocresol. Liquid Eugenol. Paracholorophenol.	Sanlor Laboratories S.A.S	Colombia
Diapex plus®	Calcium hydroxide + iodoform	Dia Dent®	Korea
Neopex	Calcium hydroxide + iodoform	Orikam Healthcare	India
Calplus™	Calcium hydroxide + iodoform	Prevest Denpro Ltd	India
e-Iodocal	Calcium hydroxide + iodoform	Kids-e-dental®	India
Calpex	Calcium hydroxide + iodoform	Ammdent	India

These commercial products have been listed after visiting the manufacturers' websites on 7th May 2025. The availability of these products may vary across different regions

- When carried off the glass slab, the mix should not be so runny that it drips off the instrument.
- A very thin consistency with more eugenol content is likely to extrude beyond the apex and cause irritation to the periapical tissues.
- A No. 25 lentulospiral is mounted on a contra-angle handpiece and is introduced up to the middle third of the canal and run in a clockwise direction at a slow speed.
- The obturating material is carried to the rotating lentulospiral with a cement carrier.
- On contacting the lentulospiral close to the canal orifices, the material is seen to run down the lentulospiral and into the canal.
- The lentulospiral is slowly moved within the canals to coat the walls. The obturation is complete once the material is filled to the orifice.

9.8.3 Thick Consistency

- Alternatively, a thick consistency of ZOE can be packed in increments with the help of pluggers.
- For a thick consistency, powder should be added to the mix, till it can be rolled on a glass slab with a spatula.
- A no. 40 K file should be wrapped with a thin wisp of moistened cotton so that the tip is covered with a plug of cotton. This can act as a modified plugger.
- The thick mix is placed in the pulp chamber and the above pluggers are used to push the material in the direction of each canal.
- A moistened cotton pellet placed in the pulp chamber can also be used to push a thick mix of ZOE with the help of tweezers or endodontic pluggers.

9.8.4 Obturation with Calcium Hydroxide–Iodoform Paste

- They can be directly dispensed into the canal, as they are available in the form of pressure syringes.
- The dispensing tip must not bind into the canal and must extend up to 2/3rds of the working length, well short of the apex.
- A rubber stop or marking should be placed on the tip provided by the manufacturers.
- The material must be expressed from the syringe, before placing into the canal to ensure there is no air incorporated in the obturation.
- As the material is expressed into the apical and middle third of the canal, the tip is slowly withdrawn till the material fills up to the orifice.
- The obturating material is compacted into the canal with a damp cotton pellet or plugger.
- The excess material is removed from the floor and walls of the pulp chamber.

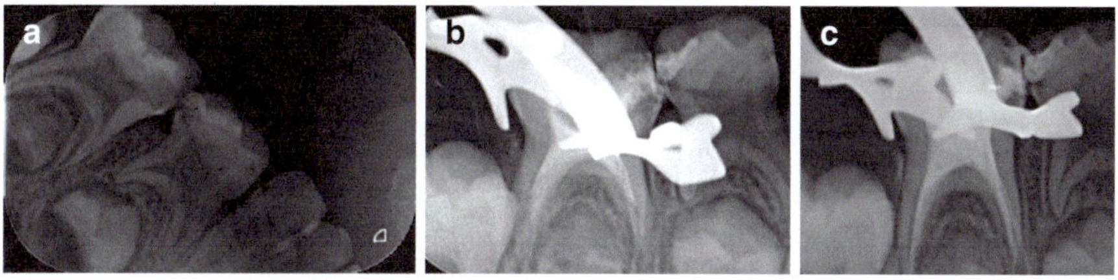

Fig. 9.11 Mandibular primary second molar indicated for pulpectomy (**a**). The immediate post-operative radiograph showed the obturation to be short by 2–3 mm in the mesial canals (**b**). The canals were re-instrumented and then re-obturated to obtain an optimal fill (**c**). (Image Courtesy: Dr. Manini Shah, India)

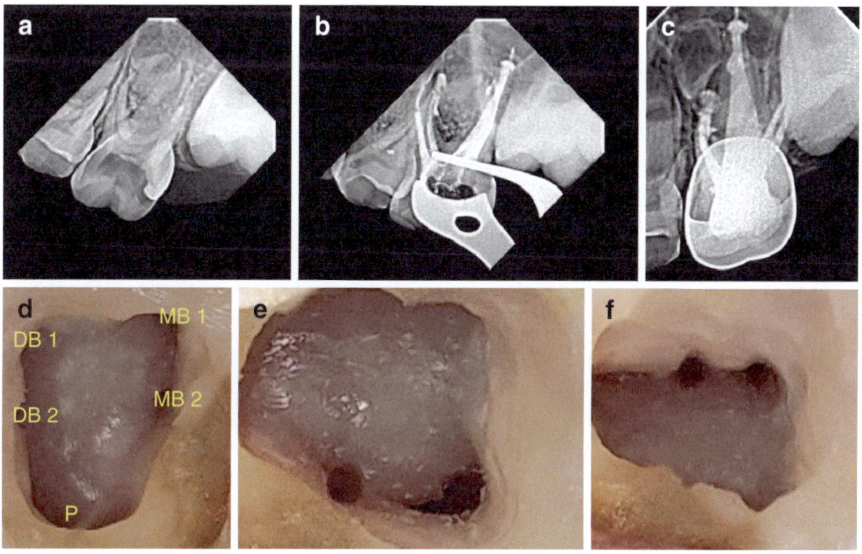

Fig. 9.12 Maxillary primary second molar showing a radiolucency involving the pulp with symptoms of irreversible pulpitis. No signs of root resorption seen (**a**). Obturation of the root canal with calcium hydroxide-iodoform paste. Five obturated canals seen with minimum extrusion of obturating material (**b, c**). Access opening revealed the presence of five orifices (**d**). Closer look at the mesial orifices (MB1 and MB2) (**e**) and distal orifices (DB1 and DB2) (**f**). (Image Courtesy: Dr. Mayur Bhattad, India)

9.8.5 Verifying the Obturation

- A radiograph is taken to determine the extent of the root canal filling. A well-prepared canal must fill without voids or should have a flush fill.

If the filling is short, re-obturation is done with the same material. A radiograph may need to be taken again to verify the obturation depending on how short the obturation was. If the obturation is still short, re-instrumentation is done as there

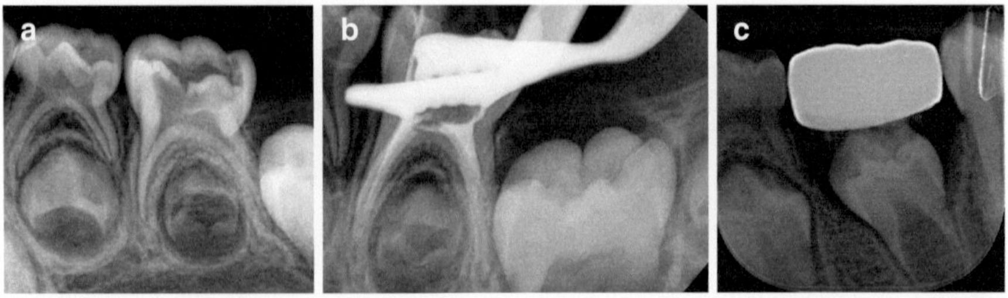

Fig. 9.13 Mandibular primary second molar indicated for pulpectomy (**a**). Pulpectomy performed and the tooth was obturated with Zinc Oxide Eugenol cement (**b**). Six-year follow-up shows uneventful exfoliation of the tooth (**c**)

may be remnant pulpal tissue, inadequate preparation of the canal or the material has set within the canal (Fig. 9.11). After verifying optimal canal fill, post obturation restoration is done with Intermediate Restorative Material (IRM) or GIC and an extracoronal restoration is placed (Fig. 9.12).

Ideally, the obturation should be flushed or remain slightly short of the apex (Fig. 9.13). Slight extrusion is acceptable, as these obturating materials will resorb over time (Fig. 9.14).

However, extrusion of the material may lead to periapical irritation, difficulty in material resorption, damage, or deflection of the succedaneous tooth (Figs. 9.14, 9.15) [62]. Excessive overfilling is unacceptable and is invariably indicative of pathological resorption around the apex, furcation or along the walls of the canal. It is advisable to perform an extraction in this clinical situation as the pulpectomy is likely to fail. The extruded material that has not hardened is irrigated and flush out of the extraction socket.

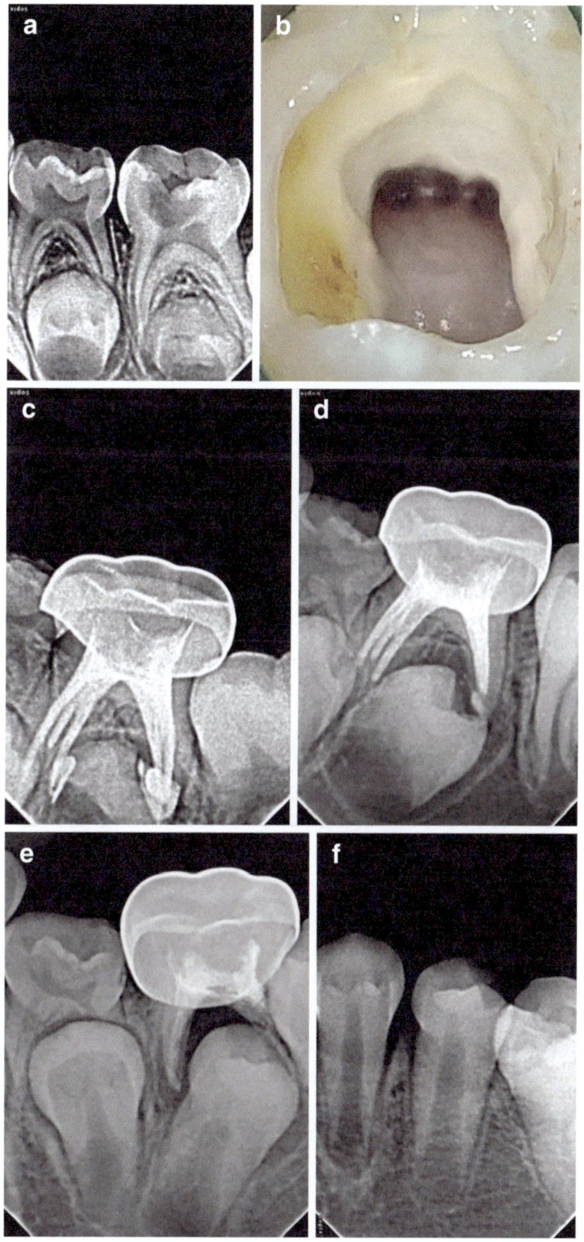

Fig. 9.14 Mandibular primary second molar showing radiolucency involving the pulp (**a**). Access opening performed and orifice of the middle mesial canal was discovered along with the mesiobuccal and mesiolingual canal orifices (**b**). Chemo-mechanical preparation was done and the tooth was obturated with calcium hydroxide-iodoform paste. Postoperative radiograph shows obturation of three mesial canals and two distal canals. Extrusion of the obturating material from mesial and distal roots seen. (**c**). Two-year follow-up shows almost complete resorption of the extruded material (**d**). Four-and-half-year follow-up shows atypical root resorption pattern with the distal root resorbing faster than medial, and deviation in the path of the succedaneous premolar (**e**). Six-year follow-up shows eruption of the premolar (**f**). (Image Courtesy: Dr. Mayur Bhattad, India)

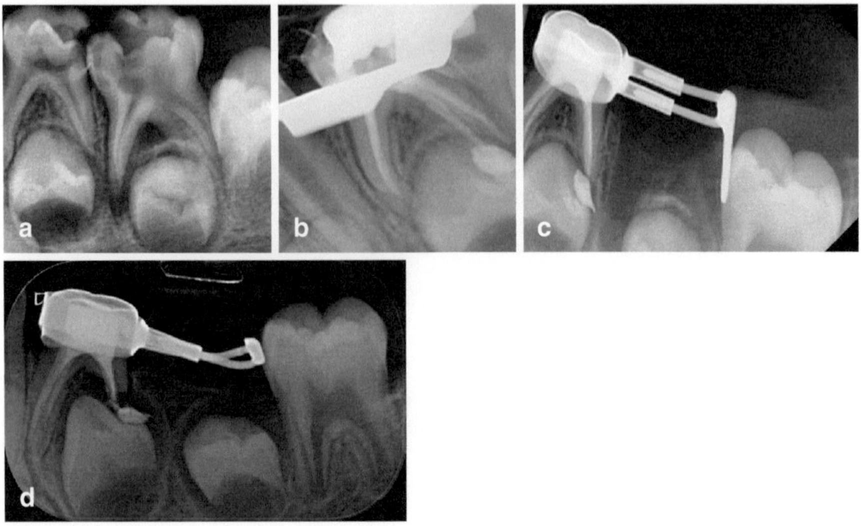

Fig. 9.15 Mandibular primary second molar had history of recurrent abscesses necessitating an extraction. The primary first molar was indicated for a pulpectomy (**a**). The tooth was obturated with Zinc Oxide Eugenol (ZOE). Extrusion of ZOE from the distal root (**b**). A Stainless Steel Crown placed on the tooth as a definitive restoration (**c**). At the 1-year follow-up, the tooth was asymptomatic and the extruded material showed some resorption (**d**)

9.9 Single Visit or Multiple Visit Pulpectomy?

Multiple visit pulpectomy involved extirpating the pulp in the first visit and in subsequent visits, the canal was instrumented and irrigated following which a closed dressing of intra-canal Calcium Hydroxide or formaldehyde was given. Overtime with better understanding and improved technique of pulpectomy backed by the successes seen in cases performed under general anesthesia, single-visit pulpectomy has become the norm [63]. Primary teeth that would have earlier been treated with multi-visit pulpectomy due to the presence of purulent exudate, recurrent abscesses, or facial swellings are no longer indicated for pulpectomy. These tooth are best treated with extraction.

9.10 The Pulpectomy Procedure Is Summarized as Below

- Anesthetize the tooth and isolate with rubber dam.
- To establish an access opening, place a straight diamond point parallel to the walls of the tooth and drill through the enamel and dentin, until a “drop” is achieved. The access should be extended until the entire chamber is deroofed and the orifice openings are identified.

- ISO No. 10 or 15 K file should be then used to scout for canals and understand the canal orientation.
- If the No. 10 or 15 K file first introduced in the canal, remains short of the provisional working length, then the canal is considered narrow. If the file can be teased to the entire working length, the canal is considered intermediate. If the file is loose throughout the working length, then the canal is considered large.
- Working length estimation must be performed using an electronic apex locator. The final working length must be kept 1–2 mm short of the estimated working length.
- In the crown down technique, coronal flaring is performed using Niti orifice openers or greater taper 4 or 6% taper files. The taper of file used, and the sequencing is based on the width of the canal and the recommendation given by the manufacturer of the chosen file system.
- For apical preparation, the files chosen should have the same taper or one taper lesser than the file used for the coronal and middle third preparation. Using rotary files with the above selected taper, apical preparation is done to a size 20. After preparation, if an ISO No. 20 file is loose in the canal, cleaning and shaping should be continued with a subsequently larger file size. Preparation is terminated at the file size, which binds in the canal.
- Intermittently, irrigation must be performed using 1% sodium hypochlorite and normal saline along with the aid of side vented needles and ultrasonic irrigation.
- After cleaning and shaping, the canal is dried with paper points and readied for obturation.
- Obturation can be done with ZOE or Calcium Hydroxide–iodoform paste or Endoflas.
- ZOE and Endoflas can be placed inside the canals using either a lentulospiral mounted on a slow-speed handpiece or with the use of hand instruments such as pluggers. Calcium Hydroxide and Iodoform are available in a pressure syringe and must be dispensed directly into the canal.
- A radiograph must be taken to assess the quality of the obturation. After verifying optimal canal fill, post-obturation restoration can be done with an Intermediate Restorative Material or Glass Ionomer Cement and a full coronal restoration must be placed.

9.11 Endodontic Mishaps

9.11.1 Intra-canal File Separation

Fracture of an endodontic file may result due to [59]:

- Complex root canal anatomy (extremely curved canals).
- Incorrect instrumentation technique (lack of lubrication, excessive torque, or speed used).
- Mechanical fatigue of endodontic file.

The separated instrument produces a mechanical obstruction of the root canal, impeding further cleansing, which significantly compromises the treatment prognosis. When an instrument fractures in the coronal or middle third of the canal, the clinician can attempt retrieval with suitable size gates glidden drills and/or ultrasonic agitation under Dental Operating Microscope (DOM). The more apically the segment is located, retrieval becomes as complicated [60, 61]. Unlike in a permanent tooth, bypassing the instrument to complete the pulpectomy is not a viable option in a primary tooth. If left behind, it may be embedded as a foreign body as the primary roots will resorb around it and also affect the eruption of the succedaneous tooth. It is advised to extract the tooth and place a space maintainer, if the instrument cannot be retrieved.

To avoid instrument breakage [64–66]:

- Ensure straight-line access to the canals to decrease the stress on the instrument; and avoid forcing the instrument.
- In case of excessively curved or cervically flared roots, it is recommended to instrument the canals with hand files, up to ISO file no. 20, before introducing rotary files.
- Assess the instrument condition before usage for unwinding, deformation, or shiny spots of wear.
- Repeat usage of files should be as per manufacturer's recommendations.

Iatrogenic perforation may occur during opening the pulp chamber or lateral or strip perforation while instrumenting the canal walls. This manifests as hemorrhaging during chemo-mechanical preparation of the canal or as excessive extrusion of the obturating material. Irrespective of the cause and presentation, such teeth should be extracted.

To avoid iatrogenic perforation:

- During access opening, a straight diamond point must remain parallel to the walls of the tooth to avoid perforating the crown.
- The straight diamond point must not extend more than half the length of its head into the coronal pulp space while unroofing the chamber,
- Alternatively, a safe end bur can be used to avoid perforating the pulpal floor.

To avoid strip or lateral perforation:

- Examine the preoperative radiograph to determine the thickness of the radicular dentin.
- The file must be used in a brush stroke motion and is directed away from the furcation.

Sodium hypochlorite accident manifests as pain and localized or wide-spread swelling [67]. While irrigation with sodium hypochlorite (NaOCl) is important to accomplish the goal of chemical shaping, one negative property of NaOCl is that it can cause soft tissue inflammation if it is expressed outside the confines of the root canal.

It is clinically manifested as severe pain and mild to moderate swelling with or without bluish purple discoloration of the skin.

To avoid sodium hypochlorite accident [68]:

- Isolation with rubber dam is mandatory.
- The irrigation needle should not bind to the canal and be kept short of the working length.
- Do not force the irrigants into the canal so as to prevent apical extrusion.
- Use a side-vent needle.
- Use negative pressure irrigation such as the EndoVac system™.

The treatment is palliative and aimed at reducing pain and swelling with the help of analgesics and antibiotics. The complete recovery will take between 2 and 6 weeks depending on the severity of the accident.

9.12 Concluding Remarks

Single visit pulpectomy is now the standard of care for treating primary teeth with extensive-stage lesions that show symptoms of irreversible pulpitis or non-vitality. The complex anatomy of primary teeth necessitates careful chemo-mechanical preparation of the root canal system. While the choice of rotary or hand instrumentation can be decided based on operator preference, rotary instrumentation reduces the working time and helps in achieving an optimal canal fill [69–71]. Zinc Oxide Eugenol cement and Calcium Hydroxide–iodoform-based obturating materials that undergo resorption along with the primary roots are used based on operator preference. In clinical situations, where the tooth in concern is associated with recurrent dentoalveolar abscesses, facial swelling, significant root resorption, extraction may be a pragmatic treatment option that immediately removes the focus of infection and safeguards the health of the developing permanent successor.

References

1. Curzon ME, Kennedy DB, Roberts JF. Kennedy's paediatric operative dentistry. John Wright; 1996.
2. Moskovitz M, Tickotsky N. Pulpectomy and Root Canal Treatment (RCT) in primary teeth. In: Fuks A, Peretz B, editors. Pediatric endodontics. Springer: Cham; 2016. https://doi.org/10.1007/978-3-319-27553-6_6.
3. Tannure PN, Barcelos R, Portela MB, Gleiser R, Primo LG. Histopathologic and SEM analysis of primary teeth with pulpectomy failure. Oral Surg Oral Med Oral Pathol Oral Radiol Endod. 2009;108:e29–33.
4. Dummett CO Jr, Kopel HM. Pediatric endodontics. In: Ingle JI, Bakland LK, editors. Endodontics. 5th ed. Hamilton: BC Decker Inc.; 2002. p. 861–902.

5. Camp JH, Fuks AB. Pediatric endodontics: endodontic treatment for the primary and young permanent dentition. In: Cohen S, Hargreaves K, editors. Pathways of the pulp. 9th ed. St. Louis: Mosby Elsevier; 2006. p. 822–82.
6. Dammaschke T, Witt M, Ott K, Schäfer E. Scanning electron microscopic investigation of incidence, location, and size of accessory foramina in primary and permanent molars. Quintessence Int. 2004 Oct;35(9):699–705.
7. Wrbas KT, Kielbassa AM, Hellwig E. Microscopic studies of accessory canals in primary molar furcations. ASDC J Dent Child. 1997;64(2):118–22.
8. Ounsi HF. Endodontic considerations in pediatric dentistry: a clinical perspective. Int Dent SA. 2009;11(2):40.
9. Marsh SJ, Largent MD. A bacteriological study of the pulp canals of infected primary molars. J Dent Child. 1967;34:460–70.
10. https://iapdworld.org/wp-content/uploads/2022/08/2022_12_pulp-therapy-for-primary-and-young-permanent-teeth.pdf
11. https://www.sdcep.org.uk/media/2zbkrdkg/sdcep-prevention-and-management-of-dental-caries-in-children-2nd-edition.pdf
12. Coll JA, Dhar V, Vargas K, Chen CY, Crystal YO, AlShamali S, Marghalani AA. Use of non-vital pulp therapies in primary teeth. Pediatr Dent. 2020;42(5):337–49.
13. American Academy of Pediatric Dentistry. Pulp therapy for primary and immature permanent teeth. The reference manual of pediatric dentistry. Chicago: American Academy of Pediatric Dentistry; 2024. p. 466–74.
14. Goerig AC, Camp JH. Root canal treatment in primary teeth: a review. Pediatr Dent. 1983;5(1):33–7.
15. McDonald RE, Avery DR. Development and morphology of the primary teeth. In: McDonald and Avery Dentistry for the Child and Adolescent-E-Book; 2010. p. 41.
16. Mathewson RJ, Primosch RE. Fundamentals of pediatric dentistry. Quintessence Books; 1995.
17. Nelson SJ, Wheeler RC. Wheeler's dental anatomy, physiology, and occlusion. Elsevier; 2010.
18. Hibbaed ED. Morphology of the root canals of the primary molar teeth. J Dent Child. 1957;24:250–7.
19. Ahmed HMA, Musale PK, El Shahawy OI, Dummer PMH. Application of a new system for classifying tooth, root and canal morphology in the primary dentition. Int Endod J. 2020 Jan;53(1):27–35.
20. Zurcher E. The anatomy of the root canals of the teeth of the deciduous dentition and of the first permanent molars. New York: William Wood & Co.; 1925.
21. Vitali FC, Santos PS, Cardoso M, Massignan C, Garcia LDFR, Bortoluzzi EA, Teixeira CDS. Are electronic apex locators accurate in determining working length in primary teeth pulpectomies? A systematic review and meta-analysis of clinical studies. Int Endod J. 2022 Oct;55(10):989–1009.
22. Ahmad IA, Pani SC. Accuracy of electronic apex locators in primary teeth: a meta-analysis. Int Endod J. 2015 Mar;48(3):298–307.
23. Paradiso D, Tullio A, Bensi C. Working length determination in primary teeth pulpectomy: a systematic review and meta-analysis. Aust Endod J. 2022;49:444.
24. George S, Anandaraj S, Issac JS, John SA, Harris A. Rotary endodontics in primary teeth – a review. Saudi Dent J. 2016 Jan;28(1):12–7.
25. Barr ES, Kleier DJ, Barr NV. Use of nickel-titanium rotary files for root canal preparation in primary teeth. Pediatr Dent. 2000;22(1):77–8.
26. Baker BCW, Parsons KC, Mills PR, Williams GL. Anatomy of root canals. IV deciduous teeth. Aust Dent J. 1975;20(101):7.
27. Ruddle C. The Protaper technique: shaping the future of endodontics. Endod Top. 2005;10:187. Available at: https://www.endoruddle.com/tc2pdfs/41/PTTechnique_Mar2005.pdf
28. http://www.endodonziamauroventuri.it/Preparazione%20rotante%20Ni-Ti/Hero%20Shaper%20-%20Brochure.pdf
29. https://vdw.pl/en/index.php?controller=attachment&id_attachment=14

30. https://www.dentsplysirona.com/content/dam/master/regions-countries/north-america/product-procedure-brand/endodontics/product-categories/files-motors-lubricants/hand-instruments/profile-iso/documents/END-DFU-ProFile-ISO-04-Hand-Files-EN.pdf
31. Ruddle C. Finishing the apical one third: endodontic considerations. Endod Top. 2005; Available at: https://www.endoruddle.com/tc2pdfs/44/ApicalOneThird_May2002.pdf
32. Zoremchhingi JT, Varma B, Mungara J. A study of root canal morphology of human primary molars using computerized tomography: an in vitro study. J Indian Soc Pedod Prev Dent. 2005;23:7–12.
33. Li G. Preparation of the root canal: equipment and technique for cleaning, shaping, and irrigation. Endod Prac. 1988:179–227.
34. Stojicic S, Zivkovic S, Qian W, Zhang H, Haapasalo M. Tissue dissolution by sodium hypochlorite: effect of concentration, temperature, agitation, and surfactant. J Endod. 2010;36:1558–62.
35. Sirtes G, Waltimo T, Schaetzle M, Zehnder M. The effects of temperature on sodium hypochlorite short-term stability, pulp dissolution capacity, and antimicrobial efficacy. J Endod. 2005;31:669–71.
36. Hülsmann M, Heckendorff M, Lennon A. Chelating agents in root canal treatment: mode of action and indications for their use. Int Endod J. 2003 Dec;36(12):810–30.
37. da Silva LA, Sanguino AC, Rocha CT, Leonardo MR, Silva RA. Scanning electron microscopic preliminary study of the efficacy of SmearClear and EDTA for smear layer removal after root canal instrumentation in permanent teeth. J Endodont. 2008;34(12):1541–4.
38. Patterson S. In vitro and in vivo studies of the effect of the disodium salt of the ethylenediamine tetra-acetate on human dentine and its endodontic implications. Oral Surg Oral Med Oral Pathol. 1963;16:83–103.
39. Kotula R, Bordacova J. Uber die wirkung der aethylendia mintetraessigsaure auf die mundflora. Dtsch Stomatol. 1969;19(9):575–81.
40. Rosenthal S, Spångberg L, Safavi K. Chlorhexidine substantivity in root canal dentin. Oral Surg Oral Med Oral Pathol Oral Radiol Endod. 2004;98(4):488–92.
41. Khademi AA, Mohammadi Z, Havaee SA. Evaluation of the antibacterial substantivity of several intra-canal agents. Aust Endod J. 2006;32(3):112–5.
42. Naenni N, Thoma K, Zehnder M. Soft tissue dissolution capacity of currently used and potential endodontic irrigants. J Endodont. 2004;30(11):785–7.
43. Okino LA, Siqueira EL, Santos M, Bombana AC, Figueiredo JA. Dissolution of pulp tissue by aqueous solution of chlorhexidine digluconate and chlorhexidine digluconate gel. Int Endod J. 2004;37(1):38–41.
44. Pozos-Guillen A, Garcia-Flores A, Esparza-Villalpando V, Garrocho-Rangel A. Intracanal irrigants for pulpectomy in primary teeth: a systematic review and meta-analysis. Int J Paediatr Dent. 2016 Nov;26(6):412–25.
45. Grossman L. Irrigants and intra-canal medicaments. In: Grossman L, editor. Endodontic practice. 10th ed. Philadelphia: Lea and Febiger; 1982. p. 343.
46. Abarajithan M, Dham S, Velmurugan N, Valerian-Albuquerque D, Ballal S, Senthilkumar H. Comparison of Endovac irrigation system with conventional irrigation for removal of intracanal smear layer: an in vitro study. Oral Surg Oral Med Oral Pathol Oral Radiol Endod. 2011 Sep;112(3):407–11.
47. Haapasalo M, Shen Y, Qian W, Gao Y. Irrigation in endodontics. Dent Clin. 2010;54(2):291–312.
48. Uroz-Torres D, González-Rodríguez MP, Ferrer-Luque CM. Effectiveness of the EndoActivator system in removing the smear layer after root canal instrumentation. J Endodont. 2010 Feb;36(2):308–11.
49. Barcelos ZOE. Paste Pulpectomues outcome in primary teeth: a systematic review. J Clin Pediatr Dent. 2011;35:241–8.
50. Ahmed HM. Pulpectomy procedures in primary molar teeth. Eur J Gen Dent. 2014;3:3–10.
51. Mortazavi M, Mesbahi M. Comparison of zinc oxide and eugenol, and Vitapex for root canal treatment of primary teeth. Int J Paediatr Dent. 2004;14:417–24.
52. Rajsheker S, Mallineni SK, Nuvvula S. Obturating materials used for Pulpectomy in primary teeth–a review. J Dent Craniofacial Res. 2018;3(1):3.

53. Nurko C, Ranly DM, García-Godoy F, Lakshmyya KN. Resorption of a calcium hydroxide/iodoform paste (Vitapex) in root canal therapy for primary teeth: a case report. Pediatr Dent. 2000;22(6):517–20.
54. Mekkriangkrai D, Nakornchai S, Jirarattanasopha V. Success rate and related factors of Vitapex Pulpectomy in primary teeth: a retrospective study. Eur J Dent. 2023 Oct;17(4):1163–9.
55. Fuks AB, Eidelman E, Pauker N. Root fillings with Endoflas in primary teeth: a retrospective study. J Clin Pediatr Dent. 2002 Fall;27(1):41–5.
56. Coll JA, Vargas K, Marghalani AA, Chen CY, AlShamali S, Dhar V, Crystal YO. A systematic review and meta-analysis of nonvital pulp therapy for primary teeth. Pediatr Dent. 2020;42(4):256–461.
57. Barja-Fidalgo F, Moutinho-Ribeiro M, Oliveira MA, de Oliveira BH. A systematic review of root canal filling materials for deciduous teeth: is there an alternative for zinc oxide-eugenol? ISRN Dent. 2011;2011:367318.
58. Fernandes MO, Matos J, Maia LC, Fidalgo TKS. Antimicrobial activity of root canal filling pastes used in pediatric dentistry. Gen Dent. 2021;69(5):34–7.
59. Najjar RS, Alamoudi NM, El-Housseiny AA, Al Tuwirqi AA, Sabbagh HJ. A comparison of calcium hydroxide/iodoform paste and zinc oxide eugenol as root filling materials for pulpectomy in primary teeth: a systematic review and meta-analysis. Clin Exp Dent Res. 2019;5(3):294–310.
60. Dalsania, et al. Obturating techniques in pediatric dentistry: literature review. J Curr Med Res Opin. 2020;16:3.
61. Nalawade HS, Lele GS, Walimbe H. Outcome of zinc oxide eugenol paste as an Obturating material in primary teeth Pulpectomy: a systematic review. J Dent Res Rev. 2017;4(4):90.
62. Coll JA, Sadrian R. Predicting pulpectomy success and its relationship to exfoliation and succedaneous dentition. Pediatr Dent. 1996;18(1):57–63.
63. Tirupathi SP, Krishna N, Rajasekhar S, Nuvvula S. Clinical efficacy of single-visit Pulpectomy over multiple-visit Pulpectomy in primary teeth: a systematic review. Int J Clin Pediatr Dent. 2019;12(5):453–9.
64. Pk M, Sc K, As S. Broken instrument retrieval with indirect ultrasonics in a primary molar. Eur Arch Paediatr Dent. 2016 Feb;17(1):71–4.
65. Parashos P, Gordon I, Messer HH. Factors influencing defects of rotary nickel titanium endodontic instruments after clinical use. JOE. 2004;30:722–5.
66. Garrocho-Rangel A, et al. Clinical management of intra-pulp canal broken endodontic files in primary teeth. Lit Rev Odovtos, San José. 2021;23(2):14–8.
67. Farook SA, Shah V, Lenouvel D, et al. Guidelines for management of sodium hypochlorite extrusion injuries. Br Dent J. 2014;271:679–84.
68. Vivekananda Pai AR. Factors influencing the occurrence and progress of sodium hypochlorite accident: a narrative and update review. J Conserv Dent. 2023;26(1):3–11.
69. Padmawar N, Pawar N, Tripathi V, Banerjee S, Tyagi G, Joshi SR. Comparative analysis of rotary versus manual instrumentation in paediatric pulpectomy procedures: a systematic review and meta-analysis. Aust Endod J. 2025 Apr;51(1):181–96.
70. Manchanda S, Sardana D, Yiu CKY. A systematic review and meta-analysis of randomized clinical trials comparing rotary canal instrumentation techniques with manual instrumentation techniques in primary teeth. Int Endod J. 2020 Mar;53(3):333–53.
71. Khadmi I, Hamrouni A, Chouchene F. Different outcomes of rotary and manual instrumentation in primary teeth pulpectomy: a systematic review and meta-analysis. Eur Arch Paediatr Dent. 2025;26:423.

Managing the Immature Tooth: Apexogenesis, Apexification, and Regenerative Endodontics

10

10.1 Introduction

Among the various challenges in treating young children, the management of pulpally involved immature permanent teeth is certainly high on the list. Continued root development is an important goal of pulp therapy in immature permanent teeth. The pulp vitality and stage of root development are critical factors in deciding the type of pulp therapy to be performed. In immature teeth with a vital pulp, apexogenesis techniques such as Indirect Pulp Treatment (IPT), Direct Pulp Capping (DPC), and pulpotomy are indicated. On the other hand, non-vital immature teeth are treated with apexification or Regenerative Endodontic Procedures [1, 2].

10.2 Apexogenesis

Apexogenesis is a Vital Pulp Therapy (VPT) procedure to encourage continued physiological development and formation of the root end. The procedure preserves pulpal vitality and encourages thickening of the radicular dentin along with root lengthening, leading to apical closure. Consequently, the crown root ratio improves, reducing the risk of root fracture [3].

10.3 What is the Rationale Behind Apexogenesis?

An open apex is found in newly erupted teeth, and apical closure appears only around 3 years after the eruption. In this duration, any injury causing pulpal degeneration could damage the viability of Hertwig's Epithelial Root Sheath (HERS) and arrest root development. Apexogenesis procedures that are minimally invasive aim to protect the vitality of the pulp, thereby allowing the epithelial root sheath to continue root development and maturation [4–8].

H. Vyas et al., *Dental Caries and Traumatic Injuries in Pediatric Dentistry*,
https://doi.org/10.1007/978-3-031-98929-2_10

10.4 What Are the Indications for Apexogenesis?

To allow for apexogenesis, procedures like IPT, DPC, and pulpotomy can be performed [9, 10].

10.4.1 In Carious Lesions

An IPT is recommended following selective caries excavation to firm or soft dentin in immature permanent teeth that are asymptomatic or those with signs and symptoms of reversible pulpitis only (Figs. 10.1, 10.2, and 10.3). If the operator encounters a pinpoint carious exposure during excavation, DPC is performed using Calcium Silicate Cements (CSCs). The tooth must be treated with a shallow pulpotomy if the carious exposure is greater than a pinpoint (Figs. 10.4 and 10.5). If the inflamed

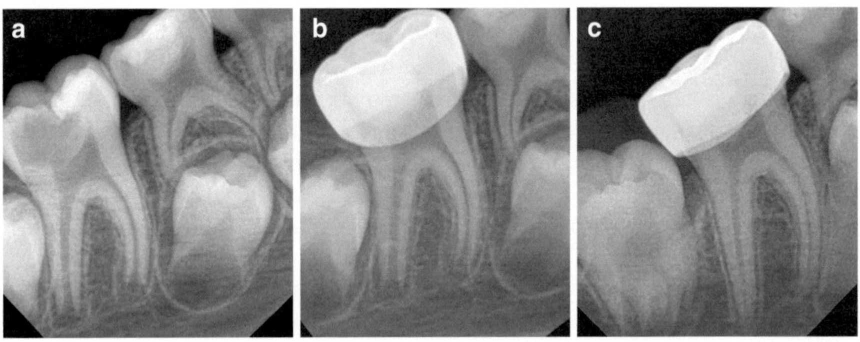

Fig. 10.1 Radiolucency involving the pulp in mandibular permanent right first molar showing Cvek's Stage 3 of root development (**a**). Selective Caries Removal performed on the floor of the lesion and Indirect Pulp Treatment done with Calcium Silicate Cement to promote apexogenesis. The tooth was restored with a Stainless Steel Crown (**b**). Complete root closure observed on the radiograph at 3-year follow-up (**c**)

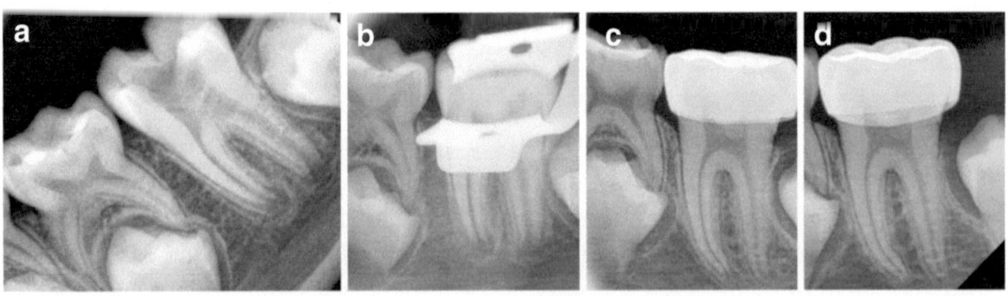

Fig. 10.2 Radiolucency involving the pulp in mandibular permanent left first molar and roots showing Cvek's Stage 4 of root development (**a**). Selective Caries Excavation performed to soft dentin on the floor of the lesion followed by placement of Calcium Silicate Cement. The tooth was restored with a Glass Ionomer Cement (GIC) and a Stainless Steel Crown (SSC) (**b**). One-year follow-up shows radicular thickening and gradual completion of root development (**c**). At 18 months follow-up, root development appears almost complete (**d**)

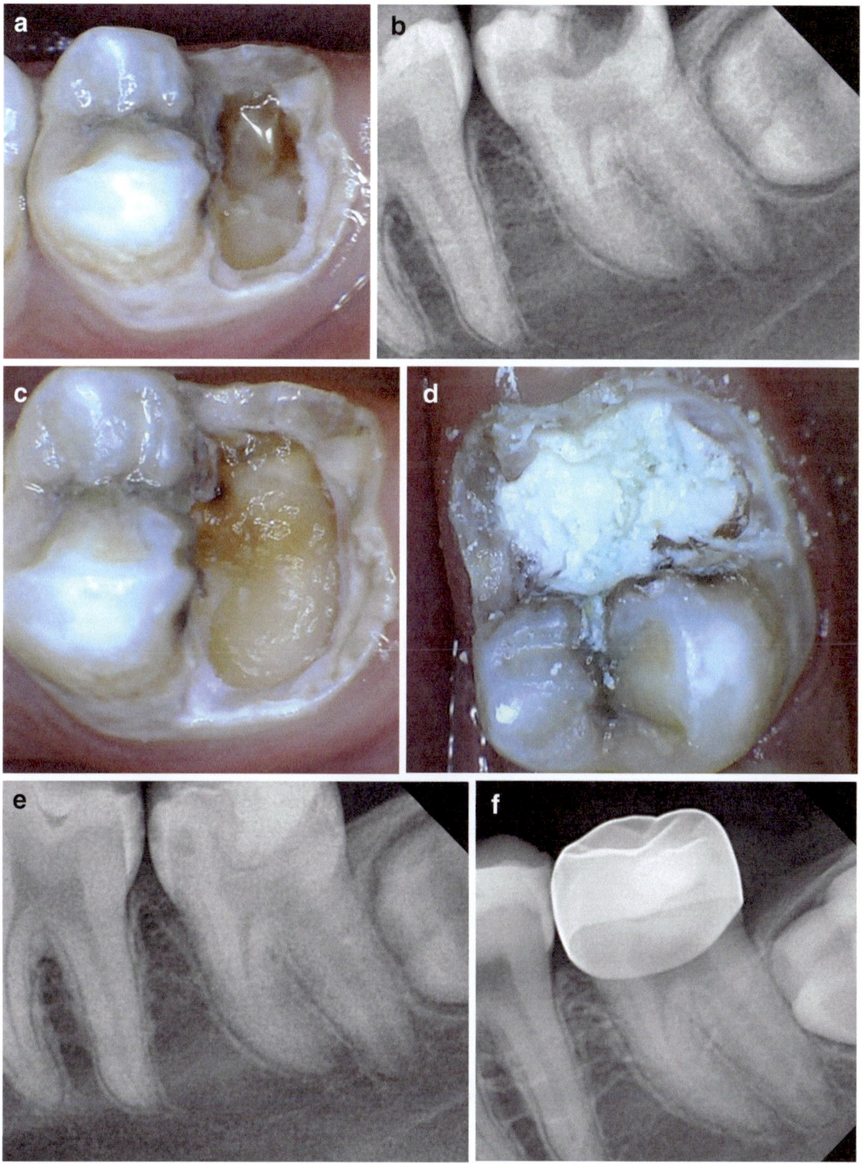

Fig. 10.3 Extensive stage lesion seen on the mandibular permanent left second molar. The tooth was asymptomatic (**a**). Radiograph showed a radiolucency approaching the pulp and the distal root showed Cvek's Stage 4 of root development (**b**). Peripheral walls were excavated to healthy tooth structure, while Selective Caries Removal was done on the floor of the lesion to firm dentin (**c**) and calcium silicate cement placed (**d**). The tooth was restored with Glass Ionomer Cement (**e**) followed by a Stainless Steel Crown. Radiograph taken at the 4-year follow-up shows closure of the apices (**f**)

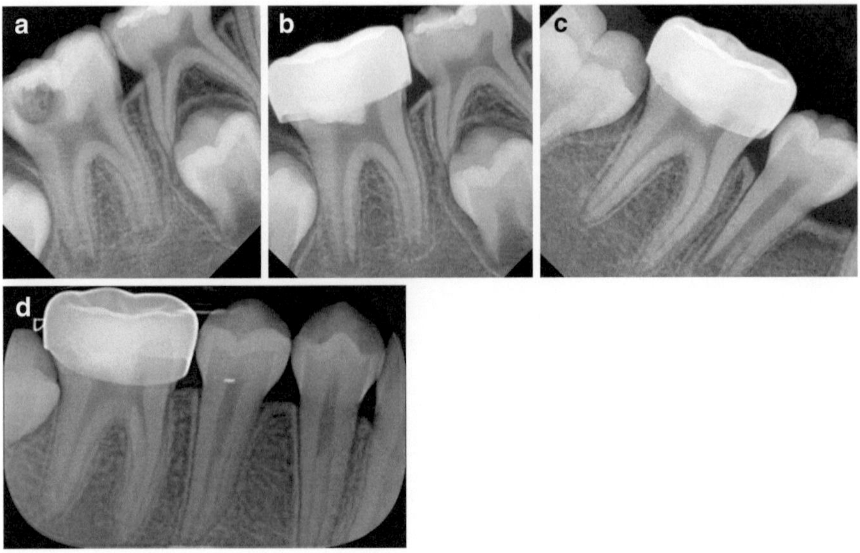

Fig. 10.4 Radiolucency approaching the pulp in mandibular permanent right first molar and Cvek's Stage 4 development of the roots seen (**a**). Partial pulpotomy performed using Calcium Silicate Cement and the tooth restored with Glass Ionomer Cement followed by a Stainless Steel Crown (**b**). Three-year follow-up shows complete closure of both apices (**c**). Five-year follow-up (**d**)

pulp continues to hemorrhage during partial pulpotomy, complete pulpotomy can be performed to reach and preserve healthy pulp tissue. In partial pulpotomy, the inflamed pulp tissue beneath a carious exposure is removed to a depth of one to four millimeters to reach healthy pulp tissue (Fig. 10.5). A complete or traditional pulpotomy involves complete surgical removal of the entire coronal vital pulp tissue. In teeth with symptoms of irreversible pulpitis with no necrotic pulp, a partial or complete pulpotomy can still be done to preserve pulp vitality and allow continued root development (apexogenesis) [1, 9, 11–13].

10.4.2 In Traumatic Dental Injuries

Indirect Pulp Capping is performed in cases of uncomplicated crown fractures. The patient often presents with a crown fracture wherein the pulpal hue is seen. If no pinpoint exposure is present, Indirect Pulp Capping is advised.

In complicated crown fractures, the approach is always conservative irrespective of the size of the exposure. While DPC can be performed for pinpoint exposures when the patient reports within a few hours of injury, a Cvek's pulpotomy is the preferred treatment [14]. The rationale is to excise around 2 mm of the contaminated and inflamed pulp that has been exposed to noxious stimuli while preserving the remaining healthy pulp that has healing and repairing potential. The remaining pulp is capped with a calcium silicate or bioceramic capping material [11, 12, 15,

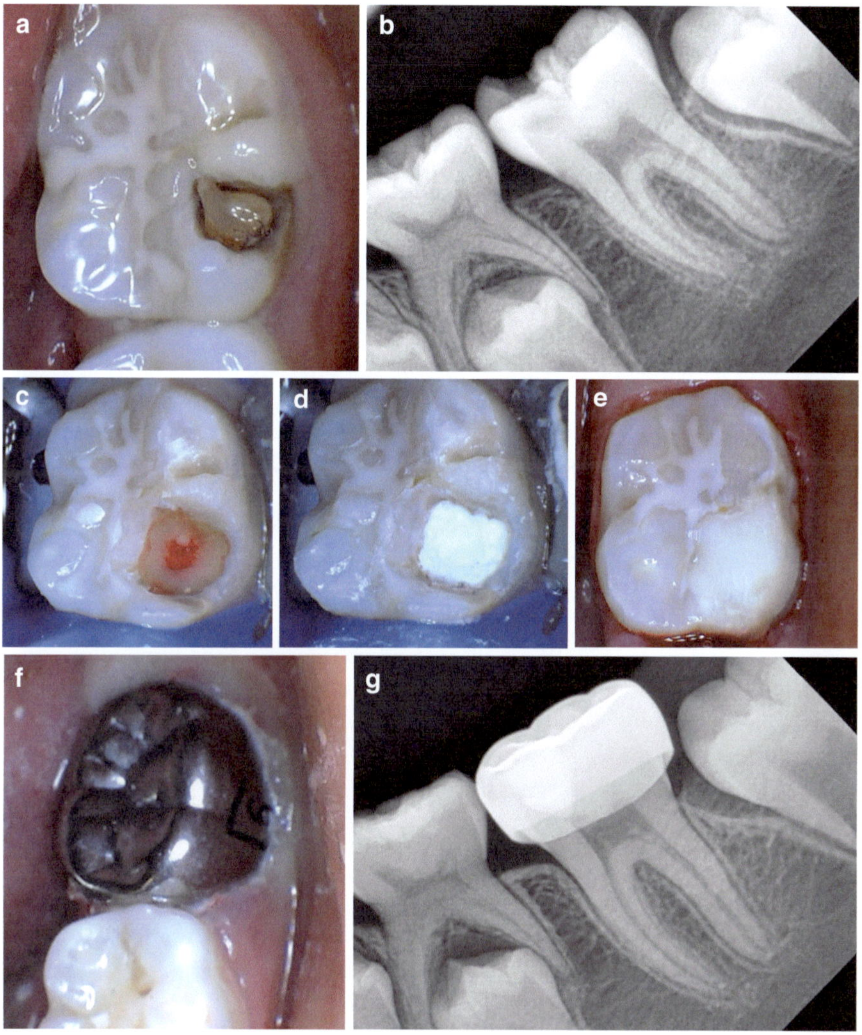

Fig. 10.5 Extensive stage lesion seen on the mandibular permanent left first molar. Tooth showed symptoms of reversible pulpitis (**a**). Radiograph showed radiolucency approaching the pulp and Cvek's Stage 4 of root development (**b**). During Selective Caries Removal, a carious exposure occurred on the floor of the lesion. The exposure was widened by 2 mm to remove inflamed tissue and a partial pulpotomy was performed (**c**). Calcium Silicate Cement was placed on the exposed pulpal tissue and floor of the lesion (**d**). The tooth was restored with Glass Ionomer Cement (**e**) followed by Stainless Steel crown (**f**). Eighteen months follow-up showed closure of both apices (**g**)

16]. Enlarging the exposure allows the Calcium Silicate Cement to be placed adequately in contact with the pulpal tissue, ensuring a better seal. Also, a larger dentinal surface is available at the fracture site to bond to the resin composite.

In larger exposures irrespective of the time elapsed, a Cvek's pulpotomy must be performed.

In complicated crown root fractures or oblique fractures extending cervically that involve a larger part of the crown, a complete pulpotomy may be done if Cvek's pulpotomy does not suffice.

10.5 Cvek's Pulpotomy or Partial Pulpotomy?

Cvek first described the partial pulpotomy in 1978 as a treatment performed on teeth affected by *complicated crown fracture*. This technique came to be known as Cvek's pulpotomy and was primarily performed on traumatized immature permanent teeth [15, 16]. Around the same time, Mejare and Cvek treated immature permanent molars with partial pulpotomy following carious exposure and reported their success in 1993. The technique known as partial or shallow pulpotomy gained popularity in treating carious teeth with incomplete root development [17]. In their respective recommendations, the American Academy of Pediatric Dentistry (AAPD) reserves the term Cvek pulpotomy for traumatized teeth and partial pulpotomy for teeth with carious exposure [12], while the International Association of Dental Traumatology (IADT) refers to the "partial pulpotomy" for treatment of traumatic pulp exposure [14]. The International Association of Pediatric Dentistry (IAPD) mentions "Cvek pulpotomy" for treatment of young permanent teeth regardless of the cause of exposure [11]. While there is no consensus on the terminology, it is understood that from a clinical perspective, there is no difference in the protocol used while performing a partial pulpotomy on a traumatized or carious tooth [16, 17].

10.6 How Does One Choose Between Performing a Partial Pulpotomy Versus a Complete Pulpotomy in Immature Permanent Teeth?

10.6.1 Traumatic and Carious Exposures

While complete pulpotomy was considered an established treatment, it is no longer the treatment of choice for complicated crown fractures or carious exposures in permanent teeth due to the more favorable prognosis of the partial pulpotomy or Cvek's pulpotomy. Partial pulpotomy involves preserving cell-rich coronal pulp tissue that is more likely to facilitate healing than the fibrous and unicellular radicular pulp tissue left behind after complete pulpotomy. The reported success rate of Cvek pulpotomy in immature permanent teeth with complicated crown fractures ranges from 87.5% to 100%. A favorable prognosis of Cvek's pulpotomy is seen in teeth with an exposure size between 0.5 and 4 mm. Studies have shown success even when the interval between the time of accident and treatment is beyond 24 h. In the presence of concomitant luxation injuries of the immature tooth, Cvek's pulpotomy is still the treatment of choice [16]. Additionally, the success rate of partial pulpotomy in carious immature permanent molars has also been shown to be around 87%–90% [18, 19].

In mature teeth with traumatic exposures, irrespective of the size of the exposure, if the patient reports within a few hours, a Cvek's or complete pulpotomy can be performed, depending on the extent of injury. Conventional root canal treatment should be preferred if significant time has elapsed since the trauma has occurred [14]. Mature permanent teeth that are *asymptomatic or show symptoms of reversible pulpitis* can be treated with IPT technique of selective caries excavation to soft or firm dentin [20]. If an exposure occurs during caries excavation, then a partial pulpotomy or a complete pulpotomy can be performed [12, 20]. Some studies suggest that mature permanent teeth showing *symptoms of irreversible pulpitis* can be treated with a full pulpotomy provided there are no signs of pulp necrosis or apical periodontitis. However, further trials are necessary to strengthen the evidence [20–22].

10.7 Apexification and Regenerative Endodontic Procedures (REPs)

Pulp necrosis of an immature permanent tooth from caries or trauma arrests further root development and leaves the tooth with thin, weak walls prone to fracture. Earlier, these teeth were treated with long-term Calcium Hydroxide (CH) intracanal medicaments to induce an apical hard tissue barrier for condensation of gutta percha. Although this method was successful, it had its limitations due to the lengthy duration of treatment, unpredictability of apical closure, and increased risk of root fracture. A one-step apexification procedure using Mineral Trioxide Aggregate (MTA) to form an apical barrier has also shown success due to its sealing of the apex, biocompatibility, and hard tissue induction potential. While this procedure has shown satisfactory results, it does not help in continued root maturation, leaving fragile dentinal walls prone to fracture. In the last two decades, regenerative endodontic treatment has been widely adopted. It refers to procedures that aim to attain organized dental pulp repair and create an environment that would allow continued root development and maturation [23, 24].

10.7.1 When to Do Apexification Or Revascularization?

Current literature shows comparable success rates for both revascularization and apexification. The criteria for success were common for both procedures in terms of infection elimination and apical barrier formation. However, Regenerative Endodontic Procedures (REPs) extended the criteria to continued root development, allowing root lengthening and thickening. Hence, the stage of root development becomes the distinguishing factor for choosing between revascularization and apexification. Cvek classified root development into the following stages based on the degree of root formation (Fig. 10.6).

Stage 1 Less than ½ of the final root length
Stage 2 Half of the final root length

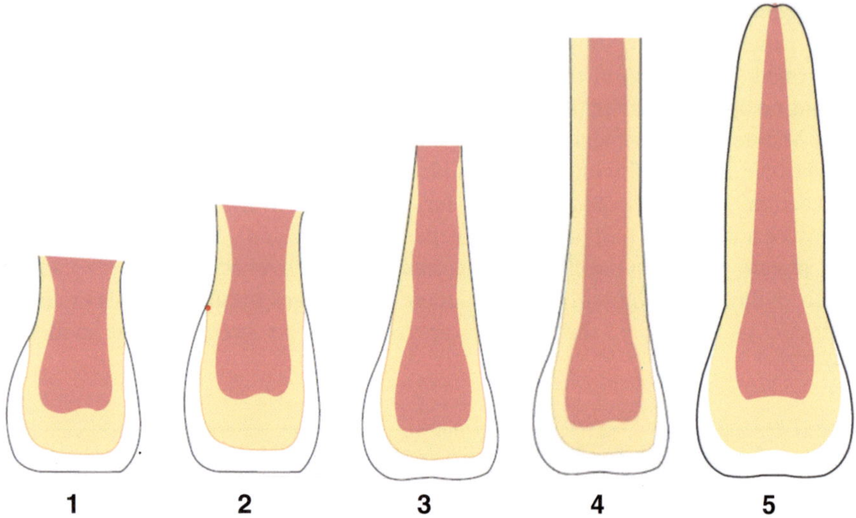

Fig. 10.6 Cvek's stages of root development: Stage 1 Less than ½ of the final root length, Stage 2 Half of the final root length, Stage 3 2/3rd of the final root length, Stage 4 Nearly complete root length, and Stage 5 Closed apical foramen and complete root development

Stage 3 2/3rd of the final root length
Stage 4 Nearly complete root length
Stage 5 Closed apical foramen and complete root development

While apexification procedures have successfully treated non-vital teeth with immature apices, blunderbuss canals with thin roots and poor crown root ratio (Cvek's Stage 1,2,3) predispose the teeth to fracture. Regenerative Endodontic Procedures (REPs) should be performed in Cvek's Stage 1, 2, and 3 of root development, as the apical foramen is more than 1.1 mm facilitating a rich blood supply and a high concentration of stem cells in the apical papilla [25–28].

From a clinical standpoint, if there is sufficient root elongation and adequate thickness of radicular dentin (Stage 4), an MTA apexification is the recommended treatment. While one assumes no continued root development with MTA apexification, a few case reports have shown continued root development in long-term follow-up. This finding can be attributed to the pluripotent stem cells surrounding the root [2].

10.7.2 Apexification Technique

Due to its limitations, the multi visit Calcium Hydroxide apexification has been replaced by the one step MTA apexification.

MTA Apexification Technique

- Under rubber dam isolation, an access cavity is prepared and working length determined by the radiographic method.
- Cleaning and shaping of the canals is done only to ensure straight line access to allow for the compaction of an apical barrier.
- Calcium Hydroxide (CH) is placed as an intracanal medicament for 7 days.
- On the second visit, CH is flushed out with saline and the canal is dried with paper points.
- MTA plug is prepared from the powder and liquid or as premixed putty, and pushed to the apical end of the canal using either an MTA carrier or endodontic pluggers.
- Several increments of MTA are condensed until the radiograph shows a plug of 4 mm thickness at the apex.
- A moist cotton pellet or paper point is placed in the access cavity, until the MTA has set.

Once the MTA apical plug has set, it simulates a barrier in non-vital teeth against which the obturating material is condensed and the tooth restored with Resin Composite or an extra-coronal restoration (Figs. 10.7 and 10.8) [29–34].

10.7.3 Which Materials with Shorter Setting Time Can Be Used for Apexification?

The formulations of MTA available earlier had a longer setting time of approximately 8 h and necessitated deferring the placement of a definitive restoration to a second visit. The newly introduced MTA formulation such as MTA Repair HP by Angelus® with a setting time of 15 min has made it possible to place a definitive restoration at the same visit. The other calcium silicate-based materials used for the apexification procedure are *Endosequence BC RRM™ fast set putty with a setting time of 20 min and Biodentine™, with a setting time of 12 min.*

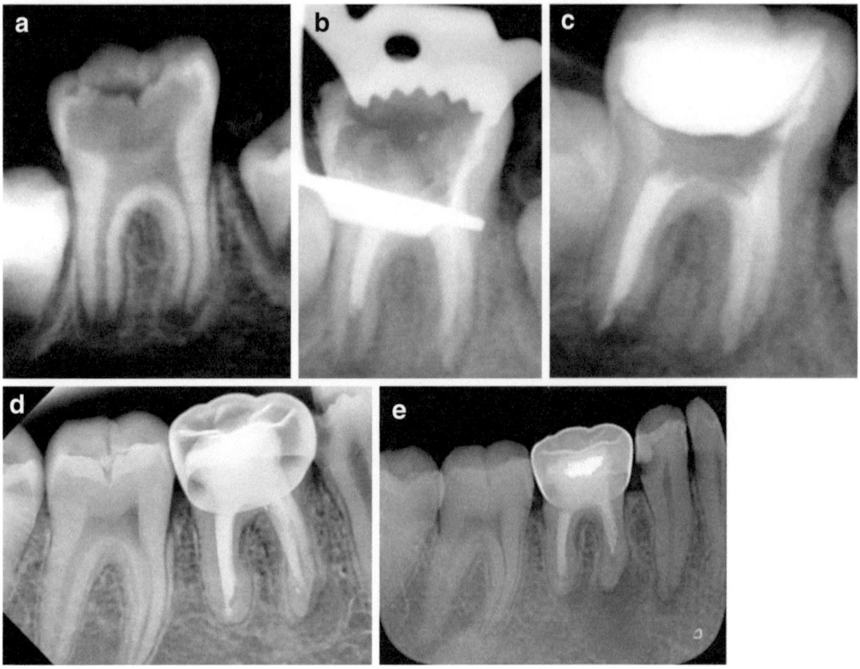

Fig. 10.7 Symptomatic mandibular permanent right first molar with radiolucency seen involving the pulp and root showing Cvek's Stage 4 of development. Calcium hydroxide placed in the canals and temporary dressing given (**a**). After 2 weeks, Calcium Hydroxide was removed and MTA obturation done as part of apexification (**b**, **c**). The tooth received a Resin Composite restoration followed by a Stainless Steel Crown. Root maturation seen at 6-year follow-up with mesial root showing periapical changes. Carious lesion seen on the mesial surface of the adjacent premolar (**d**). Sixteen-year follow-up shows a large periapical radiolucency around the mesial root and failure of restoration in the adjacent premolar (**e**)

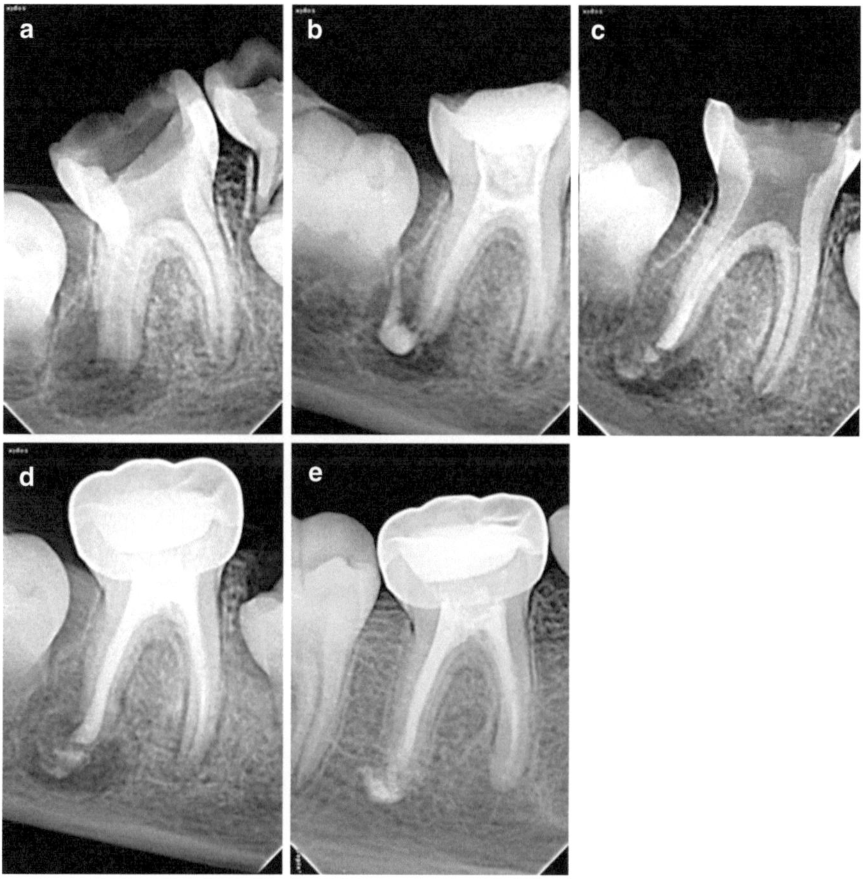

Fig. 10.8 Symptomatic mandibular permanent right first molar with radiolucency seen involving the pulp and distal root showing Cvek's Stage 4 of development. Periapical radiolucency seen around the distal root (**a**). Minimal mechanical debridement of canals performed and Calcium Hydroxide placed in the canals and temporary dressing given (**b**). After 2 weeks, Calcium Hydroxide was removed and a 3 mm MTA plug created at the apex of the distal root (**c**). All the canals were then obturated with gutta percha. The tooth received a Resin Composite restoration followed by a preformed Stainless Steel Crown. (**d**). At the four-and-half-year follow-up, complete resolution of periapical radiolucency seen (**e**). (Image Courtesy: Dr Mayur Bhattad, India)

10.8 Regenerative Endodontic Procedures (REPs)

REPs refers to biologically based procedures designed to replace damaged tooth structures, including dentin and periodontium, as well as cells of the pulp–dentine complex. In the early 1960s, reports of continued root development were seen in necrotic immature permanent teeth who's apical third were manipulated to induce bleeding. This technique, known as revascularization, is the most common form of regenerative endodontic therapy.

10.8.1 What Is the Rationale for Revascularization?

The rationale for revascularization is based on the stimulation and proliferation of the Stem Cells of the Apical Papilla (SCAP) and Periodontal Ligament Stem Cells (PDLSc) that develop from the dental papilla [24]. Due to their anatomical positioning at the site of the root development process, these cells are expected to proliferate and differentiate into cells forming dentin, pulp, and the periodontium under favorable conditions in the root canal space. The revascularization protocol ensures a reduction of bacteria and necrotic pulp tissue in the root canal system, creation of a scaffold, and placement of a tight coronal seal, thereby promoting repopulation of stem cells that cause continuation of root development and maturation [35].

10.8.2 What Are the Treatment Goals of Revascularization?

According to the American Association of Endodontists (AAE), the following are the treatment goals to be achieved for the revascularization procedure [23]:

1. Primary goal (essential): the elimination of symptoms and evidence of bony healing.
2. Secondary goal (desirable): increased root wall thickness and/or increased root length.
3. Tertiary goal: positive response to vitality testing [36].

10.8.2.1 Disinfection of the Root Canal System

Disinfection of the canals is achieved with the use of irrigants followed by placement of intracanal medicaments for 2 weeks. These disinfecting agents should ensure the elimination of infection, while maintaining the viability of the stem cells in the apical region. Mechanical preparation of the canals is avoided, as it may damage the thin dentinal walls [37, 38].

10.8.2.2 Irrigation: Sodium Hypochlorite and Ethylene Diamine Tetracetic Acid (EDTA)

A concentration of 1.5% sodium hypochlorite is recommended as a higher concentration is seen to reduce the viability of SCAP cells and a lower concentration does not effectively disinfect the root canal space. The use of sodium hypochlorite alone may interfere with the stem cell attachment to dentin; hence, it is used in combination with 17% EDTA. Conditioning of dentin with EDTA helps release growth factors that promote the adhesion, migration, and differentiation of dental pulp stem cells towards or onto dentin [39, 40].

To prevent damage to the stem cells in the periapical region, 20 ml of the solution is irrigated slowly in each canal over 5 min. The use of side-vented needles or the EndoVac™ (Kerr, USA) system is recommended. The needle should be placed no further than halfway into the canal, to prevent the extrusion of periapical debris [35, 36, 41].

10.8.3 Which Are the Intra-canal Medicaments Used in REPs?

10.8.3.1 Mixed Antibiotic Paste [31]

The Triple Anitbiotic Paste (TAP) used initially included Ciprofloxacin, Metronidazole, and Minocycline. Minocycline resulted in esthetically unacceptable bluish discoloration of teeth; hence, it was substituted with Clindamycin. Alternately, a single (Amoxicillin or Erythromycin) or double antibiotic paste (Metronidazole and Ciprofloxacin) can also be used. These antibiotic pastes allow diffusion of drugs throughout the root dentin, reliably disinfect dentin, and eliminate cultivable bacteria [42–45]. AAE recommends the use of a double (DAP) or Triple Antibiotic Paste (TAP) [35].

A typical hand-mixed slurry like consistency of antibiotic pastes results in concentrations of about 1000 mg/ml which have detrimental effects on the stem cells [46]. Antibiotic concentrations at 1 mg/ml showed a 50% survival of the SCAP cells whereas further dilution to 0.1 or 0.01 mg/ml showed no damage to these stem cells [47]. While these dilutions show low cytotoxicity, their antimicrobial efficacy is unknown. Hence, antibiotic concentrations in dilutions of around 1 mg/ml are recommended [48, 49].

10.8.3.2 Calcium Hydroxide (CH)

Calcium Hydroxide (CH) has been shown to be conducive to the survival and proliferation of SCAP cells at all concentrations. While an antibiotic paste is known to have better antimicrobial properties, one of its drawbacks is cytotoxicity. This could pose a challenge to a clinician while inducing bleeding to create a scaffold. Hence, for most cases of revascularization, CH is preferred not only due to the absence of cytotoxicity but also due to ready availability and ease of delivery into the intracanal space. It causes no discoloration but may not always resolve infected periapical lesions. However, large periapical infections may be better treated using a 1 mg/ml dilution instead of recalling the child for multiple CH dressings [50].

10.8.3.3 Preparation of Intra-canal Medicament

(a) *Antibiotic Paste*

To prepare the TAP or DAP, Ciprofloxacin (500 mg), Metronidazole (400 mg), and Minocycline (200 mg) or Clindamycin (300 mg) combinations can be used in a 1:1:1 or 1:1 ratio, respectively [40]. For a single antibiotic paste, one of the above antibiotics or Amoxicillin–Clavulanate, Erythromycin, etc., can also be used. The sugar coating on the tablets must be scraped off and the tablets reduced to a fine powder in the mortar and pestle. 1 g of antibiotic powder is mixed with 1 ml of propylene glycol or macrogol solvent to give a concentration of 1000 mg/ml. 1 ml of this mix (1000 mg/ml) is then diluted with 9 ml of solvent to give a concentration of 100 mg/ml.

1 ml of this 100 mg/ml slurry is further diluted by 9 ml of the solvent for an antibiotic concentration of 1 mg/ml. The antibiotic paste is also commercially available as a 2 in 1 or 3 in 1, 3Mix MP paste.

(b) *Calcium Hydroxide Paste*

It can be freshly prepared as 1 part of Calcium Hydroxide powder mixed with 1 part of normal saline or distilled water to attain a thin mix. This can be delivered into the canals with a lentulospiral after drying canals with paper points. Alternatively, commercially available Calcium Hydroxide dispensed as a syringe is expressed directly into the canals with a thin long tip [51–55].

Just as irrigation is done slowly, care must be taken while delivering the intra-canal medicament. The needle tip or lentulospiral must be placed only halfway into the canal. The lentulospiral must rotate at a slow speed so that the medicament does not extrude beyond the apex. It is important not to flood the periapical lesion as the antibiotics and Calcium Hydroxide cause disinfection by diffusion through the root dentin. The intra-canal medicament must be left in the canal for 2–4 weeks, or till the tooth is asymptomatic. The tooth should be sealed with Intermediate Restorative Material (IRM) or Glass Ionomer Cement (GIC).

10.8.4 Scaffolds in REP

As tissues do not grow in an empty space, a matrix or scaffold is required to deliver the cells and growth factors into the intra-canal space. The most widely researched scaffolds in REP are the Autologous Platelet Concentrates (APCs). The three APCs are blood clot revascularization (BCR), Platelet-Rich Fibrin (PRF), and Platelet-Rich Plasma (PRP) [56].

10.8.4.1 Blood Clot—As a Scaffold

Blood seeps into the canal after laceration of the periapical tissue to form a clot. This introduces stem cells with its growth factors within the root canal, aiding the in-growth of new tissue. The revascularization process is initiated by placing a no.15 or 20 K file 2–3 mm beyond the apex. The file tip is given a sharp bend to facilitate trauma to the periapical tissue and initiate bleeding. In cases where bleeding is not easily provoked, a drop of EDTA is placed in the canal and re-instrumented. While one would expect the canal space to fill with blood immediately, the entire process may take up to 15–20 min. The clot is allowed to form as close to the CEJ which will facilitate root thickening at the coronal 1/3rd that has the greatest propensity for fracture. Absence of bleeding or clot formation necessitates further instrumentation or use of alternate scaffolds.

10.8.4.2 Platelet-Rich Plasma (PRP) and Platelet-Rich Fibrin (PRF)

PRP and PRF have been recommended as alternatives to the Blood Clot Revascularization (BCR) in creating a scaffold. PRP and PRF require venous blood drawn from the arm of the patient at the time of treatment which is then put through a centrifuge. The resultant concentrate is gently introduced into the canal with a tweezer and pushed in with CollaCote® or Collaplug®. While this may add to the complexity of the procedure, these scaffolds have shown successful outcomes.

Periapical healing response was better in PRP (100%) and PRF (100%) compared to Blood Clot Revascularization (88.9%). While comparing the three scaffolds, the degree of root thickening and elongation seen was similar in all three methods. The most significant outcome was apical closure when PRF (85.1%) and PRP (85.2%) was used as compared to BCR (58.8%) [56].

The primary goal of REP is the resolution of periapical lesions. In children and young adults with smaller periapical lesions, BCR is preferred due to the relative ease of the procedure. The survival of SCAP cells is questionable in teeth with long-standing large periapical lesions. In such a clinical situation, PRP and PRF are likely to perform better than BCR due to their higher periapical healing capacity.

10.8.5 The Regenerative Endodontic Technique [35, 57–63]

At the First Appointment,

Following local anesthesia, prepare the access cavity under a rubber dam.

- Extirpate the infected or necrotic pulp with an H file with minimal instrumentation of canal walls and well short of the apical end.
- Irrigate the canals with 1.5% sodium hypochlorite alternating with saline, gently at 20 ml/canal for 5 min. This can be done with an EndoVac™ (Kerr, USA) system or a side-vent needle.
- The tooth is then irrigated with 17% EDTA at 20 ml/canal for 5 min.
- Dry the canals with paper points and place an intracanal medicament (CH or antibiotic paste).
- Seal the access cavity with 3–4 mm of temporary restorative material and recall the patient in 1–4 weeks.

At the Second Visit,

- If there are signs and symptoms, repeat the irrigation protocol and consider additional treatment time with an antibiotic paste. If the tooth is asymptomatic, anesthetize the tooth using a local anesthetic without a vasoconstrictor and isolate the tooth with a rubber dam.
- While Calcium Hydroxide is effectively removed with significantly less residual presence, it is not easy to remove the antibiotic paste from the root canal system, possibly because of their penetration and binding into the dentin.

- To remove antibiotic paste from canal walls, ultrasonic irrigation or EndoActivator® (Dentsply Sirona) with saline are more effective than needle irrigation.
- Sodium hypochlorite should not be used in this appointment. Irrigate gently with 17% EDTA after complete removal of intracanal medicament.
- Instrument the canal with a No. 15 or 20 K file that is bent at the tip. The file is inserted beyond the apical third to irritate the periapical tissue to initiate bleeding (Fig. 10.9d).
- At times, it is difficult to initiate bleeding. A drop of EDTA is placed on the file and the periapical area re-instrumented till bleeding occurs (Fig. 10.10e).
- The clot must be allowed to fill up to the Cemento Enamel Junction (CEJ). This may take anywhere from 15 to 30 min (Figs. 10.9e and 10.10f).
- Alternatively, the canal can be filled with PRP or PRF concentrate.
- A resorbable matrix such as Collaplug®, Collacote®, or CollaTape® is placed over the blood clot and capped with a calcium silicate material.
- The Calcium Silicate Cement (CSC) is removed from the walls of the orifice and a layer of Glass Ionomer Cement (GIC) placed. The access cavity is sealed with Resin Composite.
- A follow-up is advised every 3 months to assess root development and a radiograph taken every 6 months (Fig. 10.9).

Chen et al. in 2012 described five radiographic outcomes of *teeth treated with REP* [64].

Type 1—where there is increased thickening of the canal walls and continued root maturation.

Type 2—where there is no significant continuation of root development with the root apex becoming blunt and closed (Fig. 10.11).

Type 3—where there is continued root development with the apical foramen remaining open (Fig. 10.10).

Type 4—here there is severe calcification (obliteration) of the canal space (Figs. 10.9 and 10.13).

Type 5—where there is a hard tissue barrier formed in the canal between the coronal MTA plug and the root apex (Fig. 10.12).

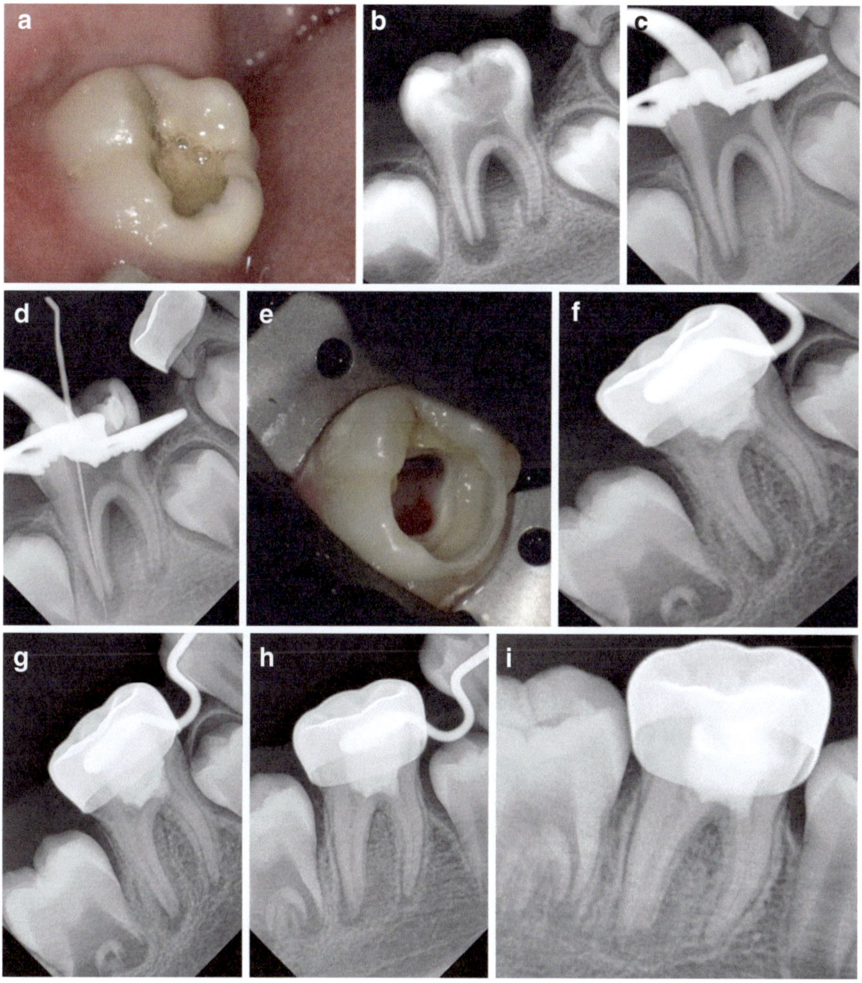

Fig. 10.9 Extensive stage lesion on the mandibular permanent right first molar with a dentoalveolar abscess (**a**). Radiograph showed radiolucency involving the pulp and Cvek's Stage 3 of root development. Periapical radiolucency seen with the mesial and distal roots (**b**). Access opening performed and root canals debrided. Calcium Hydroxide placed as an intracanal medicament for 2 weeks (**c**). After 2 weeks, the canals were irrigated, dried and periapical bleeding induced with a K file (**d**). Bleeding seen at the canal orifices (**e**). MTA placed on the orifices and the tooth restored with Stainless Steel Crown (**f**). Follow-up after 1 year shows gradual root completion and resolution of periapical radiolucency (**g**). Follow-up after 2 years (**h**). Follow-up after 3 years shows complete root development and pulp canal obliteration (Cheng Type IV) (**i**)

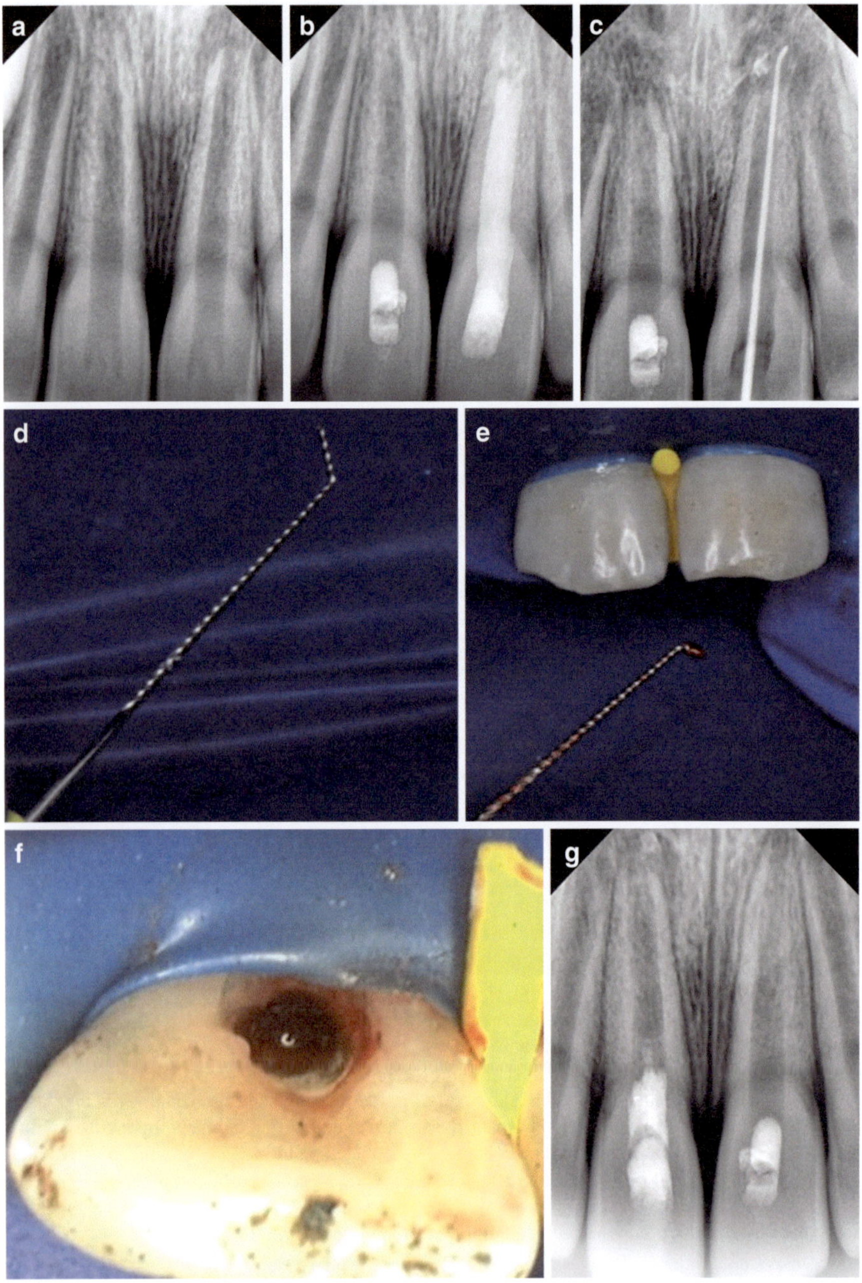

Fig. 10.10 (continued)

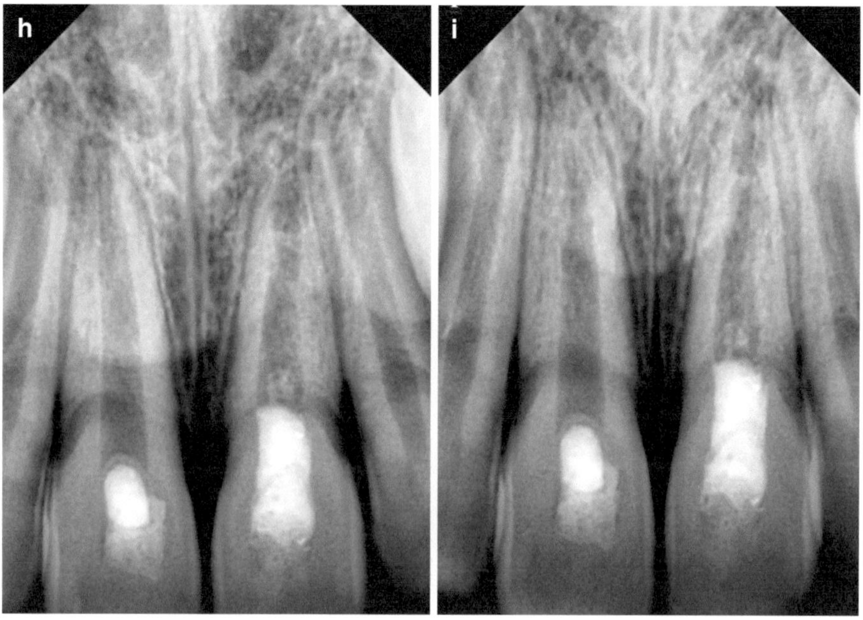

Fig. 10.10 Access opening performed on maxillary permanent left central incisor, after nonvitality was confirmed and apex showed Cvek's Stage 3 of root development. Maxillary right central incisor treated with Cvek's pulpotomy (**a**). After irrigation and minimal debridement, Calcium Hydroxide placed in the canals (**b**). At the next visit, Calcium Hydroxide removed from the canals. A 20 No K file was bent at the tip and inserted beyond working length (**c**, **d**). Since there was no bleeding initially, after piercing the periapical tissue, a drop of EDTA was placed on the file tip and the file re-inserted beyond working length (**e**). Bleeding seen at the canal orifices 2 mm beyond the CEJ (**f**). MTA placed on the canal orifices and the tooth sealed with a Resin Composite restoration (**g**). One-year follow-up (**h**). The maxillary left central incisor showed a Type 3 closure according to Chen was seen at 2-year follow-up (**i**)

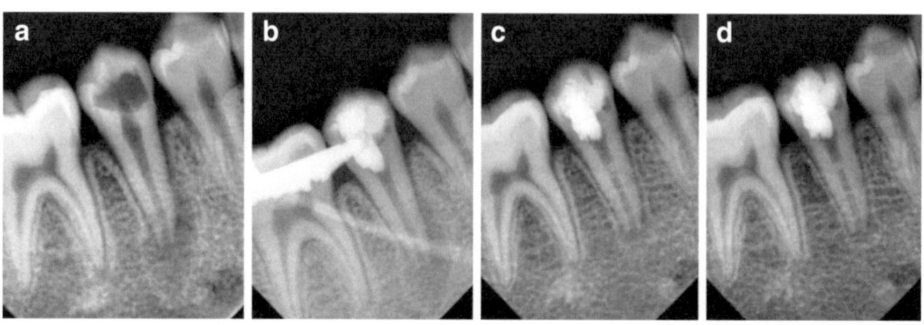

Fig. 10.11 Cvek's Stage 3 root development seen in the mandibular right second premolar (**a**). Regeneration Endodontic Procedure performed and MTA placed on the orifices (**b**). One-year follow-up showing resolution of the periapical radiolucency and radicular thickening with blunt and open apex (**c**). Two-year follow-up showing Cheng's Type 2 root closure (**d**)

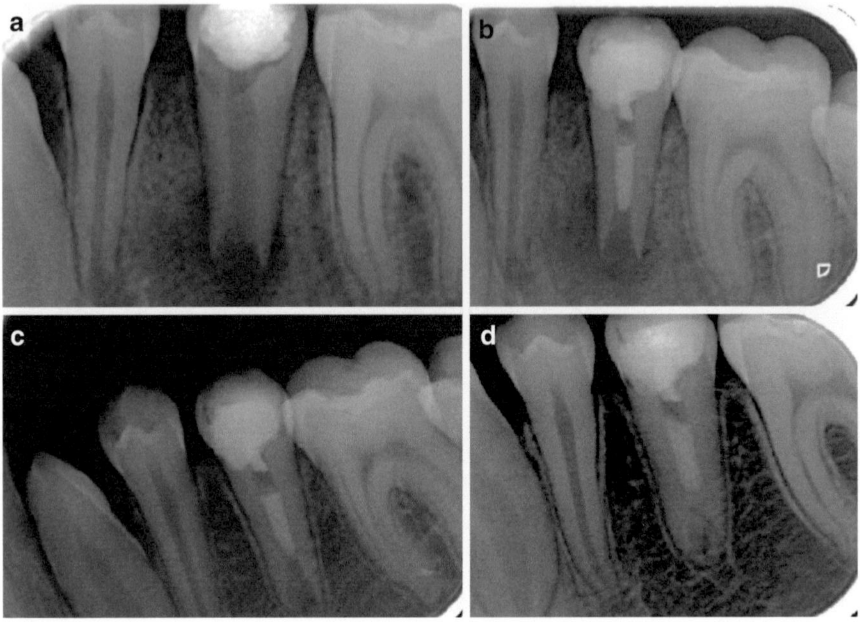

Fig. 10.12 Mandibular left second premolar with periapical radiolucency and Cvek's Stage 2 of root development (**a**). Regenerative Endodontic Procedure performed, and MTA placed (**b**). Six-month follow-up shows resolution of the periapical radiolucency (**c**). One-year follow-up shows Cheng's Type 5 root closure, where calcification is seen below the MTA plug (**d**). (Image Courtesy: Dr Manini Shah, India)

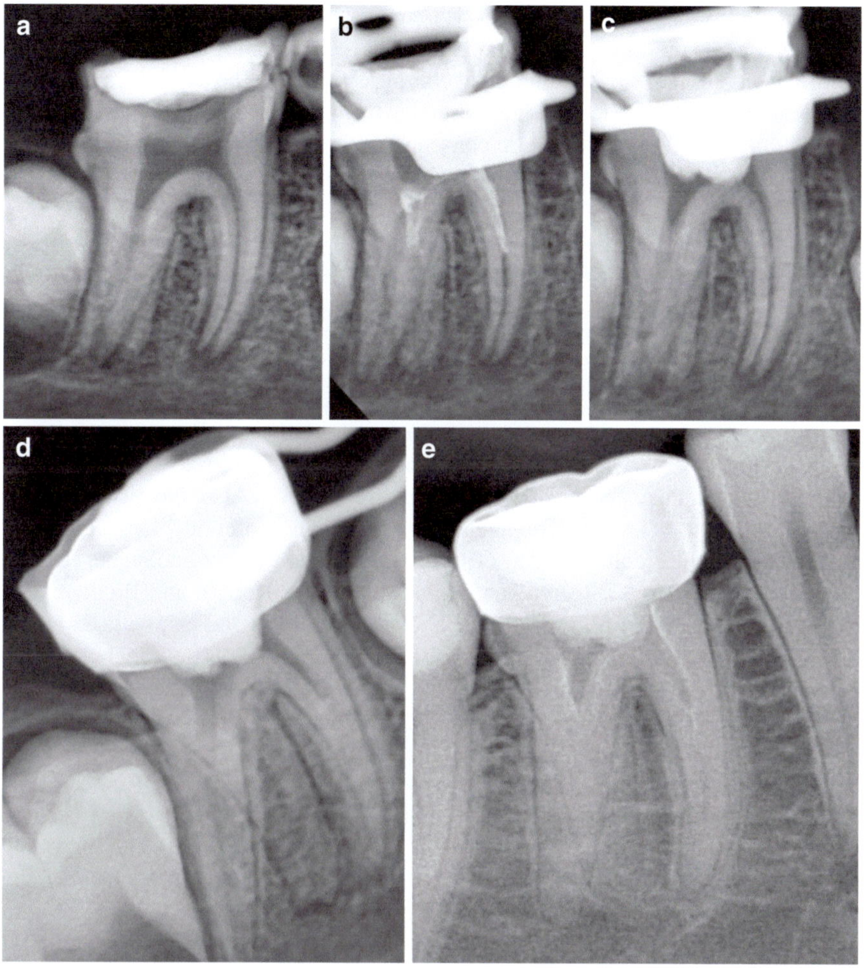

Fig. 10.13 Cvek's Stage 3 root development seen in a non-vital mandibular permanent right first molar (**a**). Access opening done and Calcium Hydroxide placed in the canals (**b**). After 2 weeks, Regenerative Endodontic Procedure performed, and MTA placed to seal the orifices (**c**). Six-year follow-up shows complete root development (**d**). Nine-year follow-up shows pulp canal obliteration (Cheng Type 4) (**e**)

10.9 What Is the Success Rate of REPs?

REPs have shown successful outcomes (up to 91.3%) in terms of resolution of symptoms and complete healing of periapical lesion. As the criteria for success with REPs also involves root thickening and lengthening, the pooled success rate for these outcomes is between 21% and 100%. This wide range shows the unpredictability of root development. It is impossible to discern the type of tissue formed based on the clinical outcome. Studies have now confirmed that the possibility of regeneration of the dentinopulpal complex is nil, and the tissue formed is less pulp like and more of cementoid and osteoid [65–68]. Whether the new vital tissue is truly pulp or pulp like is of little consequence if there is resolution of infection, continued root development, and apical closure.

10.10 What Are the Adverse Effects of REPs?

10.10.1 Discoloration

Use of Minocycline in the TAP as well as MTA placed in the coronal one third has shown to discolor teeth. This is of significance, especially for REP procedures done on anterior teeth [58]. The constituents of gray MTA such as ferrous, aluminum, and magnesium oxide have been shown to cause discoloration. Also, the bismuth oxide in gray and white MTA was seen to cause a graying discoloration when it comes in contact with dentin collagen [59, 60]. Newer materials like EndoSequence® BC putty (Brassler, USA), Bioaggregate® (DiaDent, South Korea), and Biodentine™ (Septodont, France) do not contain the above constituents and can be used where discoloration of tooth is a concern. In case of discoloration, intra-coronal bleaching is useful in treating this adverse effect and should be included when planning the treatment [69–71].

Intra-coronal Tooth Bleaching Technique

After rubber dam isolation, the access cavity is reopened leaving a 2 mm layer of GIC sealing the Calcium Silicate Cement overlying the scaffold. The bleaching agent (Opalescence™ Endo, Ultradent, USA) is expressed into the pulp chamber and a cotton pellet is placed over the bleaching agent. The access cavity is sealed with a GIC and the patient is called after 4–5 days. The procedure can be repeated until the desired color change is achieved, or no further benefit is noticed. Once the desired shade is achieved, the pulp chamber is irrigated and a Resin Composite restoration is placed.

10.10.2 Canal Obliteration

Various studies have observed that intra-canal calcification and canal obliteration is one of the possible long-term outcomes seen in teeth treated with revascularization. Revascularization following dental trauma, repeated use of CH as an intracanal medicament, or scaffold created by inducing bleeding are the probable reasons for pulp canal obliteration. Although root canal calcification is not considered a diseased state, excessive calcification will impede the vitality of revascularized tissues and can complicate endodontic treatment, if ever indicated in the future. An endodontic procedure is advised only in cases that show clinical and radiographic signs and symptoms of pulpitis [72, 73]. The tooth may need to be treated cosmetically as it is likely to appear more yellow and less life-like.

10.11 Concluding Remarks

The objective of Vital Pulp Therapy in immature permanent teeth is to maintain pulp vitality and continued root maturation. In extensive-stage lesions, Selective Caries Removal must be performed to firm or soft caries on the floor of the lesion. Similarly in traumatic injuries, IPT or Cvek's pulpotomy are performed in vital immature teeth regardless of time elapsed since injury. For the immature non-vital permanent teeth, the choice of procedure (apexification or Regenerative Endodontic Procedure) depends on the stage of root development. REP is indicated in Cvek's 1,2,3 stages of root development while MTA apexification is indicated in Cvek's Stage 4 and some cases of Stage 3. The etiology of pulp necrosis (trauma or caries) does not influence the outcome of the non-vital pulp therapy procedure. In teeth subjected to trauma, concomitant injuries to the periodontium influence the healing capacity. The long-term prognosis of teeth treated with above procedures is varied and must be followed up to monitor clinical and radiographic outcomes.

References

1. Fuks AB. Pulp therapy for the primary and young permanent dentitions. Dent Clin N Am. 2000;44(3):571–96.
2. Witherspoon DE. Vital pulp therapy with new materials: new directions and treatment perspectives—permanent teeth. Pediatr Dent. 2008;30(3):220–4.
3. Goldstein S, Sedaghat-Zandi A, Greenberg M, Friedman S. Apexification & apexogenesis. N Y State Dent J. 1999;65(5):23.
4. Andreasen JO. Pulp and periodontal tissue repair – regeneration or tissue metaplasia after dental trauma. A review. Dent Traumatol. 2012;28:19–24.
5. Friedlander LT, Cullinan MP, Love RM. Dental stem cells and their potential role in apexogenesis and apexification. Int Endod J. 2009;42(11):955–62.
6. Gronthos S, Mankani M, Brahim J, Robey PG, Shi S. Postnatal human dental pulp stem cells (DPSCs) in vitro and in vivo. Proc Natl Acad Sci. 2000;97(25):13625–30.
7. Gronthos S, Brahim J, Li W, Fisher LW, Cherman N, Boyde A, DenBesten P, Robey PG, Shi S. Stem cell properties of human dental pulp stem cells. J Dent Res. 2002;81(8):531–5.
8. Handa K, Saito M, Tsunoda A, Yamauchi M, Hattori S, Sato S, Toyoda M, Teranaka T, Narayanan AS. Progenitor cells from dental follicle are able to form cementum matrix in vivo. Connect Tissue Res. 2002;43(2–3):406–8.
9. Garcia-Godoy F, Murray PE. Recommendations for using regenerative endodontic procedures in permanent immature traumatized teeth. Dent Traumatol. 2012;28(1):33–41.
10. Trope M. Regenerative potential of dental pulp. J Endodont. 2008;34:S13–7.
11. IAPD foundational articles and consensus recommendations: pulp therapy for primary and young permanent teeth. 2022. http://www.iapdworld.org/2022_12_pulp-therapy-for-primary-and-young-permanent-teeth.
12. American Academy of Pediatric Dentistry. Pulp therapy for primary and immature permanent teeth. In: The reference manual of pediatric dentistry. Chicago: American Academy of Pediatric Dentistry; 2024. p. 466–74.

13. Schwendicke F, Frencken JE, Bjørndal L, Maltz M, Manton DJ, Ricketts D, van Landuyt K, Banerjee A, Campus G, Domejean S, Fontana M, Leal S, Machiulskiene V, Schulte A, Splieth C, Zandona A, Innes NP. Managing carious lesions: consensus recommendations on carious tissue removal. Adv Dent Res. 2016;28:58–67.
14. Bourguignon C, Cohenca N, Lauridsen E, Flores MT, O'Connell AC, Day PF, Tsilingaridis G, Abbott PV, Fouad AF, Hicks L, Andreasen JO, Cehreli ZC, Harlamb S, Kahler B, Oginni A, Semper M, Levin L. International Association of Dental Traumatology guidelines for the management of traumatic dental injuries: 1. Fractures and luxations. Dent Traumatol. 2020;36(4):314–30.
15. Krastl G, Weiger R, Filippi A, Van Waes H, Ebeleseder K, Ree M, Connert T, Widbiller M, Tjäderhane L, Dummer PMH, Galler K. Endodontic management of traumatized permanent teeth: a comprehensive review. Int Endod J. 2021;54(8):1221–45.
16. Bimstein E, Rotstein I. Cvek pulpotomy – revisited. Dent Traumatol. 2016;32(6):438–42.
17. Mejàre I, Cvek M. Partial pulpotomy in young permanent teeth with deep carious lesions. Endod Dent Traumatol. 1993;9(6):238–42.
18. Chen Y, Chen X, Zhang Y, et al. Materials for pulpotomy in immature permanent teeth: a systematic review and meta-analysis. BMC Oral Health. 2019;19:227.
19. Han S, Zhang Q. Vital pulp therapy following pulpotomy in immature permanent teeth with carious exposure. J Clin Pediatr Dent. 2023;47(5):65–72.
20. AAE position statement on vital pulp therapy. J Endodont. 2021;47(9):1340–4.
21. Wang W, Zeng Q, Li Y, Sun Y, Kim T, Tang J, Bergeron BE, Tay F, Gu L. Effectiveness of pulpotomy in managing carious exposure in mature permanent teeth: a systematic review and meta-analysis. J Dent. 2024;150:105392.
22. Ather A, Patel B, Gelfond JAL, et al. Outcome of pulpotomy in permanent teeth with irreversible pulpitis: a systematic review and meta-analysis. Sci Rep. 2022;12:19664.
23. Fuks Anna B, Peretz B. Pediatric endodontics: current concepts in pulp therapy for primary and young permanent teeth. Cham: Springer International Publishing; 2016. p. 149–61.
24. Murray PE. Review of guidance for the selection of regenerative endodontics, apexogenesis, apexification, pulpotomy, and other endodontic treatments for immature permanent teeth. Int Endod J. 2023;56:188–99.
25. Cvek M. Prognosis of luxated non-vital maxillary incisors treated with calcium hydroxide and filled with gutta-percha: a retrospective clinical study. Endod Dent Traumatol. 1992;8:45–55.
26. Xie Y, Lu F, Hong Y, He J, Lin Y. Revascularisation versus apexification for treatment of immature teeth based on periapical healing and root development: a systematic review and meta-analysis. Eur J Paediatr Dent. 2021;22(3):207–14.
27. Abada HM, Hashem AAR, Abu-Seida AM, Nagy MM. The effect of changing apical foramen diameter on regenerative potential of mature teeth with necrotic pulp and apical periodontitis. Clin Oral Investig. 2022;26:1843–53.
28. Nicoloso GF, Goldenfum GM, Pizzol TDSD, Scarparo RK, Montagner F, de Almeida Rodrigues J, Casagrande L. Pulp revascularization or apexification for the treatment of immature necrotic permanent teeth: systematic review and meta-analysis. J Clin Pediatr Dent. 2019;43(5):305–13.
29. Rafter M. Apexification: a review. Dent Traumatol. 2005;21(1):1–8.
30. Bakland LK, Andreasen JO. Will mineral trioxide aggregate replace calcium hydroxide in treating pulpal and periodontal healing complications subsequent to dental trauma? A review. Dent Traumatol. 2012;28:25–32.
31. Andreasen J, Farik B, Munksgaard E. Long term calcium hydroxide as a root canal dressing may increase risk of root fracture. Dent Traumatol. 2002;18:134–7.
32. Witherspoon DE, Ham K. One visit apexification technique for inducing root end barrier formation in apical closure. Pract Proced Aesthet Dent. 2001;13(455–60):16.
33. Shabang S, Torabinejad M. Treatment of teeth with open apices using mineral trioxide aggregate. Pract Periodontics Aesthet Dent. 2000;12:315–20.
34. Staffoli S, Plotino G, Nunez Torrijos BG, Grande NM, Bossù M, Gambarini G, Polimeni A. Regenerative endodontic procedures using contemporary endodontic materials. Materials (Basel). 2019;12(6):908.

35. Wei X, Yang M, Yue L, et al. Expert consensus on regenerative endodontic procedures. Int J Oral Sci. 2022;14:55.
36. American Association of Endodontists. AAE clinical considerations for a regenerative procedure. Available at: www.aae.org/Dental_Professional/ConsiderationsforRegenerativeProcedures.aspx.
37. Trope M. Treatment of the immature tooth with a non-vital pulp and apical periodontitis. Dent Clin N Am. 2010;54(3):313–24.
38. Law AS. Considerations for regeneratin procedures. J Endodont. 2013;39(3):S44–56.
39. Martin DE, Henry MA, Almeida JFA, Teixeira FB, Hargreaves KM, Diogenes AR. Effect of sodium hypochlorite on the odontoblastic phenotype differentiation of SCAP in cultured organotype human roots. J Endodont. 2012;(3):e26.
40. Dos Reis-Prado AH, Abreu LG, Fagundes RR, Oliveira SC, Bottino MC, Ribeiro-Sobrinho AP, Benetti F. Influence of ethylenediaminetetraacetic acid on regenerative endodontics: a systematic review. Int Endod J. 2022;55(6):579–612.
41. Elnaggar SE, El Backly RM, Zaazou AM, Morsy Elshabrawy S, Abdallah AA. Effect of different irrigation protocols for applications in regenerative endodontics on mechanical properties of root dentin. Aust Endod J. 2021;47:228–35.
42. Hoshino E, Kurihara-Ando N, Sato I, Uematsu H, Sato M, Kota K, Iwaku M. In-vitro antibacterial susceptibility of bacteria taken from infected root dentine to a mixture of ciprofloxacin, metronidazole and minocycline. Int Endod J. 1996;29(2):125–30.
43. Latham J, Fong H, Jewett A, et al. Disinfection efficacy of current regenerative endodontic protocols in simulated necrotic immature permanent teeth. J Endodont. 2016;42:1218–25.
44. Vatankhah M, Khosravi K, Zargar N, Shirvani A, Nekoofar MH, Dianat O. Antibacterial efficacy of antibiotic pastes versus calcium hydroxide intracanal dressing: a systematic review and meta-analysis of *ex vivo* studies. J Conserv Dent. 2022;25(5):463–80.
45. Ocampo PS, Lázár V, Papp B, Arnoldini M, Abel zur Wiesch P, Busa-Fekete R, Fekete G, Pál C, Ackermann M, Bonhoeffer S. Antagonism between bacteriostatic and bactericidal antibiotics is prevalent. Antimicrob Agents Chemother. 2014;58(8):4573–82.
46. Ruparel NB, Teixeira FB, Ferraz CC, Diogenes A. Direct effect of intracanal medicaments on survival of stem cells of the apical papilla. J Endodont. 2012;38(10):1372–5.
47. Parasuraman VR, Muljibhai BS. 3Mix-MP in endodontics–an overview. J Dent Med Sci. 2012;3(1):36–45.
48. Sabrah AH, Yassen GH, Liu WC, Goebel WS, Gregory RL, Platt JA. The effect of diluted triple and double antibiotic pastes on dental pulp stem cells and established Enterococcus faecalis biofilm. Clin Oral Investig. 2015;19:2059–66.
49. Khoshkhounejad M, Sharifian M, Assadian H, Afshar MS. Antibacterial effectiveness of diluted preparations of intracanal medicaments used in regenerative endodontic treatment on dentin infected by bacterial biofilm: an *ex vivo* investigation. Dent Res J (Isfahan). 2021;18:37.
50. Siqueira JF Jr, Lopes H. Mechanisms of antimicrobial activity of calcium hydroxide: a critical review. Int Endod J. 1999;32(5):361–9.
51. Banchs F, Trope M. Revascularization of immature permanent teeth with apical periodontitis: new treatment protocol? J Endodont. 2004;30(4):196–200.
52. Berkhoff JA, Chen PB, Teixeira FB, Diogenes A. Evaluation of triple antibiotic paste removal by different irrigation procedures. J Endodont. 2014;40(8):1172–7. https://doi.org/10.1016/j.joen.2013.12.027. Epub 2014 Mar 6. PMID: 25069927.
53. Alghilan MA, Windsor LJ, Palasuk J, Yassen GH. Attachment and proliferation of dental pulp stem cells on dentine treated with different regenerative endodontic protocols. Int Endod J. 2017;50(7):667–75. https://doi.org/10.1111/iej.12669. Epub 2016 Jun 27. PMID: 27272393.
54. Riaz S, Azlina A, Mahmood Z, Htun AT. Long-term treatment of dentine with triple antibiotic paste promotes stem cell viability and attachment. J Taibah Univ Med Sci. 2022;17(4):630–9. https://doi.org/10.1016/j.jtumed.2022.01.007. PMID: 35983454; PMCID: PMC9356367.
55. Capar ID, Ozcan E, Arslan H, Ertas H, Aydinbelge HA. Effect of different final irrigation methods on the removal of calcium hydroxide from an artificial standardized groove

in the apical third of root canals. J Endodont. 2014;40(3):451–4. https://doi.org/10.1016/j.joen.2013.10.019. Epub 2013 Nov 9. PMID: 24565670.
56. Murray PE. Platelet-rich plasma and platelet-rich fibrin can induce apical closure more frequently than blood-clot revascularization for the regeneration of immature permanent teeth: a meta-analysis of clinical efficacy. Front Bioeng Biotechnol. 2018;6:139.
57. Chueh LH, Huang GT. Immature teeth with periradicular periodontitis or abscess undergoing apexogenesis: a paradigm shift. J Endodont. 2006;32:1205–13.
58. Dennis J, Subramanian K, Kumar A. Management of immature permanent teeth with pulpal necrosis: a case series. Pediatr Dent. 2013;35:55–60.
59. Diogenes A, Henry MA, Teizeira FB, Hargreaves KM. An update on clinical regenerative endodontics. Endod Top. 2013;28:2–23.
60. Lin L, Kahler BA. Review of regenrative endodontics: current protocols and future directions. J Istanbul Univ Fac Dent. 2017;51(3 Suppl 1):S41–51.
61. Haung G, Sonoyama W, Liu Y. The hidden treasure in apical papilla: the potential role in dentin/pulp regeneration and bioroot engineering. J Endodont. 2008;34:645–51.
62. Kontakiotis EG, Filippatos CG, Tzanetakis GN, Agrafioti A. Regenerative endodontic therapy: a data analysis of clinical protocols. J Endodont. 2015;41(2):146–54.
63. Galler KM, Widbiller M, Buchalla W, Eidt A, Hiller KA, Hoffer PC, Schmalz G. EDTA conditioning of dentine promotes adhesion, migration and differentiation of dental pulp stem cells. Int Endod J. 2016;49(6):581–90.
64. Chen MY, Chen KL, Chen CA, Tayebaty F, Rosenberg PA, Lin LM. Responses of immature permanent teeth with infected necrotic pulp tissue and apical periodontitis/abscess to revascularization procedures. Int Endod J. 2012;45(3):294–305.
65. Zeng Q, Zhang J, Guo J, Liu S, Yang M, Lin J. Preoperative factors analysis on root development after regenerative endodontic procedures: a retrospective study. BMC Oral Health. 2022;22(1):1–7.
66. Tong HJ, Rajan S, Bhujel N, Kang J, Duggal M, Nazzal H. Regenerative endodontic therapy in the management of nonvital immature permanent teeth: a systematic review—outcome evaluation and meta-analysis. J Endodont. 2017;43(9):1453–64.
67. Shaik I, Tulli M, Unnam P, Karunakaran S, Vaddi DS, Jabeen R, Tiwari RV. Regenerative endodontic therapy in the management of nonvital immature permanent teeth: a systematic review and meta-analysis. J Pharm Bioallied Sci. 2021;13(Suppl 1):S36.
68. Koc S, Del Fabbro M. Does the etiology of pulp necrosis affect regenerative endodontic treatment outcomes? A systematic review and meta-analyses. J Evid Based Dent Pract. 2020;20(1):101400.
69. Marciano MA, Costa RM, Camilleri J, Mondelli RF, Guimarães BM, Duarte MA. Assessment of color stability of white mineral trioxide aggregate angelus and bismuth oxide in contact with tooth structure. J Endodont. 2014;40(8):1235–40.
70. Kahler B, Rossi-Fedele G. A review of tooth discoloration after regenerative endodontic therapy. J Endodont. 2016;42(4):563–9. https://doi.org/10.1016/j.joen.2015.12.022. Epub 2016 Feb 4. PMID: 26852148.
71. Santos LGPD, Chisini LA, Springmann CG, Souza BDM, Pappen FG, Demarco FF, Felippe MCS, Felippe WT. Alternative to avoid tooth discoloration after regenerative endodontic procedure: a systematic review. Braz Dent J. 2018;29(5):409–18. https://doi.org/10.1590/0103-6440201802132. PMID: 30517438.
72. Kahler B, et al. Revascularization outcomes: a prospective analysis of 16 consecutive cases. J Endodont. 2014;40:333–8.
73. Dabbagh B, Alvaro E, Vu DD, Rizkallah J, Schwartz S. Clinical complications in the revascularization of immature necrotic permanent teeth. Pediatr Dent. 2012;34(5):414–7.

Traumatic Dental Injuries to the Permanent Dentition

11

11.1 Introduction

Traumatic Dental Injuries (TDI) are one of the few true emergencies in dental practice necessitating an urgent examination followed by appropriate interventions, as indicated [1]. While these dental injuries adversely affect critical oral functions such as speech, mastication, esthetics, the shock and physical pain associated with the injury along with damage or loss of tooth structure heightens the child's anxiety, resulting in uncooperative behavior on the dental chair [2]. The lower incidence of TDIs in routine dental practice requires the dentist to refer to the guidelines for immediate treatment and the long-term management. The recommendations by the International Association of Dental Traumatology (IADT) equips clinicians with a ready blueprint on the diagnosis and management of dental trauma [3–6]. While the above provides an excellent protocol to manage most traumas, the combinations of TDI and the unpredictable outcomes make the clinical decisions and treatment a challenge.

11.2 Initial Assessment

Knowing when, where, and how the injury occurred assists the clinician in determining the severity of the trauma. It is critical to ascertain the time elapsed since the injury took place as this will determine the treatment plan and affect the prognosis of the injured tooth [1, 7–9]. Most children reporting first to the dental clinic generally present with trauma to the maxillofacial structure and dentition. However, they must be observed for the following signs and symptoms:

- Dizziness
- Headache
- Nausea/vomiting

H. Vyas et al., *Dental Caries and Traumatic Injuries in Pediatric Dentistry*,
https://doi.org/10.1007/978-3-031-98929-2_11

- Loss of memory
- Loss of consciousness
- Lethargy or irritability

The presence of any of the above signs and symptoms necessitates an immediate referral to the emergency room [1, 7–9].

11.3 Injuries to the Dental Hard Tissues and the Pulp

11.3.1 Crown Fractures

These are the most commonly occurring TDIs in the permanent dentition and the maxillary central incisor is most frequently affected [10]. When a child reports to the dental office with a crown fracture on one or more teeth, a detailed clinical examination must be carried out under a good lighting source. The affected area must be gently cleaned of debris using wet gauze to visualize the site of fracture clearly. The tooth must be inspected for additional fragments that may be subgingival or not completely dislodged. The surrounding soft tissues and lips must also be evaluated for embedded tooth fragments (Fig. 11.1) [11, 12].

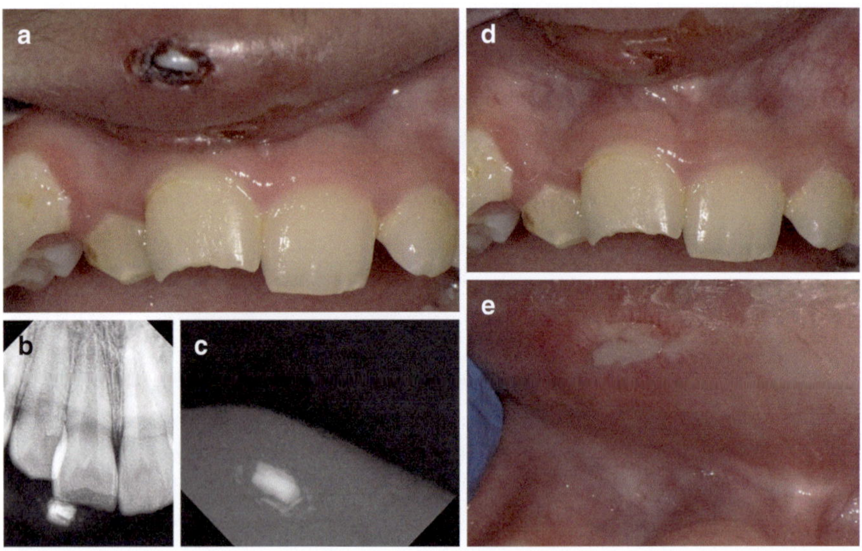

Fig. 11.1 Crown fracture of maxillary permanent right central incisor (**a**). Radiograph of the tooth with fragment embedded in the upper lip (**b**). A soft tissue radiograph taken for a closer look of the fragment (**c**). Fragment removed under local anesthesia (**d**) and the tissue was seen healing in a week (**e**)

11.3.1.1 Clinical and Radiographic Examination

The examination must focus on the following aspects, based on which the treatment protocol is decided:

- *Extent of tooth structure lost*

Crown fractures can be classified as follows:

(a) *Enamel infarction* is an incomplete fracture (crack or crazing) of the enamel, without loss of tooth structure. Enamel infarctions are best identified with trans-illumination. This is done by placing a resin curing light on either the facial or lingual surface of the tooth and viewing the area from the opposite side by either direct vision or indirect vision with a mouth mirror. In case of enamel infarctions and enamel fractures, the tooth is generally not sensitive to variations in temperature and use of an air syringe [13].

(b) *Uncomplicated Crown Fractures*
The fracture line may be horizontal or oblique. Enamel fracture involves only enamel, with loss of tooth structure (Fig. 11.2). Enamel–dentin fracture is confined to enamel and dentin without pulp exposure. If the injury is close to the pulp, *a pinkish hue* may be seen (Figs. 11.3 and 11.4) [13, 14].

(c) *Complicated crown fracture* involves enamel and dentin with pulpal involvement. The extent of pulp exposure can vary from *pinpoint to larger* (Figs. 11.8 and 11.9). In enamel–dentin fractures, both uncomplicated and complicated, the patient is likely to have sensitivity to hot and cold stimuli and react to the use of an air syringe [13, 14].

While the different type of crown fractures described above can be easily identified in *anterior teeth*, their presence may often be overlooked in the *posterior teeth* in emergency situations, especially if the tooth fragment is not displaced and the fracture line is not clearly visible. Fractures in the posterior teeth are commonly

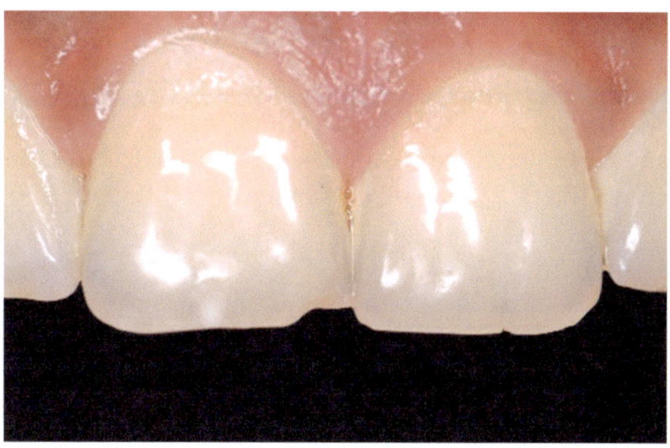

Fig. 11.2 Enamel fracture of the maxillary permanent right central incisor

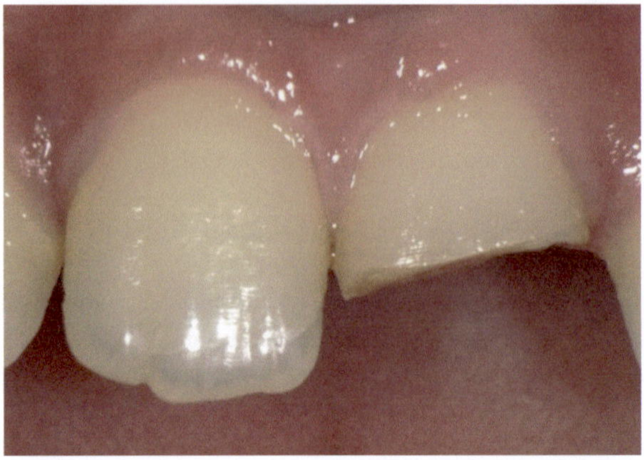

Fig. 11.3 Enamel-dentin fracture on the maxillary permanent left central incisor

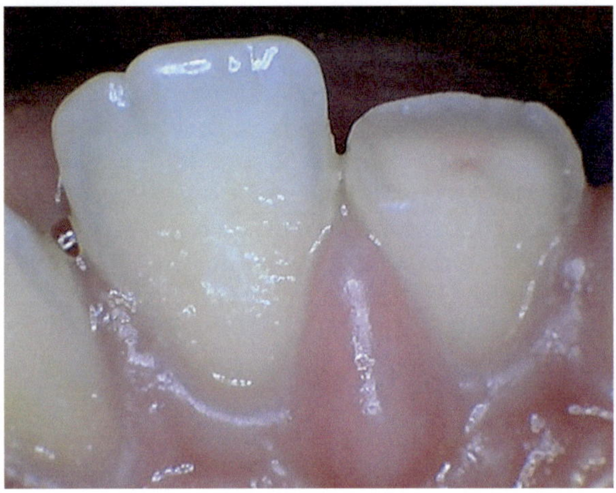

Fig. 11.4 Enamel-dentin fracture with pinkish pulpal hue seen on the maxillary permanent left central incisor

associated with trauma to the chin, wherein the mandibular teeth are forced against the maxillary teeth [15].

Vertical percussion should be performed on posterior teeth in suspected cases. The patient is asked to bite down on a cotton roll and observe for pain on chewing and movement of any fragment. A positive response to the above is indicative of a crown fracture in a posterior tooth (Figs. 11.5 and 11.6) [15–17].

- Mobility

The mobility of the tooth must be checked with the handles of two mouth mirrors placed labially and palatally. Presence of mobility along with bleeding and hemorrhage from the gingival sulcus may indicate a *luxation injury, a crown–root, or a root fracture* [18, 19]. Simultaneously, the mobility of adjacent teeth must also be

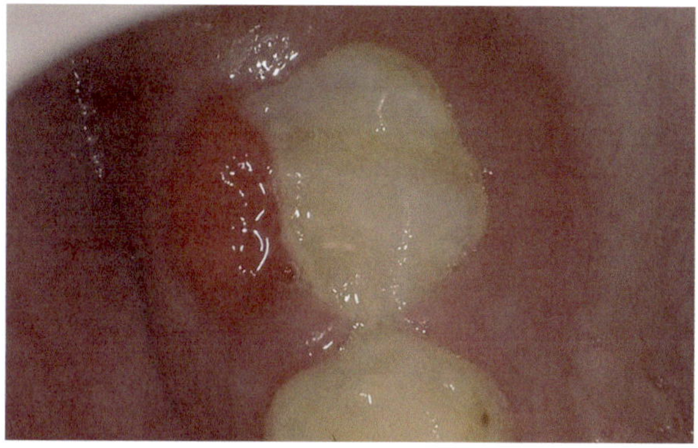

Fig. 11.5 Fracture of maxillary primary right second molar

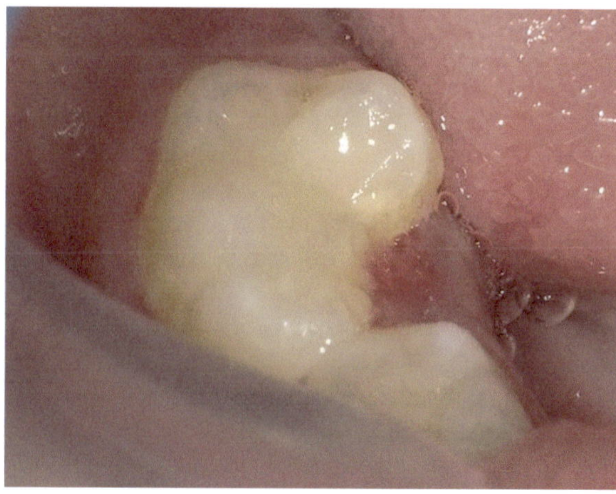

Fig. 11.6 Fracture of mandibular primary right second molar

checked. If the entire segment involving three to four teeth is mobile, it indicates an alveolar fracture [20].

- Radiographs

A paralleling radiograph must be taken as part of the initial assessment of the traumatic injury. An X-ray positioning device (Rinn XCP positioner, Dentsply Sirona, USA; EzAim® Xray Positioning System, Pac-Dent®, USA) must be used so that the baseline image and those taken during the follow-up appointments are standardized. Radiographs at an angulation of +15 and −15 to the baseline must be taken to rule out root fracture.

In *anterior teeth*, the presence of a crown fracture is self-evident on examination and a radiograph helps to ascertain the extent of the fracture line and its proximity to the pulp chamber [4, 18, 21].

In *posterior teeth* with non-displaced tooth fragments, the radiograph acts a means of diagnosis. A posterior crown fracture appears as a coronal radiolucent line on the radiograph. To rule out any overlap, the radiograph should be repeated with a change in angulation [15–17].

If the patient complains of pain on biting and the fracture line is not visible clinically or on an intraoral periapical radiograph (IOPA), an occlusal radiograph or a Cone Beam Computed Tomography (CBCT) should be advised to confirm the fracture [21].

The other aspects to be checked in the radiograph include:

Stage of root development, radicular dentinal thickness, and root length indicates whether the tooth is immature or mature. This dictates the treatment protocol and outcome. *Presence of luxation injuries and root fractures* must also be identified during the initial radiographic examination [9, 21].

- Pulp sensibility [7, 9, 18]

Trauma to the tooth may result in injury to the dental pulp. This impact may lead to pulpal degeneration over time which may affect the development of the tooth, the treatment, and its survival. Hence, it is necessary to monitor the pulpal status of a tooth following any trauma over a period. Pulp vitality is a measure of the vascularity and is assessed using tests like pulse oximetry, laser doppler flowmetry, ultrasound doppler flowmetry, and thermometry that are not commercially available for chairside usage. Clinical tests like the thermal test and the Electric Pulp Test (EPT) can elicit only a neural response [22]. As the nerve cells are known to degenerate first, the response to these tests does *indirectly* provide an assessment of the pulpal vascularity [7, 22]. They are called pulp sensibility tests and must be performed on the first appointment and repeated during follow-up visits.

Response to a pulp sensibility test is usually positive for all recent *uncomplicated crown fractures*. In case of a *complicated crown fracture*, the clinical appearance of the pulp at the site of exposure is indicative of pulp vitality. A pale pink to bright red color is suggestive of a healthier pulp while a grayish/yellowish pulp may indicate the presence of degenerative changes due to significant time elapsed since the injury. A pulp sensibility test must still be performed on the first appointment after ensuring adequate pulp protection to determine a positive or negative response at baseline [4]. The response of *immature teeth* to vitality tests is often inaccurate and they are known to give a false-negative response due to incompletely developed neural innervation [23, 24].

The heat test is performed by placing a heated gutta-core or ball-ended metallic instrument or a battery-powered heat-controlled device on the tooth. Similarly, the cold test uses CO_2 snow or dichlorodifluoromethane (DDM) (CanalPro Endo-Ice, Coltene; Roeko Endo-Frost, Coltene) which is sprayed on a cotton pellet and placed in contact with the tooth. An EPT (Digitest 3, Parkell® USA; Gentle Pulse™ Pulp Vitality Tester, Parkell® USA) comprises of an electrode which is applied to the tooth and a lip clip to complete the electric circuit [23, 25]. Pulp testing must be done before administering local anesthesia or sedation to the child. While EPT is seen to be the most accurate followed by the cold test, it is suggested that the EPT and the cold test be combined for the best results [26, 27].

For immature teeth, cold test has shown more reliability than an EPT [25].

While performing the pulp sensibility tests, the stimulus should be applied on the enamel, away from the fracture line ideally on the middle third of the tooth (Fig. 11.7). It is recommended to test the contralateral or adjacent teeth of the same dentition as this provides a control and helps in eliciting an unbiased response from the patient [23, 25].

The common responses seen to these tests are as follows:

- The pulp is deemed normal when the stimulus elicits a response, which is not pronounced or exaggerated, and does not linger as compared to the control tooth.
- The continued absence or a delayed response is usually associated with a degenerating pulp [23, 25].

All teeth irrespective of their response to pulp testing, must be retested as follows:

A tooth giving a positive response:

- Uncomplicated fractures at 6–8 weeks and 1 year.
- Complicated fractures at 6–8 weeks, 3 months, 6 months, 1 year.

A tooth giving a negative or altered response:

- Every 6–8 weeks till a definitive diagnosis of pulp status can be made.
- Must be monitored for any progressive signs of discoloration or infection [7].
- In case of repeated negative responses to the pulp test, the tooth must be deemed non-vital only after corroborating with the clinical and radiographic findings.

While pulp sensibility testing must be ideally done when the child reports with trauma, it may be difficult to perform due to the type of trauma and the cooperation of the patient. If the baseline cannot be recorded at the initial visit, the child must be recalled a few days later for pulp sensibility testing.

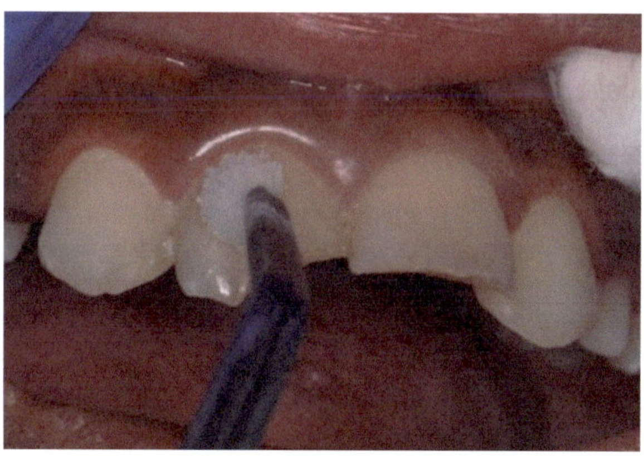

Fig. 11.7 The stimulus for pulp sensibility test must be applied on the enamel, away from the fracture line

11.3.1.2 Management of Crown Fracture (Fig. 11.15)

- *Uncomplicated crown fracture (without pulp exposure).*

The *initial management* of an uncomplicated crown fracture (without pulp exposure) remains the same irrespective of the root development.

For *crown fracture of an anterior tooth*, the parents and the child must be told to look for the tooth fragment at the site of trauma and store it in water. Fragment reattachment is the preferred definitive restoration, which should ideally be done at the same visit. Alternatively, an alginate impression of the fractured tooth may be taken to make a putty index to facilitate a resin composite buildup. If definitive treatment for an enamel dentin fracture is deferred, a Glass Ionomer Cement liner must be placed along the fracture line to ensure that the dentin is not exposed to any noxious stimuli or bacterial contamination.

If the exposed dentin is within 0.5 mm of the pulp (pinkish hue but no bleeding), a light cured Calcium Hydroxide (CH) liner or calcium silicate material can be placed followed by a Glass Ionomer Cement restoration. Teeth with concomitant luxation injuries must be splinted with the help of a resin composite and wire (upto 0.4 mm in diameter) splint or Titanium Trauma Splint for 7–14 days [4, 13, 14, 28].

The fragment must be kept hydrated in water or saline till the time of procedure. A well-hydrated fragment will not have chalky white patches. The IADT recommends a 20-min hydration protocol before the reattachment procedure [4].

In *posterior teeth* with an uncomplicated crown fracture, reattachment may be attempted if the fragment approximates well, and good isolation is achieved. In case the loose fragment extends subgingivally, the fragment is removed to assess the extent of fracture below the gingival margin before attempting reattachment.

While there are case reports showing successful fragment reattachment in posterior teeth, in areas that bear the masticatory load or the fracture extends subgingivally, an orthodontic band may be placed to reinforce the attachment [29]. If the fracture is close to the pulp, a light cured CH liner or calcium silicate material is placed followed by an interim or definitive restoration [15–17].

- *Complicated crown fractures (with pulp exposure)* (Figs. 11.8, 11.9, 11.13 and 11.14)

Due to the high cellular and vascular content in *an immature tooth*, the chances of success of vital pulp therapy are greater as compared to a tooth with completely formed roots.

The most critical factor determining the course of treatment is the *time elapsed since trauma.* Irrespective of the size of the exposure, the approach in an *immature vital tooth* must always be conservative, and procedures such as Cvek's (shallow) or complete pulpotomy must be planned [29].

While DPC can be performed for *pinpoint exposures* when the patient reports *within a few hours of injury*, a Cvek's pulpotomy is the preferred treatment [30, 31].

The rationale is to excise around 2 mm of the contaminated and inflamed pulp that has been exposed to noxious stimuli while preserving the remaining healthy

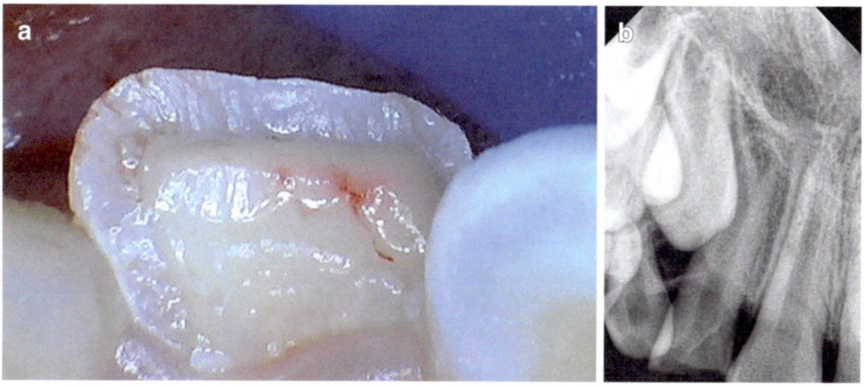

Fig. 11.8 Pinpoint pulp exposure seen clinically following a complicated crown fracture of the maxillary permanent right lateral incisor (**a**). Radiograph shows an immature root apex (**b**)

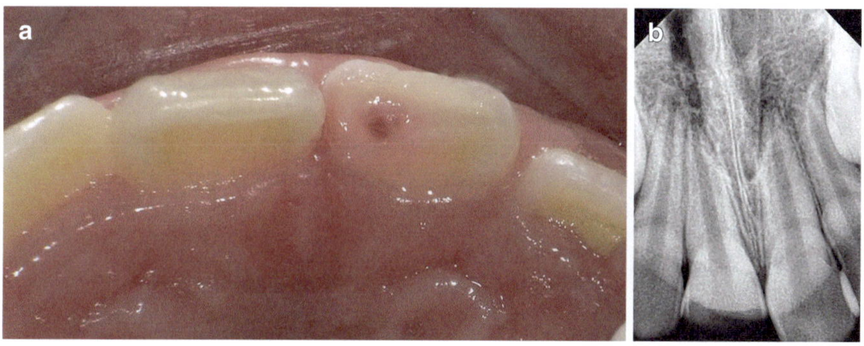

Fig. 11.9 A larger pulp exposure following complicated crown fracture to the maxillary permanent right central incisor (**a**). Radiograph shows an immature root apex (**b**)

pulp that has healing and repair potential [31, 32]. The remaining pulp is capped with a calcium silicate or bioceramic capping material and a coronal seal is provided [14, 28].

A partial pulpotomy allows the CSC to be placed adequately in contact with the pulpal tissue ensuring a better seal. Also, a larger dentinal surface is available at the fracture site to bond to the resin composite [33].

In larger exposures irrespective of the time elapsed, a Cvek's pulpotomy must be performed.

In oblique fractures extending cervically that involve a larger part of the crown, a complete pulpotomy is advised as the Cvek's pulpotomy may not suffice.

If the fracture line is such that it will not hold the pulp capping material, the exposure can be enlarged, and bleeding controlled with a cotton pellet moistened in saline for a few minutes. The exposed pulp is covered with a calcium silicate material.

The fracture line is either covered with an interim restorative material like the GIC or can be restored with fragment reattachment or resin composite buildup at the same visit.

In case of a concomitant luxation injury, the tooth must be first repositioned and stabilized with a splint followed by vital pulp therapy.

In case of complicated crown fractures in a *posterior tooth*, the same treatment protocol as discussed above is followed. An orthodontic band may be placed on the tooth to support an interim restoration. These bands can be removed when the tooth is ready to receive a definitive restoration. Alternatively, an extracoronal restoration can be placed at the same visit [15–17].

For mature anterior teeth, a Cvek's or complete pulpotomy can be performed, depending on the size of pulp exposure and extent of crown fracture, if the patient reports within a few hours [34].

A conventional endodontic therapy is better suited when

- Operator is uncertain about the pulpal health.
- Significant time elapsed since trauma.
- Presence of concomitant luxation injuries.
- A post is required to restore the tooth [4].

Definitive management for complicated and uncomplicated crown fracture involves the final restoration of the fractured tooth that can be performed at the first appointment itself. At times, the patient may need to be recalled for completing the definitive treatment. This gives the child a chance to recover from the shock and simultaneously, provides the clinician time to reassess the situation and take definitive action.

At the second appointment (anterior teeth)

- If a splint is placed, assess mobility, and remove the splint after 7 days, to prepare the tooth for restoration.
- The pulp sensibility test should be repeated and compared with baseline.
- The tooth is restored by reattaching the fragment with adhesives, or a direct composite buildup [4].

At the second appointment (posterior teeth)

Depending on the extent of sound tooth structure remaining and the number of surfaces involved, posterior teeth with crown fractures can be restored with either fragment reattachment, a direct or indirect composite restoration, or a stainless-steel crown [15–17].

Fragment reattachment of an anterior tooth offers the most esthetic outcome if the margin of the fragment approximates closely to the fractured tooth (Figs. 11.10 and 11.11). Also, it is a highly conservative procedure that requires little or no tooth preparation. Additionally, there is no discoloration as seen with a resin restoration and the wear rate, color, contour, and texture is the same as that of the adjacent natural tooth [34–36]. If inter-fragmentary space is seen or a small part is missing,

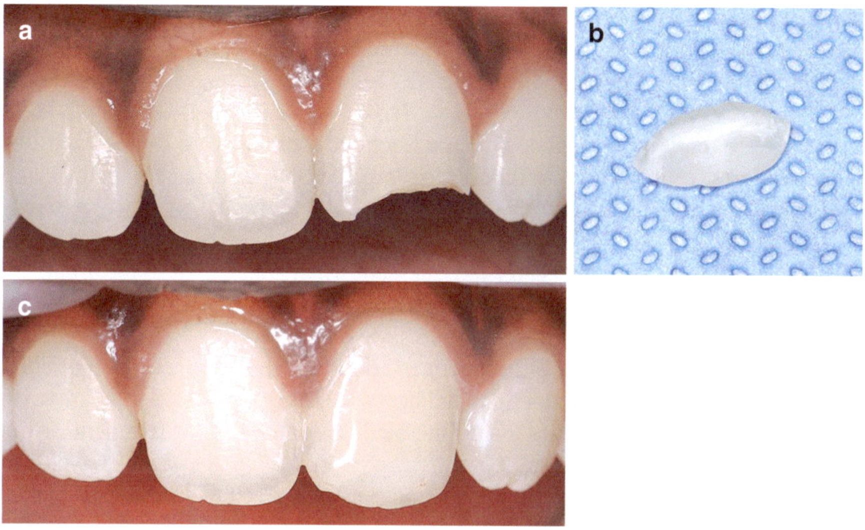

Fig. 11.10 Uncomplicated crown fracture of maxillary permanent left central incisor (**a**). Patient reported with a dry fragment. The fragment was immersed in normal saline for 20 min before reattachment (**b**). Fragment reattached to restore form and esthetics (**c**)

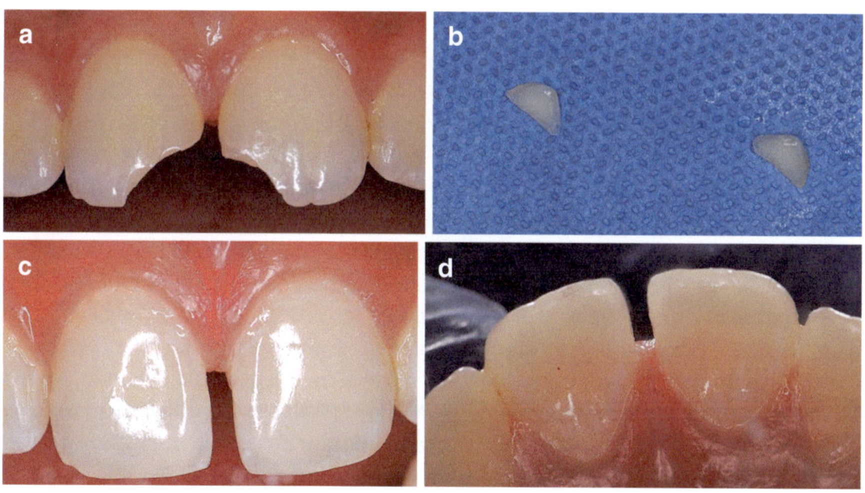

Fig. 11.11 Uncomplicated crown fracture of maxillary permanent central incisors (**a**). Patient reported within few hours, with fragments immersed in water (**b**). The fragments were reattached, labial (**c**) and palatal view (**d**)

reattachment can still be considered if there is a good amount of original tooth structure present, and the fragment can be approximated for most parts.

The fragment reattachment technique is as follows:

- Before the reattachment procedure, the fractured tooth must be cleaned and isolated with a rubber dam. A Teflon tape is placed on the adjacent teeth, if the contacts are tight to ensure separation.
- The incisal edge of the fragment could be bonded to the back end of a micro brush, so that it is easier to carry the fragment when attaching it to the tooth.
- The fragment and the fractured tooth are treated with an "etch and rinse" technique using 37% phosphoric acid for 15 s.
- Apply the bonding agent on the fractured tooth and the fragment. Do not cure, keep the fragment away from light and heat sources.
- Apply a flowable composite as an intermediary either on the fragment or the fractured tooth.
- Place the fragment on the tooth making sure the fracture line approximates correctly.
- The fractured fragment should also be checked for alignment along the long axis of the tooth. Remove excessive flowable resin and light cure for 20 s.
- The restored tooth can be finished and polished using silicon points or polishing discs immediately after the fragment reattachment [36].
- Finishing and polishing is done from resin composite restoration to the tooth.

Pulp capping materials, if needed in an uncomplicated crown fracture should be placed such that they allow for close approximation of the fragments. After placing the capping material, the fragment reattachment procedure should be performed in the same appointment so that a Glass Ionomer bandage does not need to be placed on the fractured edge. This will interfere with good approximation of the fragment to the tooth, thereby increasing the chances of failure.

Several tooth preparation techniques such as circumferential bevel, chamfer, internal grooves, and superficial over-contouring have been used in literature. There is no consensus on any one type of tooth preparation providing greater bond strength than the other. Bonding of the fragment to the tooth depends on the fit and viability of the tooth fragment. Bevelling of the tooth prior to fragment reattachment improved the retention compared to no preparation at all [37, 38].

An increase in the bond strength between tooth fragment and dentin was observed when an intermediate material like flowable composite was used [37, 38].

In cases of crown fractures *where the fragment is lost or is an improper fit*, the tooth can be restored with resin composite. The resin composite in an anterior tooth can be built up with or without a putty index, *with a stratified layering technique* [39].

Composite restorations should emulate the optical characteristics of natural teeth, which can only be achieved by the critical first step of accurate shade selection. The process of shade selection and stratification becomes easier if one is familiar with the basic morphological characteristics of an anterior tooth. For the purpose of understanding, it is important for the operator to visualize the tooth in a cross-sectional view. The enamel is the thinnest at the gingival or cervical margin and the dentin is close to the surface. As we move towards the incisal edge, the dentin reduces as the enamel thickness increases.

To obtain a life-like buildup of the resin composite, stratification should always be done using a darker composite in the inner layers and moving to a lighter shade in the outer layer. The dentinal composite in the buildup should always be sandwiched between a layer of palatal and labial enamel.

In the cervical third, there is more reflection and virtually no passage of light. As there is greater color saturation due to the underlying dentin being seen, one should use dentin shades and a very thin or no enamel layer.

The middle third will have less dentinal color as compared to the cervical third. This can be achieved by layering the dentin composite to one shade lighter than seen on the cervical third or by placing a thicker layer of overlying enamel.

The middle third also shows more reflection and prevents passage of light so as to minimize the "see through effect" which will show the demarcation between the fractured tooth and the Resin Composite buildup. Dentin composites from higher to lower opacities are placed starting from the deeper layer.

The incisal aspect of the tooth is translucent and allows more light passage and lesser reflection. When restoring this zone, it is advisable to place translucent enamel composite with minimal or no inner dentinal layer.

- *Selecting the right composite shade*

The first step during this stratification procedure is to select the base shade from the middle one-third of the tooth. Place a small amount of composite on the adjacent tooth and light cure (button dry technique). If after curing, the composite matches the adjacent enamel, then it is selected as the base shade. To give depth to the resin composite buildup, the underlying composites should be a shade darker than the outermost layer simulating the enamel. If the operator chooses to restore the tooth with resin composites having base color A2 (VITA Shade Guide®, Germany), the surface enamel on the palatal and labial surfaces should be built with A2 enamel shade and the deeper dentinal layers with darker dentin shades.

- *Step by step workflow of the composite restoration of a fractured anterior tooth (Figs. 11.12 and 11.15)*
  - At the first appointment, make a sectional impression of the fractured tooth and adjacent teeth with alginate.
  - Apply a layer of bonding agent on the stone model and do a mock composite buildup of the fractured tooth. Replicate the palatal anatomy accurately and ensure the surface is polished well.
  - Make a putty impression of the palatal surface to create a stent. The stent should extend onto the adjacent teeth on either side and up to the incisal edge taking care not to cover any portion of the labial surface.

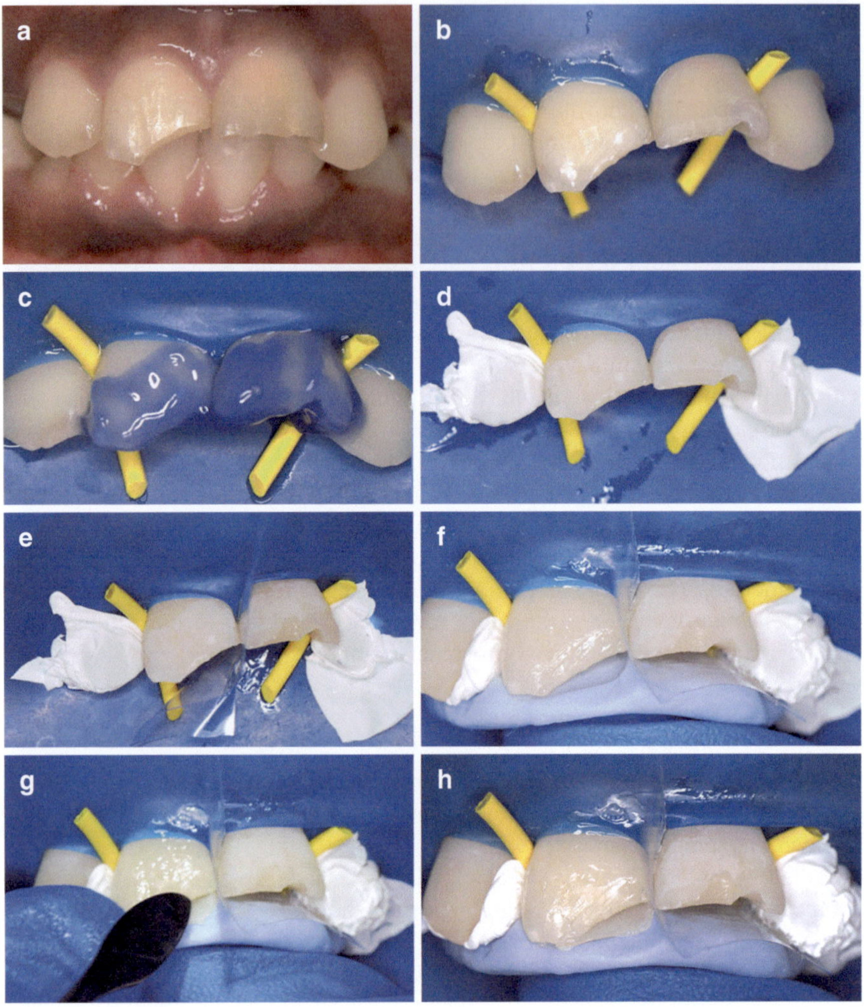

Fig. 11.12 Uncomplicated crown fracture of maxillary permanent central incisors (**a**). The teeth were isolated under rubber dam, and the fractured edges were prepared with a short bevel to improve retention of the resin composite (**b**). Both incisors were etched with 37% phosphoric acid for 15 s (**c**). The etchant was washed and air-dried such that the enamel appeared frosty (**d**). A mylar strip placed to prevent bonding agent from adhering to the adjacent tooth and to build proximal contacts. Adjacent teeth were covered with Teflon tape (**e**). Bonding agent applied on maxillary right central incisor and putty index held in place (**f**). The first increment of enamel shade built using a flat bladed instrument, to replicate the palatal shell (**g**). The palatal shell was cured (**h**). The second increment, replicating dentin was layered on the palatal shell, such that it was thick in the middle and thinned down as it approached the incisal region. The material was extended to build contact mesially (**i**). Mamelons or developmental lobes, if required should be sculpted in this layer (**j**). The third layer of a darker dentin shade built in the same manner. Internal mamelons were sculpted in this layer (**k**). The last layer of resin composite replicating enamel (same shade used to build palatal shell) placed. It should be thinnest at the cervical zone and thickest at the incisal zone, extending proximally to blend with the restoration (**l**). The left central incisor was built in a similar manner (**m**). Gross finishing of both teeth done to desired shape (**n**). Polishing done with discs and polishing paste (**o**). Teeth in palatal view showing identical contour, thickness and alignment to arch form (**p**)

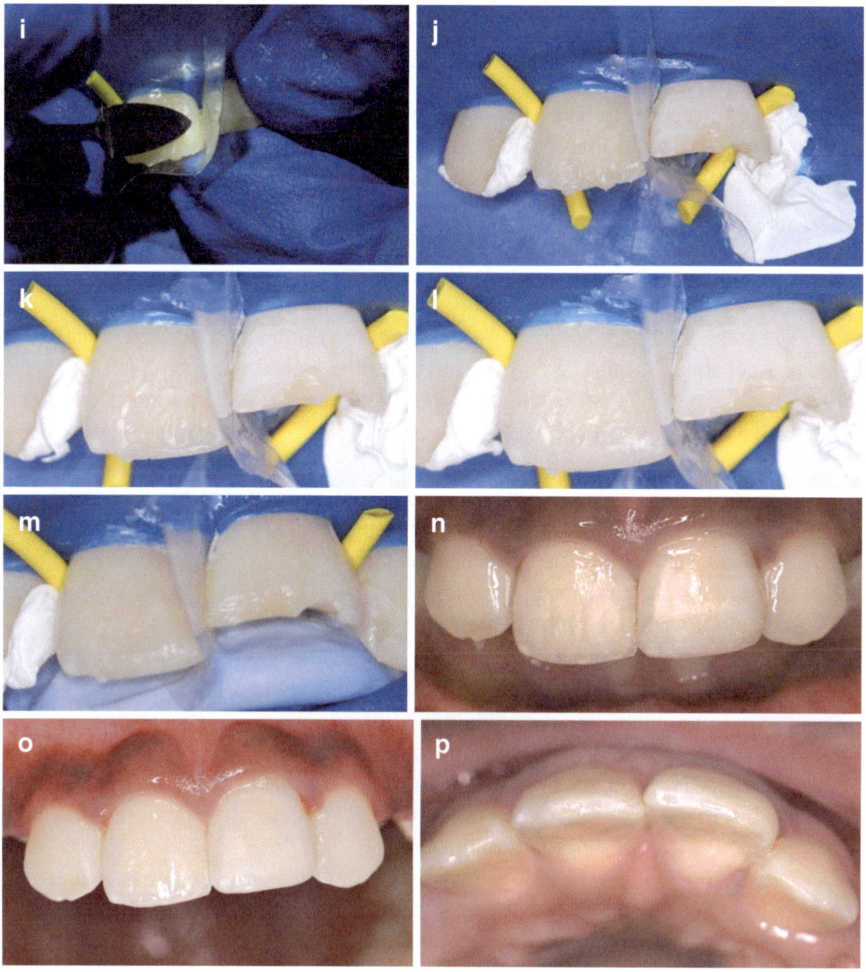

Fig. 11.12 (continued)

- This allows building of the palatal shell or first layer of stratification on which the remaining layers can be placed.
- At the second appointment, clean and polish the tooth to remove debris and plaque.
- Select the base shade using the composite button dry technique. Let us consider that we are restoring a tooth with a base shade of A2. An example of the composite stratification would be as follows:

$$\text{Base shade A2} = \text{A3 dentin shade}\left(\text{innermost layer}\right) + \text{A2 dentin shade}\left(\text{second layer}\right) + \text{A2 enamel shade}\left(\text{outermost layer}\right)$$

- Isolate the segment with a rubber dam. Additional retraction can be achieved with floss ties or gingival retraction cord. The adjacent teeth can be covered with Teflon tape.
- A 3–4 mm bevel must be placed along the fracture line to ensure a seamless and well-blended final restoration.
- Etch with 37% phosphoric acid for 20 s. Rinse and blot dry.
- Apply one or two coats of bonding agent, air dry and light cure. It is important to avoid pooling and curing of a thick layer of bonding agent, especially those containing HEMA, as this may not only compromise the bond strength but also degrade over time and lead to discoloration of the restoration.
- The stent should be held against the fractured tooth and a 0.5 mm layer of A2 enamel shade should be constructed to replicate the palatal enamel.
- Once the palatal shell is built, the stent may be removed, and matrices can be used to build proximal contours.
- Proceeding to the stratification of dentin, the first dentin layer placed should have a higher chroma (A3 dentin shade) and must be opaque. This will prevent the see through effect. It should be placed such that it is thickest cervically and thins out as it approaches the incisal.
- This layer of composite should not extend into the incisal zone. It should be sculpted to create the three developmental lobes of the incisors.
- The next layer of composite should be of a lighter shade and less opaque than the previous layer (A2 dentin shade) and is placed in a similar manner. Should internal mamelons be recreated, they must be sculpted in this layer.
- The outermost layer of composite replaces labial enamel and it should be more translucent and have lesser chroma as compared to the dentinal shades used. A thin layer of A2 enamel shade is placed cervically, increasing in thickness as it extends incisally and proximally.
- The incisal edge can be built using only enamel shades to ensure translucency. Incisal shades having a bluish gray tinge may be used to replicate the incisal esthetics [39, 40].
- The restoration should be finished using fine grit diamond points to remove gross irregularities. Polishing is done using polishing discs and interdental strips from the coarser to the finer grits.
- A surface sealant (Fortify™, BISCO, USA; PermaSeal™, Ultradent, USA) must be applied after polishing to seal microporosities.
- The final restoration should not only match the base shade chosen but also mimic the natural tooth. This is achieved by using a combination of composites with different opacities and chromas as outlined above.

11.3.1.3 Success of Fragment Reattachment Versus Direct Composite Restoration (Buildup)?

A systematic review showed that direct composite restorations had a significantly lower annual failure rate of 19.3% compared with 34.5% for the reattachment technique [37, 41, 42]. While studies show the success of composite buildup to be higher than that of fragment reattachment, in case of bonding failure, the fragment can once again be reattached to the tooth. Also, the excellent aesthetics of retaining the natural tooth makes this the procedure of choice in crown fractures when the fragment can be retrieved.

11.3.1.4 Follow-Up Period for Crown Fractures

1. Teeth with an open apex must be followed up at regular intervals with radiographic examination and pulp sensibility testing to check for root development and pulp vitality, respectively. The formation of a dentin bridge and continued root development is a possible indicator of successful vital pulp therapy (Figs. 11.13 and 11.14).
   - Complicated and uncomplicated crown fractures must have a baseline radiograph which is repeated at 6 months, 12 months, and then yearly till root completion [4].
   - Fractures with concomitant luxation injuries must be radiographed at baseline, 6–8 weeks, 3 months and 6 monthly thereafter to check for root resorption [4, 5].
2. If the root development seems arrested or there are signs of root resorption, intervention is necessary.
3. Teeth may show a varied response to pulp sensibility test:
   - If the roots are immature.
   - In complete pulpotomies or some cases of shallow pulpotomies.
   - When a large restoration or full coronal restoration is placed.
4. Lastly, in teeth showing a negative response at baseline, they must be followed up at 6–8 weeks, 3 monthly, and 6 monthly and the line of treatment decided after corroborating with clinical and radiographic evidence.
5. Pulp necrosis after treatment is usually revealed within 2–3 years and the tooth must be treated in the presence of following signs and symptoms.
   - Spontaneous pain
   - Tenderness on percussion
   - Periapical radiolucency

11.3.2 Root Fractures

Root fractures may result in complete or incomplete separation of the roots. These fractures commonly involve the dentin, cementum, as well as the pulp. Depending on the plane of fracture, they can be categorized as horizontal (mesiodistal plane), vertical, or oblique fractures. Root fractures are seen more often in mature teeth than immature teeth [43]. The developing roots and the elasticity of the alveolar socket in immature teeth make them more susceptible to luxation injuries than root fractures.

While most root fractures are seen as a transverse radiolucent line on a radiograph, incomplete or vertical fractures may often escape detection [44].

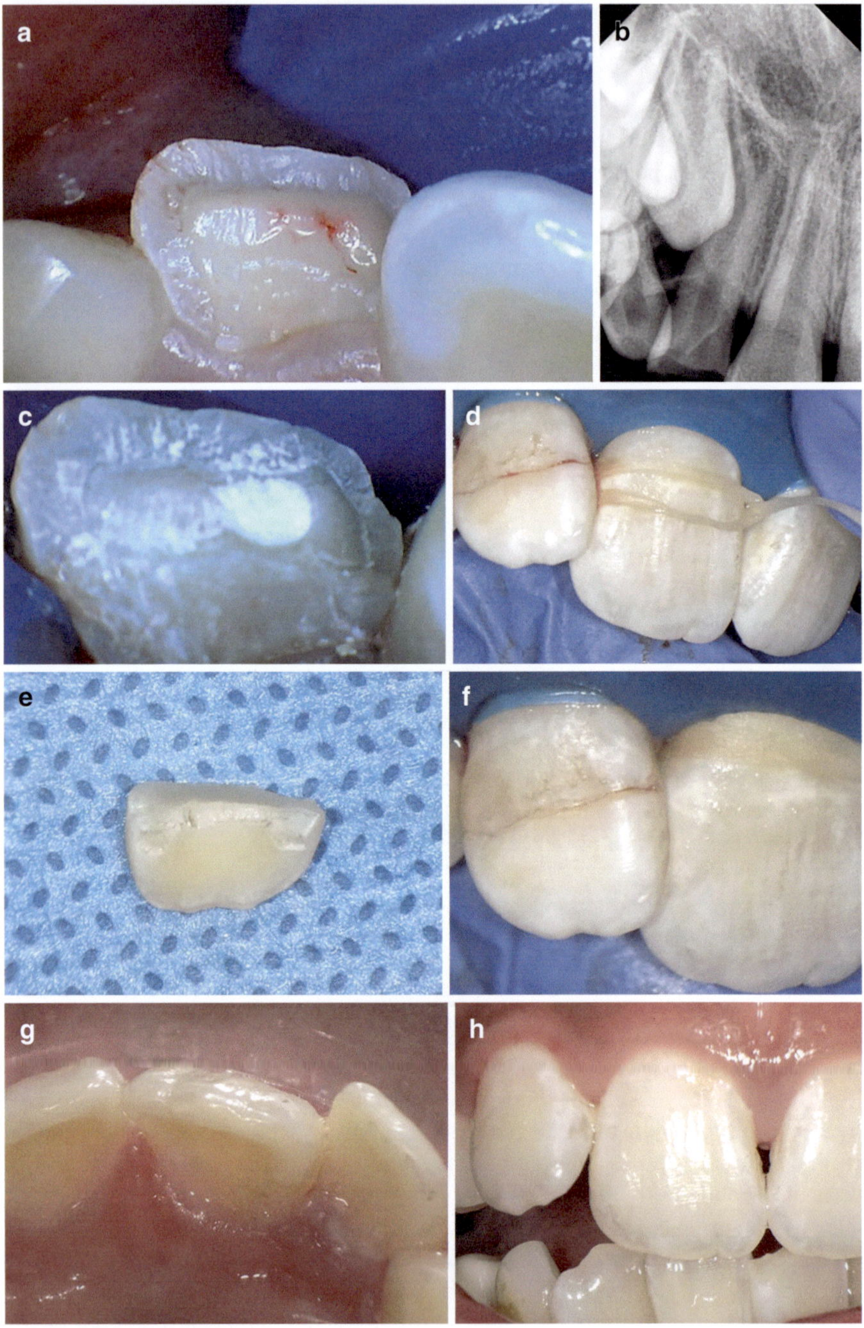

Fig. 11.13 (continued)

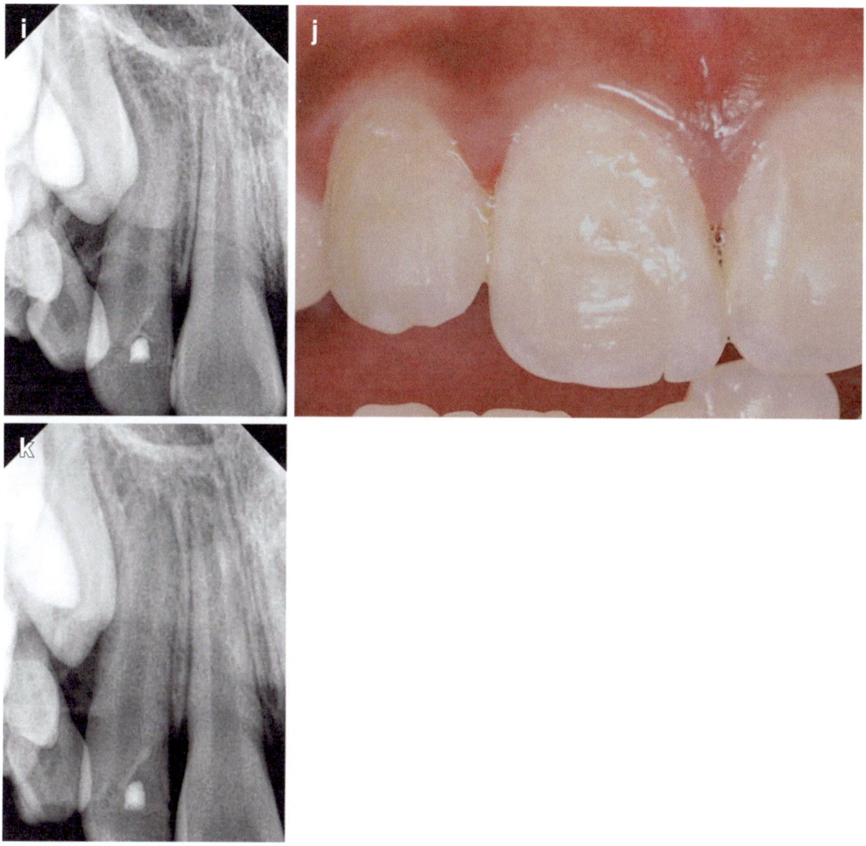

Fig. 11.13 An 8-year-old child presented with a complicated crown fracture of maxillary permanent right lateral incisor within few hours of injury. A pinpoint pulp exposure seen (**a**). Radiograph showed immature apex (**b**). The tooth was isolated under rubber dam and exposure enlarged to contain the pulp capping material. A Calcium Silicate material was used to cap the pulp (**c**). The pulp chamber was sealed with Resin Modified Glass Ionomer Cement and the fragment held in place to check fit (**d**). Broken fragment and the tooth were etched and adhesive bonding agent applied. (**e**). The fragment was held in position on the tooth and both were cured together (**f**). Palatal view showing good fit (**g**). The gap between the fragment and tooth was sealed with flowable composite and cured. The tooth was finished and polished with abrasive discs and polishing paste (**h**). Radiograph was taken immediately post treatment (**i**). Child at 1-year follow-up started with orthodontic treatment (**j**). Radiograph at 1-year recall showing further root development (**k**)

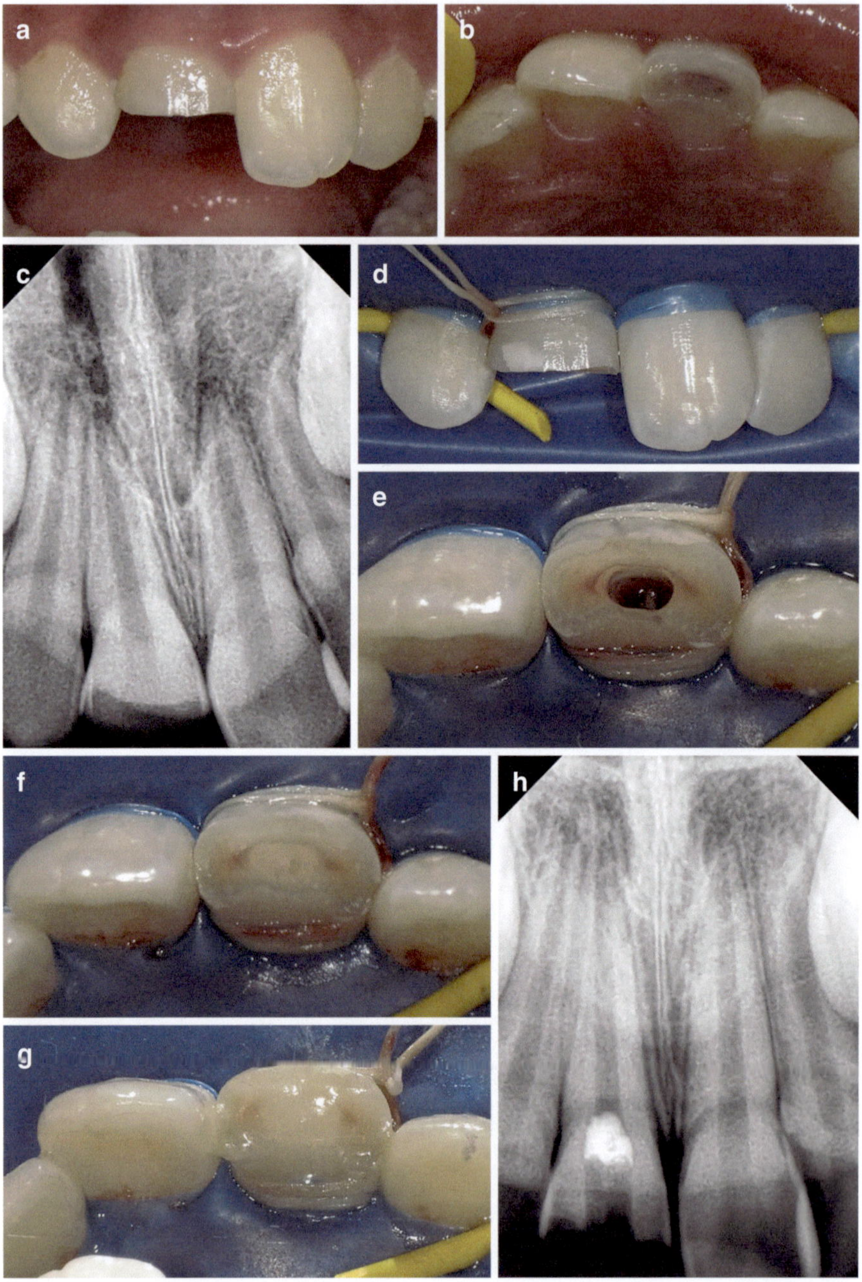

Fig. 11.14 (continued)

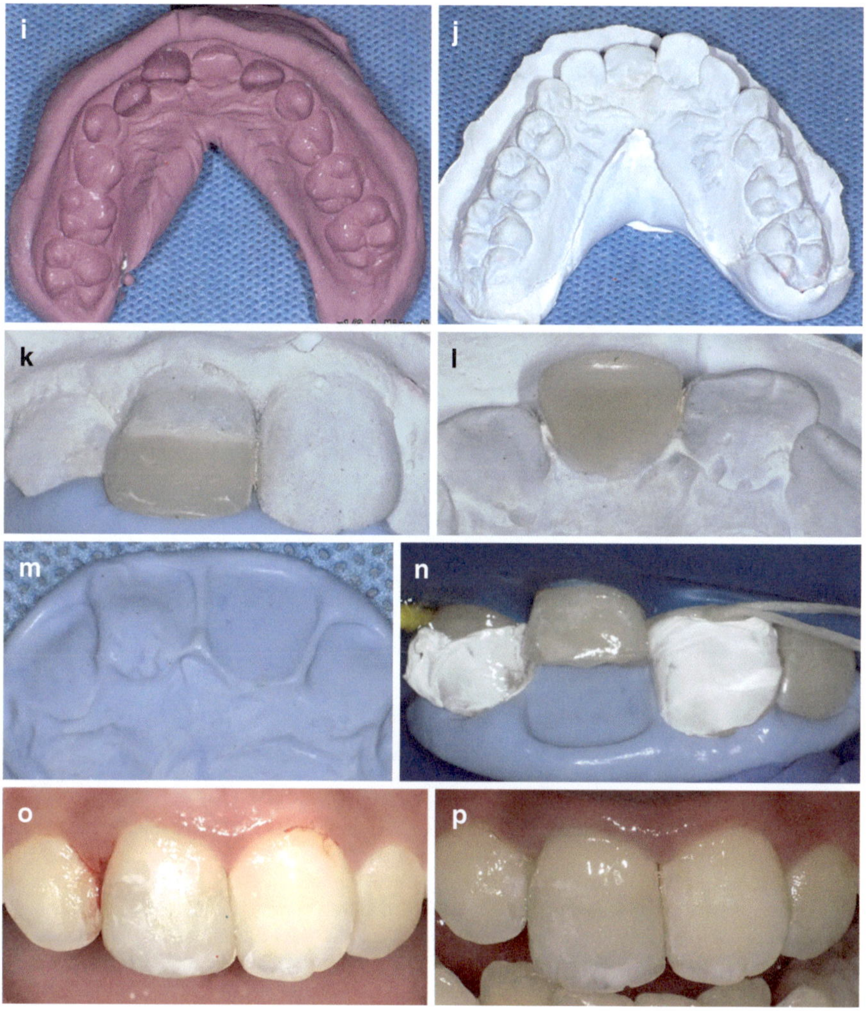

Fig. 11.14 (continued)

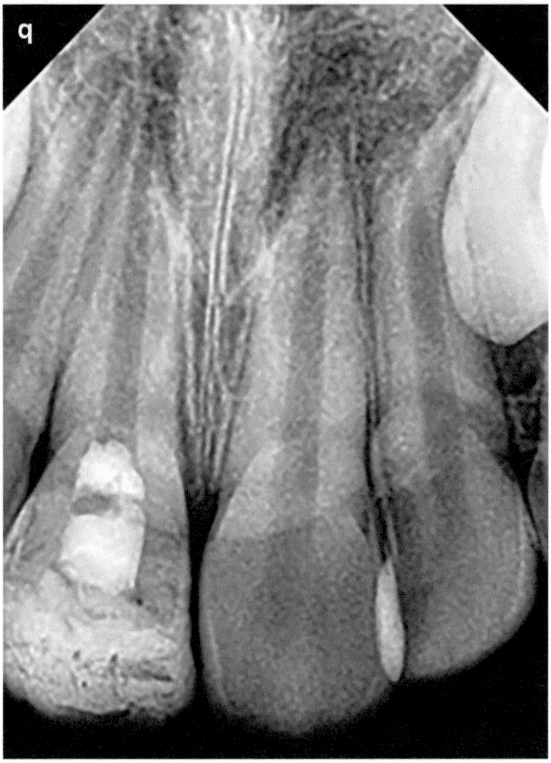

Fig. 11.14 Complicated crown fracture of maxillary permanent right central incisor (**a**). Patient presented with a larger pulp exposure few hours after trauma (**b**). The diagnostic radiograph revealed immature root apex (**c**). The tooth was anesthetized and isolated under rubber dam (**d**). Complete pulpotomy was done (**e**) and remaining pulp tissue capped with Calcium Silicate Cement (**f**). The access cavity was sealed with Resin Modified Glass Ionomer Cement and flowable resin composite (**g**). A post-pulpotomy radiograph was taken (**h**). Alginate impression was made for fabricating a putty stent for Resin Composite buildup (**i**). A dental stone model is poured for a mock tooth buildup (**j**). The mock buildup done with Resin Composite in labial (**k**) and palatal view (**l**). The material should flush with the stone model. A putty impression of the buildup made (**m**). Putty stent in place (**n**). The tooth is built with stratified composite layering technique. Immediate postoperative image (**o**). Follow-up at 6 months (**p**). Radiograph shows continued root maturation and calcific bridge formation below the Calcium Silicate Cement (**q**)

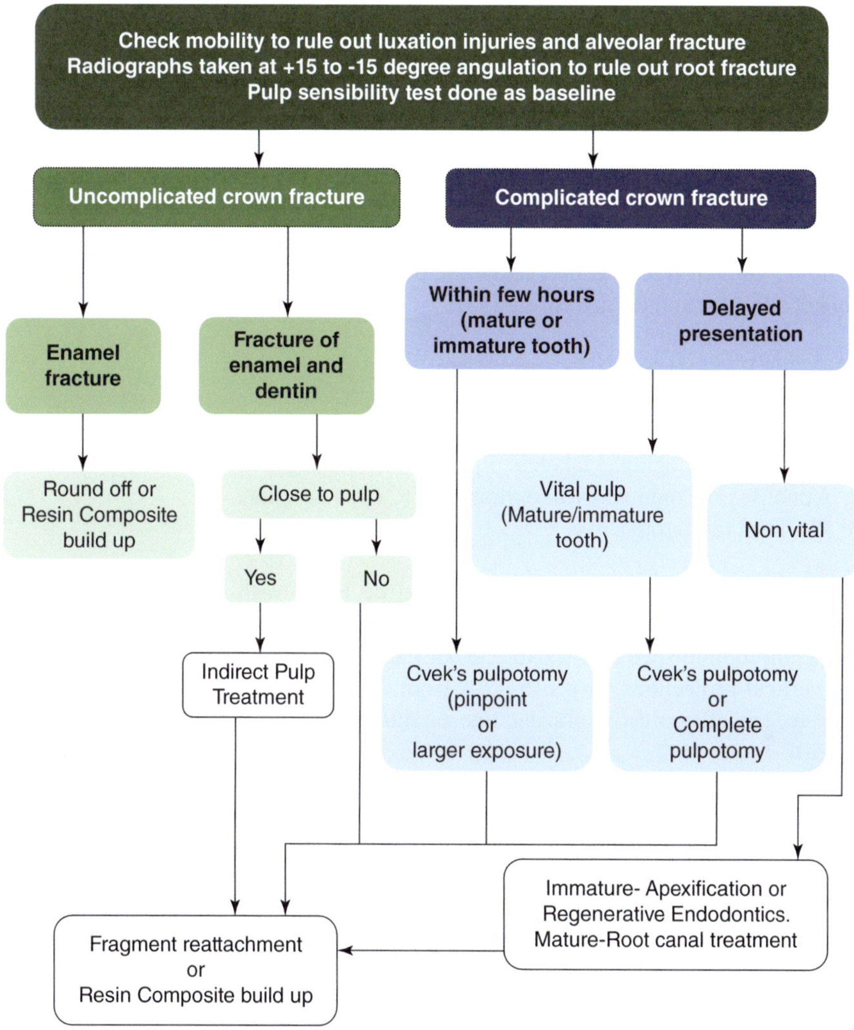

Fig. 11.15 Decision tree for crown fracture

11.3.2.1 Clinical and Radiographic Examination

The teeth most affected are the maxillary central incisors which present with horizontal or oblique fractures at the cervical, middle, or the apical third.

Cervical third fractures clinically present with increased mobility of the coronal fragment, bleeding from the gingival sulcus, possibility of extrusive or lateral luxation, or avulsion of the coronal fragment.

Middle third fractures may also present with mobility, bleeding, or hemorrhaging from the gingival sulcus.

Apical third fractures are generally asymptomatic with little or no mobility but may demonstrate tenderness on percussion.

In injuries involving multiple teeth, the alveolar process should be checked for mobility or fracture of the labial plate [45–48].

Vertical fractures are commonly seen in endodontically treated permanent posterior teeth and in children who present with trauma to the chin. The patient may present with pain on biting and/or demonstrate tenderness to percussion. Long-standing vertical fractures may show the presence of an isolated deep periodontal pocket adjacent to the fracture site [49].

11.3.2.2 Radiographic Examination

The following radiographs are recommended:

1. Periapical radiographs taken at different vertical angulations.
2. Cone Beam Computed Tomography (CBCT) as baseline.
3. Occlusal radiograph.

A baseline periapical radiograph should be taken with an X-ray positioning device. The fracture presents as a transverse radiolucent line if the central beam passes through the plane of fracture. Root fracture is detected on radiographs when the vertical projections vary ±15°–20° from the original angulation. The clinician may see an ellipsoid radiolucent line or multiple fracture lines (Fig. 11.16) [4, 48, 50].

Occlusal radiograph will detect fracture of the labial/lingual plate or a displacement of the fractured fragment in the labio-lingual direction. Root fracture of the immature tooth appears as a break in continuity of the thin root canal walls. Incomplete fractures or vertical fractures are difficult to detect. They may show a break in continuity in the root on conventional radiographic examination. If there is suspicion of root fracture or the patient is symptomatic, a CBCT is recommended to aid in the diagnosis [4].

- *What is the value of CBCT scans in root fractures?*

Radiographs may sometimes fail to detect root fractures or provide limited information about their orientation and extent. A CBCT is a three-dimensional imaging modality that can assess the extent of the fracture line and changes in root alignment or surrounding structures. A fracture line that appears horizontal on the conventional radiograph may extend in an oblique direction in the labiolingual plane. *A sagittal or oblique section of the anterior teeth* will show the labiolingual/palatal extent of the fracture line. Although CBCT does not change the initial management of root fractures, the unpredictable nature of trauma makes this imaging modality a valuable tool and provides a reference point to which scans taken during follow-up appointments can be compared. This allows for

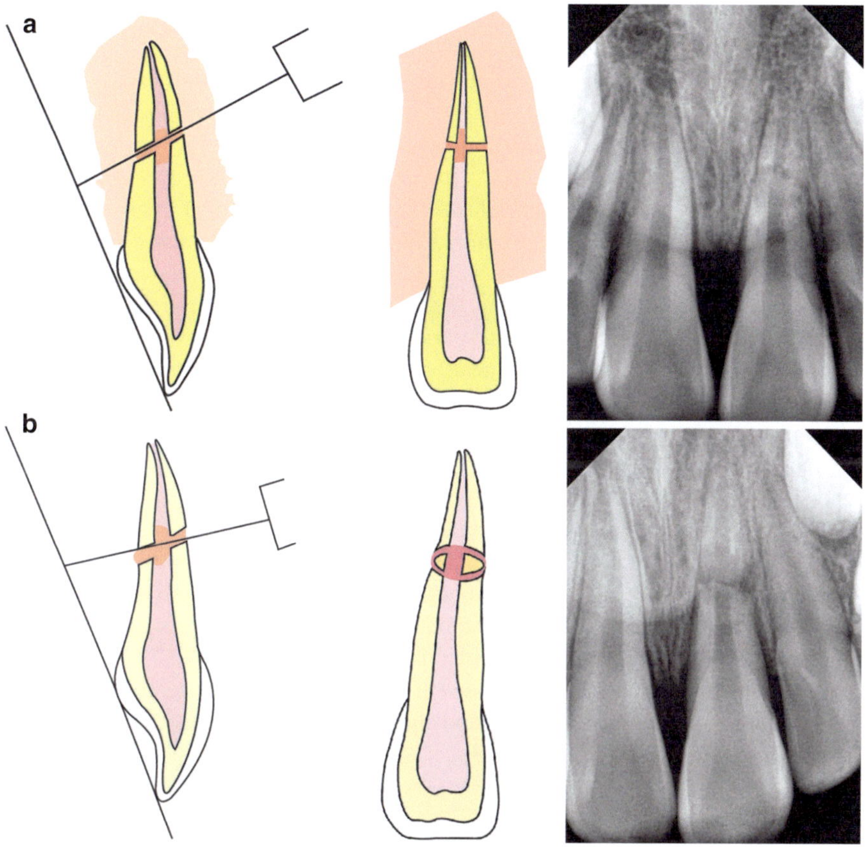

Fig. 11.16 The fracture line appears horizontal when the X-ray beam is parallel to the fracture surface. The root fracture on the maxillary left central incisor appears horizontal (**a**). The radiolucency takes on an ellipsoid appearance when the X-ray beam is angulated. The root fracture line on the maxillary left central incisor appears ellipsoid as the angulation of the beam is changed (**b**)

monitoring of complicated outcomes and helps guide further treatment decisions. CBCT scans involve a higher radiation dose compared to routine radiographs. The dose of radiation in CBCT scans can be reduced by restricting the imaging to the area of interest [48, 50].

11.3.2.3 Pulp Sensibility Test

In most cases, a positive response is noted at baseline. A negative response at baseline may indicate a transient neural damage and the teeth should not be deemed non-vital. At follow-up visits, the tooth that is healing is seen to give a positive or low response. Repeated negative response at follow-up visits may indicate permanent neural damage but does not warrant treatment unless there are unfavorable clinical and radiographic changes indicating the same [4].

11.3.2.4 Management of Root Fracture

The initial management involves *repositioning of the coronal fragment and stabilizing it with a splint.* This will approximate the fragments closer to each other and allow healing to take place.

Fracture at *the apical third and incomplete fractures* are usually not mobile and do not need splinting.

Fracture in the cervical and middle third with a mobile coronal fragment need to be immediately repositioned. The coronal fragment may have incurred *extrusive or lateral luxation injury.*

In case of *extrusive luxation injury*, the tooth must be pushed into the socket with digital pressure and stabilized with a splint.

Lateral luxation of coronal fragment often presents with a fractured labial plate. This is more common in the lower anterior region. It is important to reposition the labial plate before approximating the fractured tooth fragment.

As repositioning can be painful, local anesthesia is administered and the tooth repositioned with digital pressure.

The position of the tooth must be verified on a radiograph.

The tooth should then be splinted using a resin composite and wire splint which spans to one or two teeth on each side of the traumatized tooth/teeth (Fig. 11.17).

Endodontic treatment must not be initiated as part of the emergency management unless the tooth has a severe concomitant injury [51, 52].

If the crown has incurred complicated or uncomplicated fracture, then pulp must be protected at the same visit, after repositioning and splinting, as discussed in the section of crown fractures (Fig. 11.18).

Duration of Splint

An isolated root fracture should be splinted for at least 4 weeks.

If a concomitant alveolar plate fracture is present, then a splinting time of 1–4 months is recommended [4].

If fracture is in the cervical third of the root, below the alveolar crest, then the tooth is splinted to the adjacent tooth indefinitely with a palatal splint to potentiate healing [4, 45].

The *definitive management* involving endodontic treatment of root fracture will depend on the healing modality. A close clinical and radiographic follow-up of at least a year is required to detect the type of healing [51].

The key to successful management of root fractures is to immobilize the two fragments. It is essential to try and approximate the fragments as closely as possible but at times there may be difficulty in manipulation, poor patient cooperation or delay in reporting for treatment. The middle or apical third fractures have good prognosis independent of the type of healing if the fragments have been stabilized for at least 4 weeks.

Cervical fractures in proximity to the gingival sulcus have poor prognosis as it is difficult to immobilize the two fragments [51, 53]. They may be better managed by removal of the coronal fragment before proceeding for endodontic and prosthetic rehabilitation.

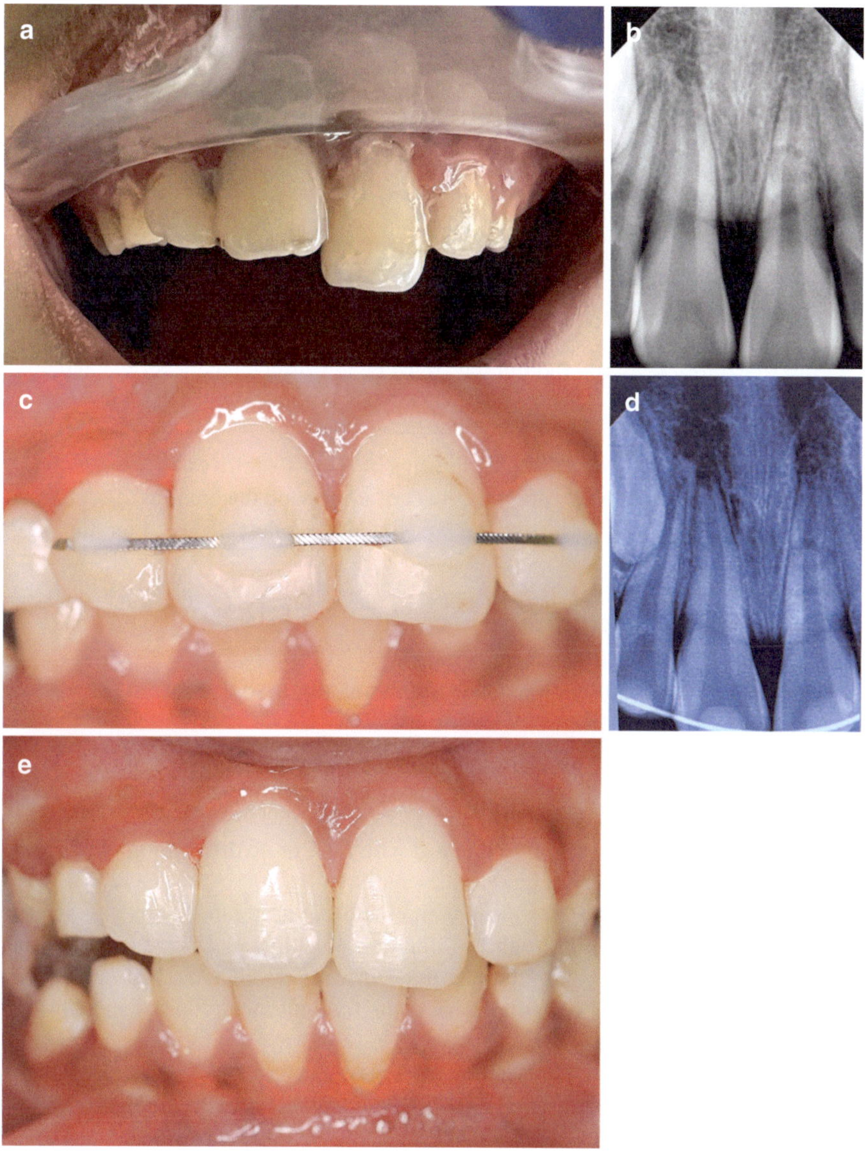

Fig. 11.17 Child presented with mobility in permanent maxillary left central incisor. Clinical and radiographic examination showed middle third root fracture, with extruded coronal fragment (**a**, **b**). The tooth was repositioned and splinted with resin composite and wire splint for 4 weeks (**c**). Radiograph taken after splinting (**d**). Follow-up at 4 weeks after splint removal (**e**)

11.3.2.5 What Is the Follow-Up Schedule for Root Fractures?

The clinician must evaluate the tooth for clinical and radiographic signs of healing or pathology at

- 4 weeks
- 6–8 weeks
- 4 months
- 6 months
- 1 year
- Then every year for at least 5 years [4].

Pulp sensibility tests and radiographs must be performed whenever the patient is recalled for follow-ups as above.

What Are the Different Healing Modalities in Root Fractures?

The mode of healing depends upon the level of injury and the amount of separation of the fractured segments. Broadly, the types of healing described in literature are:

1. Healing with hard dental tissue.
2. Healing with connective tissue.
3. Healing with bone and connective tissue.
4. No healing where granulation tissue (inflammatory tissue) forms in the fracture line [51–58].

Clinical Scenario 1: Healing with Hard Dental Tissue [51–58]

Fracture lines at the apical and middle third with little or no dislocation of the coronal fragment usually heal with hard tissue union.

If the fragments approximate closely and the tooth is splinted immediately, it is expected to heal uneventfully with proliferation of pulpal and periodontal tissues that form a callus and stabilize the fracture. *The tooth if splinted, must be in place for at least 4 weeks.* Over a 3-month period, the radiolucency reduces, and a bridge of calcified tissue is seen.

Clinically, transient discoloration may be seen that lasts up to 8 weeks. This is generally self-limiting and disappears as healing occurs between the two fractured fragments.

Clinical Scenario 2 and 3: Healing with Connective Tissue or Bone or Both [51–58]

This kind of healing is seen i*f there is luxation of the coronal part of the tooth* and/or fragments cannot be approximated closely after repositioning.

The connective tissue filling the gap between the two fragments may partially calcify over a period or be filled with bone.

In case of patients in their growing phase, the coronal fragment continues to erupt whereas the position of the apical fragment does not change. The radiograph will show an increase in gap between the fragments.

In both clinical scenarios 1 and 2, the tooth may be firm or slightly mobile. A normal reaction to percussion and normal or decreased sensibility to pulp testing is seen at baseline and follow-up visits.

The coronal fragment may have external or internal resorption that mimics pathologic root resorption and must be closely observed. This resorption is transient in nature as it is repair related and is replaced with calcified tissue in 12–24 months. The pulp canal in both fragments may obliterate at 12–24 months.

Clinical Scenario 4: Healing with Granulation Tissue [51–57]

Cervical fractures have the least favorable prognosis. The space between the fragments is filled with granulation tissue that is likely to get infected due to bacterial ingress from the gingival sulcus. The coronal fragment is tender to percussion and mobile while the apical fragment is firm and may contain vital tissue.

An abscess or draining sinus may be seen at the level of fracture, accompanied with a periodontal pocket. Radiograph shows signs of radiolucency indicating inflammatory resorption, adjacent to the fracture line within 2 months of injury.

11.3.2.6 Need for Endodontic Intervention in Cases of Root Fractures?

The objective of root fracture management is to allow the pulp to heal uneventfully and enable calcific repair at the fracture site. In case of apical and middle third root fractures, root canal obliteration of both the fragments is often seen and is considered a favorable outcome. In case of a concomitant injury such as a complicated crown fracture, the endodontic treatment should be limited to a complete or shallow pulpotomy independent of the stage of maturation of the root. This will not disturb the remaining pulpal tissue that is required for healing of the fracture site. Despite a conservative approach, the need for root canal treatment could arise within a few months after the injury. The coronal fragment becomes necrotic necessitating endodontic treatment while the apical fragment is usually unaffected. An artificial barrier such as a bioceramic plug should be placed at the apical end of the coronal fragment to prevent extrusion of the obturating material. In case of inflammatory changes in the apical fragment, either endodontic treatment of both fragments can be done, or the apical fragment is surgically removed.

Endodontic treatment is generally performed more commonly in case of cervical fractures, where the coronal fragment is sacrificed due to poor prognosis. The remaining root is treated endodontically followed by prosthetic rehabilitation with a post-retained core and crown. In case of sub crestal cervical fracture, some patients may need crown lengthening surgery or orthodontic extrusion based on the crown–root ratio (Fig. 11.18).

The tooth must be extracted if the fracture line is such that the remaining root structure compromises the crown–root ratio and the biological width, in cervical third fracture.

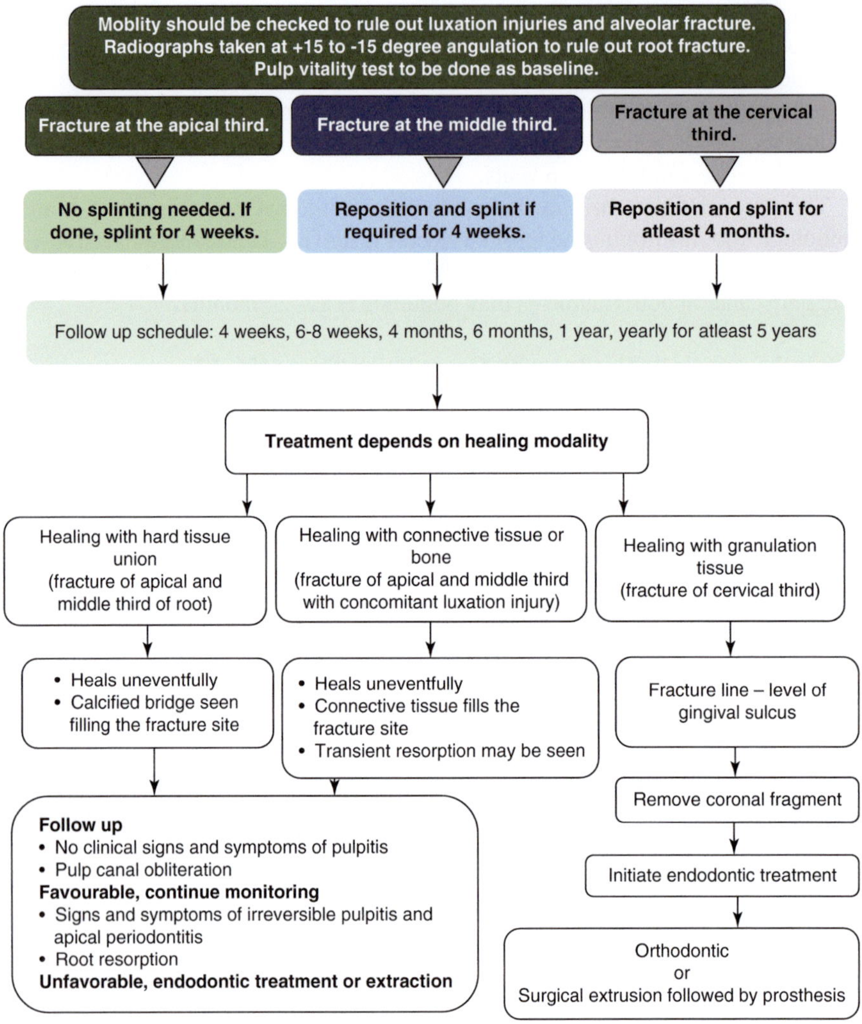

Fig. 11.18 Decision tree for root fracture

11.3.3 Crown-Root Fractures

When a fracture is seen on the labial surface of the crown and the fragment continues to remain attached, an initial diagnosis of a crown-root fracture should be suspected. A crown-root fracture involves the enamel, dentin, and cementum and can be categorized as complicated or uncomplicated. The crown-root fracture is considered complicated only when the pulp is exposed to the oral environment. As seen in root fractures, mature teeth are more susceptible to crown-root fractures as compared to immature teeth [58].

11.3.3.1 Clinical Examination

When seen from the labial aspect, the fracture line may seem to be horizontal at the level of the incisal, middle, or cervical third of the crown before extending obliquely and terminating subgingivally on the lingual/palatal surface. A vertical or oblique fracture line deviating towards the proximal surface is also a variation depending on the direction and force of impact [58]. The fragment is either partially attached or completely detached with or without pulp involvement. In case of partial attachment, the fragment is held in position by the fibers of the periodontal ligament. There may be bleeding from the gingival sulcus which maybe of pulpal or periodontal origin.

Manipulation of the attached fragment elicits a pain reaction from the patient. The patient generally complains of pain on biting and the tooth is tender on percussion.

11.3.3.2 Radiographic Examination

The primary objective of radiographic examination is *to determine the apical termination of the fracture line,* as this is crucial in deciding the treatment plan. The X-ray beam is usually perpendicular to the fracture line due to its oblique course. The apical extent of the fracture line cannot be discerned easily on a two-dimensional radiograph [58].

If the X-ray beam is perpendicular to the fracture line at any point, it will not be seen on the radiograph. Hence, it is always advisable to take two radiographs with a change in the vertical angulation of 15°. This extension of the fracture line will be seen as an ellipsoid radiolucency. Sagittal sections of CBCT reveal the apical termination in the labiolingual plane and provides additional information regarding the extent of fracture, its relation to marginal bone, and the estimated crown–root ratio [4, 59].

11.3.3.3 Assessing Pulp Status

The response to a pulp sensibility test is usually positive for crown-root fractures. While a negative response may be indicative of short-term damage to the neural supply of the tooth, sensibility testing must be repeated at follow-ups to recheck for a positive response. A repeated negative sensibility test must be corroborated with clinical and radiographic findings before initiating endodontic treatment [4].

11.3.3.4 Management of Crown-Root Fracture

A crown-root fracture *in a mature tooth* can be successfully treated, provided the subgingival termination of the fracture line can be repositioned supragingivally. This can be done in teeth wherein the fracture line does not extend beyond the cervical third, to maintain a crown–root ratio of at least 1:1 [60]. The procedure can be performed through gingivectomy, orthodontic extrusion, and surgical extrusion [4]. Prior to repositioning the fracture line, the necessary endodontic treatment should be initiated.

- *First visit*

If the patient reports with a completely dislodged or lost fragment, the clinician should perform the necessary pulp therapy on a restorable tooth.

In cases when the fragment is mobile but not completely detached, the clinician can choose one of the following:

1. Temporarily stabilize the fragment and splint to the nonmobile fractured tooth or to the adjacent teeth.
2. Remove the displaced fragment and perform the necessary pulp therapy [4].

1. *Endodontic Management*

   If pulp therapy was not performed at the first visit, it must be done at the second visit with the temporary splint in place.

A. *Uncomplicated Crown-Root Fractures*
   - The fragment is removed, and adequate isolation achieved. The exposed dentin should be protected with a calcium hydroxide liner/bio silicate material to ensure pulpal protection.

B. *Complicated Crown-Root Fractures*
   - In immature teeth, a pulpotomy is performed with a bioceramic material depending on the extent of pulp involvement.
   - In mature teeth, pulpotomy or root canal treatment is initiated. During root canal treatment, the pulp is extirpated and an intracanal Calcium Hydroxide dressing given for 2–4 weeks [34].

- *Second visit*

The *restorative management* of a crown-root fracture involves:

1. Repositioning the apical end of the crown-root fracture supragingivally.
2. Fragment reattachment or providing an extracoronal restoration.

Repositioning the apical end of the crown-root fracture supragingivally.

In an *immature tooth*, the apical end of the fracture line may move cervically due to continued tooth eruption. The coronal fragment is reattached after raising a palatal flap. The tooth should be monitored for root development and the decision to move the fracture line supragingivally must be taken after eruption and root maturation is complete.

In a *mature tooth*, the clinician can perform one or more of the following modalities depending on the level of the fracture line and the remaining root length.

- Gingivectomy and osteotomy (crown lengthening)
- Orthodontic extrusion
- Surgical extrusion
- Intentional reimplantation [4, 34, 61]

Of the above, gingivectomy and orthodontic extrusion have long-term follow-ups and have shown reasonable success.

1. *Gingivectomy and/or osteotomy (crown-lengthening procedure)* (Fig. 11.19)

Gingivectomy with or without osteotomy is primarily indicated when the fracture line lies within 2 mm of the alveolar crest. After gingivectomy, if the distance between the newly positioned gingival sulcus and the crest of the alveolar bone is less than 2 mm, the biological width will be violated. An osteotomy may need to be performed to ensure maintenance of the biological width. This will reduce the chances of gingival recession, bone loss, and periodontal pocket formation. While gingivectomy is an established crown-lengthening procedure, it is recommended only when the fracture line terminates palatally. It is not indicated on the labial gingiva as the gingival zenith will appear asymmetric, thereby compromising the aesthetics [61–63].

Technique

- After administering local anesthesia, a sulcular or internal bevel incision is made along the palatal gingival margin of the injured tooth and adjacent tooth, to raise a flap.
- If the fracture line is above the alveolar crestal bone, a gingivectomy is done and the biological width is measured.
- If the fracture line extends at the level of crestal bone or below (less than 2 mm), osteotomy is indicated along with gingivectomy.
- Osteotomy is done till at least 2–3 mm of sound root structure is seen above the alveolar bone. This will ensure that biologic width is maintained and provide a stable surface for fragment reattachment [61–63].

Fragment Reattachment (Fig. 11.19)

- The fractured fragment is positioned in place and a radiograph taken to confirm the fit.
- Adhesive reattachment must be done after achieving hemostasis under rubber dam isolation. Hemostasis can be achieved with laser or electrocautery.
- The fragment and the tooth are etched with 37% phosphoric acid for 15 s.
- A bonding agent is applied and a flowable composite used as an intermediate adhesive to improve retention.
- The attachment is light cured for 20–30 s, each labially and palatally.
- Excess material expressed from the fracture line can be finished and polished with composite polishing kit. Also, a sharp probe may be used to walk around the surgical site to remove excess cured bonding agent.
- Root planing must be done to make sure the excess material is removed before suturing the gingival flap [64, 65].

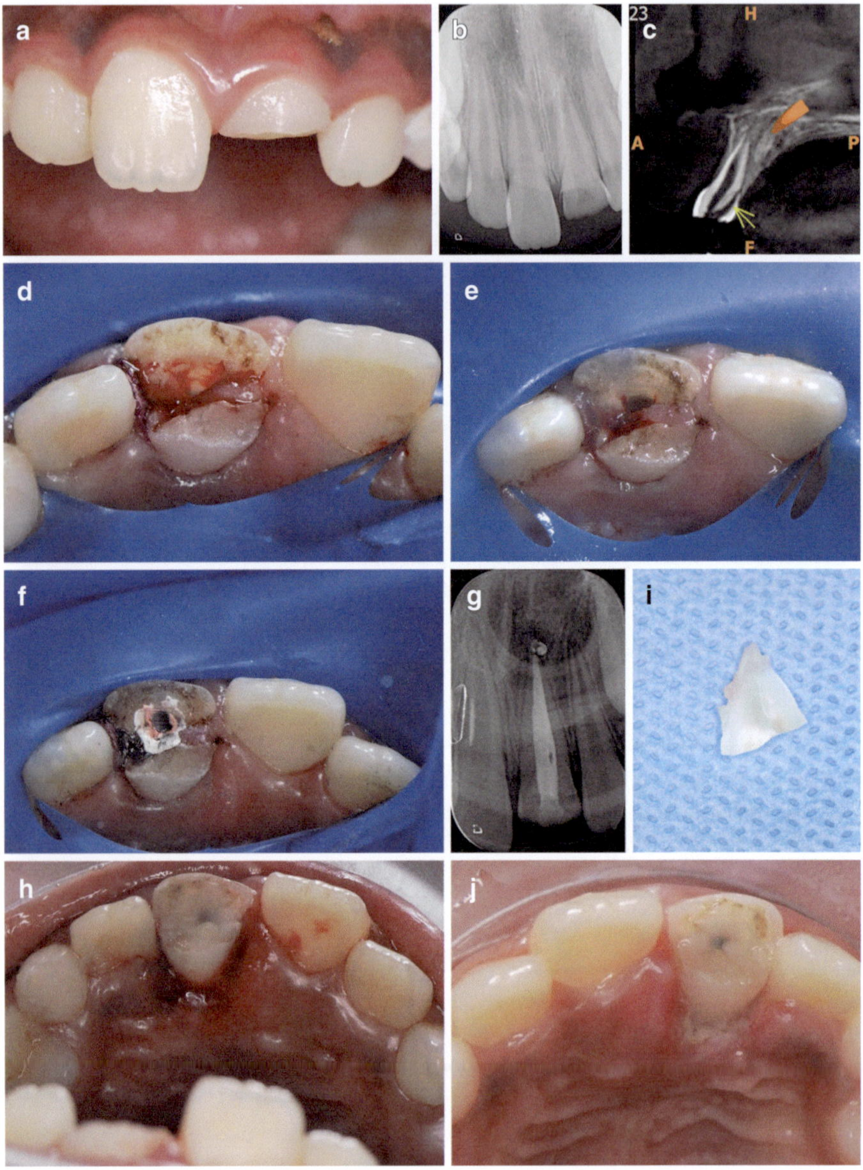

Fig. 11.19 Patient reported with a complicated crown-root fracture in maxillary permanent left central incisor, 9 months after injury (**a**). The diagnostic radiograph shows complete root formation (**b**). The CBCT revealed a crown-root fracture on sagittal cross section. The fracture line was seen to terminate at the level of alveolar crest (**c**). At the initial visit, local anesthesia was administered and tooth was isolated. The fractured fragment could not be manipulated (**d**). Root canal treatment was initiated (**e**). Adequate isolation was followed and endodontic treatment completed at the same visit (**f**). Radiograph taken after endodontic treatment (**g**). The access opening was sealed with flowable resin composite. Gingivectomy was done to access the apical extent of fracture line (**h**). The dislodged fragment was removed and stored in saline (**i**). Adequate hemostasis was achieved and the fragment reattached at the same visit (**j**). The patient was recalled in 5 days and Resin Composite buildup of the crown was completed, labial and palatal view (**k**, **l**). Follow-up after 1 week (**m**)

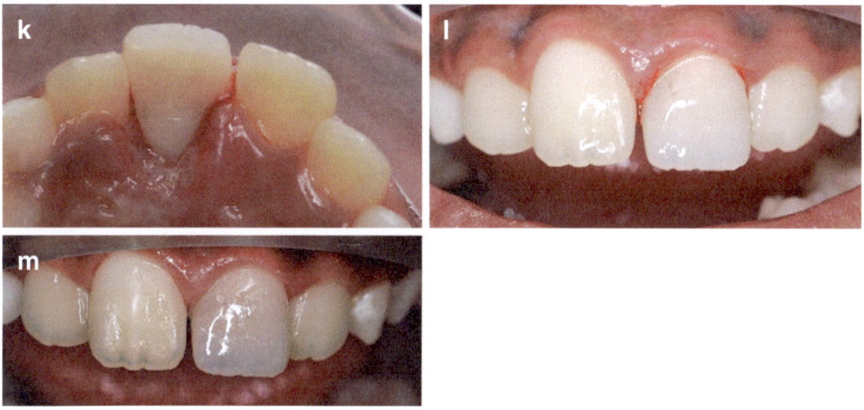

Fig. 11.19 (continued)

2. *Orthodontic Extrusion*

It is recommended in teeth, wherein the fracture line extends more than 2 mm below the alveolar crest but not more than one-third of the clinical root length to maintain a crown–root ratio of at least 1:1.

The biological basis of orthodontic extrusion lies in the principle that low, continuous orthodontic forces can induce coronal migration of the tooth and its supporting periodontal apparatus. Importantly, this movement facilitates the repositioning of the fracture line to a more favorable supragingival position, thus allowing for adequate isolation during restorative procedures and the preservation of periodontal health.

Biomechanically, extrusion is achieved using light continuous forces typically between 15 and 50 g applied through fixed appliances or auxiliary devices such as sectional archwires, elastic thread, or NiTi coil springs. The rate of extrusion generally ranges from 1 mm per week for rapid protocols to 1 mm every 2–3 weeks for more controlled movements, depending on the case complexity and root morphology. An extrusion of around 2-3 mm can be achieved with this technique. Once the desired extrusion is achieved, the tooth is stabilized for 6–8 weeks to allow for periodontal ligament reorganization and to prevent relapse. Circumferential supracrestal fiberotomy, often performed at intervals during the extrusion phase or immediately after, serves to prevent coronal migration of the gingival tissues and alveolar bone, thus maintaining the biological width.

In young patients or those with high esthetic demands, orthodontic extrusion offers the dual advantage of preserving alveolar bone and optimizing esthetic outcomes. Compared to surgical crown lengthening, it avoids apical migration of the gingival margin of adjacent teeth and preserves the natural contour of the periodontium [66–68].

3. *Surgical Extrusion*

Surgical extrusion places the fracture line supragingivally by severing the periodontal ligament attachment and moving the root coronally. Extrusion is achieved by luxation, using a periotome, a fine elevator or forcep to expose the desired length of the root, while maintaining a crown–root ratio of at least 1:1. Care must be taken not to remove or extract the tooth from the socket. The average amount of surgical extrusion that can be achieved is around 4.5 mm with a range of 2–7 mm. This is followed by placing a resin composite and wire splint to the adjacent teeth for 2 weeks.

A definitive restoration with fragment reattachment or Resin Composite buildup can be performed. The most common complication with surgical extrusion is transient surface root resorption. To mitigate the risk of adverse events, root canal treatment must be initiated before surgical extrusion with calcium hydroxide used as intracanal medicament. The medicament must be replenished for 6 months after surgical extrusion followed by obturation and placement of a final restoration [69–71].

4. *Intentional Reimplantation*

Intentional reimplantation involves extracting and repositioning the fractured tooth to facilitate a supragingival coronal restoration. It is indicated when the labial fracture is subgingival and needs to be rotated such that the supragingival palatal extension of the fracture line is made labial.

Technique

- Root canal treatment is initiated, an intracanal medicament is given and the tooth is sealed with temporary filling material.
- After a few days, the fractured tooth is extracted carefully under local anesthesia.
- Extraction must be performed with a flat-beak forcep to minimize damage to the cementum and periodontal ligament. The teeth are examined carefully to identify possible vertical root fractures.
- Then, the tooth must be reimplanted in a slightly extruded position to expose the fracture lines supragingivally.
- For initial stabilization, a resin composite and wire splint must be placed.
- After 1 week, the splint is removed.

A 180 degree rotation shifts a labial subgingival fracture, palatally. This makes it easier to restore the tooth, as the labial fracture is now supragingival. Intentional reimplantation is associated with adverse-effects of inflammatory root resorption and is seen within a year on the radiograph [72–74].

5. *Vital Root Submergence*

In teeth, where the subgingival component of the fractures involves more than 2/3rds of the root, extraction of the tooth is recommended. In young patients, it is advised to leave the apical fragment in situ to maintain the thickness of the alveolar bone [75].

11.3.3.5 How Does a Clinician Choose Among the Modalities Above?

Most cases of crown-root fractures are managed by gingivectomy or orthodontic extrusion. If the apical termination of the fracture line is <2 mm below the alveolar crest, a gingivectomy is done. If it extends beyond 2 mm but not more than 1/3rd of the root length, then an orthodontic or surgical extrusion is indicated. Gingivectomy is generally avoided on the labial gingival margin due to an undesirable esthetic outcome. In such cases, orthodontic extrusion or surgical repositioning may be preferred.

Orthodontic extrusion is more time-consuming and requires greater patient compliance. Although, surgical extrusion shows immediate results, it may lead to resorption if not performed meticulously. Studies have shown comparable success rates among the three procedures and the choice depends on the extent of fracture line, type of restoration, and the clinician's knowledge and expertise [76]. The current IADT guidelines also recommend using any one of the above treatment modalities, following which the fragment is reattached [4].

Adhesive fragment reattachment in crown-root fractured teeth is the first choice for coronal restoration. Studies with a long-term follow-up have shown that adhesive fragment reattachment (AFR) in these teeth leads to mild gingival inflammation and more significantly, a high need for re-intervention. Despite the need for re-intervention, AFR is a good long-term temporary treatment for the young patient [71].

In cases where the fracture line extends obliquely beyond 1/3rd of the root or in the presence of concomitant injuries, tooth extraction is advised. It is advisable to leave the apical fragment in situ, if it is inaccessible and removal may cause soft and hard tissue damage [4]. IADT recommends extraction followed by auto transplantation. Alternately, if the patient's age favors a fixed prosthesis, an implant replacement can be planned (Fig. 11.20) [4].

11.3.4 Luxation Injuries

Barring crown fractures, luxation injuries are the most frequently seen traumatic dental injuries in the permanent dentition. In these injuries, the damage occurs to both, the pulpal and periodontal tissues.

There are five types of luxation injuries, categorized as follows [77]:

- *Concussion* is an injury to the tooth-supporting structures without abnormal loosening or displacement but with marked reaction to percussion.
- *Subluxation (loosening)* is an injury to the tooth-supporting structures with abnormal loosening but without clinically or radiographically demonstrable displacement of the tooth.

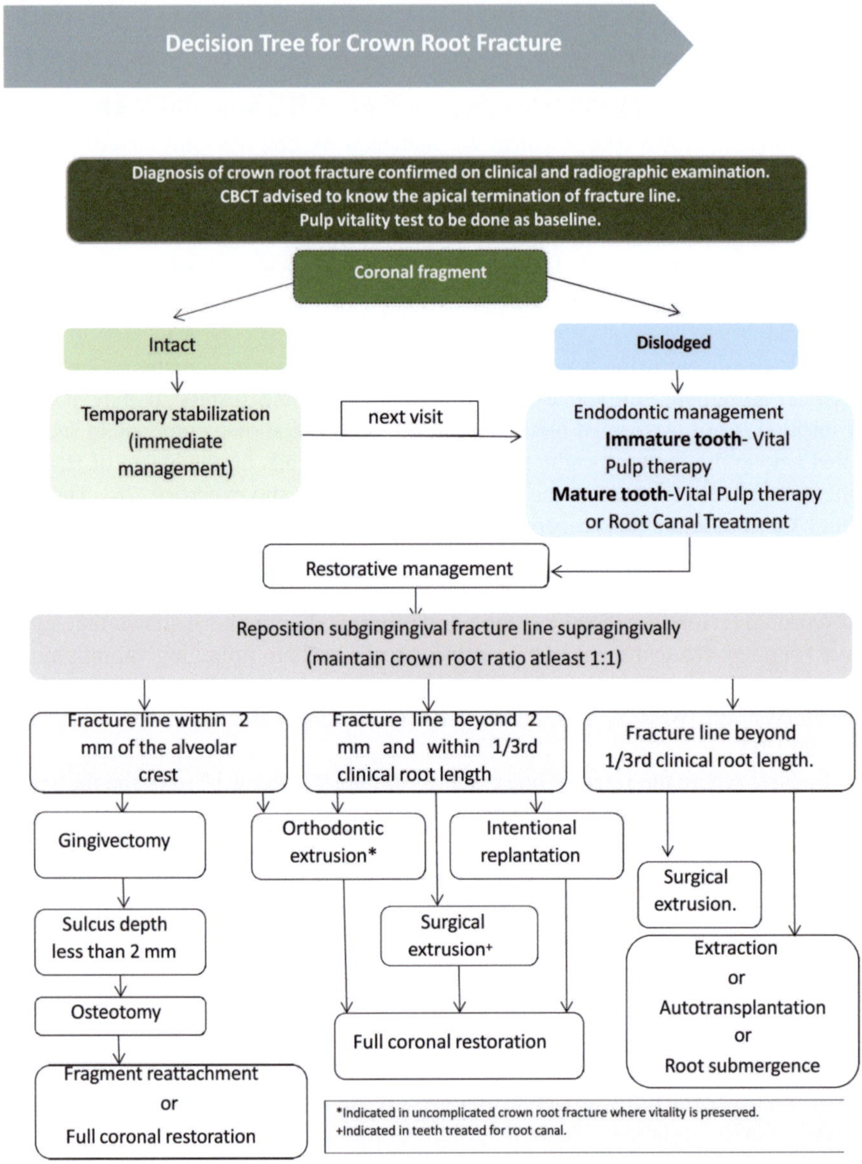

Fig. 11.20 Decision tree for crown-root fracture

- *Intrusive luxation (central dislocation)* is displacement of the tooth in an apical direction deeper into the alveolar bone.
- *Extrusive luxation (partial avulsion)* is partial displacement of the tooth out of its socket in the incisal or axial direction.
- *Lateral luxation* is the eccentric displacement (other than axial) of the tooth accompanied by comminution or fracture of the alveolar socket.

11.3.4.1 Clinical Examination

Concussion and subluxation injuries show similar clinical features and can often go unnoticed at the first glance due to their subdued clinical presentation.

The tooth is tender on palpation and the patient gives a marked reaction to percussion in a horizontal or vertical direction. The gingival margin of the tooth appears red and edematous [77].

Subluxation injuries can be distinguished from concussion by the presence of *tooth mobility*. In both these injuries, the tooth retains its normal position in the dental arch (Figs. 11.21 and 11.22).

In intrusion, the incisal edge of the tooth will be below that of the adjacent teeth. In cases of severe intrusion, the tooth may not be visible clinically and the clinician may mistake it for avulsion. Palpation of the alveolar process can often reveal the position of the displaced tooth. Intrusion may also be difficult to diagnose in the early mixed dentition period when the incisors are still erupting.

The high-pitched metallic sound elicited on percussion, like that of an ankylosed or a laterally luxated tooth, is pathognomonic of severe intrusion, too.

Extruded teeth appear elongated and partially suspended from the socket with or without deviation. The tooth shows increased mobility, percussion sound is dull and there is bleeding from the periodontal ligament space.

Due to the displacement seen in extrusive and lateral luxation, these teeth invariably interfere with occlusion, preventing the child from closing.

In ***lateral luxation*** injuries, the crown of the luxated tooth is most often, palatally displaced due to a labial impact. The injury may be associated with fracture of the labial bony plate due to penetration of the displaced root apex. As a result of this, mobility is absent, and a high-pitched metallic sound is elicited on percussion.

11.3.4.2 Radiographic Examination [4, 21]

Concussion and subluxation injuries generally do not show any radiographic changes with respect to the width of the PDL space. A widened PDL space can be appreciated in teeth showing ***lateral luxation or extrusion.***

In contrast, following ***intrusive luxation***, the PDL space will be partially or totally obliterated. If the intruded tooth has been forced through the labial bone plate, it will appear foreshortened when compared to its anti-mere. Conversely an elongated tooth implies intrusion in the palatal direction. This is particularly important for a primary tooth, where a radiographic image of an elongated tooth indicating palatal displacement is likely to impact the succedaneous tooth.

The degree of extrusion or intrusion can also be determined on the radiograph by comparing the level of CEJ or apices with that of the adjacent teeth. A CBCT is a more precise diagnostic tool in case of lateral, intrusive, and extrusive luxation to evaluate the extent of displacement in three dimensions. Additionally, it acts as a baseline for future reference [21]. In the absence of a CBCT, an occlusal radiograph will confirm the direction of the axial displacement of the tooth and reveal the presence of fracture of the alveolar process [4, 21].

A combination of occlusal and two additional intraoral periapical radiographs taken in different angulations is recommended [4].

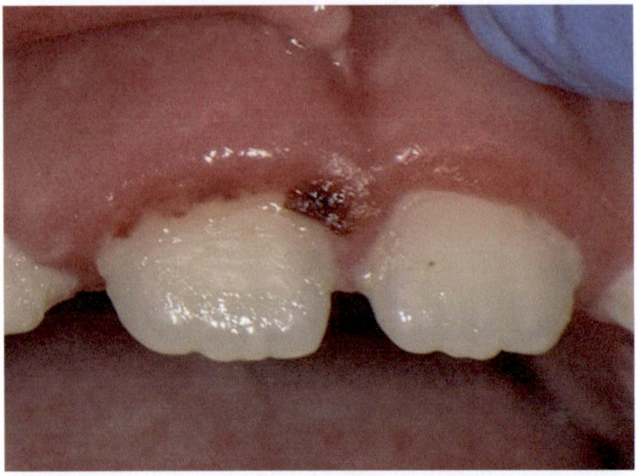

Fig. 11.21 Concussion injury to maxillary permanent right central incisor. Gingival bleeding seen without tooth mobility

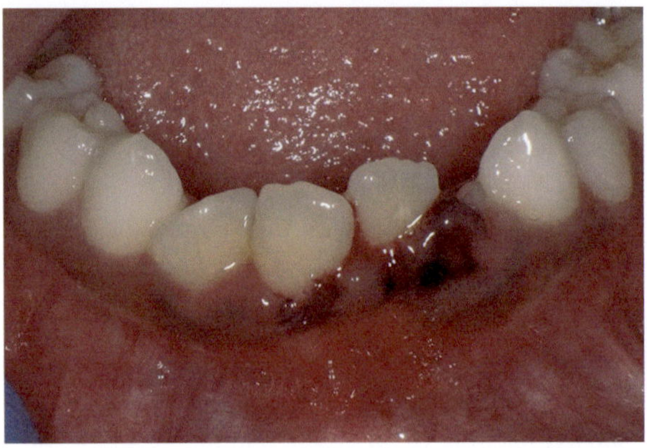

Fig. 11.22 Subluxation of mandibular permanent left central and lateral incisor

1. Change in vertical angulation of the X-ray beam for intrusive or extrusive luxation and to rule out root fractures.
2. Change in horizontal angulation of an X-ray beam detects displacement of lateral luxation injuries.

11.3.4.3 Pulp Sensibility Testing [78–82]

For all *immature teeth* that have incurred any form of luxation injury, it is important to monitor the vitality, as pulp extirpation is not indicated as part of immediate treatment. An immature tooth will often show a negative response at baseline due to incomplete neurovascular development. The tests should be repeated at follow-up visits. Continued root development should be used as a more reliable marker of vitality.

A *mature tooth* that has incurred concussion or subluxation will usually show a positive response. On the other hand, teeth with extrusive and lateral luxation may show an initial negative response. These teeth need to be monitored for pulp vitality during their follow-up schedule. Pulp sensibility testing is not of relevance to intruded teeth or severely laterally luxated teeth as the treatment involves pulp extirpation within 7 days of trauma.

It is important to ascertain pulp status at follow-up visits as necrosis of the pulp aggravates the process of root resorption, associated with luxation injuries [8, 83].

11.3.4.4 Management of Luxation Injuries

1. *Concussion and Subluxation*

There is *no active treatment recommended* for concussion injuries as these teeth most often heal uneventfully [4]. The patient can be prescribed antibiotics and analgesics, if there are concomitant shallow lacerations of the soft tissues. Deep lacerations may need suturing to facilitate secondary healing. Patient is advised a soft diet for 7–10 days. The use of 0.12% Chlorhexidine mouthwash and regular toothbrushing is advised to keep the area clean.

The injured teeth must be monitored for pulpal and periodontal healing and the patient recalled at [4]:

1. 1 month
2. 1 year

Subluxation injuries largely have a similar treatment protocol, but injuries with excessive mobility and tenderness on biting can be splinted with a resin composite and wire splint for a period of 2 weeks (Figs. 11.23 and 11.24) [4].

In these teeth, there is a greater risk of pulpal necrosis than concussed teeth. Hence, the recall interval is as follows [4]:

1. After 2 weeks, if splinted
2. 3 months
3. 6 months
4. 1 year (Fig. 11.29)

Subluxated and concussed teeth with concomitant injuries to the crown (enamel infarction, uncomplicated and complicated fracture) are at a *higher risk of experiencing pulpal necrosis and root resorption.* Therefore, the recall follow-up should be as rigorous as advised for a crown fracture [4, 83, 84].

1. 1 month
2. 3 months
3. 6 months
4. 1 year
5. Yearly for at least 5 years

Pulp sensibility tests and radiographs should be performed at every recall.

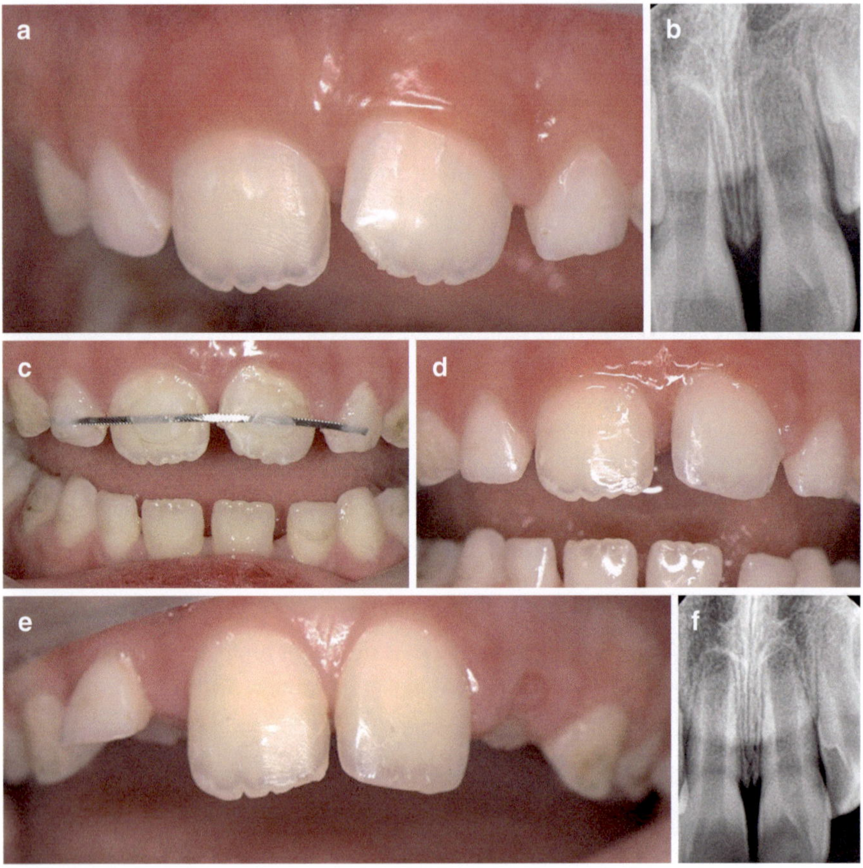

Fig. 11.23 Subluxation injury to maxillary permanent left central incisor with concomitant enamel fracture (**a**). Radiograph shows an immature root apex (**b**). The tooth was stabilized and splinted with resin composite and wire splint for 2 weeks (**c**). The splint was removed, and a resin composite buildup done after 2 weeks (**d**). Clinical and radiographic follow-up at 1 year shows continued root development (**e**, **f**)

2. *Intrusive Luxation*

The treatment protocols for intrusive luxation depend on the maturity of the tooth and severity of injury.

Immature Tooth (Fig. 11.25)

The IADT recommends allowing for spontaneous re-eruption, *irrespective of the degree of intrusion of the tooth* [4]. In cases of severe intrusion, the gingival scar tissue covering the affected tooth may need to be incised to facilitate spontaneous re-eruption. Any attempt at orthodontic repositioning should be performed

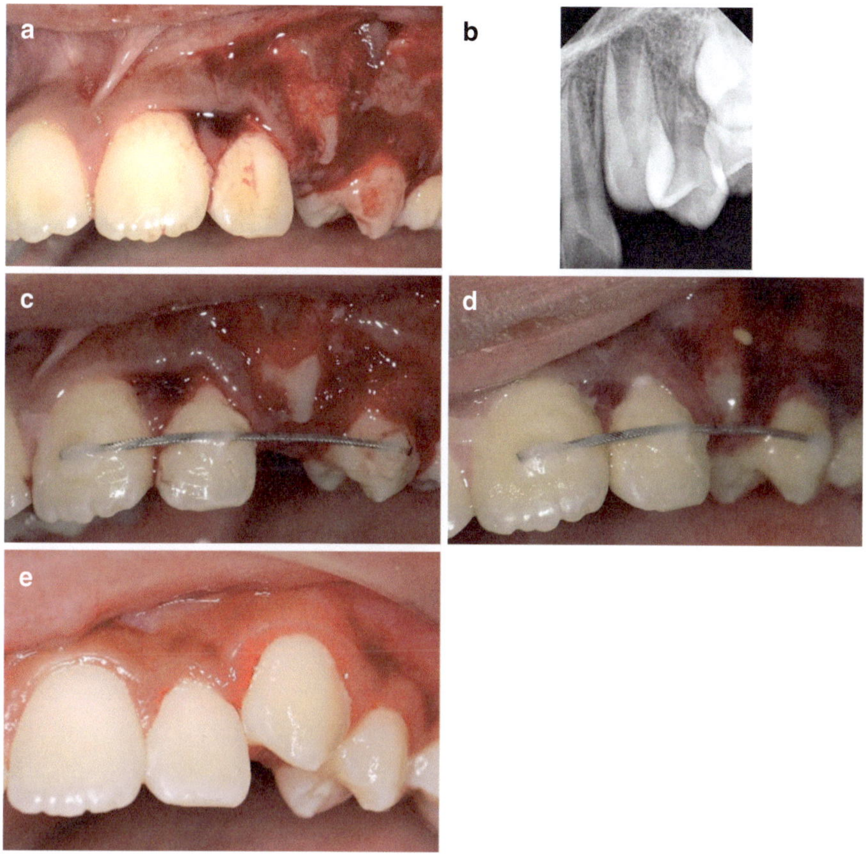

Fig. 11.24 Intrusive luxation injury of maxillary permanent left canine with gingival laceration. The maxillary left lateral incisor incurred subluxation injury and showed Grade II mobility (**a**). The diagnostic radiograph revealed Cvek's 4 and 3 stages of root development of lateral incisor and canine, respectively (**b**). A resin Composite and wire splint were placed (**c**). The child was called to remove splint after 2 weeks (**d**). The child was recalled in 3 months to check for eruption of canine. Follow-up at 3 months showed spontaneous eruption of canine (**e**)

only if no signs of re-eruption are seen even after 4 weeks [4]. Surgical repositioning of immature teeth is not advised as it increases the chances of root resorption [85, 86].

Mature Tooth

In mature teeth, the treatment protocol is dependent on the degree of intrusion. Coronal access is essential within 7–10 days of the injury as pulp needs to be extirpated to minimize the chances of root resorption.

In cases of:

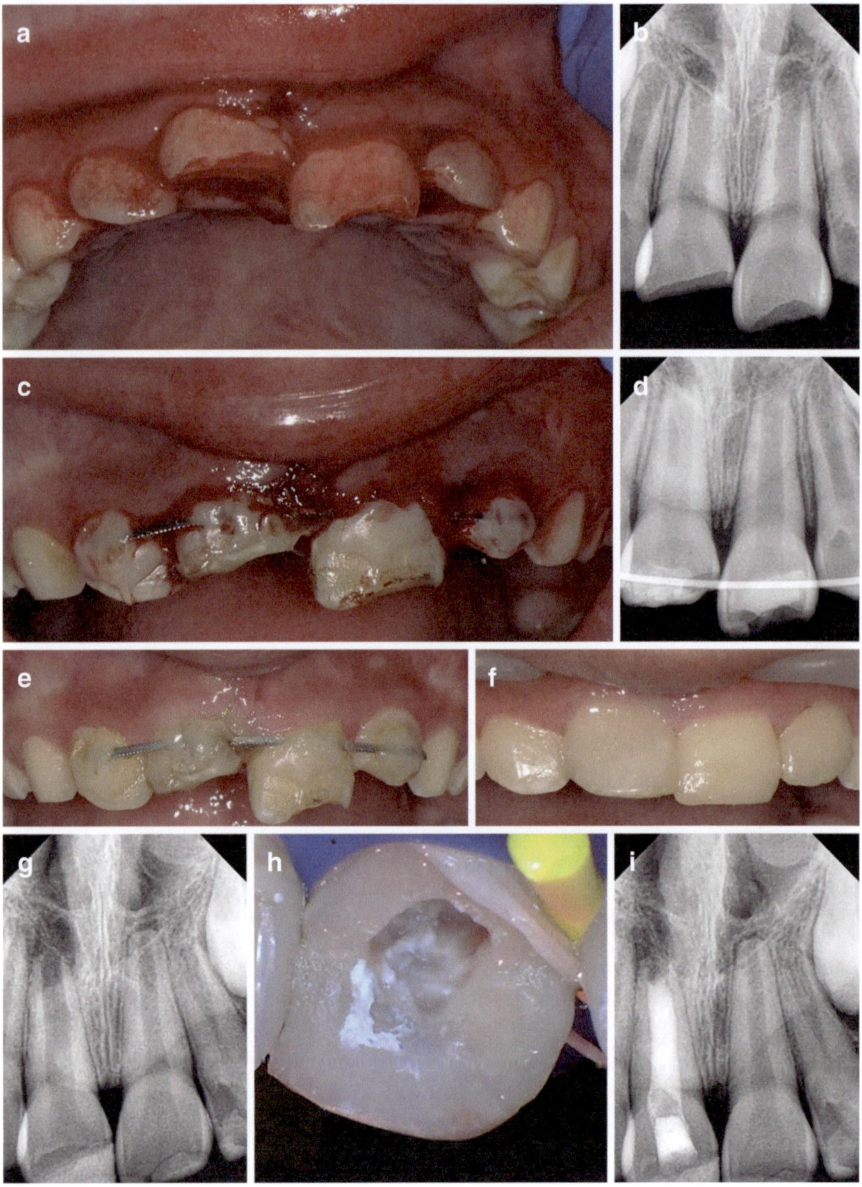

Fig. 11.25 (continued)

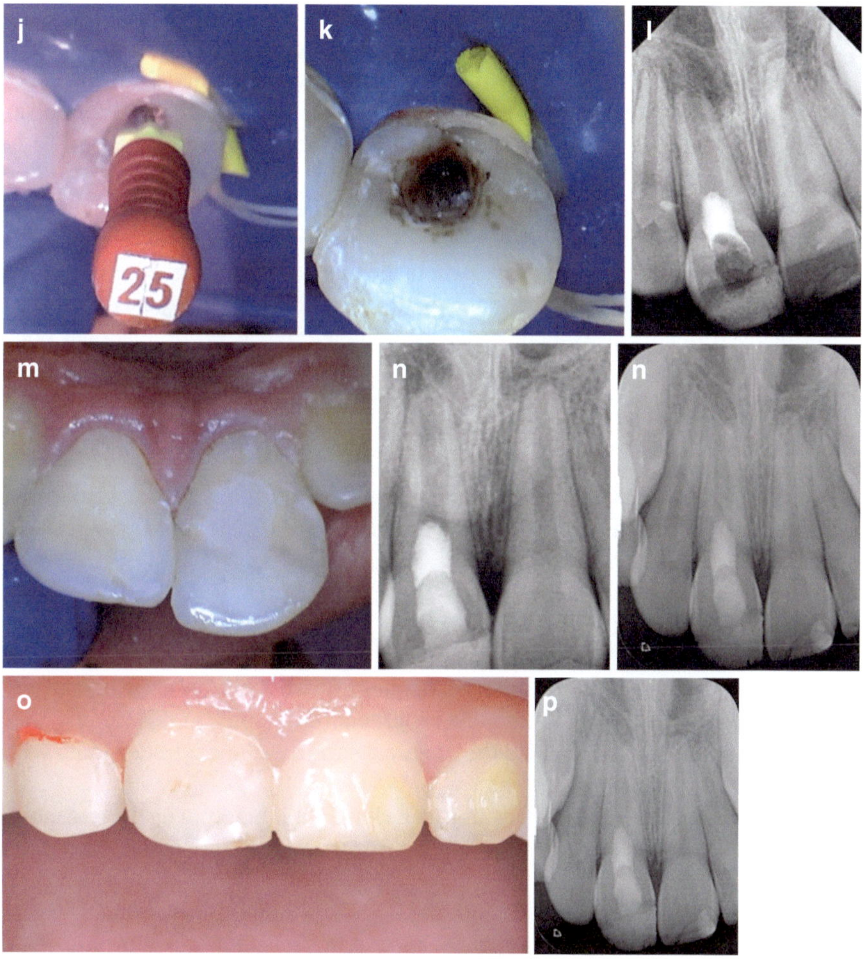

Fig. 11.25 Intrusive and mild lateral luxation of maxillary permanent central incisors with concomitant uncomplicated crown fracture (**a**). The diagnostic radiograph showed immature root apices of both incisors (**b**). The teeth were repositioned and splinted with a resin composite and wire splint. A GIC liner was used to cover the exposed dentin (**c**). A radiograph was taken after splinting and child was recalled after 2 weeks (**d**). Splint removed (**e**) and a resin composite buildup done (**f**). Arrested root development of maxillary permanent right central incisor noted after 1 year. The right central incisor showed a periapical lesion on the radiograph and negative response on vitality testing, while the left incisor showed an early response (**g**). Regenerative endodontic treatment was initiated in the maxillary right central incisor. A Calcium Hydroxide dressing was placed in the canal for 2 weeks (**h**). A radiograph was taken and patient recalled (**i**). After 2 weeks, a 25 no file was used to stimulate the periapical tissue (**j**) and a blood clot was seen to form at the canal orifices (**k**). An MTA plug was then placed at the orifice and pushed into the cervical third of the canal (**l**). The access opening was sealed with a composite restoration (**m**). The 6 monthly follow-up showed resolution of periapical lesion and formation of an apical barrier (**n**). Recall at 18 months showed resolution of symptoms clinically (**o**) and on radiograph (**p**)

- *Mild intrusion (less than 3 mm)*: It is advised to observe for spontaneous re-eruption [4]. Active repositioning via surgical or orthodontic means is advised if no coronal movement occurs within 8 weeks following trauma. With spontaneous re-eruption or orthodontic extrusion, pulp extirpation should be performed as soon as coronal access can be achieved [85, 86].
- *Moderate intrusion (3–7 mm)*: These teeth require "active repositioning" either surgically or orthodontically. The IADT recommends surgical repositioning over orthodontic repositioning in these cases [4]. Furthermore, surgical repositioning is a better treatment option in cases where the trauma is acute, i.e., it has occurred within the last few days. Orthodontic treatment is advised for patients coming in for delayed treatment as there would be complete repair of the marginal bone [87, 88].
- *Severe intrusion (more than 7 mm)*: Surgical repositioning is recommended as it also allows access to immediate endodontic treatment [4].

If the patient is delayed in reporting the injury, surgical repositioning followed by immediate pulp extirpation is still recommended *even if there are no signs of root resorption seen (Fig. 11.29)* [86, 89].

Surgical Repositioning Technique [90] (Fig. 11.26)

- Administer local anesthesia.
- Fix a resin composite wire splint, extending to two teeth on each side of the injured tooth. The injured tooth must be left out of the splint at this step.
- Once the splint is in place, hold the proximal surfaces of the intruded tooth with forceps.
- Gently loosen the tooth and reposition at the level of the adjacent unaffected tooth.
- Compress the displaced bone by applying finger pressure both labially and palatally/lingually.
- Etch rinse and dry the injured tooth crown for splinting. Apply bonding agent and a flowable composite to secure the tooth with the splint.
- If the wire splint makes access to the intruded tooth difficult, it can be placed after repositioning the tooth.
- Suture gingival lacerations, if any.
- A radiograph is taken to verify the position of the tooth and acts as a baseline.
- Monitor the tooth as per the recall schedule.

Orthodontic Repositioning [91–94]

- After administering local anesthesia, a window is created with blade and scalpel, laser or electrocautery, to expose the crown of the intruded tooth.
- Hemostasis is established and the affected tooth is isolated. The tooth's enamel surface is etched, rinsed, and dried and a bracket is bonded to it.
- Orthodontic brackets are also bonded to adjacent teeth, provided they have not incurred trauma.

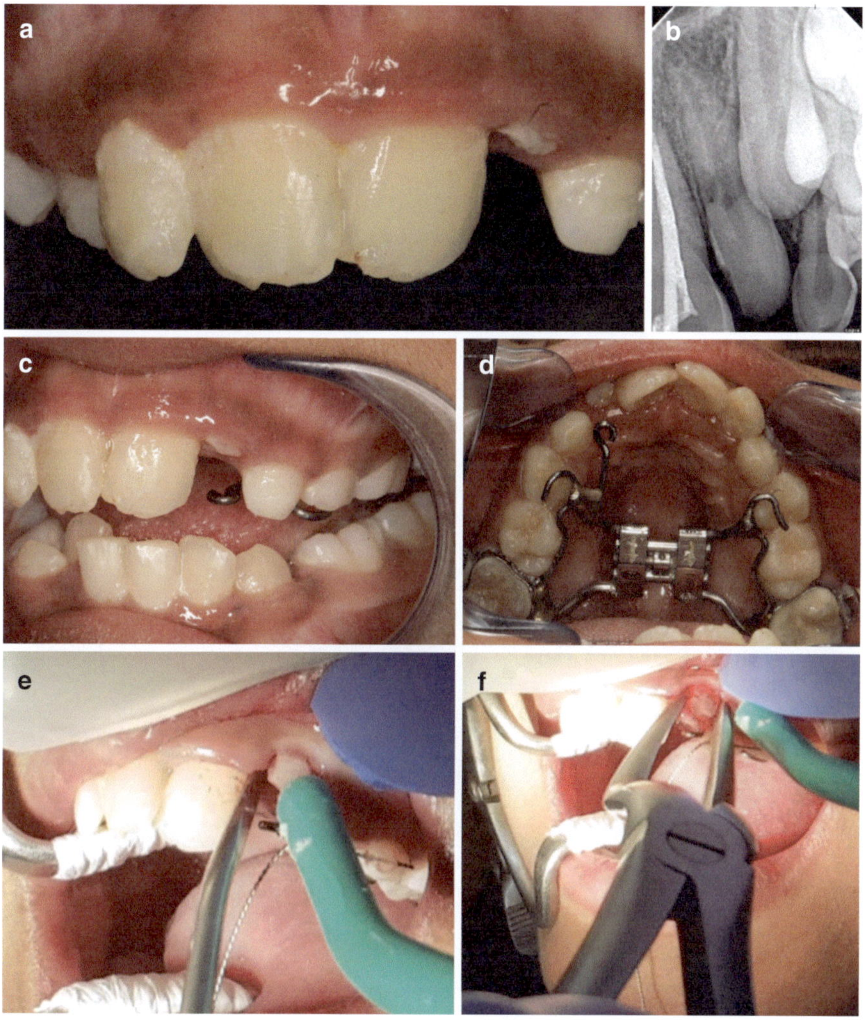

Fig. 11.26 An 11-year-old child reported with severe intrusion of maxillary permanent left lateral incisor (**a**). The diagnostic radiograph showed lateral root resorption and widened periodontal ligament space of the intruded incisor necessitating immediate pulp extirpation. The central incisors were treated for root canal earlier (**b**). The patient was given a rapid maxillary expander (**c**, **d**), to make space for the lateral incisor after extrusion. Surgical extrusion was done by gently luxating the tooth first (**e**), followed by extrusion with forceps (**f**) to a point where coronal structure was exposed feasible for endodontic access opening (**g**). The tooth was positioned in the space created by expansion and splinted for 4 weeks (**h**). Intracanal CH medicament was placed for 2 weeks (**i**). At 2 weeks, the CH medicament was removed and bleeding induced within the canal as part of revascularization procedure. An MTA plug was placed to seal the coronal third of the root canal space (**j**). The resorption had halted at 12-month recall (**k**). The child is under follow-up while undergoing simultaneous orthodontic alignment of maxillary anterior teeth (**l**). (Image courtesy: Dr Abhishek Soni, India)

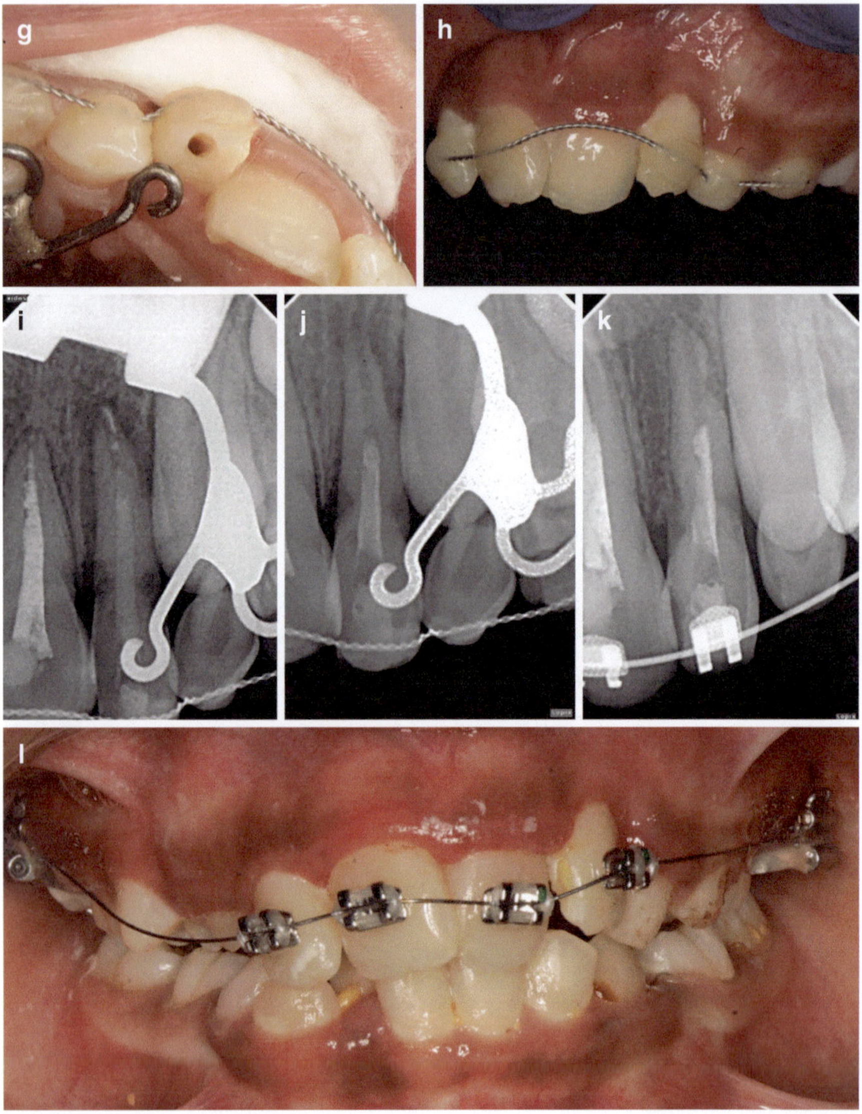

Fig. 11.26 (continued)

- A wire is placed into the brackets of adjacent teeth. To this wire, an elastic is engaged that extends to the bracket hook of the intruded tooth. The intruded tooth is gently pulled towards its proper position by means of elastics.
- The amount of extrusion would be 1.5 mm a week for 4–6 weeks. The force of extrusion must not be more than 20 g per incisor.

- A palatal bonded retainer incorporating adjacent teeth may be used for anchorage.
- Elastics should be checked and replaced once a week until successful repositioning is achieved.
- Alternately, a removable appliance such as a modified Hawley's plate with extrusion springs can be used.

3. *Extrusive Luxation*

This type of luxation injury dictates immediate repositioning of the extruded tooth followed by splinting with a resin composite and wire splint for a period of 2 weeks [4].

For immediate repositioning [95] (Fig. 11.27),

- After administering local anesthesia, one finger must rest on the incisal edge to push the tooth back into the socket and thumb on the attached gingiva or mucogingival fold.
- A continuous digital pressure needs to be applied to the tooth so that the alveolar bone expands allowing the tooth to be repositioned correctly.
- Repositioning the extruded tooth is a traumatic procedure by itself and hence must not be done repeatedly.
- Before repositioning the tooth, bonding the splint on adjacent teeth is recommended as it will be easier to fix the extruded tooth and digital pressure will be applied only once.
- If there is a delay and patient reports after the tooth has stabilized in an extruded position and repositioning is not possible using digital pressure, then
  - Repositioning using conventional orthodontic methods
  - Modification of a customized thermoformable splint
  - Intentional replantation is another method employed to reposition these teeth (Fig. 11.30)

The follow-up intervals recommended by the IADT are as follows [4]:

- 2 weeks
- 1 month
- 2 months
- 3 months
- 6 months
- 1 year
- Then yearly, for 5 years

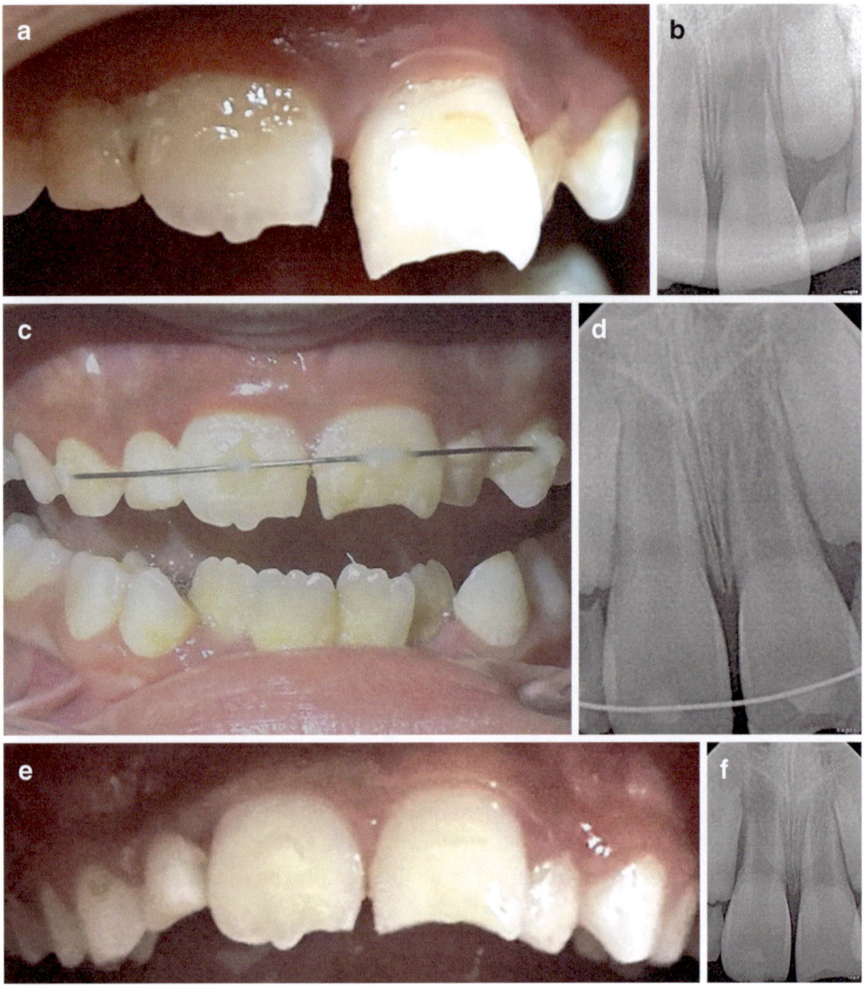

Fig. 11.27 A 9-year-old child reported with extrusive luxation injury and an uncomplicated enamel dentin fracture with maxillary permanent left central incisor and enamel fracture with right central incisor (**a**). The diagnostic radiograph confirms extrusive luxation and immature apices of both incisors (**b**). The tooth was repositioned and stabilized with a resin composite and wire splint for 2 weeks (**c**). A radiograph was taken after splinting (**d**). After 2 weeks, the splint was removed (**e**). A radiograph was taken after splint removal (**f**). Both central incisors were restored with a composite buildup (**g**). At 1-year follow-up, the right central incisor gave a negative response to pulp sensibility test (**h**). Radiograph showed arrested root development (**i**)

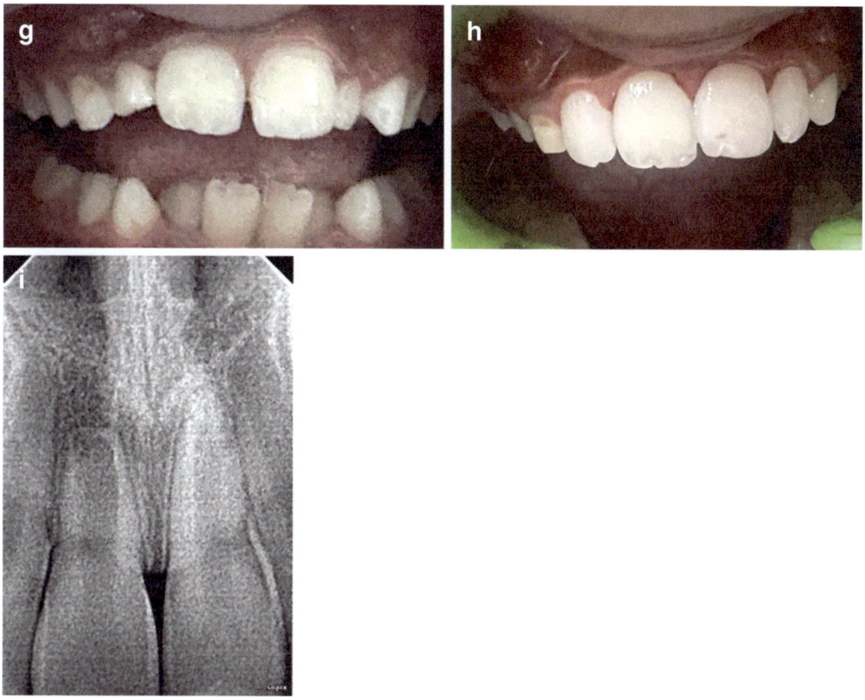

Fig. 11.27 (continued)

Customized Thermoformable Splint [96]

This form of repositioning is recommended for extruded teeth that have stabilized, are not mobile and cannot be repositioned with digital pressure. The extrusion must not be more than 2–3 mm as compared to the adjacent teeth.

- An alginate impression or a digital scan is made of the dental arch.
- The incisal edge of the extruded tooth is reduced on the model to match that of the adjacent tooth.
- A thermoformable PTEG (polyethylene terephthalate glycol) material tray is fabricated as the splint.
- The patient is instructed to always wear the splint except while eating and brushing.
- This splint will stabilize the tooth and slowly reposition it physiologically in 3–4 weeks.

Intentional Reimplantation [97, 98]

Intentional reimplantation is the purposeful extraction of the tooth followed by irrigation, curettage of the socket, and immediate replantation of the tooth back into the same socket. The success of intentional reimplantation depends on the extraoral storage time of the tooth. Thus, a shorter operative time of less than 20 min is critical for success.

Technique

After administration of local anesthesia, a scalpel and a 15 No blade must be used to detach the periodontal ligament by moving the blade around the gingival sulcus.

- The extruded tooth must be extracted in an atraumatic manner to avoid damaging the PDL cells present in the coronal portion of the root surface. To avoid damaging the gingival fibers, a sterile gauze can be placed on the tooth under the beaks of the extraction forceps.
- The extracted tooth must be kept in an appropriate storage media such as a sterile saline solution or Hank's Balanced Salt Solution (HBSS).
- Curettage and cautious irrigation of the alveolar socket with saline is performed to remove the formed clot.
- The tooth is placed back into the socket by finger pressure.
- The position can be checked by observing the alignment of its incisal edge with that of the adjacent teeth.
- A radiograph is taken to verify the position of the tooth.
- The concerned tooth must be splinted for a period of 2 weeks.
- Occlusal adjustment must be performed to prevent any occlusal interferences.
- The patient is recommended to keep the area clean with soft toothbrushing and use of 0.12% chlorohexidine mouthwash. Systemic antibiotics may be prescribed to prevent contamination.
- In case of mature teeth, root canal treatment should be initiated within 10 days of reimplantation to prevent occurrence of inflammatory root resorption.

Most cases of extrusion would report within a day or two of the injury as the mobile and extruded tooth would cause discomfort. Hence, use of digital pressure and splinting is most often the treatment of choice resulting in overall good prognosis. The other methods described above can be used depending upon the operator's preference.

4. *Lateral Luxation*

Laterally luxated teeth should be repositioned immediately and require a certain amount of force, as they need to be dislodged from their locked position [99] (Fig. 11.28).

- Local anesthesia is administered.
- If the tooth is palatally displaced, the root tip may be palpable on the labial gingiva and firm digital pressure must be applied to dislodge it from the socket.
- Depending upon the direction of the luxation, significant digital pressure is exerted on the crown of the luxated tooth, either labially or lingually, to maneuver it into its correct position.

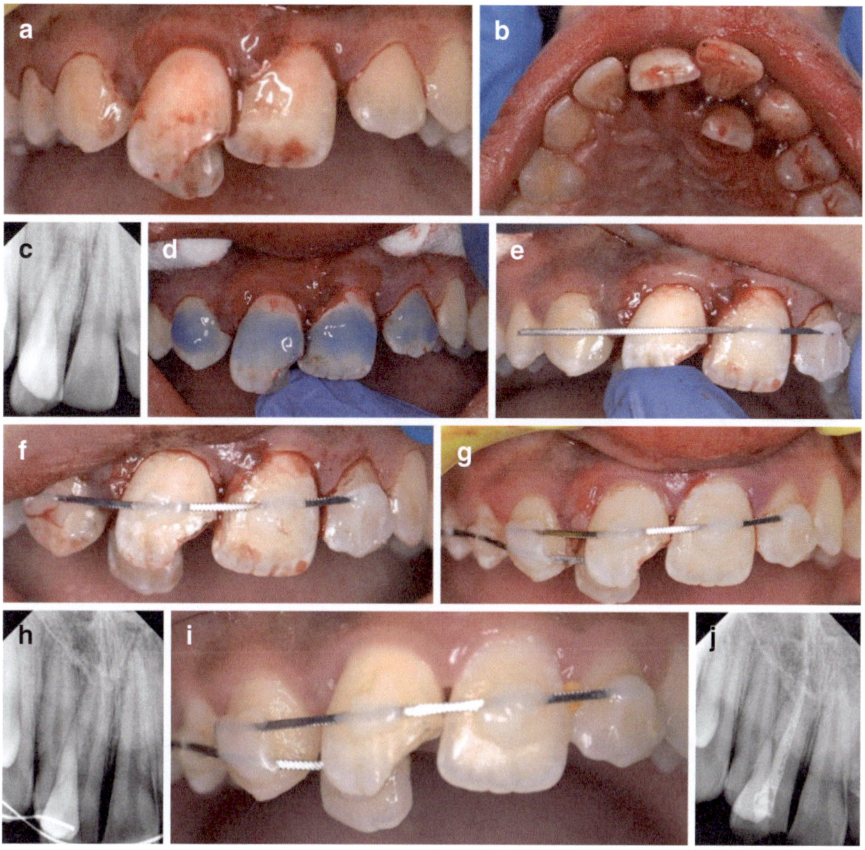

Fig. 11.28 A 10-year-old child reported with luxation injury of maxillary anterior teeth 2 h after trauma. The right central incisor had avulsed and was replanted at the primary referral center. The child was asked to bite on a cotton roll and hold the tooth in place. On clinical and radiographic examination, the maxillary right central incisor was not completely reimplanted. Lateral luxation injuries were seen with maxillary left central incisor and right lateral incisor, labial (**a**) and occlusal view (**b**). The diagnostic radiograph shows Cvek's Stage 4 of root development (**c**). The luxated teeth and those to be included in the splint were isolated, etched and dried (**d**). The laterally luxated left central incisor was first repositioned and splinted (**e**). The avulsed right central incisor was correctly repositioned and stabilized with the splint (**f**). The right lateral incisor was surgically repositioned and a separate splint was placed to stabilize it (**g**). A radiograph was taken (**h**) and patient recalled after 2 weeks (**i**). Endodontic treatment was initiated for right central incisors within 10 days. Intracanal CH dressing was given for 4 weeks followed by obturation (**j**). The maxillary permanent right central incisor was restored with a composite buildup (**k**). The child was recalled for recall every 3 months. After 3 months, the patient presented with signs of discoloration and non-vitality with left central incisor and endodontic treatment was performed for the same (**l**, **m**). The right lateral incisor showed positive response to sensibility tests. At 1-year follow-up, the right lateral incisor showed delayed response to sensibility test and pulp canal obliteration was seen on the radiograph (**n**)

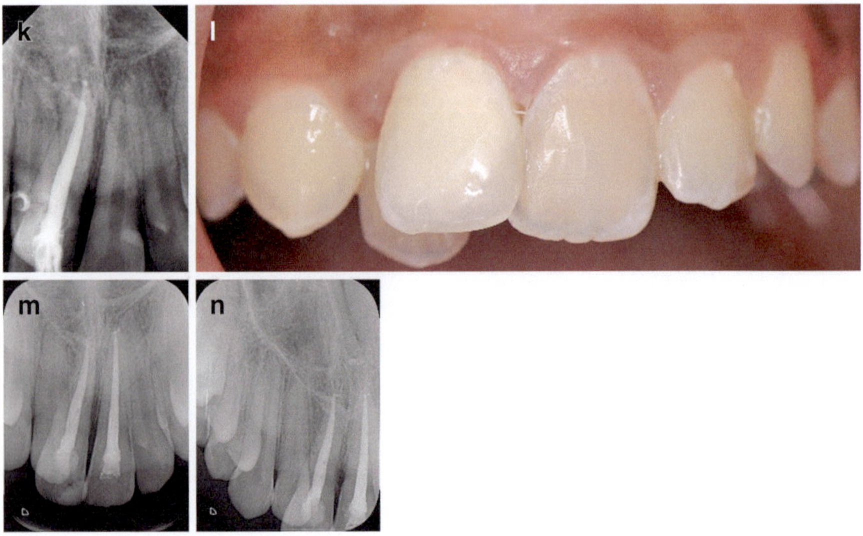

Fig. 11.28 (continued)

- If manual repositioning is not possible, the tooth can be extruded slightly with forceps to unlock it and then directed into position.
- The tooth must be splinted for 4 weeks with a resin composite and wire splint. If marginal bone loss is seen, then splinting is extended to 6–8 weeks.
- The labial and palatal bony plate must be compressed to complete the repositioning and to facilitate periodontal healing.
- Lacerated gingiva is readapted to the neck of the tooth and sutured.
- A radiograph should be taken to ensure that the tooth has been repositioned appropriately.
- The follow-up intervals suggested are similar to that of extrusive luxation (Fig. 11.30).

It is difficult to reposition a laterally luxated tooth after 3–4 days. In such situation, orthodontic forces can be used to reposition the teeth. For minor palatal luxation, a tongue blade can be used as a conservative repositioning method, that is not as forceful and causes minimal discomfort to the patient. In this technique, the tongue blade is placed lingually at an angle of 45° and the child asked to bite gently [100].

11.3.4.5 What Is the Healing Modality in Luxation Injuries?

For the last few years, the concept of *transient apical breakdown* that is seen around 2–3 weeks after trauma, has been reported in literature.

What Is Transient Apical Breakdown (TAB)?

Transient apical breakdown is seen within 2–3 weeks of trauma, when there is a complete severance of blood supply to the mature tooth. The apical breakdown is seen on the radiograph as widening of the foramen and blunting of the root apex. This improves the blood supply to the luxated tooth and is considered a favorable healing response. TAB is *not seen in cases of immature teeth* due to an already wide apical foramen. Endodontic intervention is not necessary solely on this radiographic finding. The PDL is restored in few weeks, and this is seen on the radiograph at follow-up appointments. In certain cases, TAB may continue to progressive root resorption. The early detection of root resorption will necessitate pulp tissue removal and placement of CH. Pulp canal obliteration may be seen 1–2 years after transient apical breakdown [101, 102].

11.3.4.6 Endodontic Management of Luxated Teeth

The mechanical trauma incurred by a tooth during a luxation injury indirectly subjects the dental pulp of the tooth to tension, compression, or separation at the apical constriction. In less severe cases, the trauma can cause bleeding, increased intrapulpal pressure, reduced circulation, and transient loss of sensibility. All the above can lead to pulp necrosis impacting the prognosis of the tooth.

The survival of the pulp depends on [103–106]

- *Type of luxation injury*—Teeth with intrusive luxation injuries have the highest risk of undergoing pulp necrosis followed by lateral luxation and extrusion.
- *The maturity of the tooth*—Immature teeth with wide open apices have better chances of healing than mature teeth.
- *The severity of the injury*—Presence of concomitant injuries, however small (enamel infarction or uncomplicated crown fractures), increase the risk of pulp necrosis, irrespective of the type of injury.

While concussed and subluxated teeth heal uneventfully, the chances of *pulpal necrosis* are higher if these teeth have incurred concomitant crown fractures.

Pulp canal obliteration is seen more commonly in extrusive luxation. Although this is not an unfavorable outcome, the tooth may appear discolored and less life like at follow-up visits.

The endodontic treatment protocol is based on the maturity of the tooth [4, 34].

1. *Immature Teeth*

   In immature teeth, irrespective of the type of luxation injury, endodontic treatment *should not be initiated* as there is a high chance of the tooth undergoing spontaneous revascularization. Clinically, the tooth must be monitored for discoloration and signs of mobility. Periodic radiographic examination should assess signs of arrested root development, root resorption, and periapical radiolucency. Pulp sensibility testing should be performed at each appointment and results corroborated with clinical and radiographic findings to ascertain pulpal status. If pulp necrosis is confirmed, regenerative endodontic procedures or apexification must be performed.

2. *Mature Teeth*
   While mature teeth with *concussion, subluxation and extrusive luxation injuries* usually heal uneventfully, they should be monitored at the prescribed follow-up intervals for signs of pulp necrosis and root resorption. The health of both, pulpal and PDL tissues are co-dependent and influence each other. If signs of pulp necrosis are seen at any of the follow-up appointments, then root canal treatment must be initiated, and a calcium hydroxide dressing placed to reduce the risk of root resorption. *Intruded and severely laterally luxated teeth*, if left untouched will eventually undergo necrosis. Therefore, it is imperative to remove the pulp tissue and place calcium hydroxide within 7–10 days of repositioning, so as to prevent root resorption. Calcium hydroxide dressing must be placed for at least 3–4 weeks before root canal obturation (Fig. 11.31) [34, 105–107].

In cases of root resorption seen

1. Due to non-removal of pulp
2. Post obturation even when correct protocol is followed

It is recommended to remove pulp or obturating material and place CH for at least 6 months, depending on the extent of signs and symptoms.

The clinician can identify healing of the tooth at follow-up visits as below:

Clinical signs and symptoms

- Resolution of abscess or draining sinus.
- Decrease in tooth mobility.
- Absence of tenderness on percussion.

On the radiograph,

- The resorption process must have halted or not worsened.
- Decrease or resolution of periapical radiolucency.
- Restoration of the lamina dura.

11.3.5 Avulsion

Avulsion is complete loss of tooth from its socket and the most affected teeth are the maxillary central incisors. It is commonly seen in children between 7 and 9 years of age as the short root and resilient bone makes the tooth more susceptible to avulsion [108, 109].

11.3.5.1 Clinical Examination

Avulsion is diagnosed with clinical and radiographic detection of an empty socket filled with blood clot. The gingiva and lip may be lacerated. The labial plate and the maxillary alveolar bone may be mobile indicating a fracture. When the avulsed

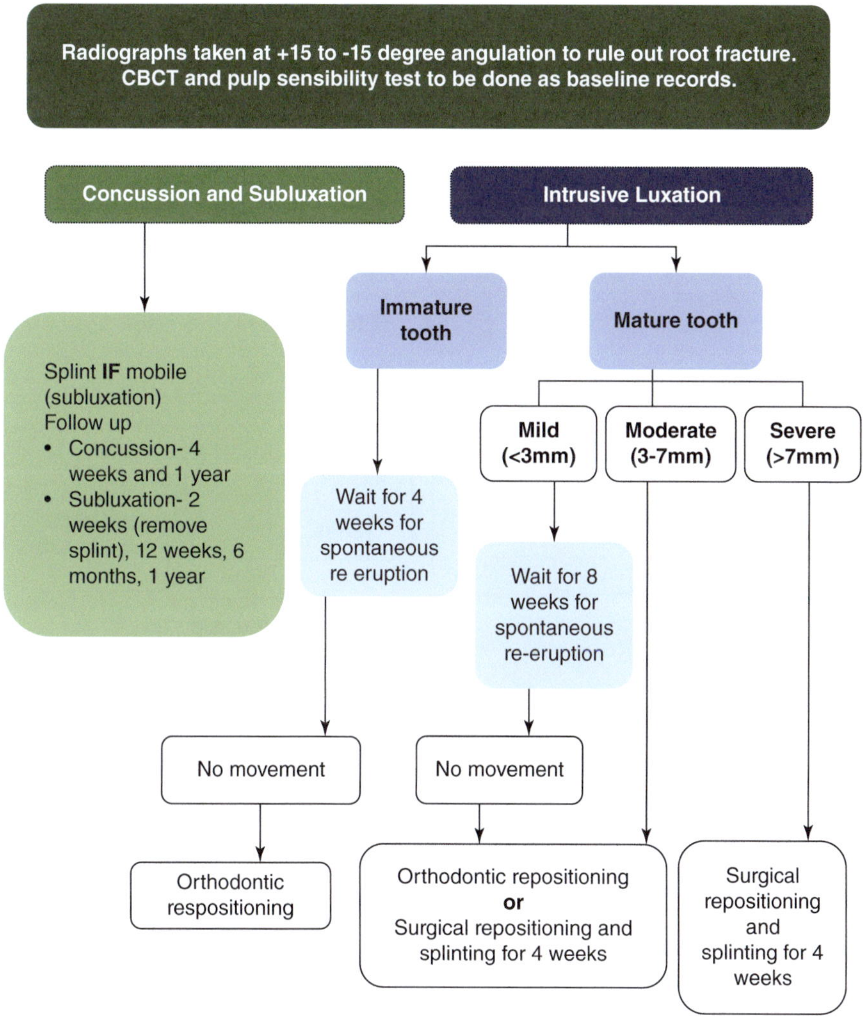

Fig. 11.29 Decision tree for luxation injuries (concussion, subluxation, and intrusive luxation)

tooth is not found, a radiographic examination is important to rule out severe intrusion or loss of coronal fragment following crown-root or root fracture. The parents and caregivers must be told to look for the tooth at the site of accident. If an avulsed tooth is retrieved, there are two possibilities of management.

1. Immediate replantation at the site of injury.
2. Tooth brought to the dentist for replantation.

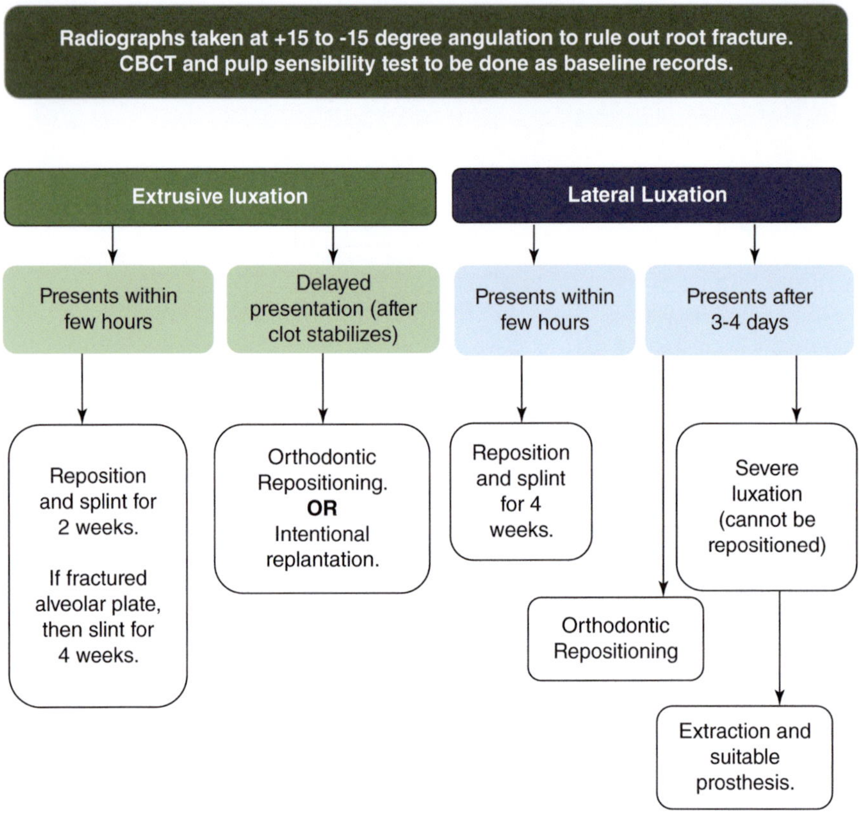

Fig. 11.30 Decision tree for luxation injuries (extrusive luxation and lateral luxation)

11.3.5.2 Management of Avulsion

1. *Immediate replantation at the site of injury* [109].

When the dental office receives a call reporting an avulsion injury, the patient or caregiver must be told to try and replant the tooth immediately. This will reduce the extra oral time and improve the prognosis or survival of the tooth. If the tooth shows visible debris, the patient or caregiver is instructed to gently rinse the tooth with milk, saline, or clean water, taking care to hold only the crown of the tooth. Once replanted, the child must be made to bite on a cotton-gauze/tissue to keep the tooth in place and visit a dentist nearby for evaluation and further treatment [109].

2. *Tooth brought to the dentist for replantation* (Figs. 11.32, 11.33, and 11.34)

If the patient or parent is unable to replant the tooth at the site of trauma, they must be told to report to the dental office immediately. The tooth must be stored in milk, HBSS (Hank's Balanced Salt Solution), patient's saliva, or saline [110–113].

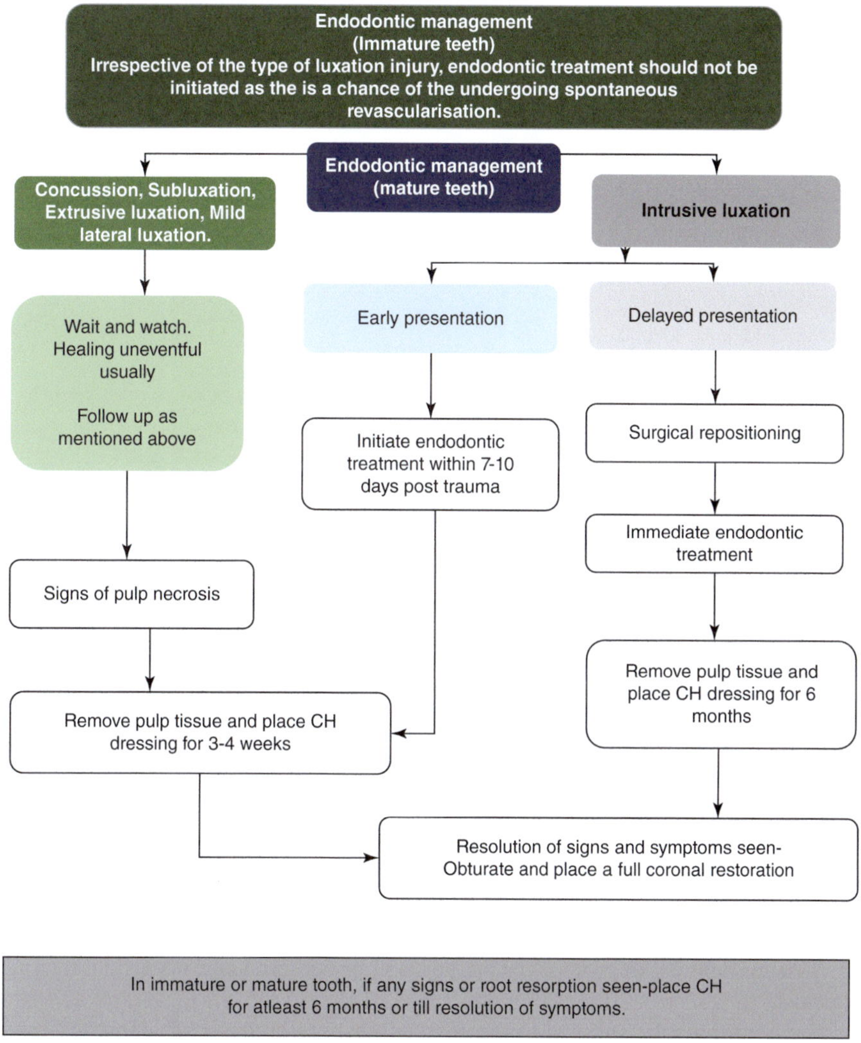

Fig. 11.31 Endodontic management of luxation injuries

At the clinic, the avulsed tooth and the alveolus are examined to rule out fracture or communition of the alveolar socket. If the alveolus is fractured, then the fractured bone must be repositioned under local anesthesia preferably without a vasoconstrictor [109].

The visible contaminants must be removed from the root surface especially around the apical foramen by rinsing under saline and the tooth must be examined for fracture.

The alveolus is irrigated with saline to remove the contaminated coagulum.

Under local anesthesia, the tooth must be replanted gently with minimal pressure.

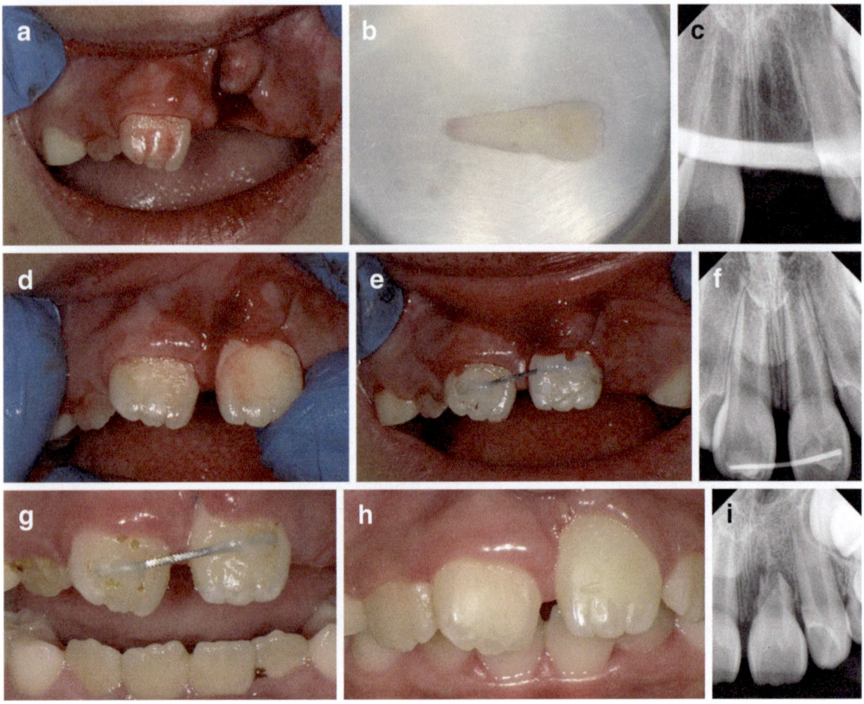

Fig. 11.32 A 7-year-old child reported with avulsed immature maxillary permanent left central incisor within an hour of injury (**a**). The tooth was transported in saline (**b**). The diagnostic radiograph showed empty socket (**c**). The tooth was replanted within an hour (**d**) and splinted with a resin composite and wire splint for 2 weeks (**e**). Radiograph was taken to verify position of tooth (**f**). Follow-up in 2 weeks (**g**). Splint was removed and patient recalled every 3 months for a follow-up (**h**). Patient reported with mobility after 1 year. Radiograph showed inflammatory root resorption (**i**)

A radiograph is taken to verify the position of the tooth and occlusion must be checked.

The tooth must be splinted to the adjacent teeth with a as resin composite and wire splint (0.4 mm in diameter) splint or a Titanium Trauma Splint (TTS) to allow physiologic movement.

Gingival laceration if present must be sutured.

Splinting is done for a week to 10 days if the tooth is mature, while an immature tooth is splinted for 14 days [2] (Fig. 11.35).

Tetanus prophylaxis is recommended based on the child's immunization history. Antibiotics are prescribed for the first week after replantation depending on the age and weight of the patient to avoid microbial infection. Additionally, chlorhexidine mouthwash may be prescribed for 7 days.

While there is great emphasis on replantation of the tooth back into the socket, the follow-up schedule is equally important to the success of the treatment. Once the initial shock of the trauma wears off and the splint is removed, parents often think

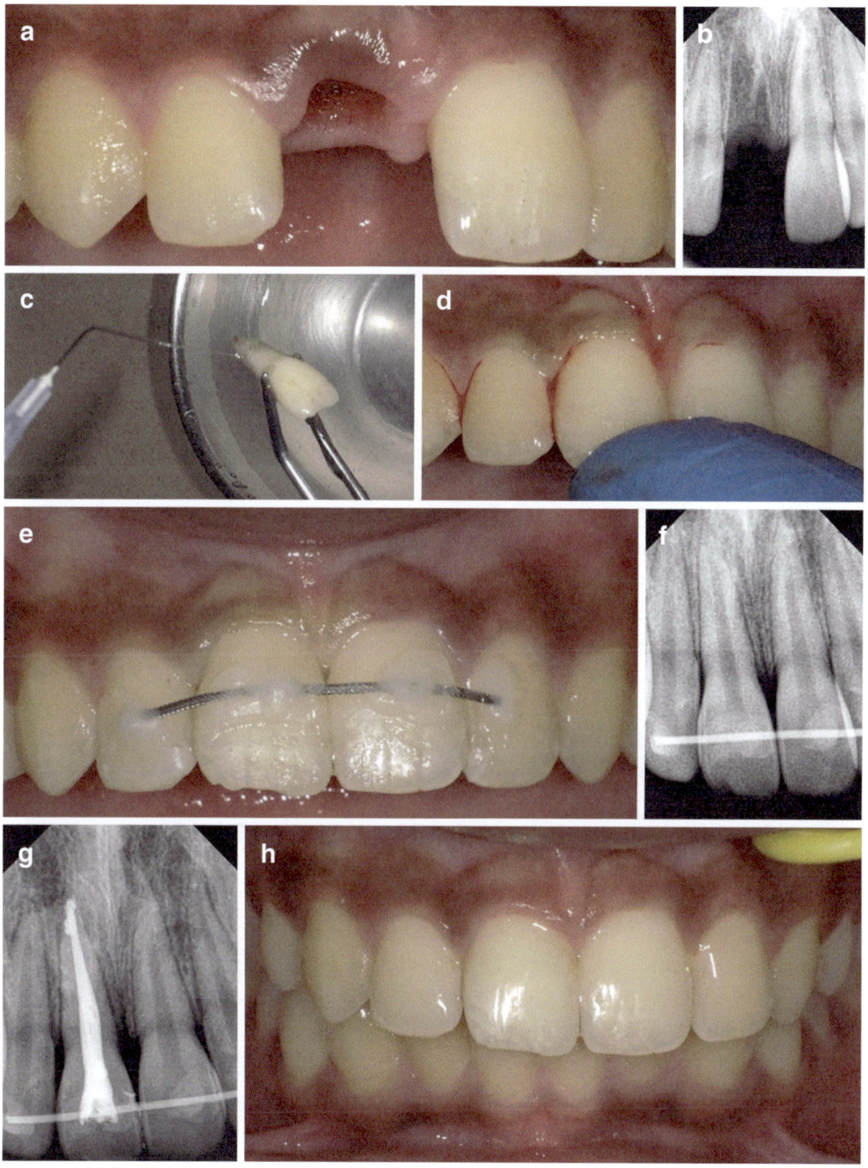

Fig. 11.33 A 10-year-old child reported with avulsion of maxillary permanent right central incisor within 1 h of trauma (**a**). Diagnostic radiograph taken to rule out injury to adjacent teeth and bone (**b**). The avulsed tooth was held gently at the crown and cleaned with a stream of normal saline (**c**). Tooth repositioned and held with digital pressure (**d**). Tooth stabilized with a resin composite and wire splint (**e**). Radiograph taken after splinting (**f**). Endodontic treatment initiated within 10 days of the trauma (**g**). Splint was removed after 2 weeks (**h**). At the first-year follow-up, the tooth appeared in infraocclusion (**i**). Radiograph shows replacement root resorption (**j**)

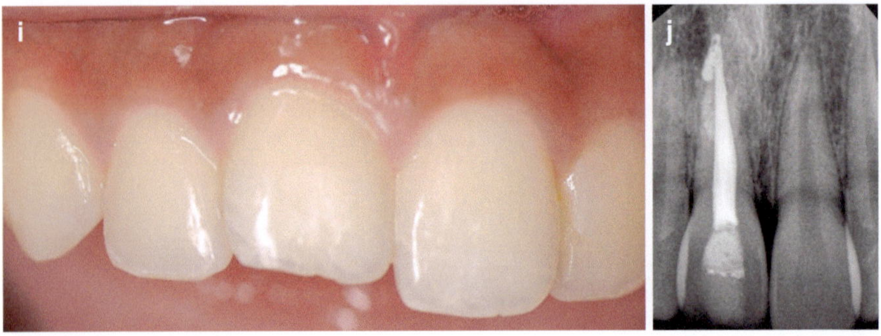

Fig. 11.33 (continued)

that the treatment is complete. It is important to counsel the parents about the need for adhering to a stringent recall schedule to ensure early detection of signs of root resorption.

11.3.5.3 What Is the Ideal Replantation Schedule?

The prognosis and survival of an avulsed tooth depends on the PDL healing, which is governed by factors such as *extraoral time and type of storage media.* The PDL survival is maximum when the tooth is replanted immediately or within 15 min of avulsion. An avulsed tooth can be replanted despite an extended extraoral time and unoptimal storage condition. The recommended storage media is milk, Hank's Balanced Salt Solution (HBSS), saliva, and saline [109–113].

11.3.5.4 What Are the Possible Clinical and Radiographic Outcomes Post Replantation? [34, 109–118]

Immature Teeth

I*rrespective of the extraoral dry time*, endodontic intervention is not recommended as replanted immature teeth have the potential to undergo spontaneous revascularization. Pulp sensibility testing can be misleading in immature teeth because complete neural innervation takes place only after root maturation. These teeth should be closely monitored clinically and radiographically including a CBCT to be taken at baseline and at follow-ups if required.

Follow-up schedule.

- *2 weeks (when the splint is removed)*
- *Radiograph at 1 month*

The tooth must stabilize while the radiograph may not show root development within 4 weeks; however, they must be recorded as baseline.

Inflammatory root resorption if seen, appears as early as 2–4 weeks on the radiograph. The process is aggressive and needs to be closely monitored. In these cases,

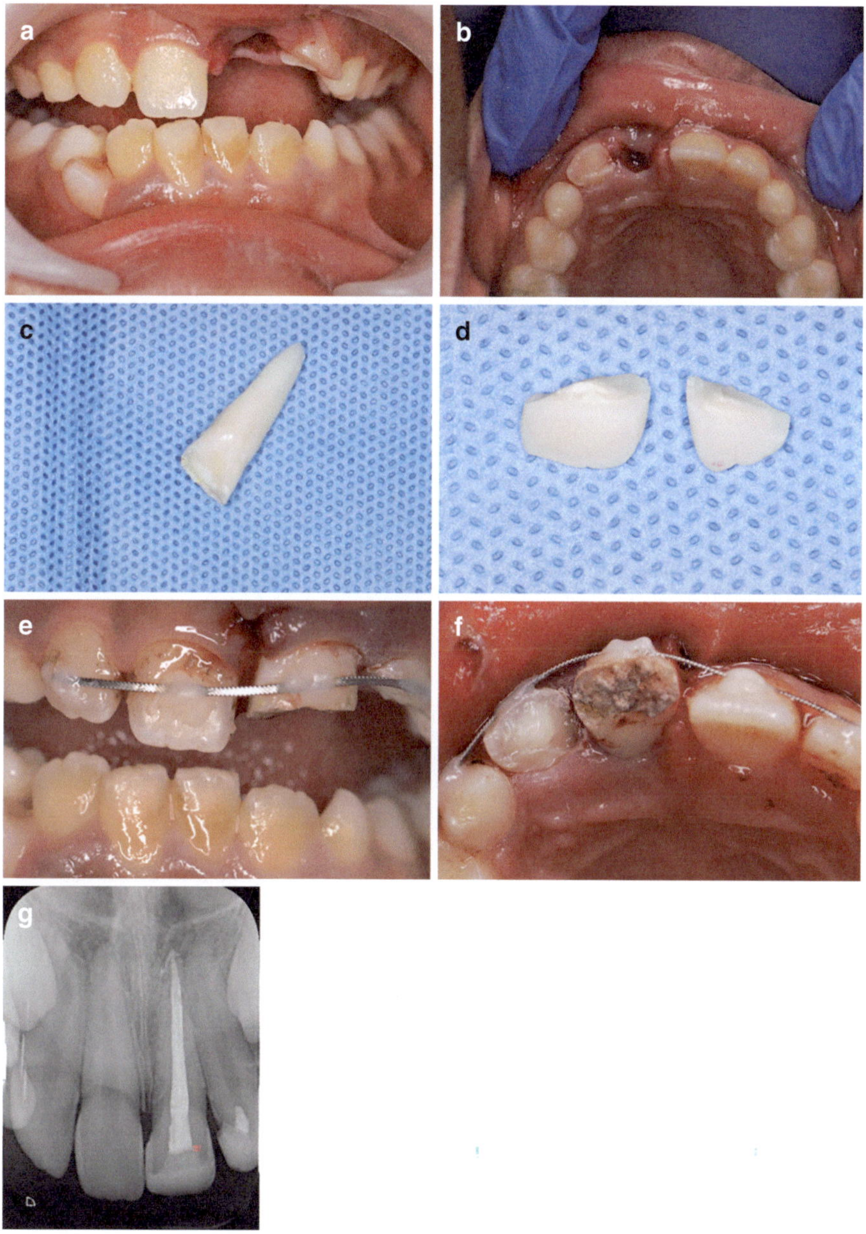

Fig. 11.34 Avulsion and crown fracture of maxillary permanent left central incisor and lateral incisor respectively, in labial (**a**) and occlusal view (**b**). The avulsed tooth had concomitant crown fracture (**c**). The fragments were kept hydrated in saline (**d**). The central incisor was repositioned and splinted for 2 weeks. The position of replanted incisor was below that of the right incisor (**e**). Endodontic treatment was initiated and CH dressing placed for 4 weeks (**f**). Cvek's pulpotomy was done on the left lateral incisor (**g**). Splint removed after 2 weeks (**h**). Endodontic treatment of the left central incisor was completed (**i**). The left central incisor appeared infraoccluded after buildup and was sent for CBCT (**j**). Occlusal view post buildup (**k**). CBCT did not show obliteration of PDL space

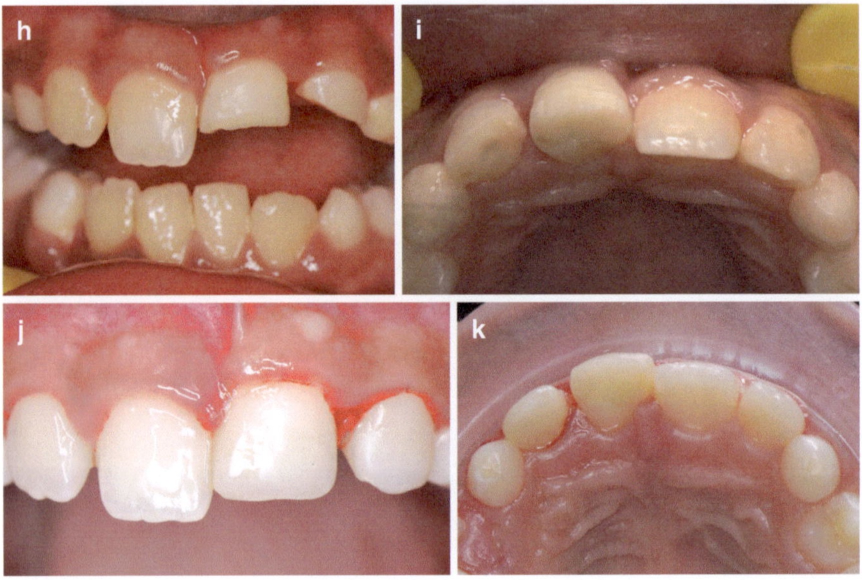

Fig. 11.34 (continued)

endodontic treatment must be initiated by completely extirpating the pulp and placing a CH intracanal dressing till the next follow-up.

- *3 months*

The tooth is evaluated radiographically for continued root development.

If inflammatory root resorption is seen as a new development or continues from before and the apical opening appears ragged with or without a periapical lesion, CH as an intracanal medicament is placed or replenished and the patient recalled at 6 months.

- *6 months*

Continued tooth eruption and root maturation are favorable outcomes at 3–6 months.

While inflammatory root resorption can continue or begin at 6 months, the radiographs may also show replacement root resorption at this interval. CH is placed or replenished and patient recalled at 6 months.

- *1 year, and yearly thereafter for at least 5 years.*

Under favorable outcomes, significant root development and maturation will be seen on the radiograph, with the tooth continuing to erupt. However, if the tooth lags in eruption, ankylosis due to replacement root resorption must be suspected as the

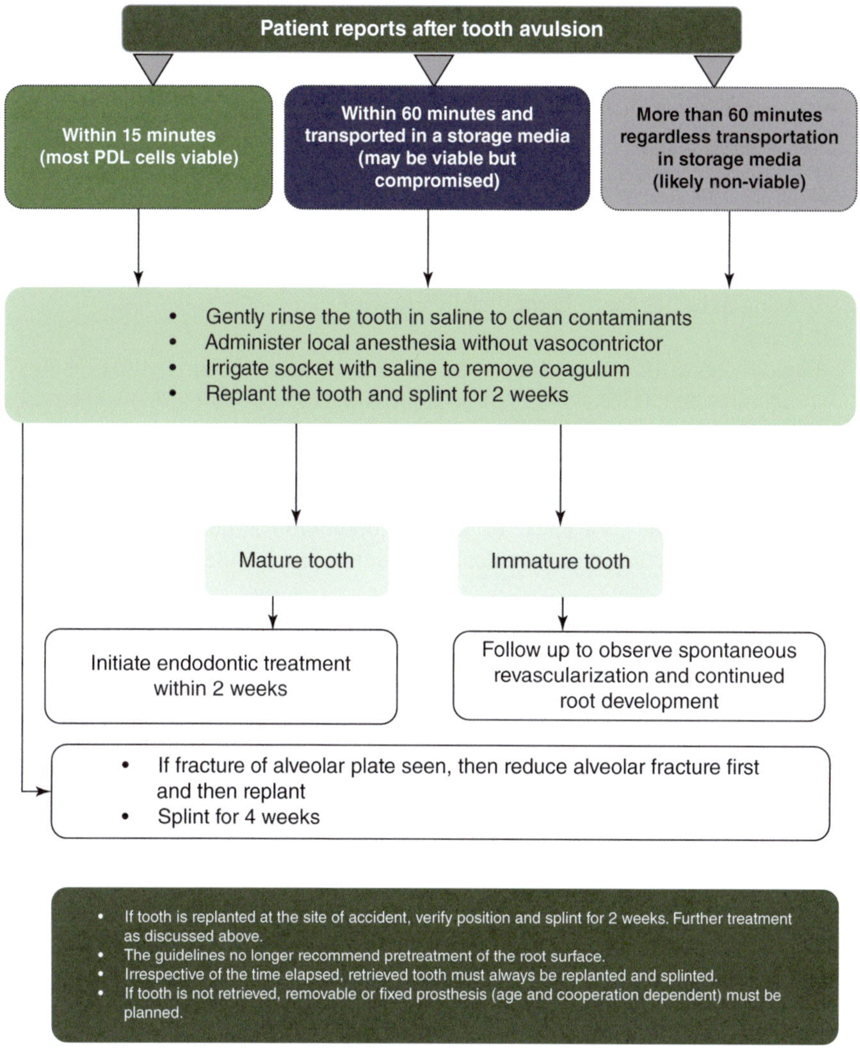

Fig. 11.35 Decision tree for avulsion injury

clinical signs of ankylosis may precede the radiographic signs. Additionally, at every follow-up appointment, recall history should be taken, and the tooth and surrounding tissues examined for clinical signs and symptoms of pulp necrosis such as dentoalveolar abscess, tooth discoloration. Apart from root resorption, the follow-up radiographs may show signs of periapical radiolucency or arrested root development.

Mature Teeth

Mature teeth are at a higher risk of root resorption, even if the extraoral time is less than one hour.

Follow-up schedule.

1. *7–10 days*
   Endodontic treatment must be initiated once initial stabilization occurs, to reduce inflammation and decrease the chances of resorption. A calcium hydroxide dressing must be placed in the canal for 4 weeks.
2. *4 weeks*
   Clinical scenario 1: According to the AAE, intracanal calcium hydroxide dressing must be left for 4 weeks. If no resorption is seen, obturation must be done and definitive restoration given.
   Clinical scenario 2: Inflammatory root resorption seen as early at 2–4 weeks on the radiograph. It appears as crater-like defects on the root wall or ragged margins of the root apex. Root canal obturation is deferred and Calcium hydroxide medicament is replenished, and patient recalled in 3 months.
3. *3 months*
   Clinical scenario 1: The obturated tooth followed up for signs of inflammatory root resorption. If no resorption is seen, the patient is recalled at 6 months for a routine follow-up.
   Clinical scenario 2: CH was placed at 4 weeks due to early signs of inflammatory root resorption and the radiograph shows resolution of resorption, then obturation must be performed. If the patient shows consistent signs and symptoms of periapical infection and radiograph reveals progressive inflammatory root resorption, then CH dressing must be replenished if the tooth is salvageable.
   Clinical scenario 3: If the obturated tooth shows inflammatory root resorption, then the gutta-percha is removed and intracanal Calcium hydroxide is placed, till the time of resolution or signs of PDL space reestablishment is seen.
4. *6 months*
   Clinical scenario 1: The tooth continues to remain asymptomatic and shows no signs of resorption. Continue follow-up as per schedule.
   Clinical scenarios 2 and 3:
   - If no further signs of inflammatory root resorption are seen at 6 months, then obturation is performed.
   - While inflammatory root resorption can continue, the first signs of replacement root resorption are simultaneously seen. Few cases of inflammatory root resorption change to replacement root resorption.
   - A dull metallic sound on percussion should raise suspicion of replacement root resorption. The radiograph may show parts of obliterated PDL space.
   - A CBCT is recommended to assess the type and extent of root resorption.
   - If either form of resorption is seen, calcium hydroxide is replenished and continued as an intracanal medicament.

5. *1 year, and yearly thereafter for at least 5 years.*

   If inflammatory root resorption is not seen in the first year after trauma, the chances of it occurring diminish with time.

   If the inflammatory root resorption is seen to resolve at these follow-ups, the decision to obturate the canal will depend upon the extent and type of root resorption. The obturating materials used may be a combination of gutta-percha and bioceramic materials such as MTA and Biodentine™.

   If the tooth continues to show inflammatory root resorption, the intracanal calcium hydroxide is replenished or the tooth extracted depending upon the amount of resorption, tooth mobility, and periapical infection.

   Infraocclusion or metallic sound on percussion is indicative of ankylosis due to replacement root resorption. Intracanal calcium hydroxide must be continued till the further treatment is planned.

The follow-up schedule including radiographs should be varied and more frequent if the extraoral time is longer and the tooth has not been transported in appropriate storage media. This is applicable to both, mature and immature teeth, as inflammatory root resorption can be seen early and is aggressive in nature. While CH can help in arresting inflammatory root resorption, it can only slow down the replacement root resorption as the process is irreversible.

11.3.5.5 What Are the Healing Modalities of Avulsion Injury?

The prognosis of a replanted tooth depends mainly on how the periodontal space heals after the tooth is replanted. The PDL space healing depends primarily on the length of extra alveolar time and extra alveolar handling. The most common unfavorable outcome is ankylosis of the replanted tooth followed by inflammatory root resorption. Ankylosis represents a fusion of cementum to the bone and occurs as early as 2 weeks (histologically) after replantation and is seen more commonly in delayed replantation or due to poor handling of the tooth that damages the PDL cells. It can be progressive or transient, depending on the extent of damage to the periodontal ligament. Progressive is when the tooth is gradually resorbed and replaced by bone; while transient ankylosis shows a minor part of the root surface in contact with the bone, but later the process reverses and the PDL space is eventually reestablished, that is, the ankylosis disappears [107, 119–122]. Inflammatory root resorption will be discussed under healing complications in Chap. 12.

11.4 Concluding Remarks

Management of Traumatic Dental Injuries in the permanent dentition requires an understanding of the healing responses, clinical judgment, and potential consequences. Clinical decision-making is governed by factors such as age of the patient, extent of injury and stage of root development. Uncomplicated crown fractures can be treated with fragment reattachment and composite build up, while fractures involving the pulp require immediate intervention to preserve vitality in both, mature and immature teeth. Regardless of the time elapsed, an immature tooth should be treated conservatively, so as to maintain pulp vitality and allow continued root maturation.

Root fractures present with a favorable prognosis when the fracture is in the apical or middle third and the coronal fragment has not incurred a concomitant luxation injury. Prognosis is questionable when the cervical third is fractured. Crown-root fracture at or above the level of alveolar crest can be treated with gingivectomy and/or osteotomy followed by buildup or fragment reattachment. For fracture lines going beyond the alveolar crest, orthodontic or surgical extrusion may be considered.

Injuries to the pulp and periodontium as in cases of intrusive luxation and avulsion of mature teeth need pulp extirpation to reduce the risk of pulp necrosis and consequent root resorption. Immediate intervention aligning with the guidelines aims at restoring the pulp and periodontal health for all TDIs. The operator must stress on the importance of follow-up as the consequences of trauma are unpredictable. Signs of tooth discoloration, mobility, non-vitality, and root resorption, if detected early, must be treated to improve the survival of the tooth.

References

1. Moule A, Cohenca N. Emergency assessment and treatment planning for traumatic dental injuries. Aust Dent J. 2016;61(Suppl 1):21–38.
2. Gassner R, Tuli T, Hachl O, et al. Craniomaxillofacial trauma in children: a review of 3,385 cases with 6,060 injuries in 10 years. J Oral Maxillofac Surg. 2004;62(4):339–407.
3. Levin L, Day PF, Hicks L, O'Connell A, Fouad AF, Bourguignon C, Abbott PV. International Association of Dental Traumatology guidelines for the management of traumatic dental injuries: general introduction. Dent Traumatol. 2020;36(4):309–13.
4. Bourguignon C, Cohenca N, Lauridsen E, Flores MT, O'Connell AC, Day PF, Tsilingaridis G, Abbott PV, Fouad AF, Hicks L, Andreasen JO, Cehreli ZC, Harlamb S, Kahler B, Oginni A, Semper M, Levin L. International Association of Dental Traumatology guidelines for the management of traumatic dental injuries: 1. Fractures and luxations. Dent Traumatol. 2020;36(4):314–30.
5. Fouad AF, Abbott PV, Tsilingaridis G, Cohenca N, Lauridsen E, Bourguignon C, O'Connell A, Flores MT, Day PF, Hicks L, Andreasen JO, Cehreli ZC, Harlamb S, Kahler B, Oginni A, Semper M, Levin L. International Association of Dental Traumatology guidelines for the management of traumatic dental injuries: 2. Avulsion of permanent teeth. Dent Traumatol. 2020;36(4):331–42.
6. Day PF, Flores MT, O'Connell AC, Abbott PV, Tsilingaridis G, Fouad AF, Cohenca N, Lauridsen E, Bourguignon C, Hicks L, Andreasen JO, Cehreli ZC, Harlamb S, Kahler B, Oginni A, Semper M, Levin L. International Association of Dental Traumatology guidelines for the management of traumatic dental injuries: 3. Injuries in the primary dentition. Dent Traumatol. 2020;36(4):343–59.
7. Andreasen JO, Andreasen FM, Andersson L. Chapter 12. Examination and diagnosis of dental injuries. In: Textbook and color atlas of traumatic injuries to the teeth. 5th ed. Copenhagen: Munksgaard; 2011. p. 295–320.
8. de Souza GM, Fernandes IA, Galvão EL, Falci SGM. Checklist for the initial evaluation of oral and maxillofacial trauma. Dent Traumatol. 2021;37(3):400–6.
9. Myers GL. Evaluation and diagnosis of the traumatized dentition. Dent Traumatol. 2019;35(6):302–8.

10. Lam R. Epidemiology and outcomes of traumatic dental injuries: a review of the literature. Aust Dent J. 2016;61(Suppl 1):4–20.
11. Bastone EB, Freer TJ, McNamara JR. Epidemiology of dental trauma: a review of the literature. Aust Dent J. 2000;45:2–9.
12. Glendor U. Epidemiology of traumatic dental injuries–a 12 year review of the literature. Dent Traumatol. 2008;24:603–11.
13. Andreasen JO, Andreasen FM, Andersson L. Chapter 13. Crown fractures. In: Textbook and color atlas of traumatic injuries to the teeth. 5th ed. Copenhagen: Munksgaard; 2011. p. 327–47.
14. Güngör HC. Management of crown-related fractures in children: an update review. Dent Traumatol. 2014;30(2):88–99.
15. Sasaki H, Ogawa T, Kawaguchi M, Sobue S, Ooshima T. Multiple fractures of primary molars caused by injuries to the chin: report of two cases. Endod Dent Traumatol. 2000;16(1):43–6.
16. Ferraz JA, Pécora JD, Saquy PC, Sousa-Neto MD. Treatment of oblique crown fractures in maxillary premolars using adhesive tooth fragment reattachment: 19 years of follow up. Dent Traumatol. 2011;27(6):455–9.
17. Canoglu H, Cehreli ZC. Reattachment of a fractured permanent molar cusp: a 12-month follow-up. Dent Traumatol. 2007;23(1):42–6.
18. Andreasen FM, Kahler B. Diagnosis of acute dental trauma: the importance of standardized documentation: a review. Dent Traumatol. 2015;31(5):340–9.
19. Bakland LK, Andreasen JO. Dental traumatology: essential diagnosis and treatment planning. Endod Top. 2004;7(1):14–34.
20. Lim L, Sirichai P. Bone fractures: assessment and management. Aust Dent J. 2016;61(Suppl 1):74–81.
21. Kullman L, Al SM. Guidelines for dental radiography immediately after a dento-alveolar trauma, a systematic literature review. Dent Traumatol. 2012;28(3):193–9.
22. Lima TFR, Dos Santos SL, da Silva Fidalgo TK, Silva EJNL. Vitality tests for pulp diagnosis of traumatized teeth: a systematic review. J Endodont. 2019;45(5):490–9.
23. Gopikrishna V, Pradeep G, Venkateshbabu N. Assessment of pulp vitality: a review. Int J Paediatr Dent. 2009;19:3–15.
24. Klein H. Pulp responses to electric pulp stimulator in the developing permanent anterior dentition. J Dent Child. 1978;45:199–202.
25. Alghaithy RA, Qualtrough AJE. Pulp sensibility and vitality tests for diagnosing pulpal health in permanent teeth: a critical review. Int Endod J. 2017;50(2):135–42.
26. Bastos JV, Goulart EM, de Souza Côrtes MI. Pulpal response to sensibility tests after traumatic dental injuries in permanent teeth. Dent Traumatol. 2014;30(3):188–92.
27. Mainkar A, Kim SG. Diagnostic accuracy of 5 dental pulp tests: a systematic review and meta-analysis. J Endodont. 2018;44(5):694–702.
28. Olsburgh S, Jacoby T, Krejci I. Crown fractures in the permanent dentition: pulpal and restorative considerations. Dent Traumatol. 2002;18(3):103–15.
29. Bimstein E, Rotstein I. Cvek pulpotomy – revisited. Dent Traumatol. 2016;32(6):438–42.
30. Krastl G, Weiger R. Vital pulp therapy after trauma. ENDO. 2014;8:293–300.
31. Krastl G, Weiger R, Filippi A, Van Waes H, Ebeleseder K, Ree M, Connert T, Widbiller M, Tjäderhane L, Dummer PMH, Galler K. Endodontic management of traumatized permanent teeth: a comprehensive review. Int Endod J. 2021;54(8):1221–45.
32. Cox CF, Bergenholtz G, Fitzgerald M, Heys DR, Heys RJ, Avery JK, et al. Capping of the dental pulp mechanically exposed to the oral microflora—a 5 week observation of wound healing in the monkey. J Oral Pathol. 1982;11:327–39.
33. Fong CD, Davis MJ. Partial pulpotomy for immature permanent teeth, its present and future. Pediatr Dent. 2002;24:29–32.
34. The recommended guidelines of the American Association of endodontists for the treatment of traumatic dental injuries. 2013. https://www.aae.org/specialty/wp-content/uploads/sites/2/2019/02/19_TraumaGuidelines.pdf.

35. Fatima S, Rahman Z. Tooth fragment reattachment: interim or a permanent solution? The Traumaxilla. 2022;4(1–3):35–9.
36. Rappelli G, Massaccesi C, Putignano A. Clinical procedures for the immediate reattachment of a tooth fragment. Dent Traumatol. 2002;18(5):281–4.
37. Tewari N, Cehreli Z, Haldar P, Atif M, Alani A, Rahul M. The risk of bonded fragment loss in crown-fractured anterior teeth managed by fragment reattachment: a systematic review and meta-analysis. Evid Based Dent. 2024;25(3):167.
38. Garcia FC, Poubel DL, Almeida JC, Toledo IP, Poi WR, Guerra EN, Rezende LV. Tooth fragment reattachment techniques—a systematic review. Dent Traumatol. 2018;34(3):135–43.
39. Manuata J, Salat A. Layers: an atlas of composite resin stratification. Milan: Style Italiano; 2013.
40. Leven A. Layers: an atlas of composite resin stratification. Br Dent J. 2013;214:319.
41. Haupt F, Meyerdiercks C, Kanzow P, Wiegand A. Survival analysis of fragment reattachments and direct composite restorations in permanent teeth after dental traumatic injuries. Dent Traumatol. 2023;39:49–56.
42. Bissinger R, Müller DD, Reymus M, Khazaei Y, Hickel R, Bücher K, Kühnisch J. Treatment outcomes after uncomplicated and complicated crown fractures in permanent teeth. Clin Oral Investig. 2021;25(1):133–43.
43. Andreasen JO, Andreasen FM, Andersson L. Chapter 15. Root fractures. In: Textbook and color atlas of traumatic injuries to the teeth. 5th ed. Copenhagen: Munksgaard; 2011. p. 377–412.
44. Molina JR, Vann WF Jr, McIntyre JD, Trope M, Lee JY. Root fractures in children and adolescents: diagnostic considerations. Dent Traumatol. 2008;24(5):503–9.
45. Abbott PV. Diagnosis and management of transverse root fractures. Dent Traumatol. 2019;35(6):333–47.
46. Malhotra N, et al. A review of root fractures: diagnosis, treatment and prognosis. Dent Update. 2011;38(9):615–6, 619–20, 623–4 passim.
47. Özler CÖ, Cehreli ZC. Conservative management of a cervical horizontal root fracture by long-term stabilisation: a case report. Aust Endod J. 2022;48(2):338–41.
48. Andreasen JO, Ahrensburg SS, Tsilingaridis G. Root fractures: the influence of type of healing and location of fracture on tooth survival rates – an analysis of 492 cases. Dent Traumatol. 2012;28(5):404–9.
49. Khasnis SA, Kidiyoor KH, Patil AB, Kenganal SB. Vertical root fractures and their management. J Conserv Dent. 2014;17(2):103–10.
50. Salineiro FC, Kobayashi-Velasco S, Braga MM, Cavalcanti MG. Radiographic diagnosis of root fractures: a systematic review, meta-analyses and sources of heterogeneity. Dentomaxillofac Radiol. 2017;46(8):20170400.
51. Lindahl B. Transverse intra-alveolar root fractures: roentgen diagnosis and prognosis. Odont Revy. 1963;9:10–24.
52. Jacobsen I, Kerekes K. Diagnosis and treatment of pulp necrosis in permanent anterior teeth with root fracture. Scand J Dent Res. 1980;88:370–6.
53. Andreasen FM, Andreasen JO. Resorption and mineralization processes following root fracture of permanent incisors. Endod Dent Traumatol. 1988;4:202–14.
54. Andreasen FM, Andreasen JO, Bayer T. Prognosis of root-fractured permanent incisors–prediction of healing modalities. Endod Dent Traumatol. 1989;5:11–22.
55. Cvek M, Andreasen JO, Borum MK. Healing of 208 intra-alveolar root fractures in patients aged 7–17 years. Dent Traumatol. 2001;17:53–62.
56. Andreasen JO, Andreasen FM, Mejàre I, Cvek M. Healing of 400 intra-alveolar root fractures. 1. Effect of pre-injury and injury factors such as sex, age, stage of root development, fracture type, location of fracture and severity of dislocation. Dent Traumatol. 2004;20:192–202.
57. Andreasen JO, Andreasen FM, Mejàre I, Cvek M. Healing of 400 intra-alveolar fractures. 2. Effect of treatment factors, such as treatment delay, repositioning, splinting type and period and antibiotics. Dent Traumatol. 2004;20:203–11.

58. Andreasen JO, Andreasen FM, Andersson L. Chapter 14. Crown-root fractures. In: Textbook and color atlas of traumatic injuries to the teeth. 5th ed. Copenhagen: Munksgaard; 2011. p. 355–75.
59. May JJ, Cohenca N, Peters OA. Contemporary management of horizontal root fractures to the permanent dentition: diagnosis—radiologic assessment to include cone-beam computed tomography. Pediatr Dent. 2013;35(2):120–4.
60. Heithersay GS. Combined endodontic-orthodontic treatment of transverse root fractures in the region of the alveolar crest. Oral Surg Oral Med Oral Pathol. 1973;36:404–15.
61. Vignesh R, Sharmin D, Rekha CV, Annamalai S, Baghkomeh PN. Management of complicated crown-root fracture by extraoral fragment reattachment and intentional reimplantation with 2 years review. Contemp Clin Dent. 2019;10(2):397.
62. Zhen M, Wang C, Hu WJ, Zhang H, Li LS, Wei YP, Chung KH. Periodontal evaluation of crown-root fractured teeth following modified crown lengthening surgery. Br Dent J. 2017;222(1):21–5.
63. Andreasen JO, Andreasen FM, Andersson L. Chapter 36. Esthetics concerns in restoring the traumatised dentition: a biologic approach. In: Textbook and color atlas of traumatic injuries to the teeth. 5th ed. Copenhagen: Munksgaard; 2011. p. 912–32.
64. Khandelwal P, Srinivasan S, Arul B, Natanasabapathy V. Fragment reattachment after complicated crown-root fractures of anterior teeth: a systematic review. Dent Traumatol. 2021;37(1):37–52.
65. Naudi AB, Fung DE. Tooth fragment reattachment in multiple complicated permanent incisor crown-root fractures – a report of two cases. Dent Traumatol. 2008;24(2):248–52.
66. Reichardt E, Krug R, Bornstein MM, Tomasch J, Verna C, Krastl G. Orthodontic forced eruption of permanent anterior teeth with subgingival fractures: a systematic review. Int J Environ Res Public Health. 2021;18(23):12580.
67. Faria LP, Almeida MM, Amaral MF, Pellizzer EP, Okamoto R, Mendonça MR. Orthodontic extrusion as treatment option for crown-root fracture: literature review with systematic criteria. J Contemp Dent Pract. 2015;16(9):758–62.
68. Malmgren O, Malmgren B, Frykholm A. Rapid orthodontic extrusion of crown root and cervical root fractured teeth. Endod Dent Traumatol. 1991;7(2):49–54.
69. Elkhadem A, Mickan S, Richards D. Adverse events of surgical extrusion in treatment for crown–root and cervical root fractures: a systematic review of case series/reports. Dent Traumatol. 2014;30(1):1–4.
70. Das B, Muthu MS. Surgical extrusion as a treatment option for crown–root fracture in permanent anterior teeth: a systematic review. Dent Traumatol. 2013;29(6):423–31.
71. Çalişkan MK, Türkün M, Gomel M. Surgical extrusion of crown-root-fractured teeth: a clinical review. Int Endod J. 1999;32(2):146–51.
72. Fariniuk LF, Ferreira EL, Soresini GC, Cavali AE, Baratto FF. Intentional replantation with 180 degrees rotation of a crown-root fracture: a case report. Dent Traumatol. 2003;19(6):321–5.
73. Ganapathy S, Vedam V, Rajeev V, Nair SV. Intentional replantation with 180° rotation of a complicated crown-root fracture: a case report. Trauma Case Rep. 2020;27:100306.
74. Mokhtari S, Hajian S, Sanati I. Complicated crown-root fracture management using the 180-degree rotation method. Int J Clin Pediatr Dent. 2019;12(3):247–50.
75. Crowder L, Colloc T, Surendran S, McGregor S, Kilgariff J. Endodontic management of submerged roots following complicated traumatic dental injury (TDI) in children and adolescents: a systematic review. Int J Paediatr Dent. 2024;34(5):608–20.
76. Cordaro M, Staderini E, Torsello F, Grande NM, Turchi M, Cordaro M. Orthodontic extrusion vs. surgical extrusion to rehabilitate severely damaged teeth: a literature review. Int J Environ Res Public Health. 2021;18(18):9530.
77. Andreasen FM, Laurindsen E, Concussion AJO. Concussion and subluxation. In: Andreasen JO, Andreasen FM, Andersson L, editors. Textbook and color atlas of traumatic injuries to the teeth. 5th ed. Oxford: Wiley-Blackwell; 2018. p. 454.
78. Rock WP, Grundy MC. The effect of luxation and subluxation upon the prognosis of traumatized incisor teeth. J Dent. 1981;9:224–30.

79. Bastos JV, Goulart EM, de Souza Cortes MI. Pulpal response to sensibility tests after traumatic dental injuries in permanent teeth. Dent Traumatol. 2014;30:188–92.
80. Schendel KU, Schwartz O, Andreasen JO, Hoffmeister B. Reinnervation of autotransplanted teeth. A histological investigation in monkeys. Int J Oral Maxillofac Surg. 1990;19:247–9.
81. Fulling HJ, Andreasen JO. Influence of maturation status and tooth type of permanent teeth upon electrometric and thermal pulp testing. Scand J Dent Res. 1976;84:286–90.
82. Kvinnsland I, Heyeraas KJ, Byers MR. Effects of dental trauma on pulpal and periodontal nerve morphology. Proc Finn Dent Soc. 1992;88:125–32.
83. Lauridsen E, Hermann NV, Gerds TA, Ahrensburg SS, Kreiborg S, Andreasen JO. Combination injuries 1. The risk of pulp necrosis in permanent teeth with concussion injuries and concomitant crown fractures. Dent Traumatol. 2012;28(5):364–70.
84. Tewari N, Lauridsen E, Atif M, Srivastav S, Tsilingaridis G, Haldar P, Andersson L. Risk of pulp necrosis and related complications in the permanent anterior teeth with lateral luxation: a systematic review and meta-analysis. Dent Traumatol. 2024;40(5):482–98.
85. Humphrey JM, Kenny DJ, Barret EJ. Clinical outcomes for permanent incisor luxations in a pediatric population I intrusions. Dent Traumatol. 2003;19:266–73.
86. Elkhadem A, Mickan S, Richards D. Adverse events of surgical extrusion in treatment for crown-root and cervical root fractures: a systematic review of case series/reports. Dent Traumatol. 2014;30:1–14.
87. Sandler C, Al-Musfir T, Barry S, Duggal MS, Kindelan S, Kindelan J, Littlewood S, Nazzal H. Guidelines for the orthodontic management of the traumatised tooth. J Orthod. 2021;48(1):74–81.
88. Medeiros RB, Mucha JN. Immediate vs late orthodontic extrusion of traumatically intruded teeth. Dent Traumatol. 2009;25(4):380–5.
89. Caliskan MK, Turkun M, Gomel M. Surgical extrusion of crown-root-fractured teeth: a clinical review. Int Endod J. 1999;32:146–51.
90. Belevcikli M, Altan H, Altan A. Surgical extrusion of anterior teeth with intrusion traumatic injury: a report of two cases. Eur Endod J. 2020;5(3):295–9.
91. Zhang J, Qin M. Orthodontic extrusion treatment of intrusive maxillary incisors: two case reports with either incomplete or complete root formation. AJO-DO Clin Companion. 2022;2(5):439–48.
92. Calasans-Maia JA, Calasans-Maia MD, Matta ENR, Ruellas ACO. Orthodontic movement in traumatically intruded teeth: a case report. Dent Traumatol. 2003;19:292–5.
93. De Alencar AH, Lustosa-Pereira A, de Souza HA, Figueiredo JH. Intrusive luxation: a case report. Dent Traumatol. 2007;23:307–12.
94. Mamber EK. Treatment of intruded permanent incisors: a multidisciplinary approach. Endod Dent Traumatol. 1994;10:98–104.
95. Amaral MF, De Almeida MM, De Faria LP, Brandini DA, Poi WR, Okamoto R. Treatment of extrusive luxation in permanent teeth: literature review with systematic criteria. J Contemp Dent Pract. 2017;18(3):241–5.
96. Lago L, da Silva L, Fernandez-Formoso N, Rilo B. Extrusive luxation. Therapeutic procedure. Clin Case Reports. 2023;11(5):e7289.
97. Wang L, Jiang H, Bai Y, Luo Q, Wu H, Liu H. Clinical outcomes after intentional replantation of permanent teeth: a systematic review. Bosn J Basic Med Sci. 2020;20(1):13–20.
98. Asgary S, Alim Marvasti L, Kolahdouzan A. Indications and case series of intentional replantation of teeth. Iran Endod J. 2014;9(1):71–8.
99. Spinas E, Zangani A, Mallus T, Marogna G, Carboni L. Extrusive and lateral luxation injuries in permanent teeth: literature review and treatment complications update. Eur J Paediatr Dent. 2024;25(2):163–7.
100. Sharma A, Hegde AM. Use of tongue blade to reposition palatally luxated tooth due to trauma: a novel technique. Int J Clin Pediatr Dent. 2012;5:207–8.
101. Andreasen FM. Transient apical breakdown and its relation to color and sensibility changes after luxation injuries to teeth. Endod Dent Traumatol. 1986;2:9–19.

102. Cohenca N, Karni S, Rotstein I. Transient apical breakdown following tooth luxation. Dent Traumatol. 2003;19(5):289–91.
103. Andreasen FM. Prognosis of luxated permanent teeth the development of pulp necrosis. Endod Dent Traumatol. 1985;1:207–20.
104. Andreasen FM. Pulpal healing after luxation injuries and root fracture in the permanent dentition. Endod Dent Traumatol. 1989;5:111–31.
105. Clark D, Levin L. Prognosis and complications of mature teeth after lateral luxation: a systematic review. J Am Dent Assoc. 2019;150(8):649–55.
106. Kallel I, Lagha M, Moussaoui E, Douki N. Lateral luxation: is root resorption an unavoidable complication? Clin Case Rep. 2022;10(5):e05880.
107. Abbott PV. Prevention and management of external inflammatory resorption following trauma to teeth. Aust Dent J. 2016;61:82–94.
108. McTigue DJ. Managing traumatic injuries in the young permanent dentition. In: Pinkham JR, Casamassimo PS, Fields HW, McTigue DJ, Nowak A, editors. Pediatric dentistry: infancy through adolescence. 4th ed. St. Louis: Elsevier Saunders; 2005. p. 593–607.
109. Fouad AF, Abbott PV, Tsilingaridis G, Cohenca N, Lauridsen E, Bourguignon C, O'Connell A, Flores MT, Day PF, Hicks L, Andreasen JO. International Association of Dental Traumatology guidelines for the management of traumatic dental injuries: 2. Avulsion of permanent teeth. Dent Traumatol. 2020;36(4):331–42.
110. Adnan S, Lone MM, Khan FR, Hussain SM, Nagi SE. Which is the most recommended medium for the storage and transport of avulsed teeth? A systematic review. Dent Traumatol. 2018;34(2):59–70.
111. Zhang N, Cheng Y, Li F, Kang Q. Network meta-analysis of 10 storage mediums for preserving avulsed teeth. Front Med (Lausanne). 2021;8:749278.
112. De Brier N, Dorien O, Borra V, Singletary EM, Zideman DA, De Buck E, Bendall JC, Berry DC, Carlson JN, Cassan P, International Liaison Committee on Resuscitation First Aid Task Force. Storage of an avulsed tooth prior to replantation: a systematic review and meta-analysis. Dent Traumatol. 2020;36(5):453–76.
113. American Association of Endodontists. Recommended guidelines of the AAE for the treatment of traumatic dental injuries (revised 2013). American Association of Endodontists; 2013.
114. Fulling HJ, Andreasen JO. Influence of maturation status and tooth type of permanent teeth upon electrometric and thermal pulp testing. Eur J Oral Sci. 1976;84(5):286–90.
115. Hammarström L, Blomlöf L, Lindskog S. Dynamics of dentoalveolar ankylosis and associated root resorption. Endod Dent Traumatol. 1989;5(4):163–75.
116. Kenny KP, Day PF, Sharif MO, Parashos P, Lauridsen E, Feldens CA, Cohenca N, Skapetis T, Levin L, Kenny DJ, Djemal S. What are the important outcomes in traumatic dental injuries? An international approach to the development of a core outcome set. Dent Traumatol. 2018;34(1):4–11.
117. Galler KM, Grätz EM, Widbiller M, Buchalla W, Knüttel H. Pathophysiological mechanisms of root resorption after dental trauma: a systematic scoping review. BMC Oral Health. 2021;21(1):163.
118. Andreasen JO, Farik B, Munksgaard EC. Long-term calcium hydroxide as a root canal dressing may increase risk of root fracture. Dent Traumatol. 2002;18:134–7.
119. Rosenberg B, Murray PE, Namerow K. The effect of calcium hydroxide root filling on dentin fracture strength. Dent Traumatol. 2007;23:26–9.
120. Souza BD, Dutra KL, Kuntze MM, Bortoluzzi EA, Flores-Mir C, Reyes-Carmona J, Felippe WT, Porporatti AL, Canto GD. Incidence of root resorption after the replantation of avulsed teeth: a meta-analysis. J Endodont. 2018;44:1216–27.
121. Lauridsen E, Andreasen JO, Bouaziz O, Andersson L. Risk of ankylosis of 400 avulsed and replanted human teeth in relation to length of dry storage: a re-evaluation of a long-term clinical study. Dent Traumatol. 2020;36(2):108–16.
122. Patel S, Saberi N. The ins and outs of root resorption. Br Dent J. 2018;224(9):691–9.

Consequences and Management of Traumatic Dental Injuries in the Permanent Dentition

12

12.1 Introduction

Traumatic dental injuries (TDIs) to the permanent dentition pose a significant clinical challenge due to their complex biological consequences and long-term impact on oral health. While immediate management often focuses on repositioning and stabilizing injured teeth, the true success lies in anticipating and addressing the sequelae that manifest weeks, months, or even years after the injury. Complications such as pulp necrosis, root resorption, pulp canal obliteration, and ankylosis are not uncommon and may compromise the tooth's function, esthetics, and longevity. This chapter discusses the various healing complications associated with TDIs in permanent teeth, highlighting their clinical presentation, diagnostic challenges, and current best practices for management.

12.2 What Are the Healing Complications Anticipated at Follow-Up of Traumatic Dental Injuries?

12.2.1 Pulp Necrosis

The risk of developing pulp necrosis depends on the severity of injury, stage of root development, and presence of concomitant injuries. Pulp necrosis is seen as an early complication, and if untreated can lead to periapical lesions further progressing to inflammatory root resorption in mature permanent teeth [1–6]. This complication is most frequently encountered in *intrusive luxation followed by lateral and extrusive luxation.* It is also observed in long-standing untreated complicated crown fractures and uncomplicated crown fractures that are close to the pulp space in mature teeth. [3, 7] While it is least observed in teeth with concussion and subluxation injuries, the risk of necrosis increases with the presence of concomitant trauma.

H. Vyas et al., *Dental Caries and Traumatic Injuries in Pediatric Dentistry*,
https://doi.org/10.1007/978-3-031-98929-2_12

12.2.1.1 What Are the Signs and Symptoms of Pulp Necrosis in a Traumatized Tooth?

Pulp necrosis is seen due to severance of blood vessels at the apical foramen that results in seepage of blood into the extravascular pulp space and into the dentinal tubules. The color of the tooth changes from red to gray to black over a period. On a radiograph, periapical rarefaction observed as early as 2–3 weeks is significantly associated with pulp necrosis. Following a traumatic injury, the tooth may not always show a positive response, especially when there is pressure or severance of the neurovascular bundle at the apical foramen, as seen in luxation and avulsion injuries. While the immature tooth may take up to 3 months to reveal a positive response, a mature tooth may take up to a year. A diagnosis of pulp necrosis should be made only after corroborating patient history with clinical and radiographic signs [3–5].

12.2.1.2 When Should Endodontic Treatment Be Initiated?

Intrusion and severe lateral luxation injuries in mature teeth necessitate immediate endodontic treatment as they are associated with highest risk of root resorption, if the pulp is not extirpated. Other injuries in both mature and immature teeth must also be monitored for signs of pulp necrosis and/or root resorption. The diagnosis of pulp necrosis is never straightforward, especially in cases where there are no signs of irreversible pulpal and periapical changes. If the clinician suspects early root resorption on the radiograph, without the presence of other clinical signs and symptoms, a CBCT is advised to confirm the diagnosis. The first sign of root resorption should prompt the clinician to initiate endodontic treatment and place a medicament of intracanal calcium hydroxide, in both mature and immature teeth.

It is important to differentiate root resorption from Transient Apical Breakdown (TAB) which is seen as widening of the apical opening in cases of luxation injuries in mature teeth. A delay in endodontic treatment is advised for extrusive and mild lateral luxation with the objective to wait for TAB to resolve. TAB is seen as early as 2–3 weeks and may take from 3 months to a year to resolve. The tooth must be monitored on radiographs and endodontic treatment initiated if signs of progression are seen.

12.2.2 Root Resorption

12.2.2.1 What Are the Types of Root Resorption? (Fig. 12.1)

12.2.2.2 What Are the Factors That Cause Root Resorption?

For root resorption to occur, two important factors mentioned below must be present [8, 9]:

- *Breakdown of the natural barriers in the tissues.*

The external natural barriers are the periodontal ligament (PDL) and the cementum, while the internal natural barriers are the odontoblasts and predentin.

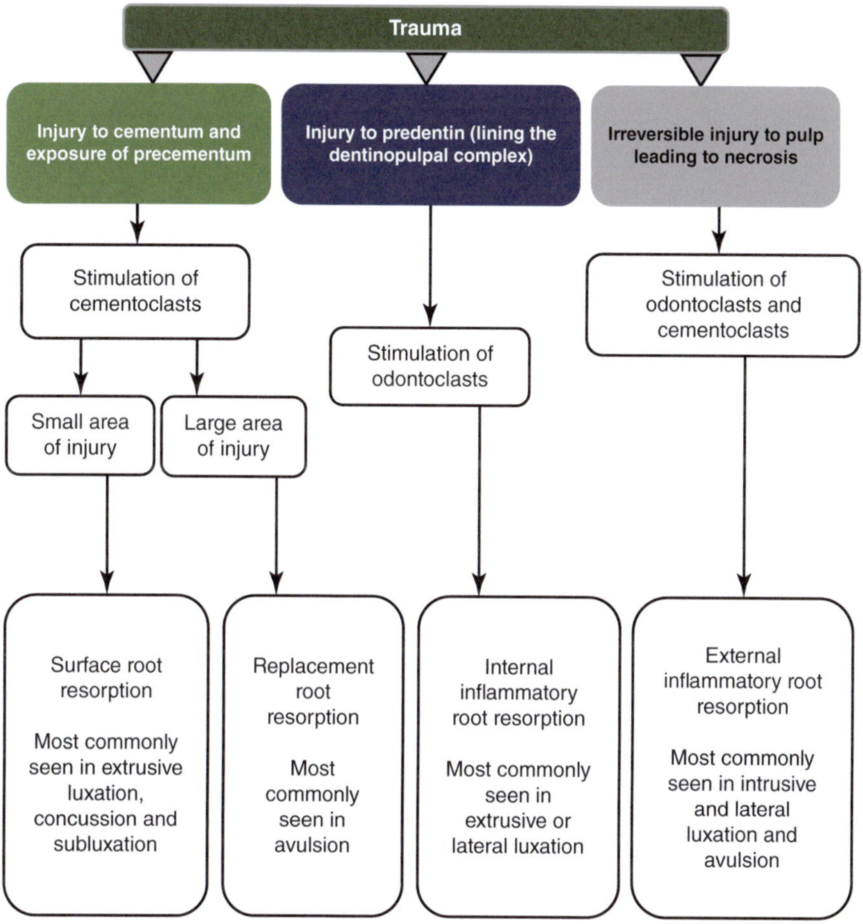

Fig. 12.1 Classification of root resorption

- *Continuous stimulating factor* for root resorption is the presence of bacteria leading to necrosis of pulp and PDL tissues. Thus, the management of root resorption post trauma is directed at controlling the above variables. Patients with a history of trauma require regular monitoring as resorption process begins 2 weeks post trauma and will be evident on a radiograph as early as 3 months.

Once pulp extirpation is done following intrusive luxation, avulsion or severe lateral luxation in mature teeth, they still need to be followed closely for signs of root resorption.

Immature teeth having similar injuries are expected to undergo spontaneous revascularization. However, resorption may still occur and if early signs go undetected, then the root resorption seen is aggressive in nature.

12.2.2.3 What Are the Types of Root Resorption?

- *Surface/Transient/Repair-Related Root Resorption* [10].

This type of resorption is seen in concussion, subluxation, and extrusive luxation. The process is self-limiting and seen as small areas of resorption of the cementum (*external surface resorption)* or dentin (*internal surface resorption*) [10]. Clinically, there are no signs or symptoms. Radiographically, resorption will not always be seen but at times may reveal blunting of the root apex [11]. Radiographs taken at different angulations may reveal crater-like defects along the root surface and this is more evident on a Cone Beam Computed Tomography (CBCT) scan [12]. There is no active intervention recommended in these cases, as it is seen to heal uneventfully in two to 3 weeks. Presence of even minor concomitant injury such as an enamel fracture significantly increases the risk of both pulpal necrosis and root resorption [3, 4].

- *Inflammatory Root Resorption (IRR).*

This is more commonly seen in mature teeth that incur intrusive and lateral luxation injuries. The incidence of this pattern of root resorption is also higher with respect to avulsion injuries associated with delayed replantation of teeth that were stored in a dry environment. The sole factor escalating the inflammatory resorption process is the necrosed and infected pulp and this underscores the need for pulp extirpation within 7–10 days of trauma.

The root resorption is initiated at a denuded area of the root surface (breach in cementum or predentin) and progresses due to pulp necrosis following severance of the blood supply. The necrosed pulp attracts resorbing cells such as macrophages and osteoclasts to the site leading to *progressive resorption* and destruction of the root. Types of Inflammatory Root Resorption (IRR) [13, 14].

1. External Inflammatory Root Resorption (EIRR).
2. Internal Inflammatory Root Resorption (IIRR).
3. Cervical Inflammatory Root Resorption (CIRR).

1. *External Inflammatory Root Resorption (EIRR).*

EIRR can occur either at the apex or along the root length (lateral inflammatory resorption), with the latter being the most common resorption pattern seen following trauma. Early stages of this resorption are asymptomatic whereas extensive root resorption may show mobility and pain on chewing. Some cases may present with a draining sinus, indicative of a chronic apical abscess. Increased mobility may indicate attachment loss or pathological root fracture. On a radiograph, early EIRR is characterized by a ragged appearance of the external root surface with loss of lamina dura. At the apical region, resorption leads to blunting of the apex and radiolucency extending to the surrounding bone [15–17]. (Figs. 12.2 and 12.3).

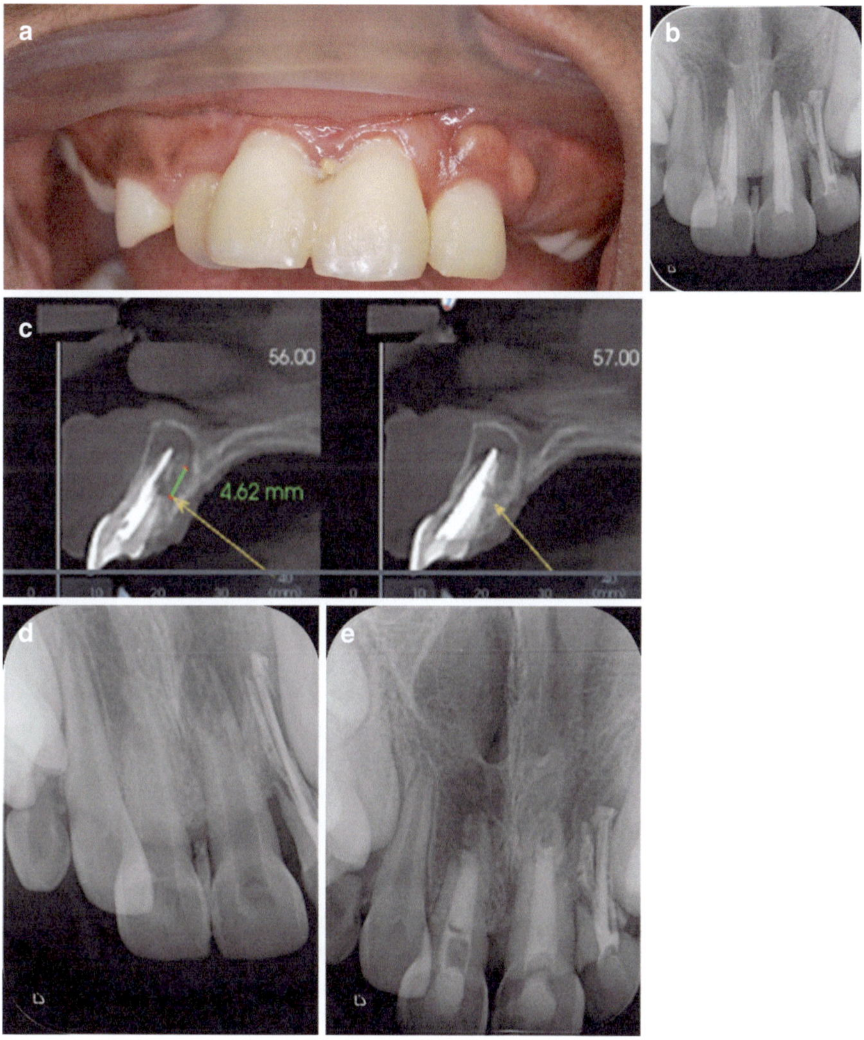

Fig. 12.2 Patient reported 1 year after avulsion of maxillary permanent central incisors and left lateral incisor. The teeth were replanted, splinted, and treated for root canal at the time of trauma at another center. The extraoral time before replantation was more than 60 min. Lateral incisor showed Grade III mobility and a dentoalveolar abscess (**a**). Severe external inflammatory resorption was seen with the replanted teeth on the radiograph (**b**). Sagittal section of the maxillary central incisor showed the extent of resorption (**c**). The obturating material was removed from the central incisors and the canals debrided and irrigated (**d**). Calcium Hydroxide was placed as a medicament. Gutta-percha was removed from the lateral incisor and the tooth was extracted (**e**)

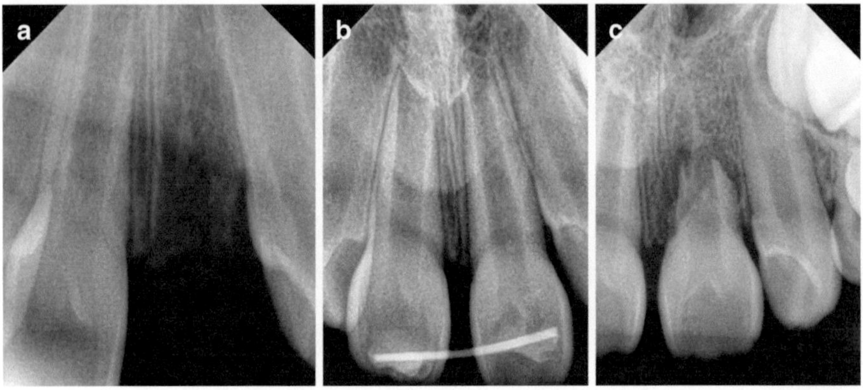

Fig. 12.3 Avulsion injury with maxillary permanent left central incisor (**a**). Tooth was replanted and splinted for 2 weeks (**b**). As apex was immature, the tooth was monitored for spontaneous revascularization. Patient did not report for follow-up till 15 months. Radiograph showed inflammatory resorption at the 15-month follow-up (**c**)

2. *Internal Inflammatory Root Resorption (IIRR).*

IIRR occurs within a section of the pulp or root canal space resulting in loss of dentin. The resorption begins at the root canal wall and progresses towards the cementum. Early stages of this resorption reveal no clinical signs or symptoms. Resorption is seen clinically only if it progresses towards the coronal 1/3rd, appearing as a pinkish discoloration due to the highly vascularized connective tissue. As the pulp becomes necrotic, the color turns gray. Radiographically, a characteristic oval-shaped increase in the size of the pulp chamber or the root canal is seen. It is important to differentiate between internal and external inflammatory root resorption. At times, resorption on the labial or lingual external root surface may superimpose on the canal and falsely appear as internal root resorption. Therefore, it is advisable to take radiographs from different mesial or distal angulations. Alternately, the sagittal slice of a CBCT scan will accurately identify the resorptive defect [18–20].

12.2.2.4 How Is External and Internal Inflammatory Root Resorption Managed? [21–25]

In both immature and mature teeth, Calcium Hydroxide (CH) intracanal dressings (pH 12.5) placed for at least 6 months can result in an arrest of the resorptive process and promote healing of periodontal lesions. While the initial management is the same, the definitive management and prognosis of each differs.

12.2.2.5 External Inflammatory Root Resorption

For Mature Teeth

- Administer local anesthesia, apply a rubber dam, and initiate access opening.
- The pulp chamber and canal must be irrigated with copious amounts of 1.5% sodium hypochlorite.
- Ultrasonic activation of sodium hypochlorite is advised.
- In mature teeth, instrumentation can be performed as per regular protocols taking care to direct the file away from the resorption site.
- The canal should then be irrigated with saline solution, dried with paper points, and medicated with Calcium Hydroxide paste.
- The duration of intracanal medicament varies from 4 weeks to several months, depending on the severity of resorption and healing seen at follow-ups.
- The tooth in question must be monitored every 3 weeks and the dressing replaced every 3 months until resorptive lesions disappear and the outline of the PDL space is reestablished.
- Once this is achieved, the root canal space can be obturated with gutta-percha and bioceramic sealer (Endosequence BC, Brassler® USA; Bio-C® Sealer Ion⁺, Angelus®, Brazil; CeraSeal™, Meta Biomed, South Korea) or obturated completely with MTA.

For Immature Teeth

- In immature teeth, the same protocol as above is followed.
- Instrumentation is minimal keeping in mind the thin radicular dentin, and must be kept short of the apex.
- Calcium Hydroxide is placed as an intracanal medicament from 4 weeks to several months.
- Once the EIRR is seen to resolve, further treatment is needed for root end formation either by MTA apexification or Regenerative Endodontic Procedures.

12.2.2.6 For Internal Inflammatory Root Resorption [26, 27]

- Administer local anesthesia and apply a rubber dam before initiating access opening.
- The pulp chamber and canal must be irrigated with copious amounts of 1.5% sodium hypochlorite.
- The resorptive defect is inaccessible to mechanical instrumentation, therefore greater emphasis must be placed on the chemical dissolution of pulp tissue with sodium hypochlorite.
- Ultrasonic activation of sodium hypochlorite is recommended.
- The canal should then be irrigated with saline solution, dried with paper points, and medicated with a paste of calcium hydroxide.
- The permanent root canal filling needs to be flowable to seal the resorptive defect and hence, thermoplastic gutta-percha techniques are recommended.

- When the root wall has been perforated by the internal resorption process, a calcium silicate cement should be used to seal the perforation.
- In case of immature teeth, the apical third and resorption lacunae are both filled with Calcium Silicate Cement.

12.2.2.7 When Is Surgical Endodontics Recommended for IRR?

A surgical approach is recommended in cases, where the defect has breached the periodontium and bone thereby communicating with the oral cavity. This is evidently seen on sagittal slices or the 3D construction image on a CBCT. Raising the flap will expose the defect and allow direct access to perform mechanical cleaning.

12.2.2.8 Technique

- Following local anesthesia, endodontic treatment is completed after which a mucoperiosteal flap is raised.
- The exposed defect is curetted and the intraradicular dentin cavity is prepared under a dental operating microscope. The area is cleaned and dried.
- The defect is filled with calcium silicate cement and the flap is repositioned and sutured.
- Alternately, the entire canal can be filled with MTA to ensure the seal of the resorption area [28, 29].

3. *Cervical Inflammatory Root Resorption or External Invasive Resorption (CIRR).*

This form of resorption occurs after injury to an area on the cervical root surface (cementum) below the gingival sulcus. The damaged root surface is colonized by resorbing cells. Most often, the resorption is transient and cemental repair will occur within 2–3 weeks without treatment. If the process continues, the resorbing cells will burrow into the dentin. Due to the defensive abilities of the predentin, at first the resorptive process will not penetrate the pulp but spread vertically around the root canal in an irregular fashion. With time, the resorptive process usually will penetrate the root canal space [30].

12.2.2.9 Clinical and Radiographic Features

Cervical resorption can be diagnosed clinically only after the resorptive process reaches the supragingival area of the crown. It is seen as a pinkish hue, when the vascularized granulation tissue becomes visible through the enamel. Radiographically, this defect is usually an irregular radiolucency that starts cervically and spreads along the external surface of the roots. As the defect becomes larger, it may appear to surround the pulp leaving the root canal walls intact. In the more advanced stages, the invading tissue creates a communication between the pulp and the periodontium along the length of the canal [31, 32].

12.2.2.10 How Is Cervical Root Resorption Managed?

The management depends on whether the cervical root resorptive lesion has perforated the pulp canal space.

Resorptive defects that have not penetrated the root canal space can be treated by periodontal flap reflection alone. There are differing views on the necessity of performing endodontic treatment to remove the bacteria and halt the progress of the infection [33–35].

- If endodontic treatment is being performed, it should be initiated at the first appointment.
- Local anesthesia is administered, a rubber dam placed, and an access opening done.
- After working length determination, mechanical instrumentation is performed as per regular protocol.
- During the cleaning and shaping process, the clinician is likely to encounter profuse bleeding, possibly from the perforated area.
- Thus, complete biomechanical preparation and obturation may not be possible at the first visit.
- Canal patency must be maintained with either a calcium hydroxide medicament or a gutta-percha cone and the access cavity is sealed.
- At the second appointment, after local anesthesia administration, a full-thickness flap should be raised to allow maximum visualization and access to the resorbed site.
- The area should be thoroughly curetted until no bleeding is present and the cavity walls are sound. This will ensure that the vascular supply is not maintained, and remaining resorptive cell front is removed and there is less likelihood of recurrence.
- The resorbed cavity may be conditioned with 90% trichloroacetic acid. Lavage with sodium hypochlorite and scrubbing with Ethylenediaminetetraacetic Acid has also been advocated [36].
- An intracanal medicament is given and temporary restorative material is placed in the resorptive cavity.
- The site is reopened 10–14 days later. Further curettage is performed, if necessary, endodontic treatment completed and resorption cavity sealed with Calcium Silicate material [37].

Orthodontic extrusion is also recommended in certain cases to access the resorbed site. If the lesion is perforating the canal, the resorptive defect is generally accessed through the root canal space.

- *Replacement Root Resorption (RRR)*

Ankylosis represents a fusion of cementum to the bone and is generally seen to occur 6 months following trauma. It can be progressive or transient depending on the extent of damage to the periodontal ligament. Progressive is when the tooth is gradually resorbed and replaced by bone; while transient ankylosis shows a minor part of the root surface in contact with the bone; but later the process reverses and the PDL space is eventually reestablished such that the ankylosis disappears. It is the most common unfavorable outcome after delayed reimplantation of an avulsed tooth and in teeth that have incurred severe intrusion [38, 39].

12.2.2.11 How Is Replacement Resorption Diagnosed and Managed?

The degree of development of crestal bone is associated with the process of tooth eruption and growth of the patient. Ankylosis due to replacement resorption prevents vertical growth of the crestal bone involving the traumatized tooth, especially in a growing child.

The first clinical sign of replacement resorption is a high metallic sound on percussion followed by a decrease in tooth mobility. Over time, the replacement resorption results in infraocclusion causing tilting of the adjacent teeth over the ankylosed tooth. Ankylosis is visible on conventional X-ray images when 20% of the root area is affected. It manifests as partial or total obliteration of the periodontal ligament space [40] (Fig. 12.4).

A CBCT must be considered as it shows a higher number of foci of replacement resorption at earlier stages which conventional X-ray images fail to reveal [41].

Progressive ankylosis is an irreversible process and cannot be controlled with traditional endodontic treatment. However, the consequences of ankylosis can be reduced in children and adolescents with timely intervention by performing procedures like decoronation and autotransplantation.

12.2.2.12 Decoronation

Decoronation is the treatment of choice for teeth that are undergoing replacement resorption in growing children. It maintains the existing bone volume and preserves the vertical bone growth. At times, replacement resorption can cause transient ankylosis that reverses within 8 weeks to a year to reestablish a normal PDL space. Therefore, the clinician is advised to wait till a definitive diagnosis of progressive ankylosis is made before initiating treatment [42].

While it is impossible to stop replacement resorption, decoronation halts progressive infraocclusion and helps to restore vertical bone growth. Extraction of the ankylosed tooth followed by prosthetic replacement is not recommended, as it can damage the buccal plate causing loss of attached bone and poor development of bucco-palatal arch width.

12.2.2.13 Rationale and Timing [42–45]

The rate at which the replacement resorption process occurs, varies based on the age.

If it occurs in a young patient (8–16 years), the tooth will resorb and be replaced by bone in 3–7 years. In older patients (17 years and above), the tooth will be retained much longer.

Thus, decoronation must be planned as follows:

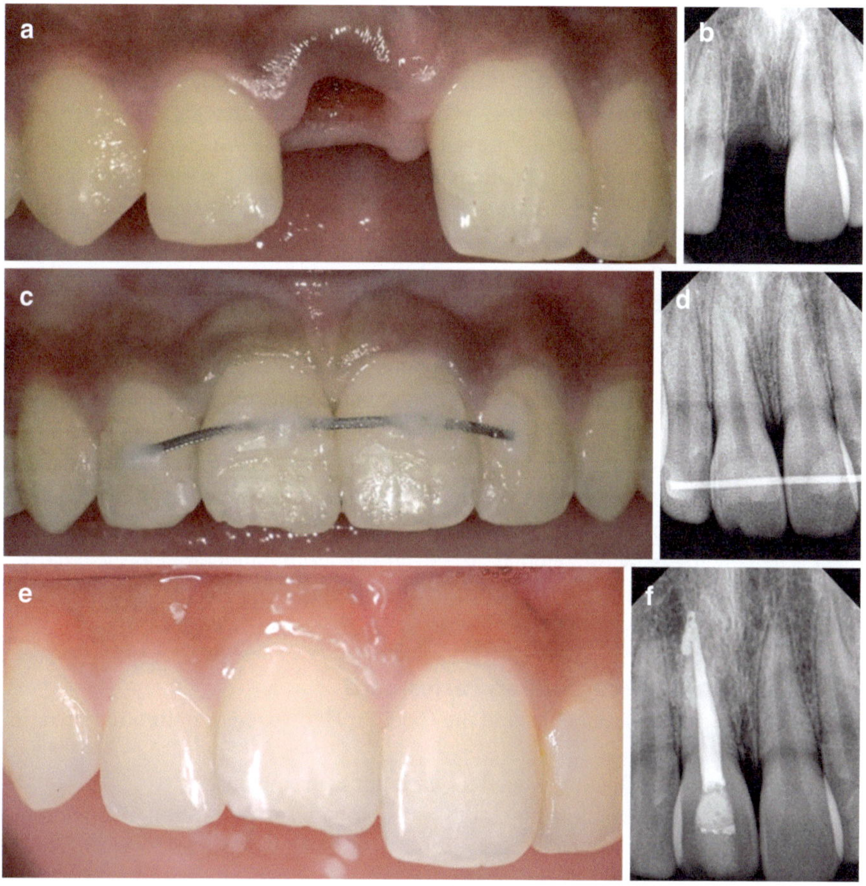

Fig. 12.4 A 10-year-old child reported with avulsion of maxillary permanent right central incisor within 1 h of trauma (**a**). Diagnostic radiograph taken to rule out injury to adjacent teeth and bone (**b**). Tooth replanted and stabilized with a resin composite and wire splint (**c**). Radiograph taken after splinting. Endodontic treatment initiated within 10 days of trauma (**d**). The tooth at 1-year follow-up appeared in infraocclusion (**e**). Radiograph shows Replacement Root Resorption (**f**)

1. *In the early mixed dentition (7–10 years)*

Replacement root resorption is seen to occur slowly, as this is the period prior to the growth spurt. Decoronation should be performed within 2 years of the diagnosis or before the growth spurt begins.

2. *In the late mixed dentition (10–12 years)*

The rate of replacement resorption will be accelerated, as this period coincides with the growth spurt. Decoronation should be performed as soon as progressive ankylosis is confirmed.

3. *In the permanent dentition (more than 12 years)*

The process of resorption and infraocclusion slows down. If untreated by this age, there is significant infraocclusion and bone deformation seen. Decoronation must still be performed as it will prevent further bone deformation even though it may not increase the bone height and volume. If replacement resorption occurs after growth spurt, the tooth can be kept under observation and decoronated when infraposition is between 1/4th to less than 1/2 the length of the adjacent tooth.

12.2.2.14 How Does Decoronation Help in Maintaining the Bone Height and Width?

The marginal gingival and periodontal fibers formed during eruption of teeth play an important role in the development of the alveolar ridge. When a tooth becomes ankylosed, the periodontal fibers are partly or totally replaced by bone in the ankylosed area, and tooth eruption is arrested. These fibers are also linked to the adjacent teeth causing them to tip as they continue to erupt. As the root is submerged after decoronation, new periosteum and gingival fibers are formed on top of the alveolar crest. The new fibers facilitate bone growth and undergo remodeling as the adjacent teeth continue to erupt. This maintains the height and width of the alveolus at the decoronation site [46–49].

12.2.2.15 How Is Decoronation Performed?

- The access cavity is reopened and the Calcium Hydroxide or obturating material is removed.
- The canal is cleaned and irrigated to wash out the remnants.
- After raising a gingival flap, the tooth is decoronated at the level of alveolar bone and the root is then further submerged 1.5–2 mm below the alveolar crest. This is done with water-cooled diamond bur taking care not to damage the alveolar bone.
- This also allows for new periosteal and gingival fibers to be formed.
- The resultant bleeding must be allowed to fill the root canal space as this will act as foci to facilitate replacement resorption.
- The gingival flap is sutured to cover the remaining root.
- The decoronated tooth will be replaced by bone over a period of 1–10 years.
- An esthetic prosthesis must be planned based on patient's age and treatment needs.

12.2.2.16 What Are the Options for Replacing the Coronal Tooth Space Following Avulsion or Decoronation?

In a young growing patient, if the avulsed tooth is not reimplanted, then the following treatment options can be considered [46–49].

Clinical Scenario 1: The Patient Is Between 6 and 8 Years of Age and the Premolars Have Completed Only ¼ Root Development

In such patients, a removable partial denture is the easiest and most common prosthetic replacement given. Alternatively, a maxillary expansion plate may be given with a pontic attached that will act as an interim prosthesis and facilitate maxillary expansion. A lingual wire soldered to the molar bands with an artificial tooth as a pontic can be given.

If no interceptive orthodontic treatment is required, a Maryland bridge with a tooth, natural (same as the decoronated tooth) or artificial, is attached to the adjacent tooth on each side from the palatal surface with resin composite.

Parents must be informed that the above options fulfill only the esthetic needs and prevent space loss in the growing child. They do not allow for alveolar bone growth and development and have questionable retention.

Clinical Scenario 2: The Patient Is 8–12 Years of Age and the Premolars Have Completed Only ½ to 2/3rd Root Development

Once the child reaches the mixed dentition phase, the premolars must be monitored for root development. The 9–12-year window is ideal for autotransplantation, particularly in a crowded dentition with Class II malocclusion; wherein orthodontic treatment would necessitate the extraction of a premolar. The tooth is transplanted directly to the extraction site. If the procedure is timed correctly, then it allows alveolar bone growth and development.

Clinical Scenario 3: The Avulsed Tooth Is Reimplanted and Shows Signs of Progressive Ankylosis and Infraocclusion After Growth Spurt

Post decoronation, if the patient is below 18 years of age, the tooth can be prosthetically rehabilitated with a removable partial denture or a Maryland bridge.

An implant can be placed after the patient turns 18 years, even before the resorbing tooth is completely replaced by bone. If an implant is placed immediately after decoronation, the bone will continue to remodel. Resorption of the tooth and its replacement with bone will continue for several years before completely integrating with the implant.

The cavity space for an implant can be prepared and the implant placed with the same angulation and alignment as it would be placed in an ideal situation [50, 51]. One of the advantages of the decoronation followed by dental implant placement in teeth with ankylosis and replacement resorption is the maintenance of the bone volume in the region, both vertical and horizontal.

12.2.2.17 Should Decoronation Be Performed Before or After Orthodontic Treatment?

Orthodontic treatment may be needed for the entire dentition due to preexisting malocclusion or to manage the ensuing malalignment following progressive ankylosis. Therefore, decoronation can be performed before or after orthodontic treatment depending on the growth of the child, extent of replacement resorption, and severity of malocclusion. If orthodontic treatment is initiated before decoronation, the ankylosed tooth should be left off the archwire or can be utilized for anchorage. If decoronation is done during orthodontic treatment, an interim prosthesis can be made with a pontic attached to the archwire with a bracket [52, 53].

12.2.2.18 Autotransplantation

Autotransplantation refers to "transplantation of an unerupted or erupted tooth in the same individual, from one site to another extraction site or a new surgically prepared socket". Like decoronation, this procedure too facilitates the growth of alveolar bone and additionally, ensures regeneration of normal periodontal ligament (PDL) that is needed for proprioception and orthodontic movement. It is recommended in patients having an ankylosed tooth and a crowded dentition with Class II malocclusion, wherein orthodontic treatment would necessitate the extraction of a premolar. The treatment plan must be formulated with the help of a multidisciplinary team comprising of a pediatric dentist, oral surgeon, and orthodontist [54].

12.2.2.19 Selection of Donor Teeth [54–56]

The best results are obtained when root development of the donor tooth is one-half to two-thirds of the total root length. Transplantation of donor tooth bud with roots formed less than one-half may be too traumatic and could compromise further root development. If a tooth with a complete root formation is transplanted, it will generally require root canal therapy performed 2 weeks after transplantation. Prior to the surgery, a CBCT of the donor tooth is taken. This will aid in surgical simulation and development of 3D printed donor teeth replicas and surgical stents prior to the procedure. The replicas allow clinicians to evaluate the adequacy of the prepared socket before carrying out the actual transplant. Surgical stents allow for accurate preparation of the socket and positioning of donor teeth at the recipient site. This minimizes trauma and extra-alveolar time of the donor teeth.

- The recipient socket prepared must be larger than the dimensions of the donor tooth root to prevent forceful or multiple attempts to insert it into the socket, as this will compromise PDL healing.
- The 3D tooth replica should be used to ensure the preparation of the surgical site is adequate.
- The donor tooth is extracted and transplanted to the surgical site.
- A radiograph is taken to verify the position.
- A resin composite splint is placed for 4 weeks to ensure healing of the periodontal ligament.
- The donor tooth should be restored to match the morphology and esthetics of the adjacent teeth, once the splint is removed.
- Orthodontic treatment should be deferred until 6 months post-transplant.
- In case of any signs of pulpal necrosis and non-vitality of the donor tooth, MTA apexification or regenerative endodontics may need to be performed.

12.2.3 Pulp Canal Obliteration

Most commonly related to lateral luxation injuries or injuries that disrupt the neurovascular supply to the tooth. It is also seen in injuries sustained by immature permanent teeth and rarely seen in injuries where there is no dislocation of the tooth [57].

12.2.3.1 Clinical and Radiographic Signs

There is accelerated deposition of dentin within the root canal space causing the crown to appear yellow and less life like. The response to pulp sensibility test is low or absent. Radiographically, there is reduction in size of the pulp chamber compared to adjacent teeth that have not incurred trauma. There is gradual reduction in the root canal space leading to partial or total obliteration of the root canal. It appears 3–12 months after injury. Pulp canal obliteration may develop secondary pulp necrosis and periapical changes. Teeth undergoing rapid canal obliteration (within 2 years of trauma) were seen to be associated with pulp necrosis (Figs. 12.5 and 12.6).

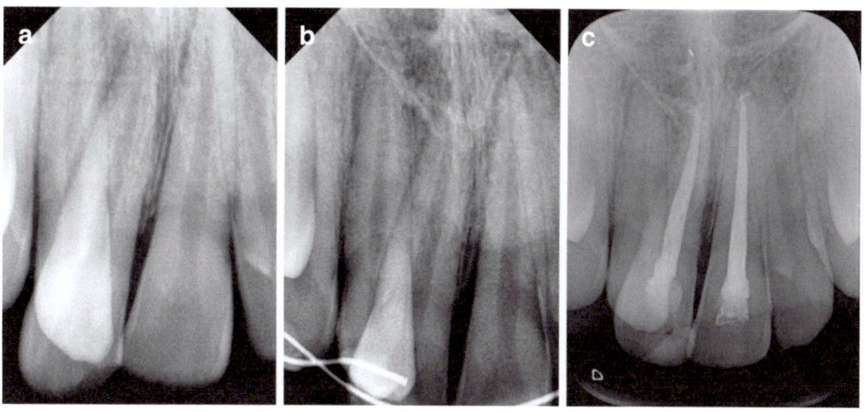

Fig. 12.5 Avulsion injury with maxillary permanent right central incisor and lateral luxation with left central incisor and right lateral incisor (**a**). The teeth were repositioned and splinted for 2 weeks (**b**). Root canal treatment completed in both central incisors, while the right lateral incisor was monitored clinically and on radiographic follow-up. At the 1-year follow-up, the lateral incisor showed delayed response to sensibility testing and pulp canal obliteration was observed on the radiograph (**c**)

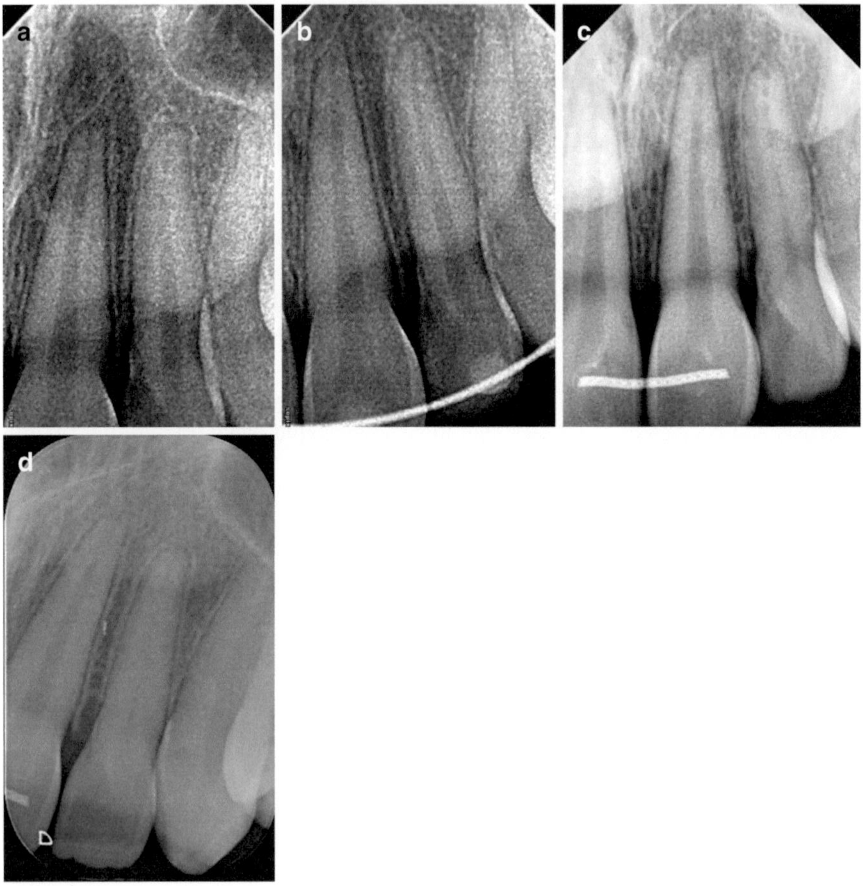

Fig. 12.6 Lateral luxation injury with maxillary permanent left lateral incisor (**a**). The tooth was repositioned and splinted for 4 weeks (**b**). At the 1-year follow-up, the child had a retainer on the central incisors after frenectomy. Clinical and radiographic examination showed no abnormality (**c**). At 2-year follow-up, the left central incisor showed a delayed response to pulp sensibility test and pulp canal obliteration was noted on the radiograph (**d**)

12.2.3.2 Management

Pulp canal obliteration is not considered as an unfavorable outcome and management depends on the clinical and radiographic findings. If the findings are limited to only coronal discoloration, cosmetic intervention is suggested with or without prophylactic endodontic intervention. In case of secondary periapical changes, endodontic treatment under a microscope may be required [58, 59].

12.3 Concluding Remarks

Traumatic Dental Injuries (TDIs) in permanent teeth present complications such as pulp necrosis, root resorption, and pulp canal obliteration. Early identification and intervention are crucial to preserving tooth function, esthetics, and improving survival. Pulp necrosis is a common complication following luxation injuries and untreated fractures, requiring careful monitoring and timely endodontic intervention. The different types of root resorption have a distinct pathophysiology and while initial management is palliative or symptomatic, the definitive management differs. The definitive treatment for inflammatory root resorption depends on the type and extent of resorption and stage of root development. Whereas, management of ankylosis is governed by the age and growth of the patient. Pulp canal obliteration is not always considered an unfavorable outcome. Management of complications of TDI is multidisciplinary, emphasizing timely intervention based on growth phases and radiographic findings.

References

1. Andreasen FM, Vestergaard PB. Prognosis of luxated permanent teeth—the development of pulp necrosis. Endod Dent Traumatol. 1985;1:207–20.
2. Oikarinen K, Gundlach KKH, Pfeifer G. Late complications of luxation injuries to teeth. Endod Dent Traumatol. 1987;3:296–303.
3. Lauridsen E, Hermann NV, Gerds TA, Ahrensburg SS, Kreiborg S, Andreasen JO. Combination injuries 1. The risk of pulp necrosis in permanent teeth with concussion injuries and concomitant crown fractures. Dent Traumatol. 2012;28:364–70.
4. Lauridsen E, Hermann NV, Gerds TA, Ahrensburg SS, Kreiborg S, Andreasen JO. Combination injuries 2. The risk of pulp necrosis in permanent teeth with subluxation injuries and concomitant crown fractures. Dent Traumatol. 2012;28:371–8.
5. Lauridsen E, Hermann NV, Gerds TA, Ahrensburg SS, Kreiborg S, Andreasen JO. Combination injuries 3. The risk of pulp necrosis in permanent teeth with extrusion or lateral luxation and concomitant crown fractures without pulp exposure. Dent Traumatol. 2012;28:379–85.
6. Hermann NV, Lauridsen E, Ahrensburg SS, Gerds TA, Andreasen JO. Periodontal healing complications following extrusive and laterial luxation in the permanent dentition: a longitudinal cohort study. Dent Traumatol. 2012;28:394–403.
7. Andreasen FM. Pulpal healing after luxation injuries and root fracture in the permanent dentition. Endod Dent Traumatol. 1989;5:111–31.
8. Tronstad L. Root resorption—etiology, terminology and clinical manifestations. Dent Traumatol. 1988 Dec;4(6):241–52.
9. Al-Badri S, Kinirons M, Cole B, Welbury R. Factors affecting resorption in traumatically intruded permanent incisors in children. Dent Traumatol. 2002 Apr;18(2):73–6.
10. Fuss Z, Tsesis I, Lin S. Root resorption – diagnosis, classification and treatment choices based on stimulation factors. Dent Traumatol. 2003;19(4):175–82.
11. Laux M, Abbott PV, Pajarola G, Nair PN. Apical inflammatory root resorption: a correlative radiographic and histological assessment. Int Endod J. 2000;33:483–93.
12. Estrela C, Bueno MR, de Alencar AHG, et al. Method to evaluate inflammatory root resorption by using cone beam computed tomography. J Endodont. 2009;35(11):1491–7.
13. Patel S, Durack C, Ricucci D. Chapter 20, root resorption. In: Hargreaves KM, Berman LH, editors. Cohen's pathways of the pulp. 11th ed. St Louis: Elsevier; 2016a. p. 660–83.

14. Heboyan A, Avetisyan A, Karobari MI, Marya A, Khurshid Z, Rokaya D, Zafar MS, Fernandes GV. Tooth root resorption: a review. Sci Prog. 2022 Jul;105(3):00368504221109217.
15. Wedenberg C, Zetterqvist L. Internal resorption in human teeth—a histological, scanning electron microscopic, and enzyme histochemical study. J Endodont. 1987;13:255–9.
16. Ahangari Z, Nasser M, Mahdian M, Fedorowicz Z, Marchesan MA. Interventions for the management of external root resorption. Cochrane Database Syst Rev. 2015;11:CD008003.
17. Abbott PV. Prevention and management of external inflammatory resorption following trauma to teeth. Aust Dent J. 2016 Mar;61:82–94.
18. Haapasalo M, Endal U. Internal inflammatory root resorption: the unknown resorption of the tooth. Endod Top. 2006;14:60–79.
19. Patel S, Kanagasingam S, Pitt Ford T. External cervical resorption: a review. J Endodont. 2009a;35:616–25.
20. Gartner AH, Mack T, Somerlott RG, Walsh LC. Differential diagnosis of internal and external root resorption. J Endodont. 1976;2:329–34.
21. Estrela C, Sydney GB, Bammann LL, Felippe JO. Mechanism of action of calcium and hydroxyl ions of calcium hydroxide on tissue and bacteria. Braz Dent J. 1995;6:85–90.
22. Carrotte P. Endodontics: Part 9. Calcium hydroxide, root resorption, endo-perio lesions. Br Dent J. 2004;197:735–43.
23. Cai C, Chen X, Li Y, Jiang Q. Advances in the role of sodium hypochlorite irrigant in chemical preparation of root canal treatment. Biomed Res Int. 2023;2023:8858283.
24. Zare Jahromi M, Kalantar Motamedi MR. Effect of calcium hydroxide on inflammatory root resorption and ankylosis in replanted teeth compared with other intracanal materials: a review. Restor Dent Endod. 2019;44(3):e32.
25. Mohammadi Z, Dummer PM. Properties and applications of calcium hydroxide in endodontics and dental traumatology. Int Endod J. 2011;44:697–730.
26. Nilsson E, Bonte E, Bayet F, Lasfargues JJ. Management of internal root resorption on permanent teeth. Int J Dent. 2013;2013:929486.
27. Main C, Mirzayan N, Shabahang S, Torabinejad M. Repair of root perforations using mineral trioxide aggregate: a long-term study. J Endodont. 2004;30(2):80–3.
28. Fernandes M, de Ataide I, Wagle R. Tooth resorption part I-pathogenesis and case series of internal resorption. J Conserv Dent. 2013;16(1):4–8.
29. Hsien HC, Cheng YA, Lee YL, Lan WH, Lin CP. Repair of perforating internal resorption with mineral trioxide aggregate: a case report. J Endod. 29(8):538–9.
30. Chen Y, Huang Y, Deng X. External cervical resorption—a review of pathogenesis and potential predisposing factors. Int J Oral Sci. 2021 Dec;13(1):19.
31. Heithersay GS. Clinical, radiologic, and histopathologic features of invasive cervical resorption. Quintessence Int. 1999;30:27–37.
32. Mavridou AM, et al. Understanding external cervical resorption in vital teeth. J Endodont. 2016;42:1737–51.
33. Patel J, Beddis HP. How to assess and manage external cervical resorption. Br Dent J. 2019;227:695–701.
34. Gulsahi A. Clinical and radiologic appearances of invasive cervical resorption. J Oral Health Dent Manag. 2014;13:934–9.
35. Frank AL, Torabinejad M. Diagnosis and treatment of extracanal invasive resorption. J Endodont. 1998;24:500–4.
36. Heithersay GS. Treatment of invasive cervical resorption: an analysis of results using topical application of trichloroacetic acid, curettage, and restoration. Quintessence Int. 1999;30:96–110.
37. Torabinejad M, Parirokh M. Mineral trioxide aggregate: a comprehensive literature review—part II: leakage and biocompatibility investigations. J Endodont. 2010;36:190–202.
38. Andersson L, Blomlöf L, Lindskog S, Feiglin B, Hammarström L. Tooth ankylosis: clinical, radiographic and histological assessments. Int J Oral Surg. 1984;13:423–31.

39. Souza BDM, Dutra KL, Kuntze MM, Bortoluzzi EA, Flores-Mir C, Reyes-Carmona J, et al. Incidence of root resorption after the replantation of avulsed teeth: a meta-analysis. J Endodont. 2018;44:1216–27.
40. Lin S, Ashkenazi M, Karawan M, Teich ST, Gutmacher Z. Management of ankylotic root resorption following dental trauma: a short review and proposal of a treatment protocol. Oral Health Prev Dent. 2017;15(5):467–74.
41. Rege IC, de Lucena BT, Martins AF, Leles CR, Mendonça EF. Pixel gray measurement for the diagnosis of dental ankylosis in cone beam computed tomography images. Oral Surg Oral Med Oral Pathol Oral Radiol. 2021;131(6):721–9.
42. Malmgren B. Decoronation: how, why, and when? J Calif Dent Assoc. 2000;28:846–54.
43. Sala M, Mendoza-Mendoza A, Yañez-Vico RM. Decoronation: an alternative treatment for replacement root resorption. Case Rep Dent. 2017;2017:2826948.
44. Malmgren B, Cvek M, Lundberg M, Frykholm A. Surgical treatment of ankylosed and infra-positioned reimplanted incisors in adolescents. Scand J Dent Res. 1984;92(5):391–9.
45. Sapir S. Decoronation: indications and treatment timing. Refuat Hapeh Vehashinayim (1993). 2006;23(1):19–26. 68
46. Einy S, Kridin K, Kaufman A, Cohenca N. Immediate post-operative rehabilitation after decoronation a systematic review. Dent Traumatol. 2020;36(2):141–50.
47. Mohadeb J, Somar M, He H. Effectiveness of decoronation technique in the treatment of ankylosis a systematic review. Dent Traumatol. 2015;32(4):255–63.
48. Malmgren B. Ridge preservation/decoronation. J Endodont. 2013;39(3):S67–72.
49. Lin S, Schwarz-Arad D, Ashkenazi M. Alveolar bone width preservation after decoronation of ankylosed anterior incisors. J Endodont. 2013 Dec;39(12):1542–4.
50. Davarpanah M, Szmukler-Moncler S. Unconventional implant treatment: I. Implant placement in contact with ankylosed root fragments. A series of five case reports. Clin Oral Implants Res. 2009;20:851–6.
51. Scheuber S, Bosshardt D, Bragger U, Von Arx T. Implant therapy following trauma of the anterior teeth – a new method for alveolar ridge preservation after post-traumatic ankylosis and external root resorption. Schweiz Monatsschr Zahnmed. 2013;123:417–39.
52. Sandler C, Al-Musfir T, Barry S, et al. Guidelines for the orthodontic management of the traumatised tooth. J Orthod. 2021;48:74–81.
53. Bakkari A, Salamah FB. Updated guidelines for the orthodontic management of traumatized and endodontically treated teeth: a review study. Cureus. 2022;14(9):e28943.
54. Tsukiboshi M, Tsukiboshi C, Levin L. A step-by step guide for autotransplantation of teeth. Dent Traumatol. 2023 Jul;39:70–80.
55. Jang Y, Choi YJ, Lee SJ, Roh BD, Park SH, Kim E. Prognostic factors for clinical outcomes in autotransplantation of teeth with complete root formation: survival analysis for up to 12 years. J Endodont. 2016;42(2):198–205.
56. Anssari Moin D, Verweij JP, Waars H, van Merkesteyn R, Wismeijer D. Accuracy of computer-assisted template-guided autotransplantation of teeth with custom three-dimensional designed/printed surgical tooling: a cadaveric study. J Oral Maxillofac Surg. 2017;75(5):925.e1–7.
57. Andreasen FM, Zhjie Y, Thomsen BL, Andersen PK. Occurrence of pulp canal obliteration after luxation injuries in the permanent dentition. Dent Traumatol. 1987 Jun;3(3):103–15.
58. Vinagre A, Castanheira C, Messias A, Palma PJ, Ramos JC. Management of pulp canal obliteration—systematic review of case reports. Medicina. 2021;57(11):1237.
59. McCabe PS, Dummer PM. Pulp canal obliteration: an endodontic diagnosis and treatment challenge. Int Endod J. 2012 Feb;45(2):177–97.

Traumatic Injuries to the Primary Dentition and Sequelae to Permanent Dentition

13

13.1 Introduction

The management of traumatic dental injuries (TDIs) in the primary dentition differs from that in the permanent dentition due to the shorter life span of primary teeth and their proximity to the developing permanent successors [1, 2]. In young children, traumatic dental injuries (TDIs) commonly affect the maxillary deciduous incisors between 18 and 30 months of age [3–5], at which time the permanent tooth germs below are undergoing calcification of their crowns [6]. While the impact of the injury often causes damage to the succedaneous tooth [1, 2, 7], the focus of injury management must be to eliminate the child's discomfort along with preventing further iatrogenic damage to the tooth bud. Children who have suffered dental trauma often report to emergency rooms of hospitals due to the presence of concomitant external or internal soft tissue injuries [8]. At such times, the resident physician examining the child must ensure that the dentist on call is part of the care team. The treatment approach is further complicated by the child's anxiety, fear, and the degree of cognitive development as these injuries often occur in the pre-cooperative group [9]. Procedural sedation or general anesthesia if needed should be done for both, dental and medical management of the injury.

13.2 Crown Fractures

13.2.1 Clinical and Radiographic Examination

In the primary dentition, crown fractures commonly involve the line angles or the incisal edges of the upper central incisors. These injuries may be associated with damage to surrounding soft tissues, such as laceration, erosion, or contusion of lips, gingiva, internal mucosa, or tongue. Before examining the teeth, it is necessary to clean the area and remove any debris with the help of a wet gauze and establish hemostasis, if needed.

H. Vyas et al., *Dental Caries and Traumatic Injuries in Pediatric Dentistry*,
https://doi.org/10.1007/978-3-031-98929-2_13

As seen in the permanent dentition, crown fractures if present can be of the following types:

- Enamel infarction.
- Uncomplicated crown fractures: Enamel fracture or enamel-dentin fracture without pulp exposure.
- Complicated crown fractures wherein the fracture exposes the dental pulp.

Examination of complicated crown fractures of primary teeth must assess size of the pulp exposure, the time elapsed since trauma and the quality of pulp tissue [7, 10]. Presence of early childhood caries may contribute to the severity of the injury and is another factor that influences treatment planning.

A periapical radiograph for enamel infarctions/enamel fractures is not recommended; [11] however, a radiograph of enamel-dentin and complicated crown fractures should be taken as baseline. The stage of root development, presence of root resorption and any other injuries such as root fracture or luxation must be assessed on the radiograph [7]. Often, radiographs taken may reveal changes, consequent of an earlier trauma. In pre-cooperative children, radiographs may be difficult, and the diagnosis and treatment may need to be decided based on clinical signs and symptoms.

Pulp sensibility testing by electric or thermal methods is not reliable in the primary dentition and is not routinely performed [11].

13.2.2 Management

A. *Uncomplicated Crown Fractures*

- *Enamel infarctions*: These cracks in enamel are mostly limited to the dentinoenamel junction and require no treatment [8–11].
- *Enamel fractures:* The sharp edges of the fractured tooth can be simply smoothened and polished using abrasive discs or diamond burs (Fig. 13.1) [8–11].
- *Enamel-Dentin fractures:* Injuries involving the crowns of primary teeth need to be managed conservatively with minimal treatment. Depending on the age of the child, enamel-dentin fractures may be left untreated if the fracture line is not close to the pulp. If the fracture line appears very close to the pulp, a light-cured calcium hydroxide liner or a biosilicate cement like MTA or Biodentine followed by a GIC bandage must be placed as part of emergency management [12]. Restorations should be placed with the main objective of protecting the pulp and ensuring retention of the capping agent or if there are esthetic requirements. Zirconia and strip crowns provide better esthetics and longevity than composite buildups or fragment reattachment [13]. A Strip crown can be used if it is a single tooth fracture as it will be easier to match the shade and contour with the adjacent teeth.

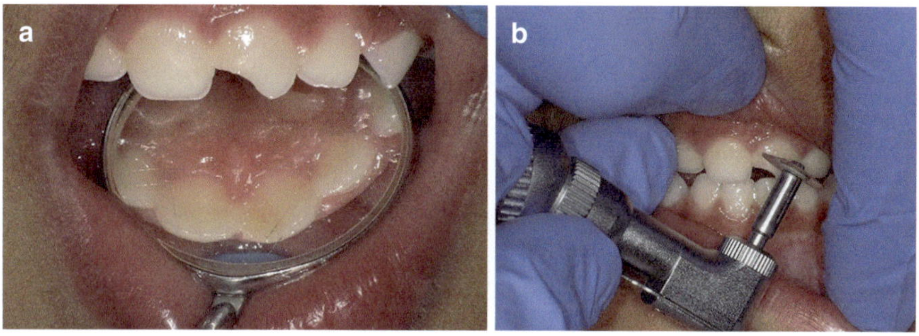

Fig. 13.1 Enamel-dentin fracture of maxillary primary left central incisor (**a**). The sharp incisal edge was rounded with finishing and polishing discs (**b**)

B. *Complicated Crown Fractures*

These injuries are especially difficult to manage in young anxious children, as they necessitate the administration of local anesthesia. If the child is uncooperative, the need for procedural sedation or general anesthesia must be considered. Irrespective of the size of pulpal exposure, a partial or complete pulpotomy can be performed in vital teeth. These vital pulp procedures encourage continued root development of immature primary teeth [12, 13]. Pulpectomy can be performed for non-vital teeth. These teeth need to be restored with an extra-coronal restoration, i.e., strip crowns or zirconia crown [14, 15]. In teeth which are close to exfoliation or show signs of significant root resorption, extraction is indicated (Fig. 13.2).

In case of enamel fractures, there is no *follow-up* schedule recommended. For enamel-dentin fractures, only a clinical examination is recommended at 6–8 weeks followed by 1 year. Considering the aggressive nature of the resorption process in the primary dentition, it still may be prudent to monitor these teeth even after 6–8 weeks, as part of the child's routine dental follow-ups, especially if there are concomitant dental injuries such as concussion or subluxation. Coronal discoloration is a known outcome that generally occurs within 10 to 14 days of the injury and is seen to be transient. If the discoloration persists or occurs at a later stage, endodontic treatment should not be initiated unless there are other signs of pulp necrosis. A radiograph must be taken if signs of pulp pathosis such as dentoalveolar abscess, mobility is noted. If the tooth becomes symptomatic, pulpectomy or extraction is advised [15–18]. Teeth with complicated crown fractures must be monitored clinically at 1 week, 6–8 weeks, and 1 year.

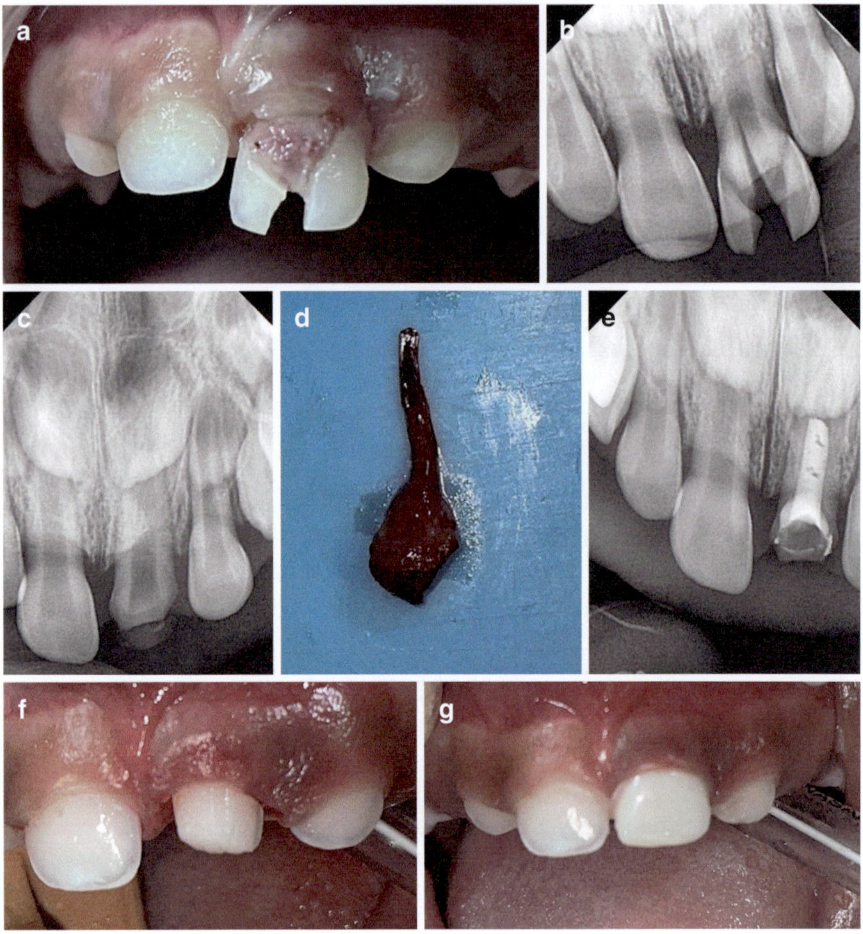

Fig. 13.2 Child reported with complicated crown fracture of maxillary primary left central incisor 24 h after trauma (**a**). The radiograph showed multiple fracture lines (**b**). The dislodged fragment was removed under General Anesthesia (**c**) and the tooth treated for pulpectomy (**d**). A radiograph was taken after pulpectomy (**e**) and the tooth prepared to receive a preformed zirconia crown (**f**). Immediate post-operative photograph (**g**) (Image courtesy: Dr Gopika Sharma, India)

13.3 Crown-Root Fractures

13.3.1 Clinical and Radiographic Examination

These are fractures involving the enamel, dentin, and cementum are among the least observed traumatic dental injuries in the primary dentition. Depending on the pulpal involvement, these injuries can be classified as uncomplicated and complicated.

On clinical examination, the fracture line originates in the crown portion of the tooth and extends apically into the root in an oblique direction.

The coronal fragment is generally seen attached to the gingiva by the gingival and periodontal fibers and there is little to moderate displacement of the crown. The patient may experience transitory pain on mastication [8–10].

Trauma to the chin can lead to crown-root fractures in primary molars and injury to the mandibular condyle. A periapical radiograph taken at different vertical angulations will reveal the fracture line. An occlusal radiograph will detect labial or palatal displacement of the coronal fragment. The radiographic examination determines the apical termination of the fracture line and assesses the restorability of the tooth [8–10].

13.3.2 Management

The treatment plan is influenced by whether there is significant displacement of the coronal fragment. If no displacement is seen, the tooth can be left in situ and no treatment is instituted.

Loose and displaced coronal fragments should be extracted as part of emergency management. The injury site should then be closely examined for the presence of pulp exposure and restorability of the tooth.

If the tooth is restorable:

- In the absence of an exposure, a light-cured calcium hydroxide liner or Calcium Silicate Cement liner (MTA, Biodentine) can be placed on the fracture line followed by a Glass Ionomer Cement bandage.
- If an exposure is present, a pulpotomy or pulpectomy must be performed.
- Later, these teeth will need to be restored by a full crown coverage.

If the tooth is unrestorable, extraction is the preferred treatment [19]. The retained tooth is followed up at 1 week, 6–8 weeks, and 1 year. Any clinical sign of pathosis warrants a radiographic examination [11].

13.4 Root Fractures

13.4.1 Clinical and Radiographic Examination

Root fractures in primary teeth are relatively rare. They are detected on radiographic examination and are usually located mid-root or in the apical third.

Periapical X-rays with different angulations may need to be taken to locate the fracture line.

Clinically, the tooth demonstrates mobility, and the coronal fragment may or may not be displaced.

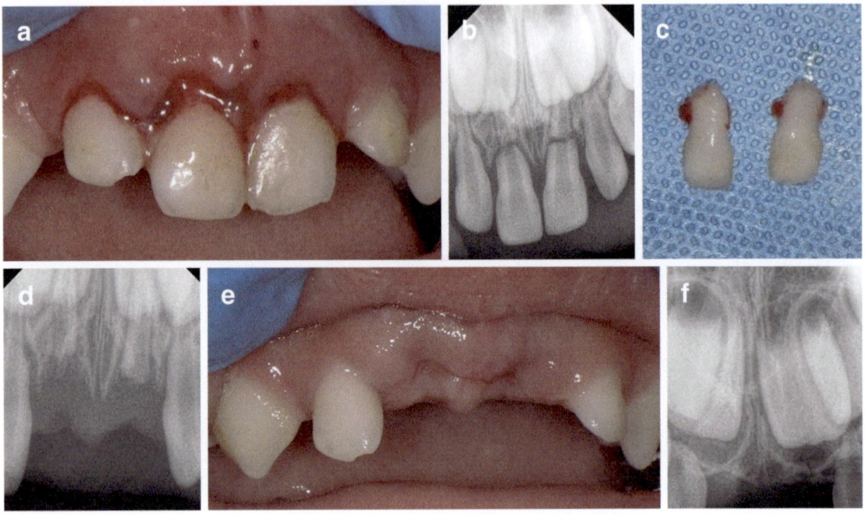

Fig. 13.3 Clinical and radiographic examination show cervical third root fracture of the maxillary primary central incisors with extrusion of coronal fragments (**a**, **b**). The mobile coronal fragments were extracted (**c**), and the apical fragments were left behind to resorb (**d**). Clinical photo at follow-up (**e**) and resorption of both apical fragments seen on radiograph in 6 months (**f**)

13.4.2 Management (Figs. 13.3 and 13.4)

With respect to apical third and mid-root fractures:

If there is minimal or no displacement of the coronal fragment, the tooth can be left untreated and will resorb at the expected time. If the fragment is displaced and interferes with occlusion, it may be repositioned, and a wire-composite splint placed for 4 weeks [11]. Splinted teeth with root fractures must be followed up clinically and radiographically at 1 week, 4 weeks, 8 weeks, and 1 year.

Cervical third root fractures and loose coronal fragments should be extracted to prevent aspiration. The apical fragment can be left behind to undergo physiologic resorption, as any attempt to remove it may damage the developing permanent successor. If the coronal fragment in cervical fractures is not extracted, there is a greater risk of pulpal necrosis and root resorption [20, 21].

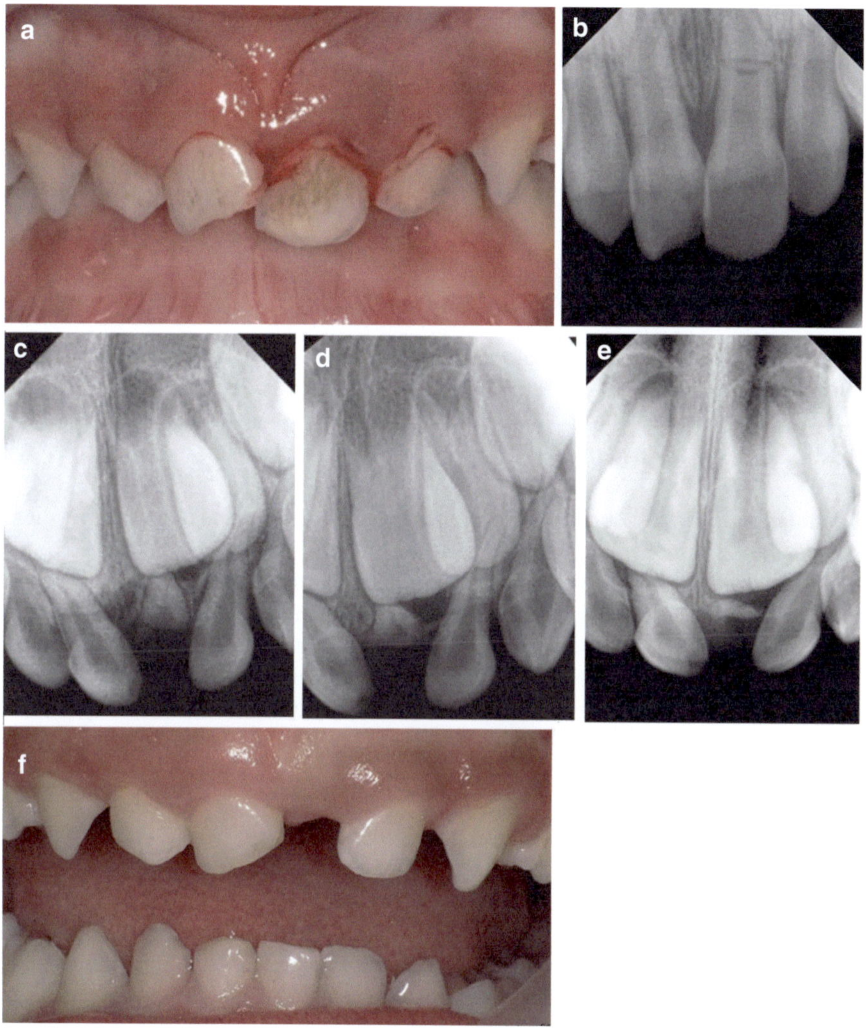

Fig. 13.4 Luxation injury and mobility of maxillary primary left central incisor (**a**). Radiograph shows the middle third root fracture line and clear separation of the fragments. The coronal fragment was extracted and apical fragment left to resorb (**b**). Follow-up in 8 months showing root resorption (**c**). Follow-up in 17 months showing further resorption of the apical fragment (**d**). Follow-up after 24 months showing almost complete resorption of the apical fragment (**e**). Space loss seen after 3 years in the anterior segment (**f**)

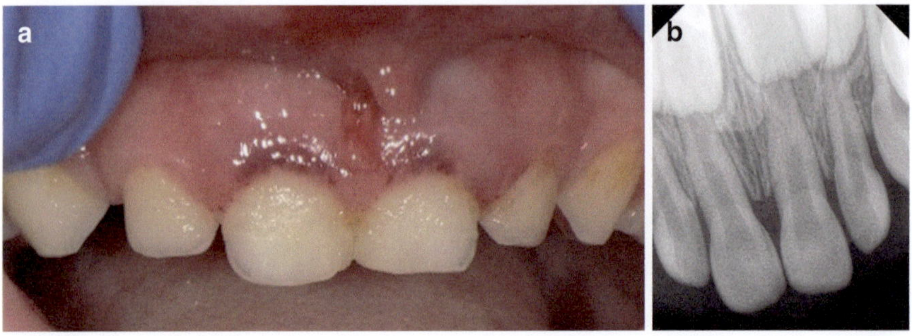

Fig. 13.5 Subluxation injury of maxillary primary central incisors (**a**). Radiograph taken as baseline record and to rule out concomitant injury (**b**)

13.5 Luxation Injuries

Luxation injuries are a common occurrence in primary teeth due to the soft resilient bone and the short root lengths of primary teeth.

Concussion is an injury to the tooth supporting structures *without abnormal tooth displacement and mobility*. In *subluxation*, there is loosening of the tooth seen with *mobility but no marked displacement* in the socket (Fig. 13.5).

In *intrusive luxation*, the tooth displaces into the apical bone. *Extrusive luxation* displaces the tooth out of its socket while in *lateral luxation*, the tooth displaces in a direction other than axial [8–11].

13.5.1 Clinical and Radiographic Examination

Concussion: The tooth is tender on percussion and there is no bleeding seen from the gingival sulcus.

Subluxation: The parent usually gives history of bleeding from the gingival sulcus and on clinical examination, there is abnormal tooth mobility. There may be slight periapical widening seen on the baseline radiograph.

Extrusive luxation: The tooth appears elongated, mobile, and usually displaced in the palatal or lingual direction. There is occlusal interference seen. There is apical widening of the PDL space on a periapical or occlusal radiograph.

Lateral luxation: The tooth is displaced and locked into the socket in a direction other than axial (palatal/labial or lingual). Commonly in lateral luxations, the crowns are displaced in the palatal direction. The root apex will most often penetrate the thin labial plate and be palpated through the gingiva (Fig. 13.6).

The tooth is immobile and will interfere with occlusion. A periapical radiograph will reveal widening of the PDL space. An occlusal radiograph will determine the direction of tooth displacement and fracture of the alveolar process.

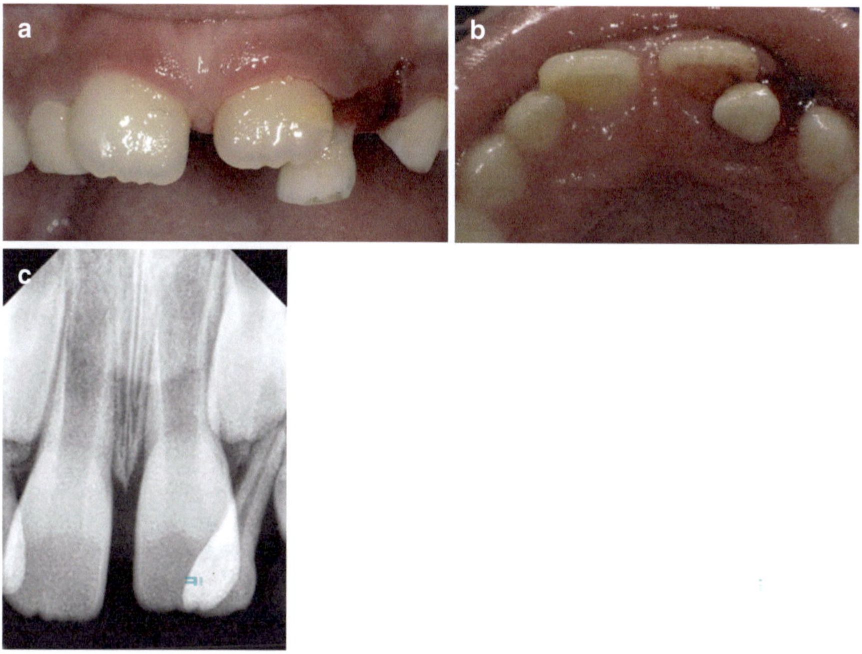

Fig. 13.6 Lateral luxation of maxillary primary left lateral incisor, displaced in the palatal direction, front view (**a**), palatal view, (**b**) and radiograph (**c**)

Intrusion: The tooth is displaced into its socket. This type of injury is seen to have the most severe consequences due to its proximity to the succedaneous tooth. If the tooth is displaced labially, the root apex may be palpated in the vestibule. There may be swelling of the upper lip due to hematoma.

A periapical and occlusal radiograph is recommended to identity the degree and direction of intrusion. It also helps to distinguish severe intrusion from avulsion injuries. *The tooth appears shortened when it is displaced buccally away from the succedaneous tooth.*

If it appears elongated and the apical third cannot be visualized, the tooth is displaced in the direction of the succedaneous tooth [11].

Although rare, all luxation injuries must be ruled out for accompanying root fractures.

13.5.2 Management of Luxation Injuries

- *Concussion and subluxation*

Usually, concussion and subluxation do not require any specific treatment. These types of luxation injuries have a good prognosis.

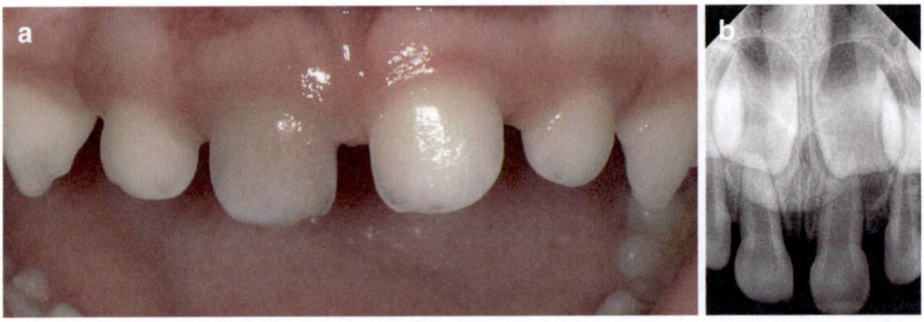

Fig. 13.7 Discolored maxillary primary right central incisor with history of concussion injury (**a**). Clinical picture and radiograph show no pathology requiring intervention and the tooth was kept under follow-up (**b**)

The patient must be advised a soft diet and to avoid biting with the affected teeth for 7–10 days. Brushing twice daily is recommended. If brushing around the injured teeth is difficult, then use of 0.12% Chlorhexidine mouthwash twice daily is advised. In younger children, the injured teeth and gums can be cleaned with a cotton swab dipped in mouthwash or Chlorhexidine wipes. Concussed and subluxated teeth must be evaluated clinically at 4–6 weeks and1 year [11]. The tooth may appear discolored on follow-up; however endodontic treatment must not be initiated without the presence of other indications of non-vitality (Fig. 13.7).

- *Lateral luxation*

Management of lateral luxation depends on the severity of injury, time elapsed since injury, position of the injured tooth in relation to its successor and cooperation of the child.

No treatment—When the injury is minor and there is no occlusal interference, repositioning is not advised [8–11].

Repositioning—If the luxation injury interferes with occlusion and the patient reports within a few hours of trauma, repositioning is advised. Under local anesthesia, the tooth is held at the crown using forceps and a slight extrusive force is applied before repositioning the tooth back into its socket. Alternatively, the tooth can be repositioned using digital pressure. The teeth are stabilized with a flexible splint for 4 weeks [11].

Extraction—If the root of the laterally luxated tooth is in proximity to its successor or has penetrated the buccal bone and gingiva, extraction is advised to prevent further damage to the succedaneous tooth. When significant time has elapsed since injury and occlusal interference is seen, the tooth should be extracted as repositioning will not be possible [22, 23].

A clinical follow-up is recommended at 1 week, 4 weeks (only if splint is to be removed), 6–8 weeks, 6 months, and 1 year [11]. A radiographic follow-up is taken annually to determine the development and eruption pattern of the permanent tooth, especially in cases of luxation that required splinting.

- *Extrusive luxation*

No treatment: In extrusive luxation less than 3 mm and that does not interfere with occlusion, no repositioning is advised. Immature primary teeth should be allowed to spontaneously reposition themselves [11].

Repositioning: If the tooth is mildly extruded (<3 mm) *but interferes with occlusion*, it can be repositioned, if the patient reports within a few hours of the injury. Delay in reporting after the injury results in the formation of a coagulum which makes repositioning difficult and traumatic. Occlusal adjustment may be performed to relieve the interference. If the tooth is mobile, it is splinted for 4 weeks [11, 24–26].

Extraction: If repositioning or occlusal adjustment is not possible, then extraction is advised. A tooth that has extruded beyond 3 mm would be mobile and must be extracted (Figs. 13.8 and 13.9). [11]

Fig. 13.8 Extrusive luxation of maxillary right central incisor

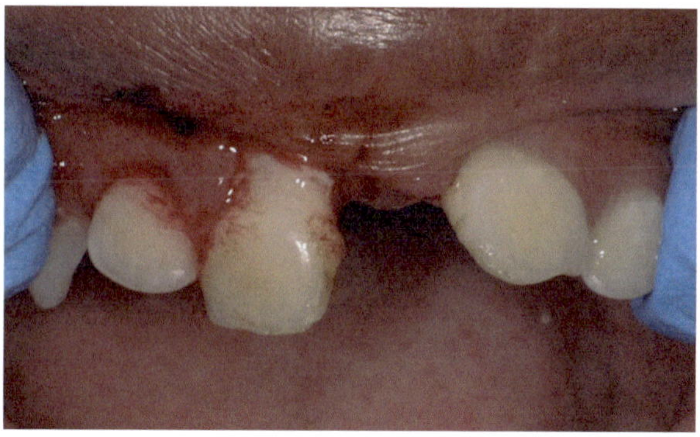

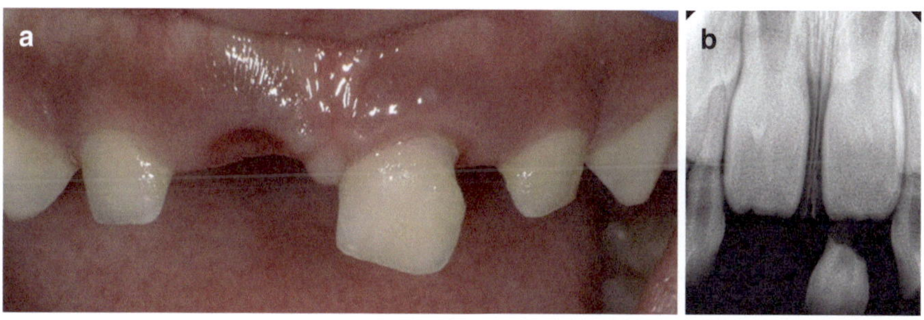

Fig. 13.9 Extrusion of maxillary primary left central incisor and avulsion of right central incisor (**a**). Radiograph shows the tooth was close to exfoliation (**b**)

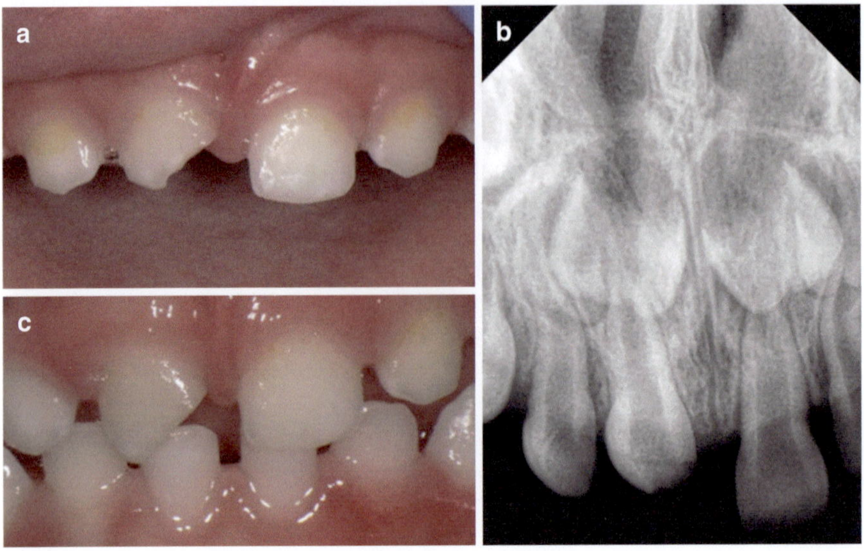

Fig. 13.10 Intrusion of maxillary right central incisor (**a**). Foreshortening of the tooth is appreciated on radiograph (**b**). Re-eruption seen in 6 months (**c**)

A follow-up at 1 week, 4 weeks (only if splint is to be removed), 6–8 weeks, and 1 year is recommended [11]. The clinician must stress on the possibility of consequences and recall the patient for annual follow-ups, till the permanent tooth erupts.

- *Intrusive luxation*

No treatment: The tooth must be allowed to spontaneously re-erupt irrespective of the extent and direction of displacement. This may take up to 6 months and at times even up to 1 year (Figs. 13.10 and 13.11).

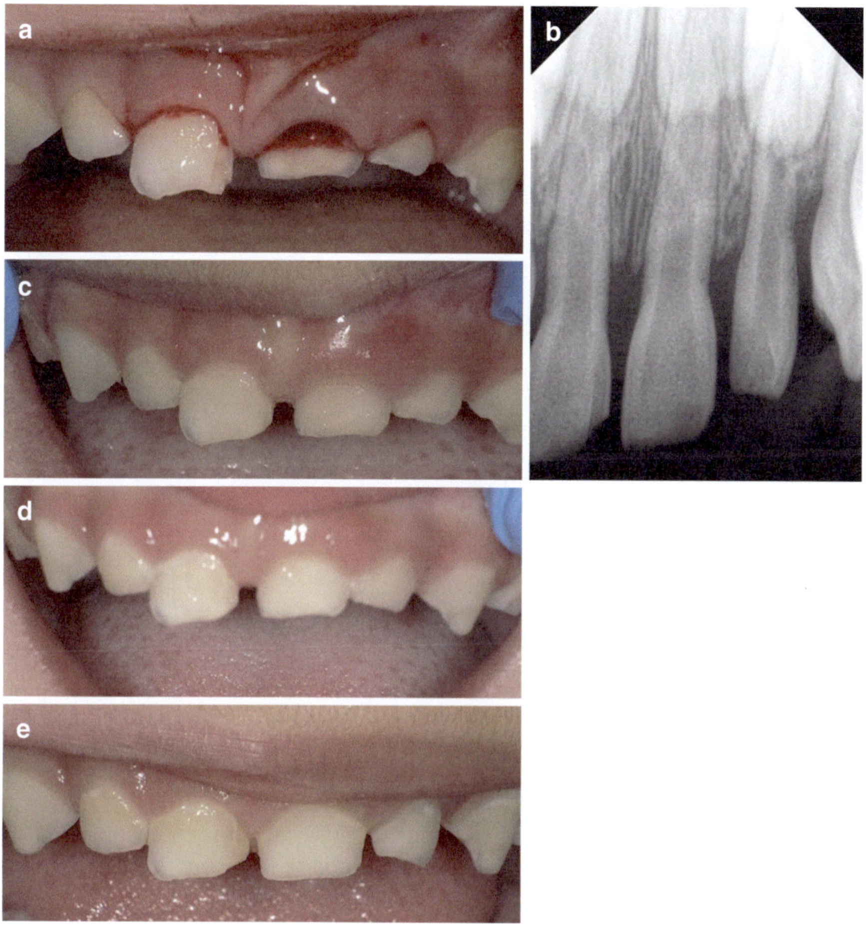

Fig. 13.11 Intrusive luxation injury of maxillary primary left central and lateral incisor seen clinically (**a**) and on a radiograph (**b**). Partial re-eruption seen after 1 week (**c**). Follow-up after 1 month shows further eruption (**d**). Complete re-eruption seen at 1 year (**e**)

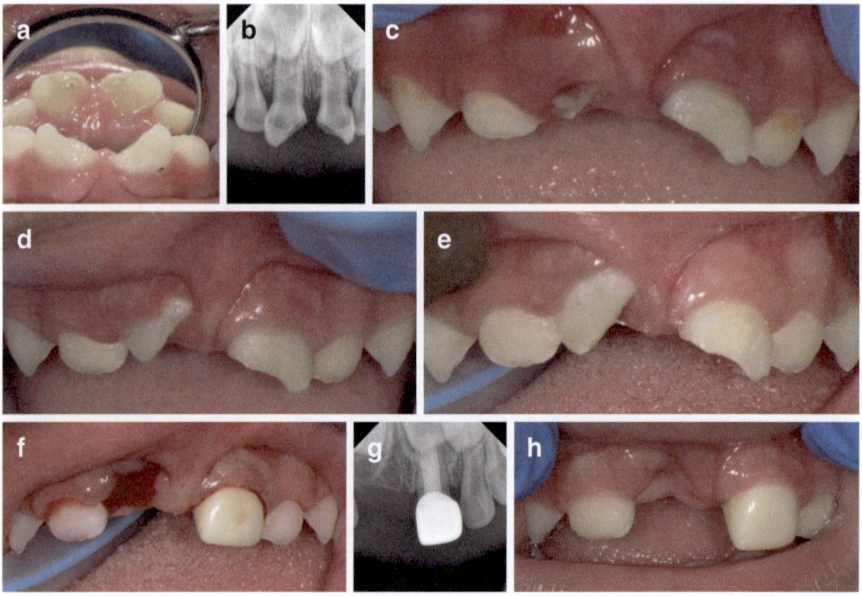

Fig. 13.12 Child with a history of enamel-dentin fracture of maxillary primary central incisors (**a**). Radiograph taken to rule out concomitant injury (**b**). A repeat trauma episode after 20 days caused intrusion of the right central incisor (**c**). The central incisor showed signs of re-eruption in 1 week (**d**). After 1 month with further eruption seen in a mesial angulation (**e**), the right central incisor was extracted and left central incisor treated for pulpectomy and restored with a preformed zirconia crown (**f**). Radiograph taken after pulpectomy (**g**). Follow-up at 1 week (**h**)

Repositioning: Repositioning of an intruded primary tooth is not recommended.

Extraction: If the tooth is intruded such that it is seen penetrating the gingiva, then extraction is advised (Figs. 13.12, 13.13, and 13.14) [11, 27].

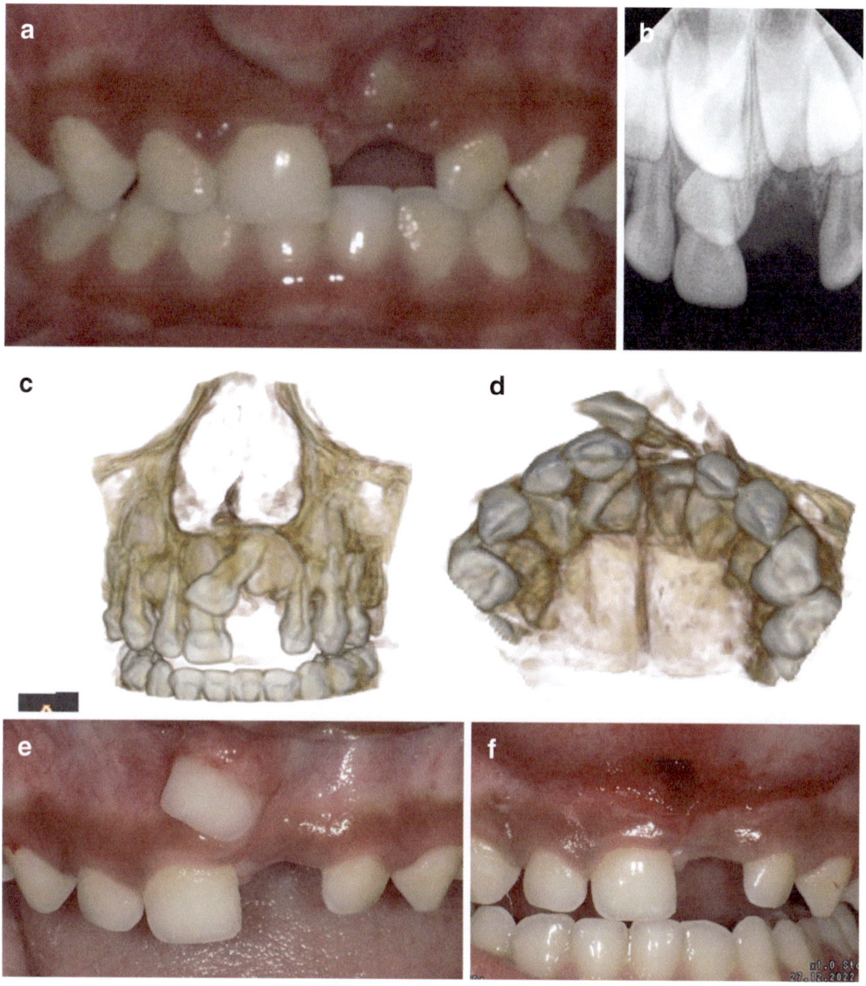

Fig. 13.13 Intrusion of maxillary primary left central incisor (**a**). Radiograph showing mesial angulation of the intruded tooth (**b**). The CBCT volumetric image showed mesial (**c**) and labial direction of intrusion (**d**). Re-eruption of the tooth seen at 3-month follow-up (**e**). The tooth was extracted due to unfavorable path of eruption (**f**)

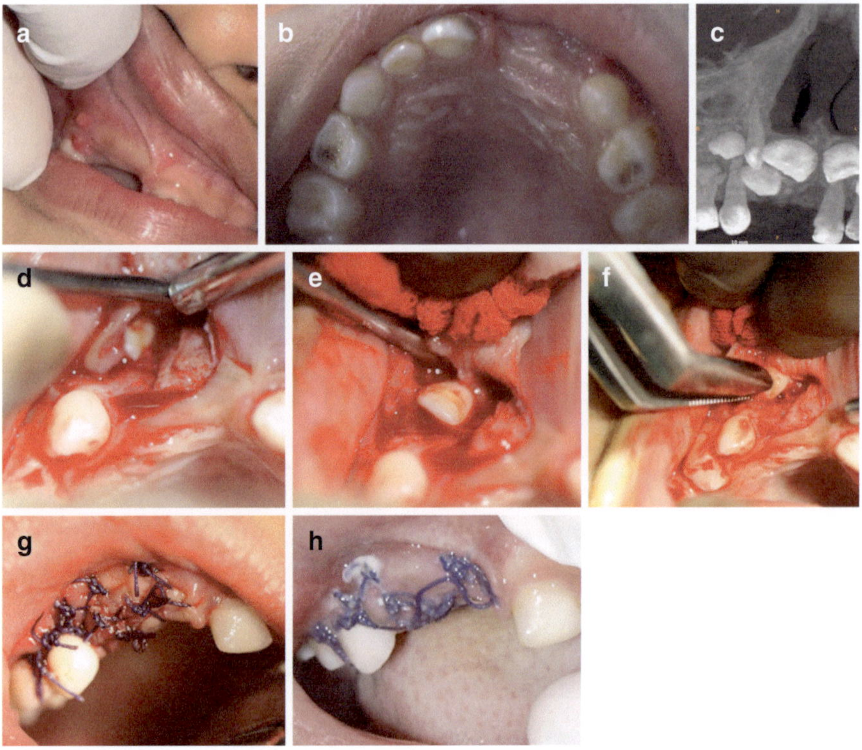

Fig. 13.14 Child reported with a history of trauma 2 months ago. Parent gave the history of avulsion of maxillary primary right central incisor. On clinical and radiographic examination, the maxillary right incisors were absent. The vestibule appeared obliterated on the right side with palpable hard tissue suspected of an intruded tooth. Draining sinuses were seen in the same region (**a**, **b**). The CBCT showed severe intrusion of lateral incisor into the canine space (**c**). The tooth was extracted surgically under General Anesthesia, as part of full mouth rehabilitation. An incision was made to raise a buccal gingival flap. Reactive fibrous tissue overlying the intruded tooth was removed and the tooth exposed (**d**). The tooth was elevated (**e**) and extracted (**f**). The gingival flap approximated and sutured (**g**). The child was recalled in a week (**h**)

13.6 Avulsion

Avulsion is complete loss of tooth from its socket.

13.6.1 Clinical and Radiographic Examination

The socket appears empty both clinically and radiographically. Avulsion injuries must be distinguished from severe intrusion and loss of crown in crown-root fractures, with the help of radiographs (Fig. 13.15).

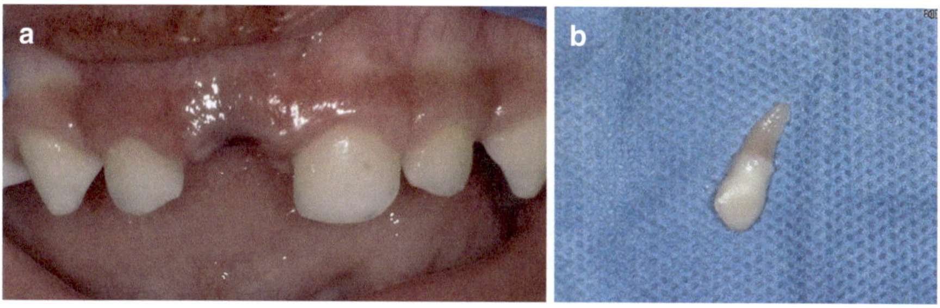

Fig. 13.15 Avulsion of maxillary primary right central incisor (**a**). The tooth showed resorbing root (**b**)

If the lost tooth is not located, a radiograph of the lacerated soft tissue must be taken to locate the tooth or its fragments [8–11]. Another possibility is inhaling the tooth in which case the child will express symptoms of distress and must be referred to the emergency department [14]. It is important to find the avulsed tooth even though it is not to be replanted.

13.6.2 Management

It is not recommended to replant an avulsed primary tooth as the risks outweigh the benefits. Replantation would involve splinting and endodontic management under local or general anesthesia. While ankylosis is commonly seen following replantation of permanent teeth, there is insufficient literature to suggest the same for primary teeth. However, the outcomes of replanting primary teeth even under ideal situations is too unpredictable to justify the esthetic rehabilitation and this treatment only adds to the burden of care [28, 29].

13.7 Sequelae to Permanent Dentition

The severity of sequelae depends on the degree of development of the permanent successor and the proximity of the primary roots to the permanent crown at the time of trauma. The type of trauma to the primary tooth and its direction of displacement can also alter the development and eruption of the permanent tooth.

The greatest number of aberrations in the development of permanent teeth are seen with *intrusion and avulsion injuries to primary teeth.* The severity of malformation was greatest when trauma occurred *below age three* [30].

The main consequences seen in the permanent teeth are [30–37]

- *Enamel discoloration*—These lesions are sharply demarcated and often located on the labial surface of the crown. The size varies spots to large patches. The most commonly affected teeth are the maxillary central incisors, with the age of patients at the time of injury ranging from 1 to 3.5 years. This sequelae is unrelated to a specific type of injury to the primary dentition.
- *Enamel hypoplasia*—The lesion is white to yellow in color on the labial surface. A horizontal groove is seen encircling the tooth cervical to the discolored area, which may or may not be detected on the radiograph before eruption. The maxillary central incisors are most commonly affected and the age of the patient at the time of injury is 2 years. Injuries such as extrusion, intrusion, or avulsion of the primary teeth result in such sequelae (Fig. 13.16).

- *Alterations in eruption*

Injuries to the primary tooth that cause changes in the connective tissue overlying the permanent tooth resulting in deviated eruption. Eruption may be delayed by at least a year following premature loss of primary incisors.

- *Crown and root dilaceration*

The injury displaces either the crown or the root of the already formed permanent tooth in a direction away from the long axis of the tooth. On the radiograph, the crown appears foreshortened (crown dilaceration) and the root shows a mesial or distal bend (root dilaceration). A CBCT may be needed to ascertain the position and extent of the anomaly, before intervention. Around half of these teeth fail to erupt or erupt ectopically, in a facial or lingual direction relative to adjacent teeth. The teeth commonly involved are the maxillary and mandibular permanent central incisors. Injury to the primary dentition usually occurs around the age of 2–5 years. This sequelae is associated with avulsion and intrusion of the primary tooth (Fig. 13.17).

- *Odontoma-like malformations*

Clinically, there may be delayed eruption of the odontoma and impaction or ectopic eruption of the adjacent tooth. A radio-opaque mass with little resemblance to a tooth germ is seen on the radiograph. The age at the time of injury ranges from 1 to 3 years. The type of injury affecting the primary dentition appears to be intrusive luxation or avulsion (Fig. 13.18).

13.7.1 Root Duplication

Root duplication occurs when half or less than half of the permanent crown is formed. An extra root is seen mesially or distally extending from the partially formed crown, on radiographic examination. It is a rare sequela associated with intrusion injury.

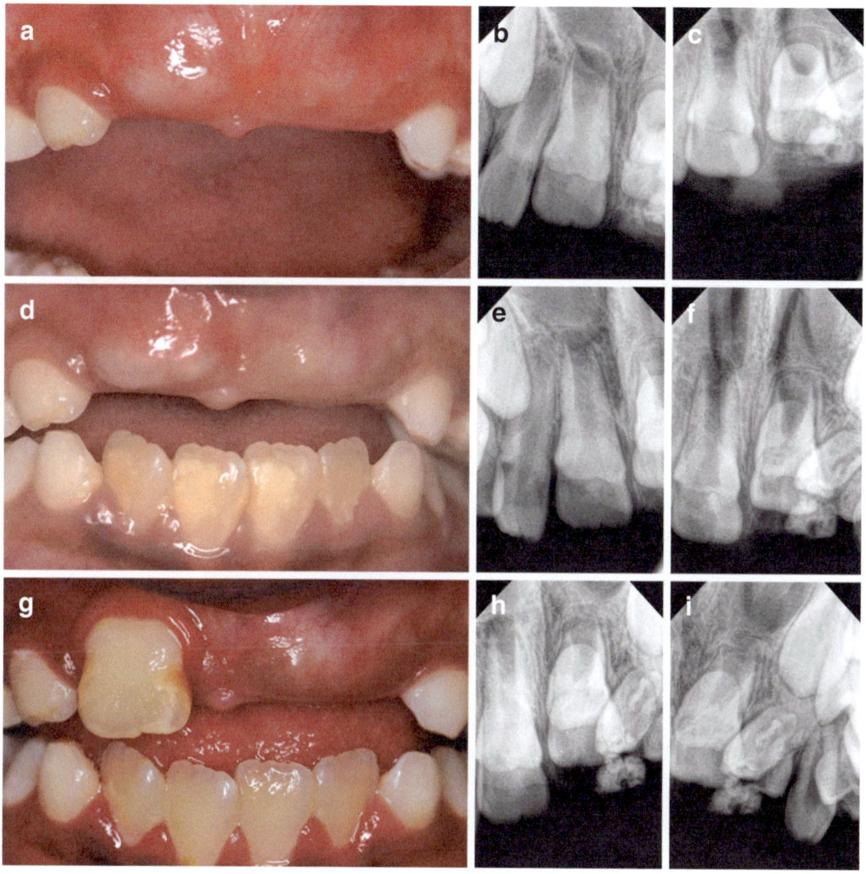

Fig. 13.16 Delayed eruption of maxillary permanent central incisors at age 9. Patient gives a history of avulsion of maxillary primary incisors when he was 18 months old. The right lateral incisor had erupted showing hypoplasia of incisal third (**a**). Radiograph taken at first visit shows malformed central incisors and left lateral incisor (**b**). Odontoma-like structures were seen overlying the left central and lateral incisors (**c**). A CBCT was advised and child recalled in 6 months. Pre-eruption bulge was noticed in the region of central incisors (**d**). Radiograph showed incisal movement of the right central incisor with further root maturation (**e**) and no movement of left incisors (**f**). Patient recalled in 6 months. The right central incisor had erupted and shows hypomineralized patches and hypoplastic tooth structure (**g**). The radiograph shows root development (**h**) and ectopic eruption of left lateral incisor and odontoma-like structure in the same region (**i**). The child is scheduled for surgical removal of odontoma and orthodontic re-evaluation

- *Partial or complete arrest of root formation*

The sequela commonly affects the permanent maxillary central incisors which either erupts normally with short roots and may be lost due to poor periodontal support. The tooth appears foreshortened or is seen to undergo resorption on the radiograph. It is seen after an avulsion injury sustained by the primary dentition between 5 and 7 years of age.

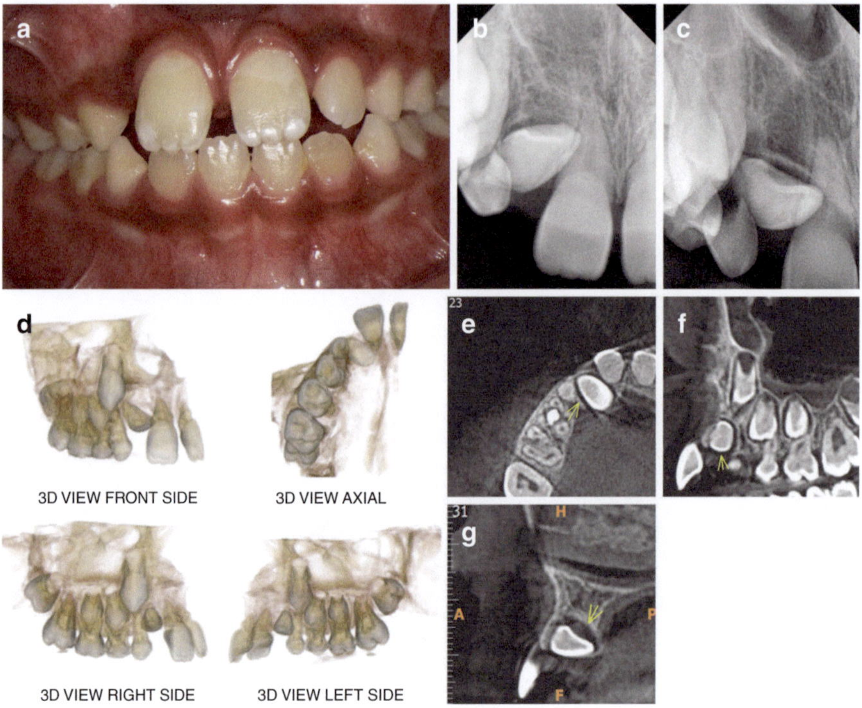

Fig. 13.17 Child reported with proclined anterior teeth. History of avulsion of maxillary central incisors when child was 5 years old. Clinically, the maxillary right lateral incisor is missing (**a**). Radiograph taken at two different angulation shows ectopic position of the lateral incisor without visible root structure (**b** and **c**). CBCT shows mesio-palatal positioning of the tooth within the alveolus with possible curvature at the cervical third of the root and arrested root development (**d**). Axial (**e**), sagittal (**f**), and coronal section (**g**) showing the possible shape and location of the impacted tooth

The management of sequela requires an interdisciplinary approach. Discoloration and hypoplasia of enamel is treated by a combination of tooth whitening, Resin Infiltration, or veneers. Eruption guidance of deflected or impacted permanent teeth can be performed through orthodontic treatment. Additionally, impacted teeth or malformed teeth such as odontoma require surgical removal.

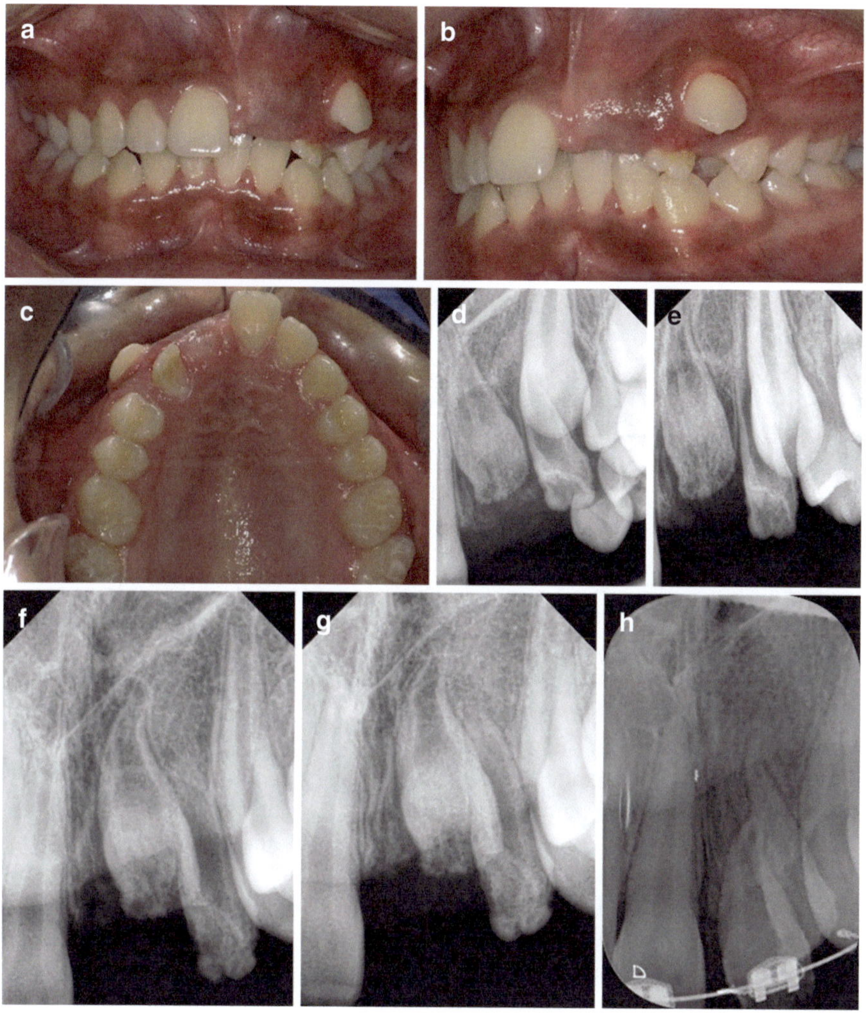

Fig. 13.18 A 11-year-old patient with delayed eruption of maxillary permanent left central incisor and ectopic eruption and hypoplasia of left lateral incisor in frontal (**a**), lateral (**b**), and occlusal view (**c**). History of trauma when child was 3 years old. Radiograph taken at age 9 (**d**), 10 (**e**), 11 (**f**), and 13 (**g**) years shows incisal movement of left central and lateral incisor. The left incisors show further root development with root dilaceration. The central and lateral incisors showed complete root development (**h**). Initial phase of orthodontic treatment was started. At age 15, the central incisor emerged ectopically from the labial attached gingiva and the lateral incisor was seen in crossbite due to alignment of lower anterior teeth (**i**). The central incisor was surgically exposed, and a button bonded to its labial surface (**j**). The tooth is being brought in position orthodontically (**k**)

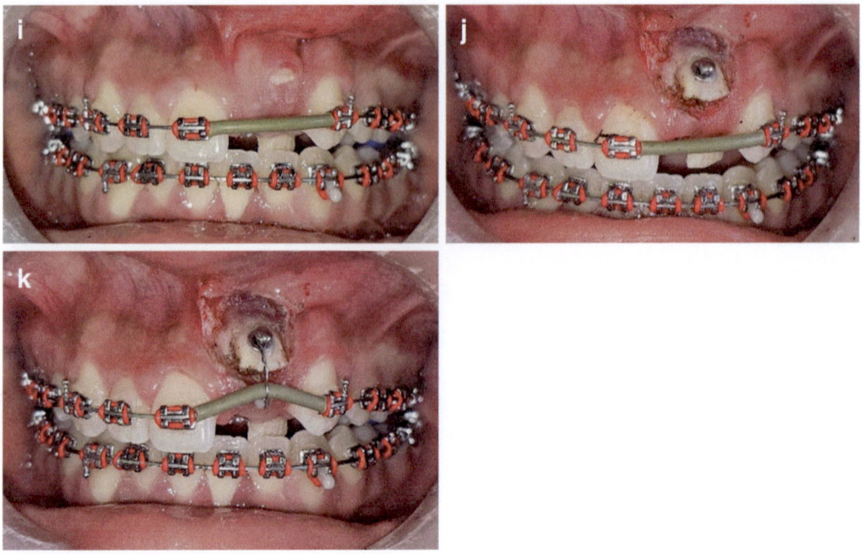

Fig. 13.18 (continued)

13.8 Concluding Remarks

The management of traumatic injuries in the primary dentition necessitates maintaining a balance between immediate clinical intervention and safeguarding the permanent successors. Given the age of presentation and limited cooperation in young children, a conservative approach is vital. Crown fractures without pulpal involvement require only smoothening of the sharp incisal margins. Teeth with traumatic pulp exposures should be treated with a pulpotomy for maintaining pulp vitality. Teeth with minor luxation injuries such as mild intrusion, lateral luxation may reposition themselves without any active intervention. Avulsed primary teeth should not be repositioned to avoid damaging the successor. Some injuries to primary teeth may lead to significant developmental disturbances in the permanent dentition. Clinical and radiographic follow-up is essential for monitoring healing and identifying early signs of pulpal pathology or sequelae to the succedaneous tooth. Interdisciplinary coordination, especially for managing delayed eruption, malformations, or impactions in the permanent teeth is critical for achieving both functional and esthetic rehabilitation.

References

1. Andreasen JO, Ravn JJ. The effect of traumatic injuries to primary teeth on their permanent successors. II. A clinical and radiographic follow-up study of 213 teeth. Scand J Dent Res. 1971;79(4):284–94.

2. Lenzi MM, da Silva Fidalgo TK, Luiz RR, Maia LC. Trauma in primary teeth and its effect on the development of permanent successors: a controlled study. Acta Odontol Scand. 2019;77(1):76–81.
3. Galea H. An investigation of dental injuries treated in an acute care general hospital. J Am Dent Assoc. 1984;109:434–9.
4. Garcia-Godoy F, Garcia-Godoy F, Garcia-Godoy FM. Primary teeth traumatic injuries at a private pediatric dental center. Endod Dent Traumatol. 1987;3(3):126–9.
5. Petti S, Glendor U, Andersson L. World traumatic dental injury prevalence and incidence, a meta-analysis-one billion living people have had traumatic dental injuries. Dent Traumatol. 2018;34(2):71–86.
6. Logan WHG, Kronfeld R. Development of the human jaws and surrounding structures from birth to the age of fifteen years. J Am Dent Assoc. 1933;20(3):379–427.
7. Flores MT, Onetto JE. How does orofacial trauma in children affect the developing dentition? Long-term treatment and associated complications. Dent Traumatol. 2019;35(6):312–23.
8. Flores MT. Traumatic injuries in the primary dentition. Dent Traumatol. 2002;18(6):287–98.
9. Dummett CO Jr. Dental management of traumatic injuries to the primary dentition. J Calif Dent Assoc. 2000;28:838–45.
10. Andreasen JO, Andreasen FM, Andersson L. Textbook and color atlas of traumatic injuries to the teeth. 5th ed. Copenhagen: Munksgaard; 2011; Chapter 22, Injuries to the Primary Dentition. p. 556–88.
11. Day PF, Flores MT, O'Connell AC, Abbott PV, Tsilingaridis G, Fouad AF, Cohenca N, Lauridsen E, Bourguignon C, Hicks L, Andreasen JO, Cehreli ZC, Harlamb S, Kahler B, Oginni A, Semper M, Levin L. International Association of Dental Traumatology guidelines for the management of traumatic dental injuries: 3. Injuries in the primary dentition. Dent Traumatol. 2020;36(4):343–59.
12. Turkistani J, Hanno A. Recent trends in the management of dentoalveolar traumatic injuries to primary and young permanent teeth. Dent Traumatol. 2011;27(1):46–54.
13. Kapoor H, Srivastava N, Panthri P. Reattachment of broken tooth fragment in primary teeth-a report of two cases. Ann Ess Dent. 2014;6(2):22–5.
14. Fuks AB. Current concepts in vital primary pulp therapy. Eur J Paediatr Dent. 2002;3(3):115–20.
15. Kupietzky A, Holan G. Treatment of crown fractures with pulp exposure in primary incisors. Pediatr Dent. 2003;25(3):241–7.
16. Ajayakumar LP, Chowdhary N, Reddy VR, Chowdhary R. Use of restorative full crowns made with zirconia in children: a systematic review. Int J Clin Pediatr Dent. 2020;13(5):551–8.
17. American Academy of Pediatric Dentistry. Pulp therapy for primary and immature permanent teeth. The reference manual of pediatric dentistry. Chicago: American Academy of Pediatric Dentistry; 2023. p. 457–6.
18. Holan G. Pulp aspects of traumatic dental injuries in primary incisors: dark coronal discoloration. Dent Traumatol. 2019;35(6):309–11.
19. Costa VP, Oliveira LJ, Rosa DP, Cademartori MG, Torriani DD. Crown-root fractures in primary teeth: a case series study of 28 cases. Braz Dent J. 2016;27(2):234–8.
20. Spinas E, Di Giorgio G, Murgia MS, Garau V, Pinna M, Zerman N. Root fractures in the primary teeth and their management: a scoping review. Dent J (Basel). 2022;10(5):74.
21. Kevci M, Gerds TA, Lauridsen E, Andersson L. The risk of healing complications in primary teeth with root fractures: a retrospective cohort study. Dent Traumatol. 2023;39(5):455–61.
22. Das S, Thosar NR, Khubchandani M, Malviya NS, Ragit R. Management of laterally luxated primary teeth: a case report. Cureus. 2023;15(2):e35218.
23. Cunha RF, Delbem AC, de Mello Vieira AE, Pugliesi DM. Treatment of a severe dental lateral luxation associated with extrusion in an 8-month-old baby: a conservative approach. Dent Traumatol. 2005;21(1):54–6.
24. Holan G. Conservative treatment of severely luxated maxillary primary central incisors: case report. Pediatr Dent. 1999;21:459–62.

25. Faria LV, Chaves HGDS, Silva EAB, Antunes LDS, Antunes LAA. Minimally invasive treatment of an extruded deciduous tooth-case report. Dent Traumatol. 2019;36:303–6.
26. Di Giorgio G, Zumbo G, Saccucci M, Luzzi V, Ierardo G, Biagi R, Bossù M. Root fracture and extrusive luxation in primary teeth and their management: a case report. Dent J (Basel). 2021;9(9):107.
27. Gurunathan D, Murugan M, Somasundaram S. Management and sequelae of intruded anterior primary teeth: a systematic review. Int J Clin Pediatr Dent. 2016;9(3):240–50.
28. Martins-Júnior PA, Franco FA, de Barcelos RV, Marques LS, Ramos-Jorge ML. Replantation of avulsed primary teeth: a systematic review. Int J Paediatr Dent. 2014;24(2):77–83.
29. Holan G. Replantation of avulsed primary incisors: a critical review of a controversial treatment. Dent Traumatol. 2013;29(3):178–84.
30. Andreasen JO, Andreasen FM, Andersson L. Textbook and color atlas of traumatic injuries to the teeth. 5th ed. Copenhagen: Munksgaard; 2011; Chapter 23, Injuries to Developing Teeth. p. 589–624.
31. Lenzi MM, Alexandria AK, Ferreira DM, Maia LC. Does trauma in the primary dentition cause sequelae in permanent successors? A systematic review Dental traumatology. 2015;31(2):79–88.
32. Sandhu M, Gulia S, Nagpal M, Sachdev V. Circular enamel hypoplasia: a rare enamel developmental disturbance in permanent teeth. J Clin Diagn Res. 2014;8(8):ZD39–40.
33. Goswami M, Rahman B, Singh S. Outcomes of luxation injuries to primary teeth-a systematic review. J Oral Biol Craniofac Res. 2020;10(2):227–32.
34. de Amorim LF, Estrela C, da Costa LR. Effects of traumatic dental injuries to primary teeth on permanent teeth–a clinical follow-up study. Dent Traumatol. 2011;27(2):117–21.
35. La Monaca G, Pranno N, Vozza I, Annibali S, Polimeni A, Bossù M, Cristalli MP. Sequelae in permanent teeth after traumatic injuries to primary dentition. Minerva Stomatol. 2019;68(6):332–40.
36. Andreasen JO, Ravin JJ. Enamel changes in permanent teeth after trauma to their primary predecessors. Scand J Dent Res. 1973;81(3):203–9.
37. de Amorim CS, Americano GCA, Moliterno LFM, de Marsillac MWS, Andrade MRTC, Campos V. Frequency of crown and root dilaceration of permanent incisors after dental trauma to their predecessor teeth. Dent Traumatol. 2018;34(6):401–5.

Role of Cone Beam Computed Tomography in Traumatic Dental Injuries

14

14.1 Introduction

Cone Beam Computed Tomography (CBCT) has become an increasingly common investigation tool in Pediatric Dentistry. It is specifically designed to give high-resolution three-dimensional images of oral and maxillofacial structures to aid in diagnosis and treatment planning. It allows precise assessment of the location, extent, and orientation of fractures, resorptive defects, and periapical pathologies following Traumatic Dental Injuries (TDIs). Due to the higher radiation dose compared with conventional periapical imaging, the use of CBCT must be reserved for cases where detailed anatomical information is essential, that cannot be obtained through conventional means.

14.2 What Are the Indications of a CBCT?

Periapical radiographs and Orthopantomogram combined with a thorough clinical examination remain the standard of care and is always a part of the initial evaluation. A conventional radiograph renders a two-dimensional image while a CBCT allows for multiple images in the sagittal, axial, and coronal planes, providing a three-dimensional representation of the area of interest.

The DIMITRA (dentomaxillofacial pediatric imaging: an investigation towards low-dose radiation-induced risks) position statement provides recommendations regarding applications of CBCT in Pediatric Dentistry [1]. The TDIs that benefit from a CBCT in terms of diagnosis and treatment planning are as follows:

- Luxation injuries
- Alveolar fractures
- Impact of tooth displacement to surrounding teeth
- Crown-Root fractures

H. Vyas et al., *Dental Caries and Traumatic Injuries in Pediatric Dentistry*,
https://doi.org/10.1007/978-3-031-98929-2_14

It allows monitoring of healing and detecting complications such as root resorption or thinning of Periodontal Ligament (PDL) space, even in early stages. CBCT is seen to improve the diagnosis of periapical pathologies arising from TDIs compared to conventional radiographs [2–4]. It also plays a critical role in assessing dentoalveolar fractures, maxillary and mandibular fractures and displacements, zygomatic fracture, and temporomandibular joint (TMJ) injuries [1]. In cases of severe orofacial trauma or when young patients require sedation in a hospital setup, advanced imaging modalities such as Magnetic Resonance Imaging (MRI) and Computed Tomography (CT) are better suited for a comprehensive evaluation.

14.3 What Are the Terminologies in CBCT?

The *Field of View (FOV)* refers to the area of interest that is captured by the imaging system during a single scan. Larger FOVs are suitable for capturing larger anatomical regions or multiple structures simultaneously such as jaw fractures or larger pathologies. Smaller FOVs are ideal for focusing on specific areas of interest such as root resorptions or root fractures. Some machines have a fixed FOV while others can change their FOV. The newer CBCT machines can capture smaller FOV (4 × 4cm) for one or two teeth or larger FOV (5 × 5 cm, 8 × 5 cm, 10 × 5 cm, 10 × 8 cm or the entire face) depending on the area to be evaluated.

The *resolution* depends on the indication of the CBCT and must be communicated with the radiologist before taking the image. A high resolution means a higher radiation dose as there will be an increase in the exposure time. A high-resolution image is indicated for detection of initial resorptive defects or for endodontic purposes while a low-resolution image is sufficient for cysts or impacted teeth.

The final image is built of *voxels*, the size of which is inversely proportional to the resolution of the image. A high-resolution image will be made of smaller voxels.

A CBCT shows images in three reference planes. *Axial section* is obtained in a horizontal plane, parallel to the ground. These slices provide a cross-sectional view of the scanned area, with structures appearing as they would if you were looking from the top down (Fig. 14.1).

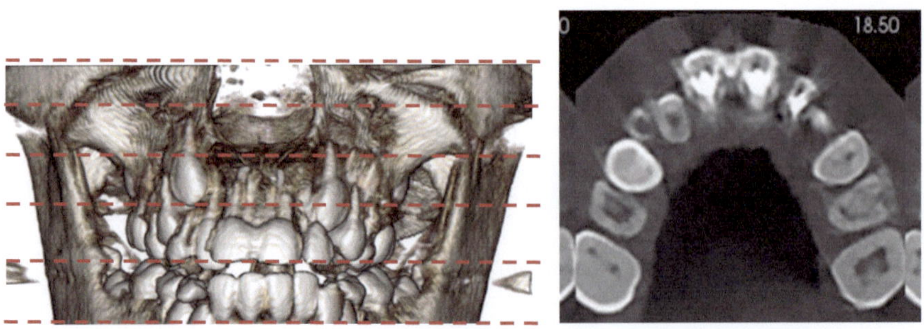

Fig. 14.1 The dotted lines moving from top to bottom reveal sections in the axial plane

Sagittal section is obtained in a vertical plane, from the patient's right to left or vice versa. These slices provide a lateral view, allowing for the evaluation of structures from the side. For the anterior teeth, a sagittal view will reveal the pathology in the buccolingual plane, whereas for posterior teeth, a sagittal view will reveal the pathology in a mesio-distal plane, similar to a periapical radiograph (Fig. 14.2).

Coronal section is also obtained in a vertical plane, providing a front to back view of the scanned area. These slices are useful for assessing the anatomy mesio-distally, similar to a periapical radiograph for anterior teeth. For posterior teeth, a coronal slice reveals the tooth and surrounding structures in a buccolingual view (Fig. 14.3).

A *volume renderer* stacks images in all three planes (axial, coronal and sagittal) to reconstruct a three-dimensional image that can be assessed by the operator (Fig. 14.4).

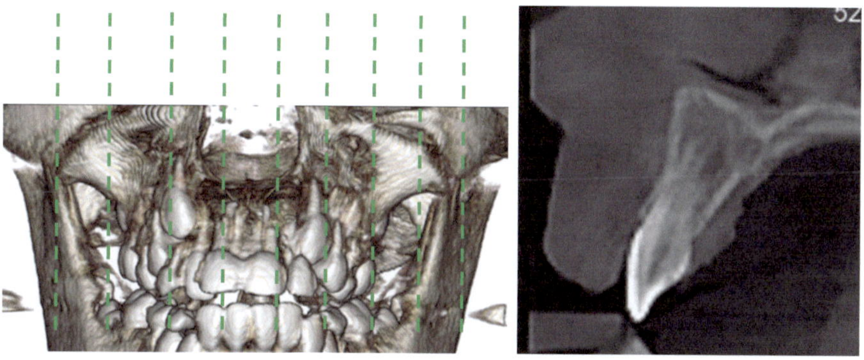

Fig. 14.2 The dotted lines moving from right to left or vice versa reveal sections in the sagittal plane

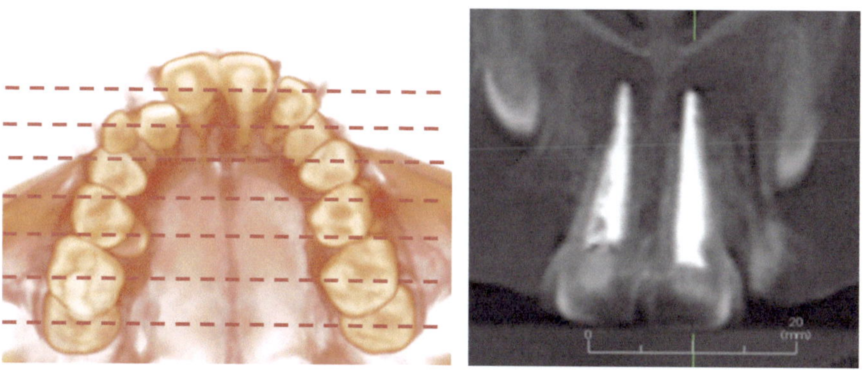

Fig. 14.3 The dotted lines moving from front to back reveal sections in the coronal plane

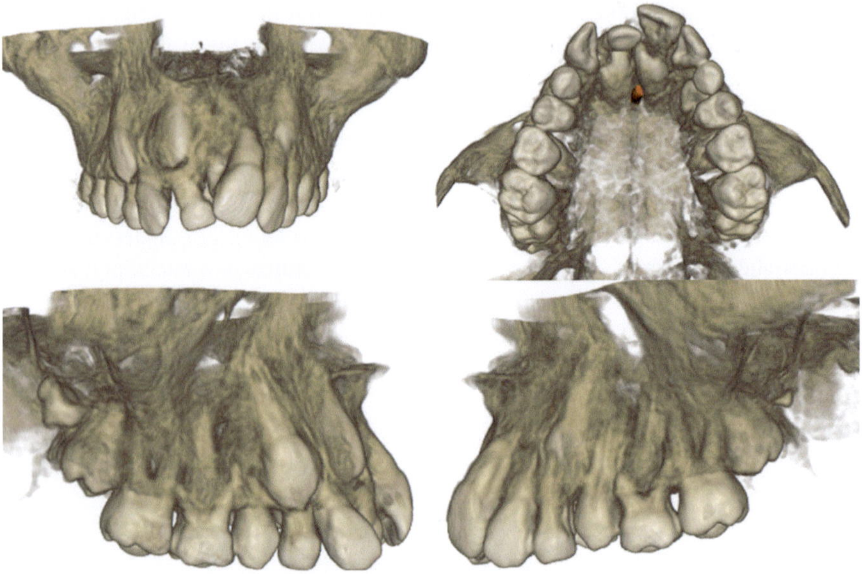

Fig. 14.4 Reconstructed three-dimensional image showing an impacted maxillary permanent right central incisor and presence of a mesiodens

14.4 How to Prescribe a CBCT?

Prepare a written prescription for the CBCT scan including essential information such as:

- Name and age of the patient.
- Clinical and radiographic indication for the scan: This should include patient history, signs and symptoms, radiographic images, and findings of the suspected pathology.
- Specific anatomical region or structures to be imaged.
- Desired FOV: Operators must select an appropriate FOV based on the indication and the size and location of the area of interest. For studying a smaller lesion or pathology (root resorption), a smaller FOV should be prescribed. Any additional instructions or preferences such as contrast enhancement or specific

reconstruction images must be noted in the prescription. After the CBCT, the images can be reviewed on hard copies or soft copies which may have a volume renderer if requested.

14.5 How to Read a CBCT?

A CBCT report begins with the volume renderer or the three- dimensional image of the scanned area. The software allows for the reconstruction of three-dimensional images from the acquired cross sections. These images provide a holistic view of the anatomy, offering a better understanding of the spatial relationships between structures (Fig. 14.4).

The report will show views (sagittal, axial, or coronal) of the scanned area which has multiple lines that are numbered. The distance between these numbers can be changed to get thicker or thinner sections. This allows users to navigate through the volume and locate specific sections with ease. When the report gives an overview in sagittal and coronal orientation, the sections shown are always in the third dimension, that is, in the axial plane. Similarly, an overview in axial and sagittal orientation will show sections in the coronal plane (Figs. 14.5, 14.6, 14.7, 14.8, 14.9, and 14.10).

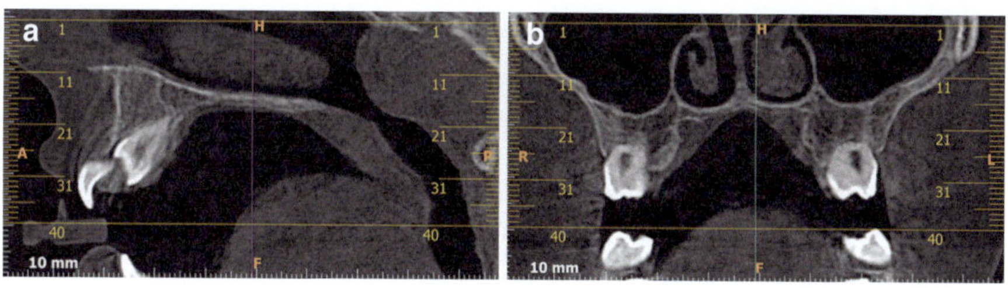

Fig. 14.5 The sagittal (**a**) and coronal views (**b**) show sections that are numbered between 1 and 40. Each number corresponds to an axial cross section

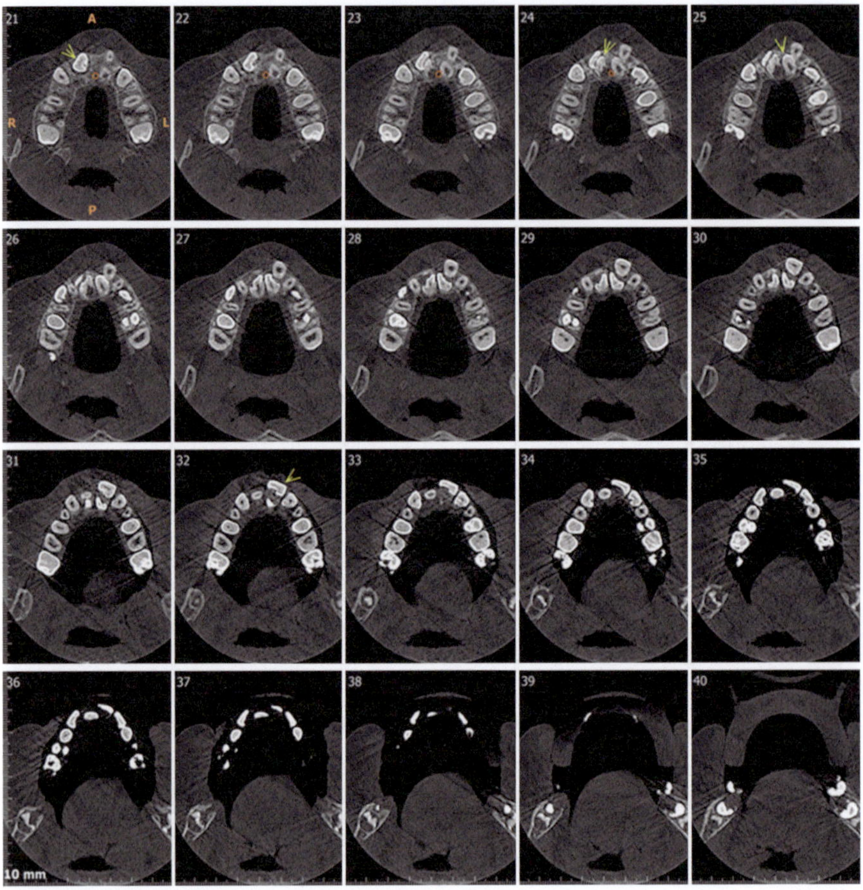

Fig. 14.6 The axial sections between 21 and 40 show pathology marked in yellow and clinical landmarks in orange

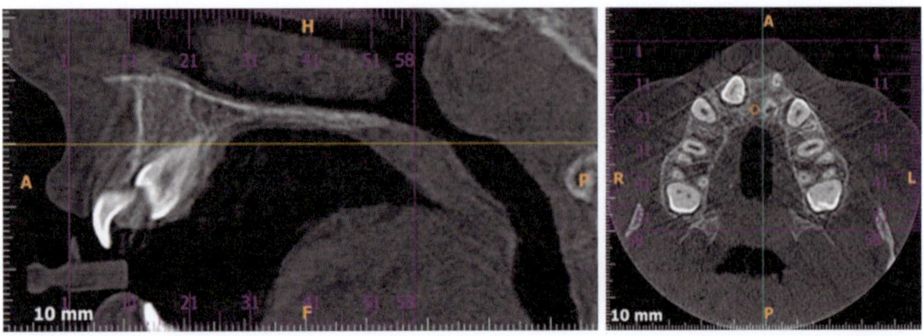

Fig. 14.7 The sagittal and axial views have slices numbered from 1 to 58. Each number corresponds to a coronal section. The area between 6 and 20 is where the pathology is located

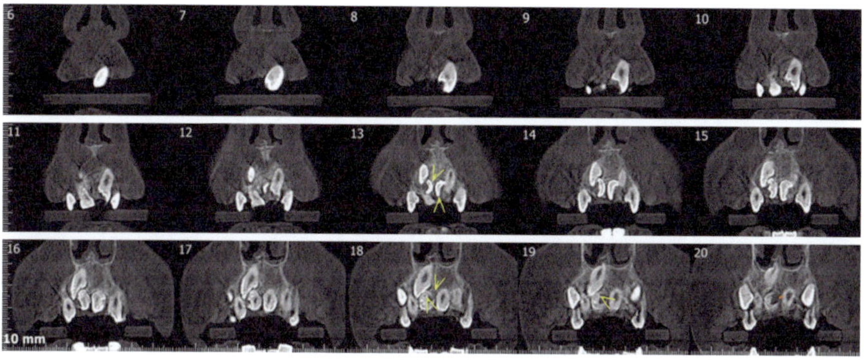

Fig. 14.8 The coronal sections between 6 and 20 show pathology marked in yellow and clinical landmarks in orange

Fig. 14.9 The axial view of the scanned maxilla has sections numbered from 1 to 106. For example, on the right side posteriorly, the scan will give coronal sections up to the curvature of the arch (numbers 1–31). The scan will reveal oblique sections (numbers 31–41) and moving ahead to the anterior maxilla, the scan will show sagittal sections (numbers 41–71). Similarly, the left side will show oblique sections (numbers 71–81) and coronal sections (numbers 81–106). The area 51 and 75 is where the pathology is located

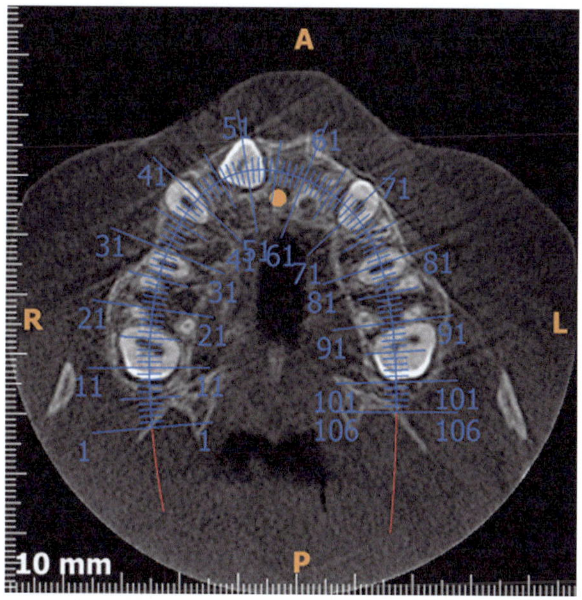

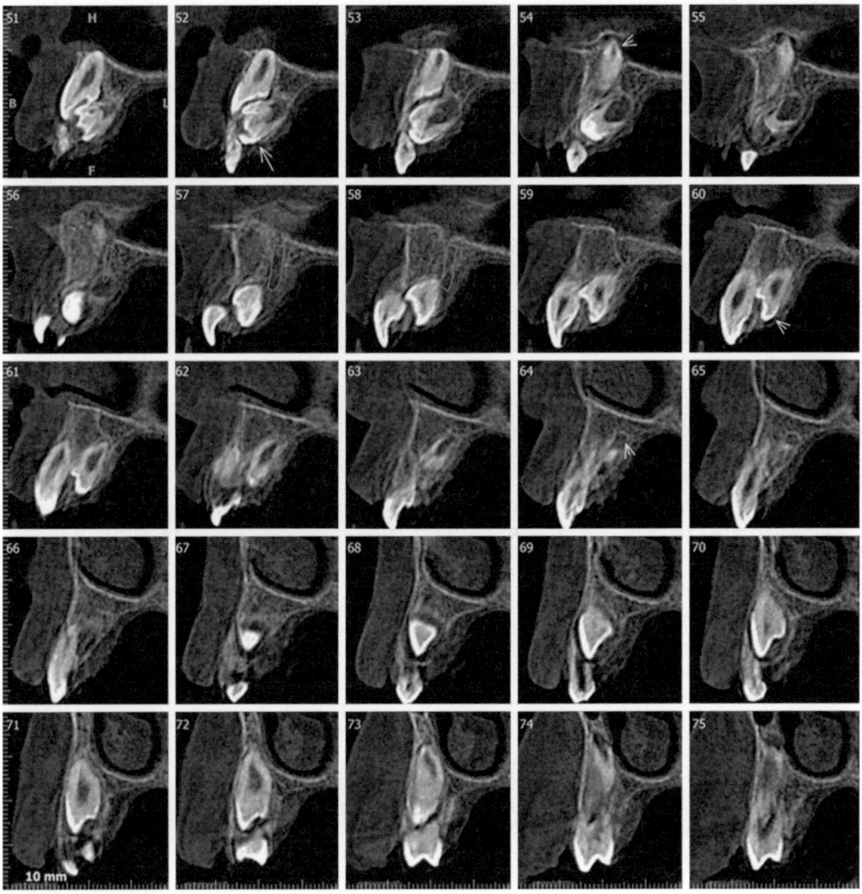

Fig. 14.10 The sagittal sections between 52 and 60 show pathology marked in yellow and clinical landmarks in orange

14.6 Reading CBCT in Traumatic Dental Injuries

14.6.1 Crown-Root Fractures and Root Fractures

The International Association of Dental Traumatology (IADT) recommends taking three intraoral radiographs to detect crown-root fractures or root fractures. The detection of root fracture depends on the separation between the fractured segments, direction of the fracture line, and angulation of the X-ray beam [5]. The fracture line is detected on the radiograph only if the X-ray beam passes through it. On a periapical radiograph of an anterior tooth, the root fracture may appear as a horizontal or an ellipsoidal line (Fig. 14.11a, b) [6]. A coronal cross section on

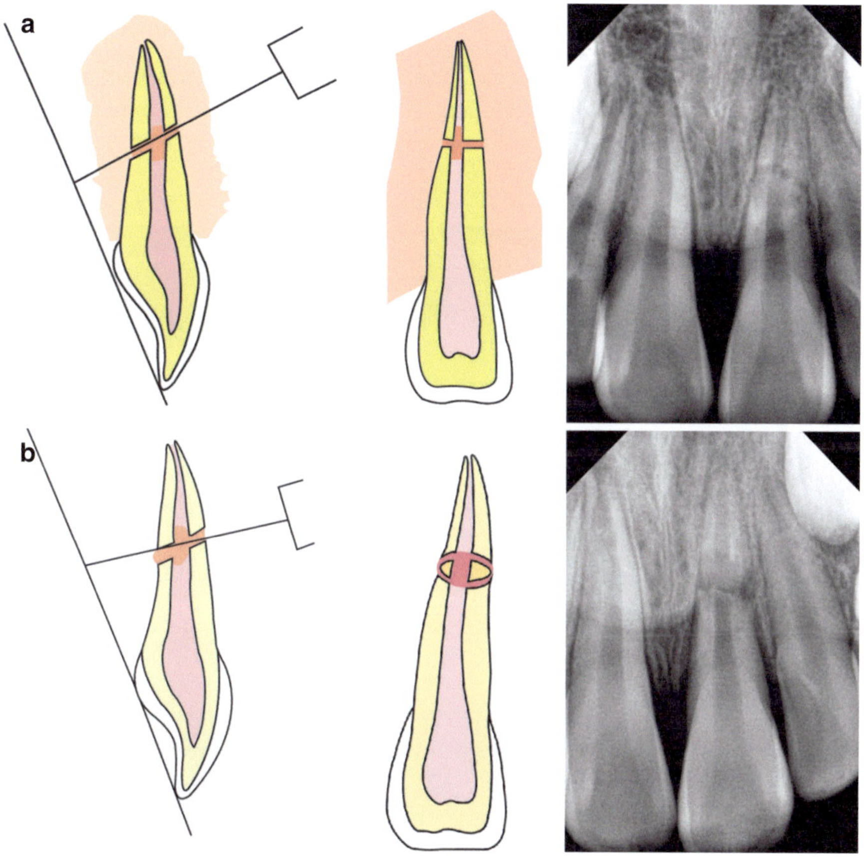

Fig. 14.11 Fracture line appears horizontal when the X-ray beam is parallel to the plane of fracture (**a**). An angulated beam will appear as an ellipsoid on the radiograph (**b**)

a CBCT will show a similar fracture line as seen on the periapical radiograph. A sagittal cross section will reveal the oblique extension of the fracture in the bucco-lingual dimension (Fig. 14.15). *As the treatment of apical and middle third root fractures in permanent anterior teeth usually do not require active intervention, prescribing a CBCT is not likely to change the treatment course.*

However, for crown-root fractures, prescribing a CBCT for diagnosis is going to influence the treatment plan. The treatment of a crown-root fracture depends on the apical extent of the fracture line that is captured on the sagittal section of the CBCT [5, 6]. This is not possible to read on a conventional radiograph.

- *Case*

Patient reported with a complicated crown-root fracture in permanent maxillary left central incisor, 9 months after injury. A CBCT was advised as the radiograph did not reveal the extent of fracture line (Figs. 14.12, 14.13, 14.14, 14.15, and 14.16).

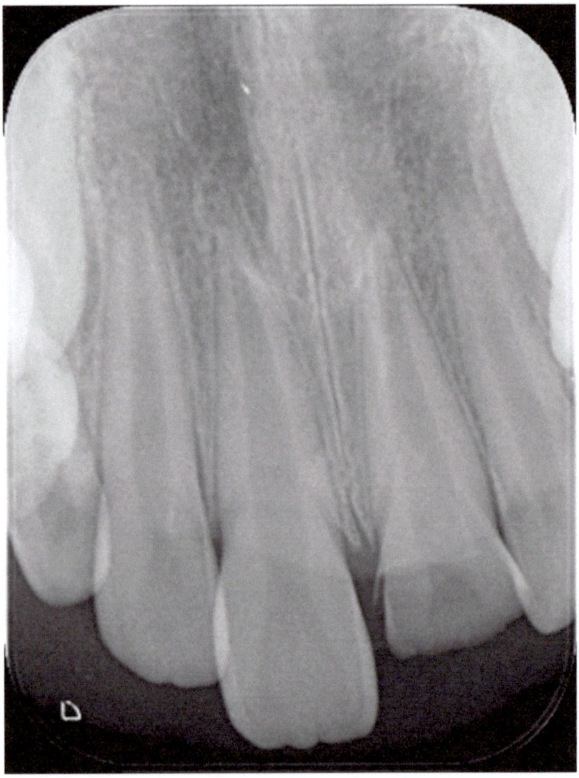

Fig. 14.12 Crown root fracture of maxillary left central incisor

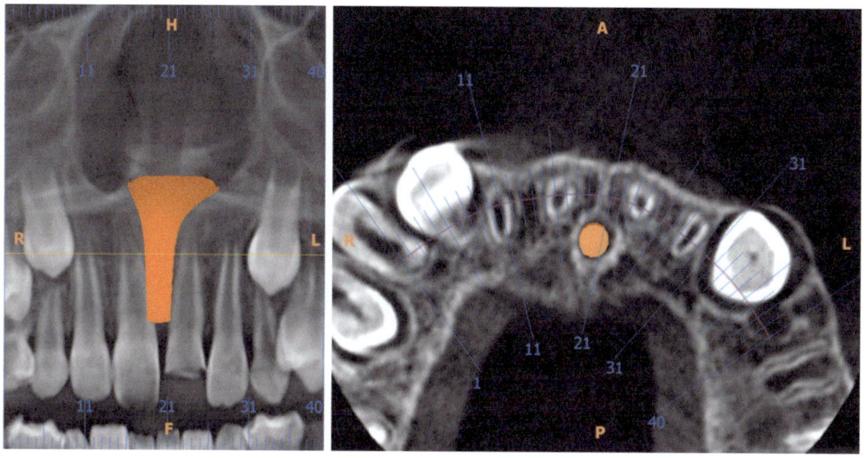

Fig. 14.13 The coronal and axial views have sections numbered from 1 to 40. The area between 20 and 30 is where the traumatized tooth is located. These slices will show the sagittal cross sections of the tooth

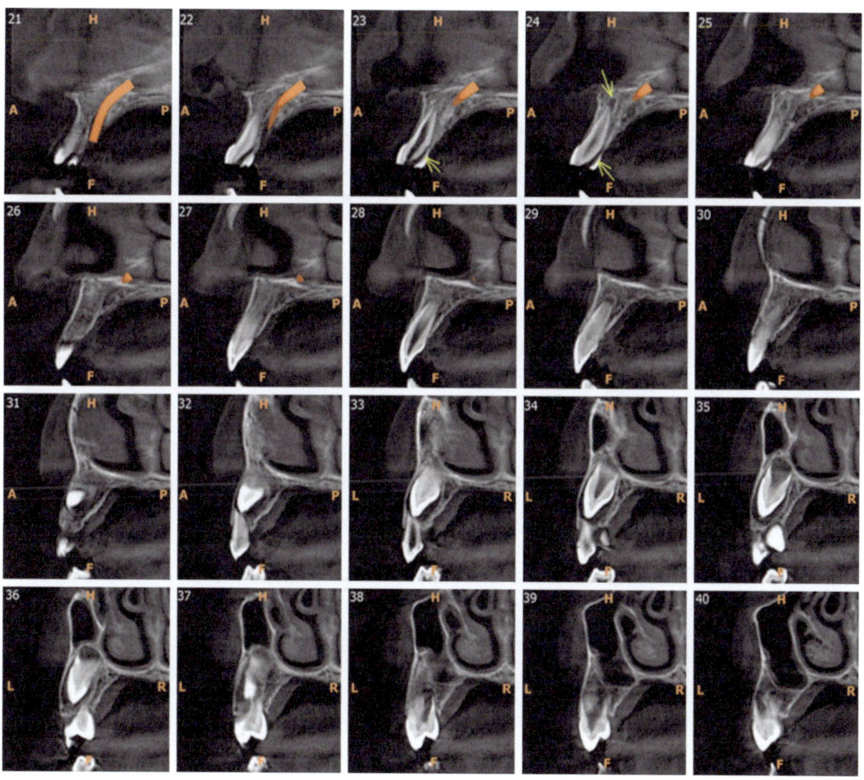

Fig. 14.14 The sagittal sections between 21 and 25 reveal the fracture line

Fig. 14.15 A close-up of section number 24 reveals the apical extent of the fracture line at the level of alveolar crest and apical radiolucency suggestive of periapical pathology. This information helps the clinician decide the course of treatment

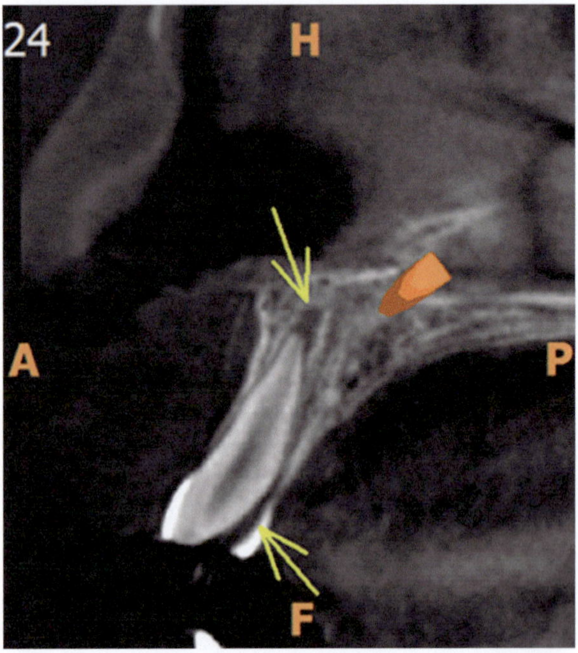

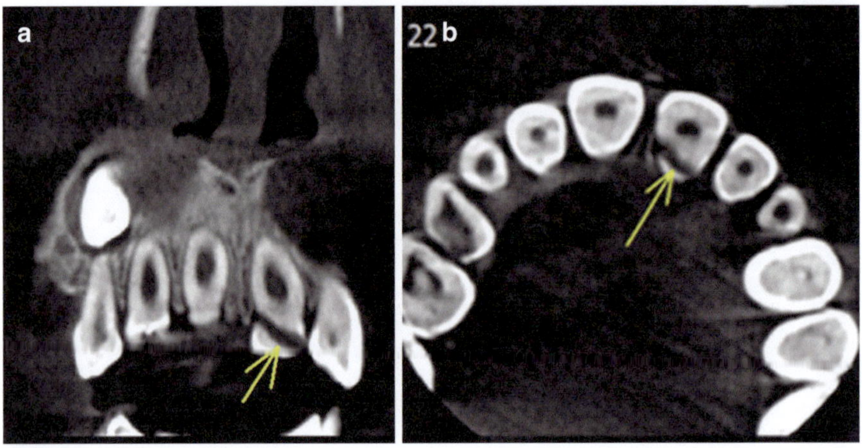

Fig. 14.16 While the coronal (**a**) and axial sections (**b**) reveal the fracture line and are given in the report, the apical extent of a crown root fracture which determines the course of treatment is best viewed on the sagittal section

14.6.2 CBCT in Luxation Injuries

In lateral luxation injury, the crown is usually displaced lingually or palatally and the apical third is displaced buccally. On a periapical radiograph, the luxated tooth will appear elongated or foreshortened compared to its adjacent teeth. The coronal cross section of the tooth on the CBCT will provide a view similar to that of a periapical radiograph. As the movements are mostly in the buccolingual plane, the axial and the sagittal slices of the CBCT will best reveal the labiolingual displacement of the tooth and a breach in the cortical plate, if any. A volume renderer will provide a three-dimensional view of the displacement or locking of the root tip through the alveolar plate [7].

- *Case*

Child reported with history of trauma 2 months ago. Parent gives history of avulsion of maxillary primary central incisor. On clinical and radiographic examination, the maxillary primary right central and lateral incisors were missing. A CBCT was advised as a tooth-like structure was palpable deep in the vestibular region of maxillary right canine, which was not captured on the radiograph (Figs. 14.17, 14.18, 14.19, 14.20, 14.21, 14.22, 14.23, 14.24, and 14.25).

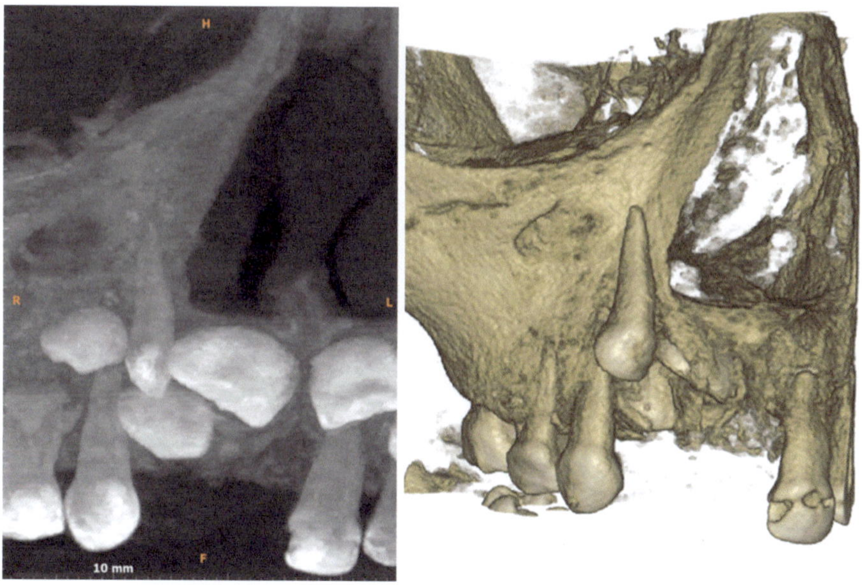

Fig. 14.17 The volume renderer shows severe intrusion of the maxillary primary right lateral incisor into the canine space

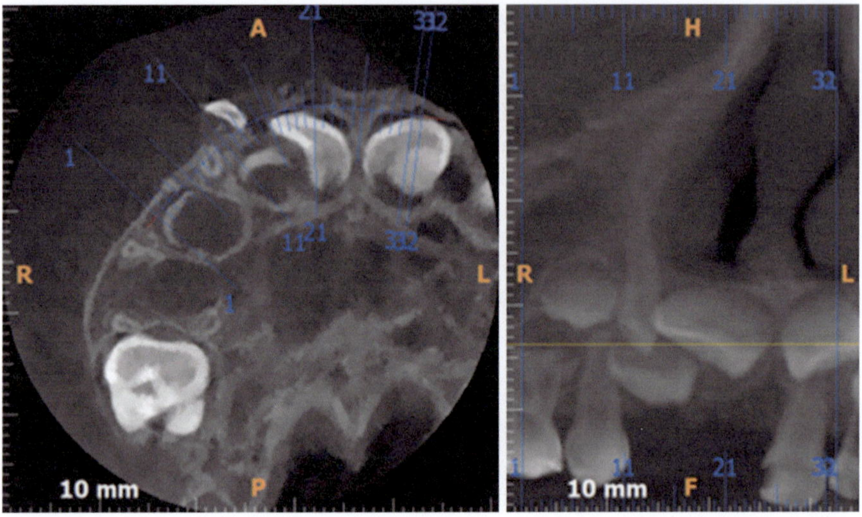

Fig. 14.18 The axial and coronal views have sections numbered from 1 to 32. The area between slices 10 and 20 is where the intruded lateral incisor is located. These slices will show the oblique sagittal cross sections of the tooth

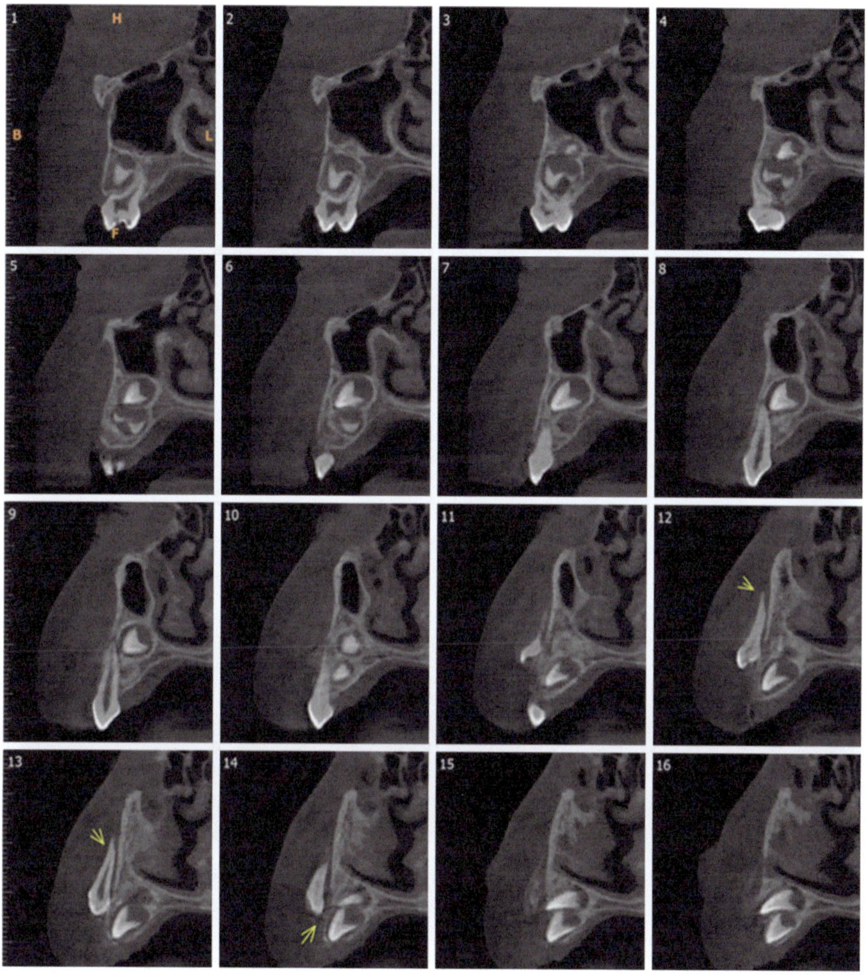

Fig. 14.19 The sagittal sections between 11 and 14 reveal the intruded tooth

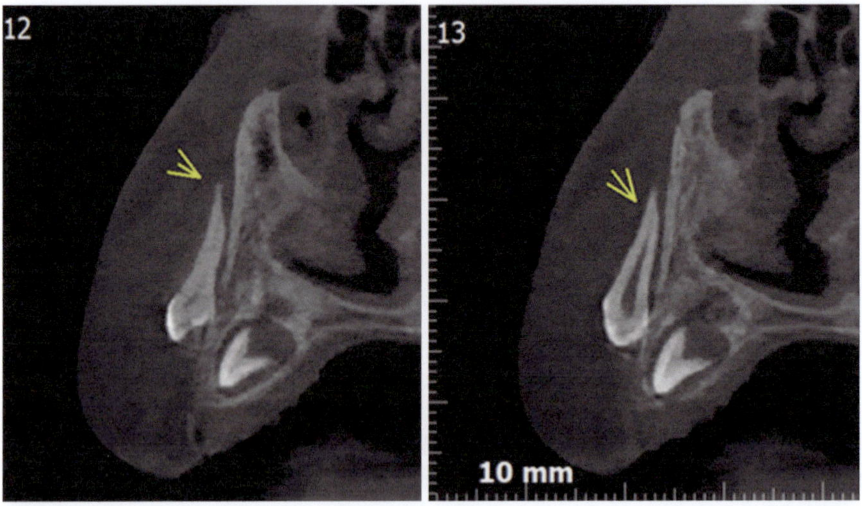

Fig. 14.20 The sections 12 and 13 reveal the proximity of the intruded tooth to the labial cortical plate and relation to the succedaneous tooth

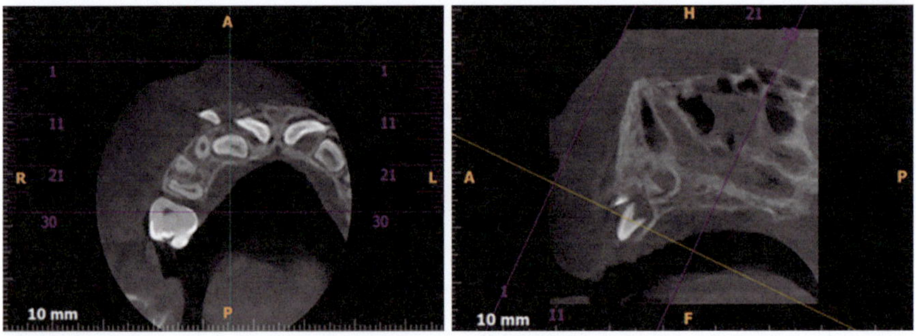

Fig. 14.21 The axial and sagittal views have sections numbered from 1 to 30. The area between slices 5 and 15 is where the intruded lateral incisor is located. These slices will show the coronal cross sections of the tooth

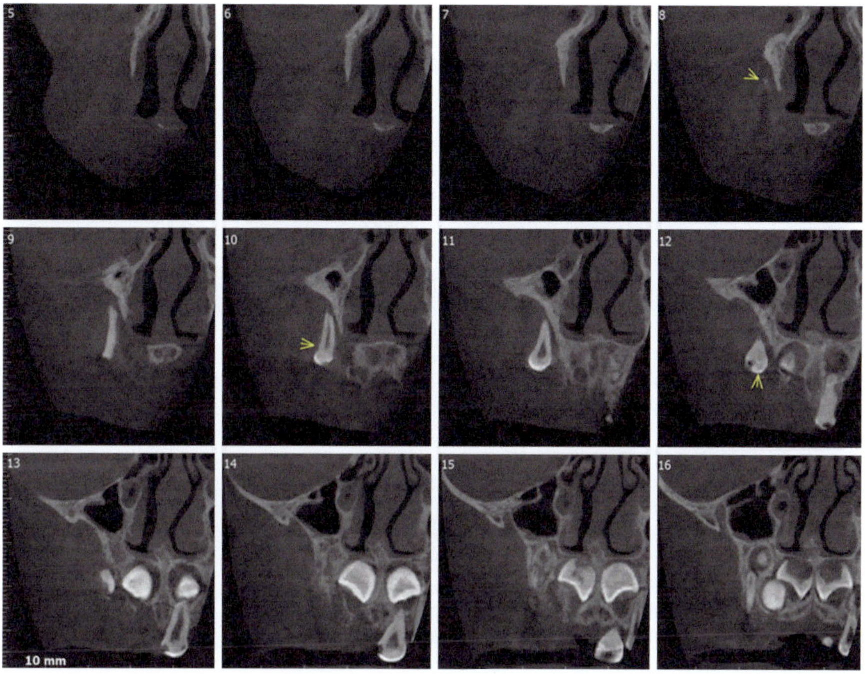

Fig. 14.22 The coronal sections between 9 and 12 reveal intruded tooth

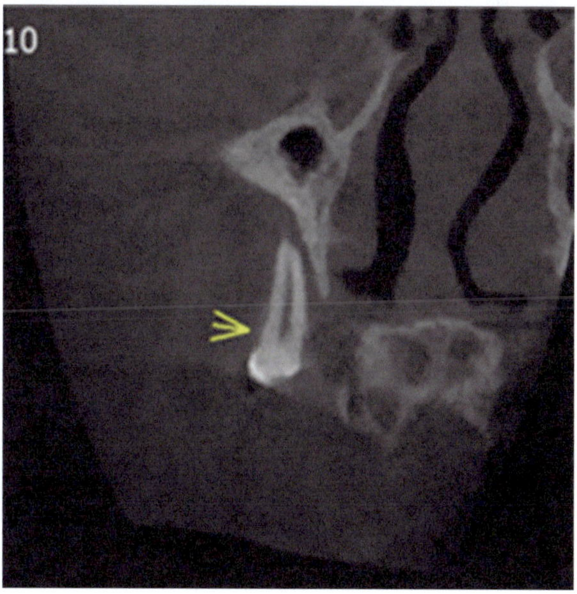

Fig. 14.23 The section 10 reveals the relation of the intruded tooth with the floor and lateral wall of the nasal cavity

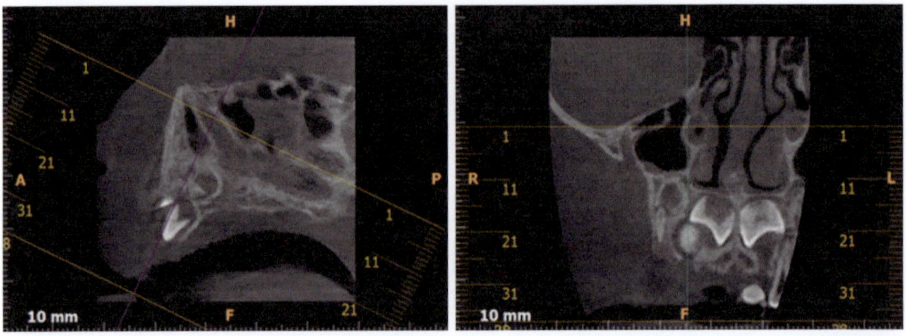

Fig. 14.24 The sagittal and coronal views have sections numbered from 1 to 31. The area between slices 11 and 20 is where the intruded lateral incisor is located. These slices will show the axial cross sections of the tooth

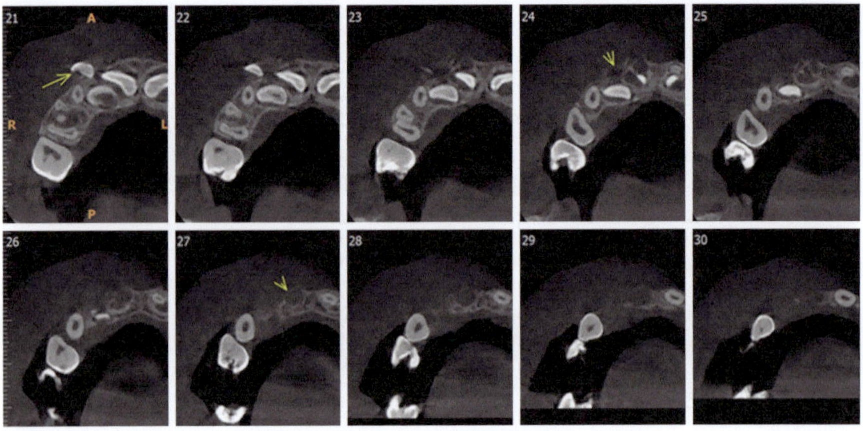

Fig. 14.25 Sections 21 and 24 show the labio-lingual relation of the tooth with the surrounding structures

14.6.3 CBCT in Root Resorption

CBCT allows to take a clear view of root resorption, quantifies the lesion and its relation to the surrounding bone. While resorption on the mesial and distal surfaces of the root may be seen on the periapical radiograph, it does not reveal resorption on the labial surface. Resorption on the labial or palatal root surfaces can be seen in the sagittal cross section of a CBCT. When early signs of resorption are suspected, the clinician must inform the CBCT provider, the area of interest that will require a smaller FOV and a high-resolution image [8, 9].

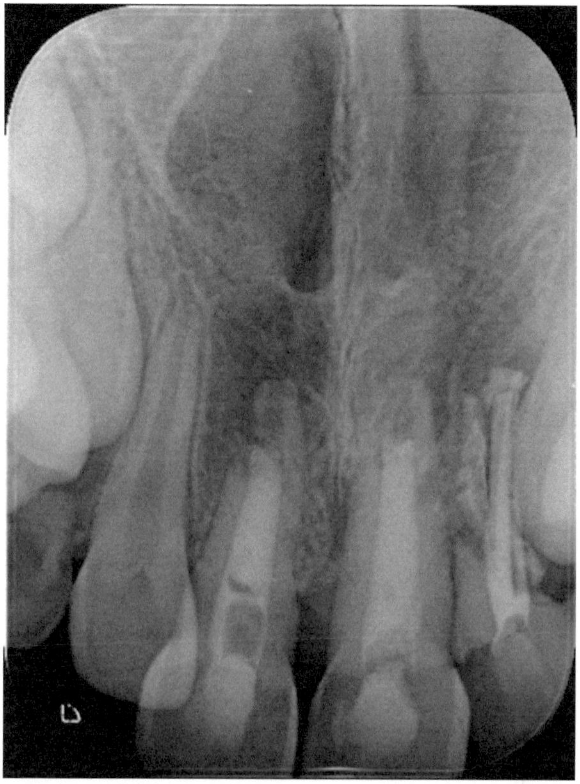

Fig. 14.26 Radiographs of permanent maxillary central incisors showing external inflammatory root resorption

Patient reported 1 year after replantation of avulsed maxillary permanent central incisors and left lateral incisor. The teeth had been repositioned, splinted, and treated endodontically at the time of trauma at another center. Severe external inflammatory root resorption was seen in relation to the endodontically treated teeth on the radiograph (Fig. 14.26). A CBCT was advised to determine the areas of pathology (Figs. 14.27, 14.28, 14.29, 14.30, 14.31, 14.32, 14.33, and 14.34).

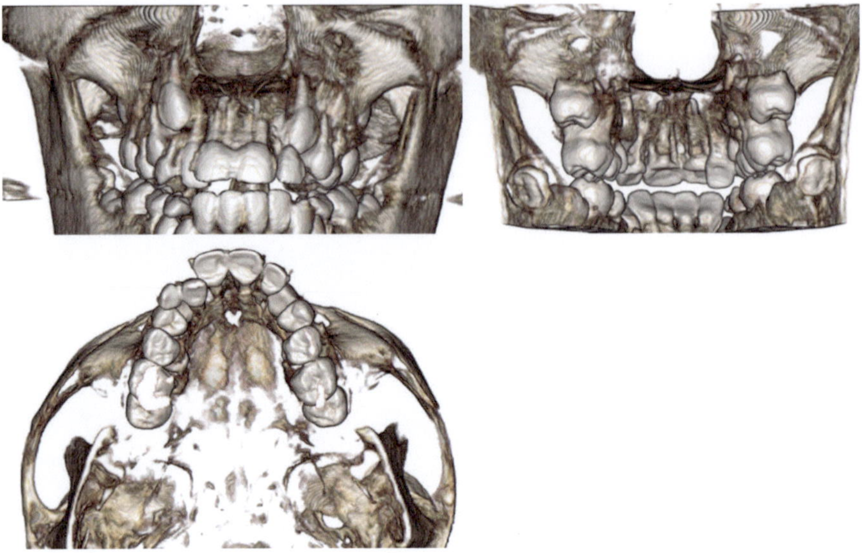

Fig. 14.27 Reconstructed three-dimensional image of the scanned area when seen from front (labial view), inside (palatal view), and top (axial view)

Fig. 14.28 CBCT of full maxillary arch was taken. The blue lines indicate the sections numbered from 0 to 120. The slices between 40 and 60 (green lines) show oblique to sagittal sections of the area of pathology on patient's right

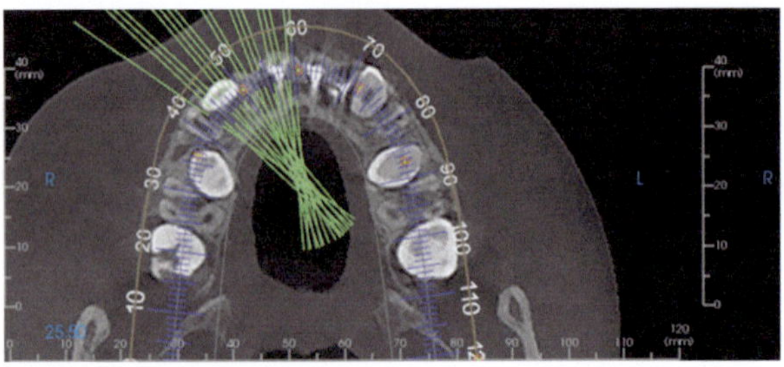

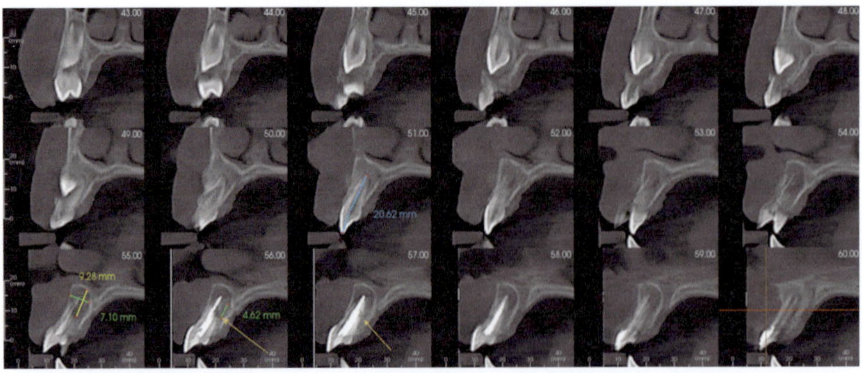

Fig. 14.29 The sagittal sections between 55 and 59 reveal the periapical lesion

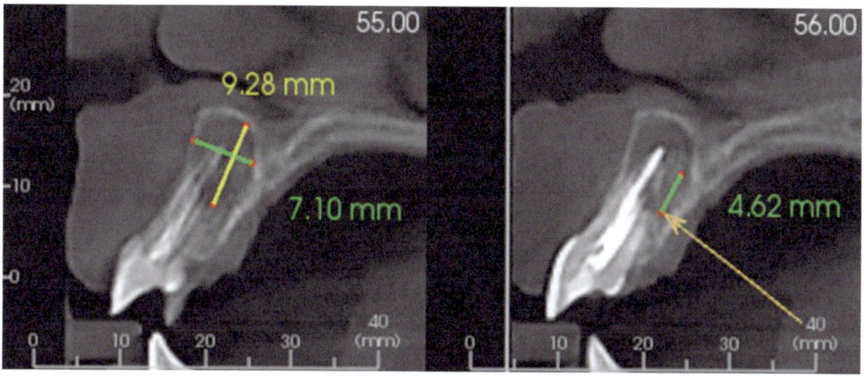

Fig. 14.30 Sagittal sections 55 and 56 measure the extent of external inflammatory root resorption in cervico-apical and labiopalatal aspect of right central incisor

Fig. 14.31 The area between 60 and 75 (green lines) shows oblique to sagittal sections of the area of pathology on patient's left

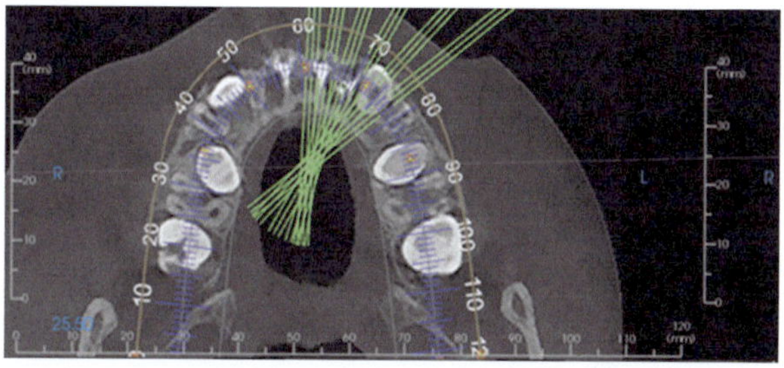

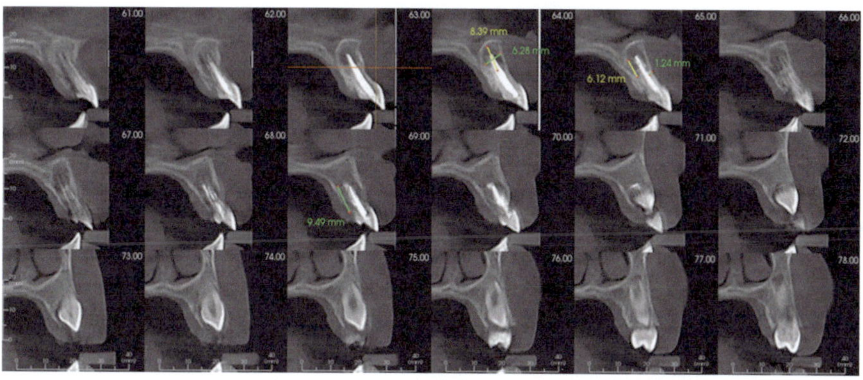

Fig. 14.32 The sagittal sections between 63 and 64 reveal the periapical lesion

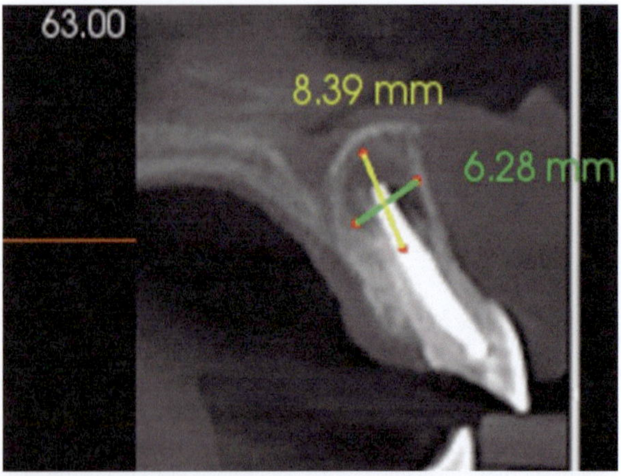

Fig. 14.33 Sagittal section 63 shows the extent of root resorption in the cervico-apical and labiopalatal aspect of left central incisor

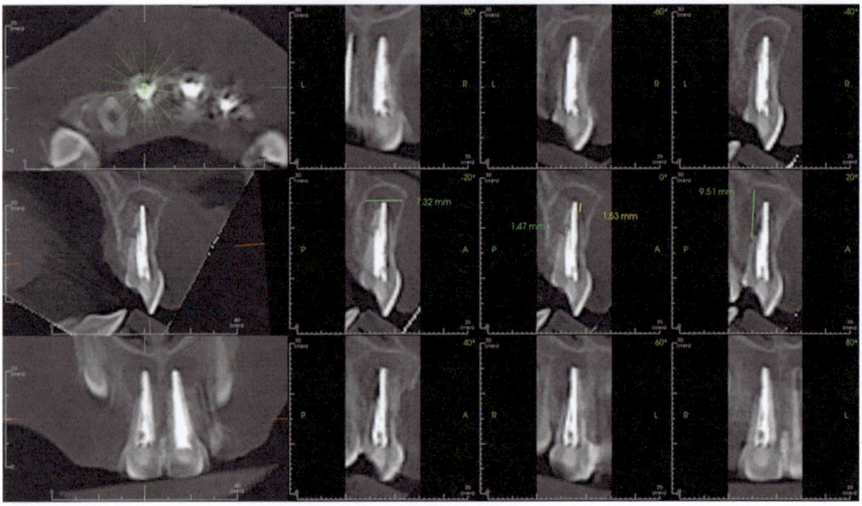

Fig. 14.34 A 360° scan of the central incisors. The images show cross sections in coronal and sagittal plane

14.6.4 Traumatic Dental Injuries Sequelae to Permanent Dentition

The sequelae of TDI in permanent teeth can range from minor manifestations, such as enamel opacities, to more severe outcomes like arrested tooth development. The variability in sequelae depends on the severity of trauma to the primary teeth or the maxillofacial region and the age at which the trauma occurred. CBCT enables detailed assessment of the nature, extent, and location of aberrant development, thereby aiding in planning of interventions, particularly in severe cases.

- *Case*

Delayed eruption of maxillary permanent central incisors at age 9. Patient gives a history of avulsion of maxillary primary incisors when he was 18 months old. Radiograph taken at first visit shows malformed central incisors and left lateral incisor. Odontom-like structures were seen overlying the left central and lateral incisors. A CBCT of the maxilla was advised (Figs. 14.35, 14.36, 14.37, 14.38, 14.39, and 14.40).

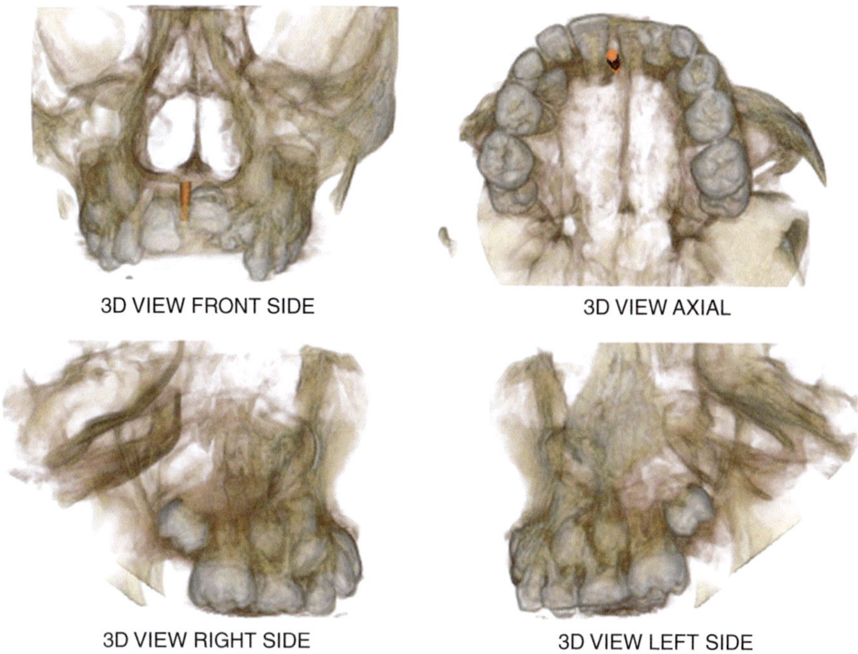

Fig. 14.35 The three-dimensional view shows the maxillary right central incisor on path of eruption in front view. The position of the left central incisor is below that of the right central incisor. Complex odontome suspected on the left lateral incisor as seen in front and axial views

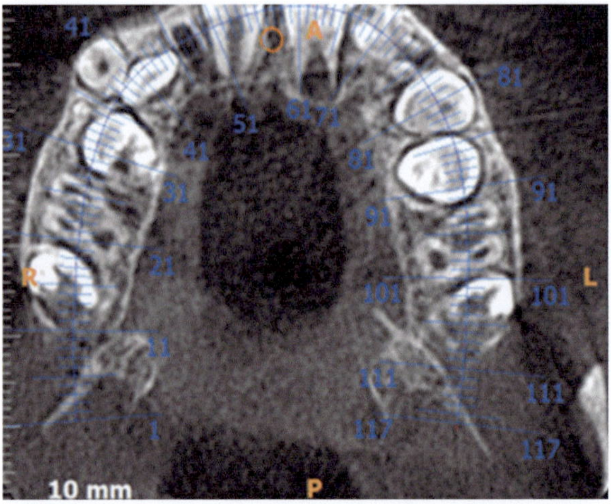

Fig. 14.36 The maxillary arch is divided into multiple sections between 1 and 117. The area of pathology is between 40 and 70

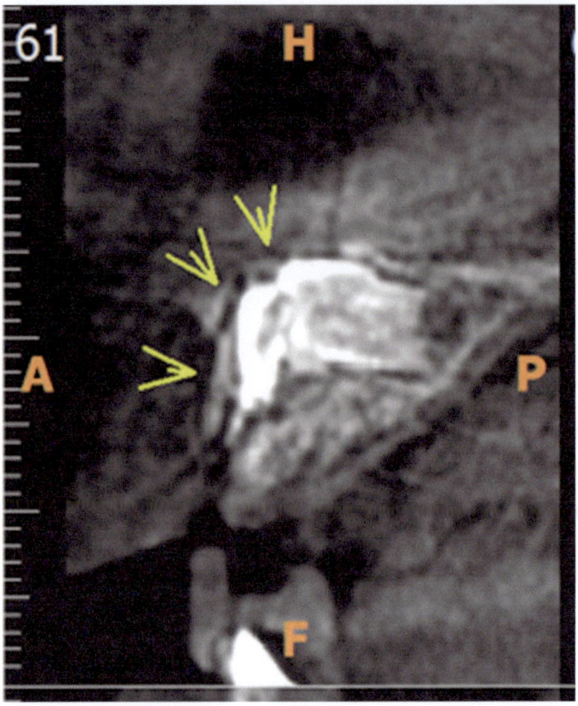

Fig. 14.37 Section 61 is in sagittal plane showing complex tooth like structures suggestive of odontome, placed labially in the region of left central and lateral incisors

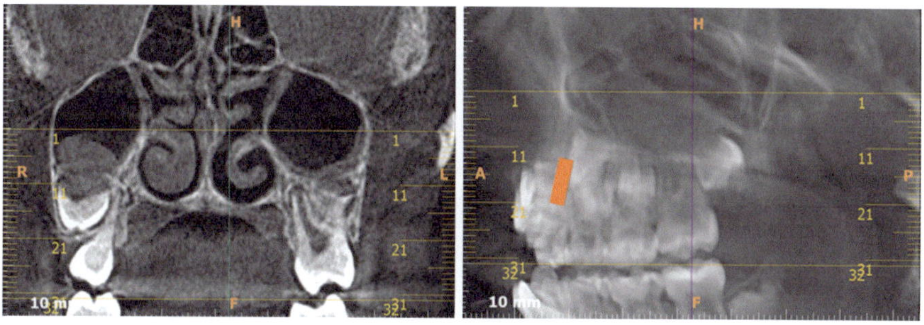

Fig. 14.38 The coronal and sagittal views have sections numbered from 1 to 32. The area between slices 15 and 25 is where the odontome is located. These slices will show the axial cross sections of the tooth

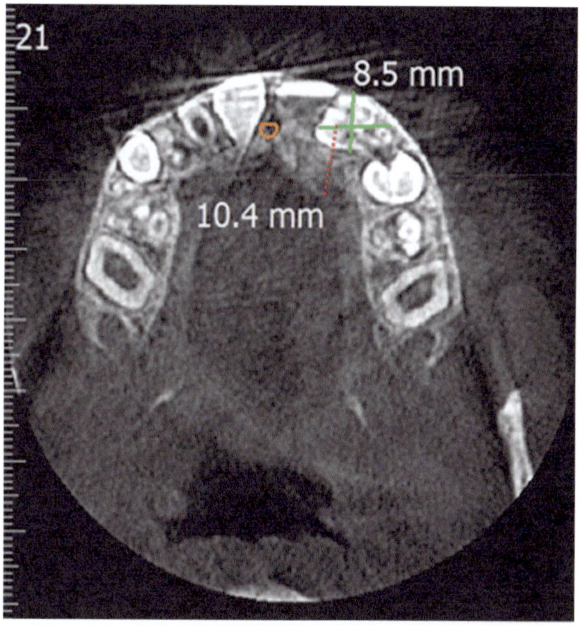

Fig. 14.39 Axial section number 21 shows the odontome in labiopalatal plane. The approximate size of the lesion is marked in this axial section

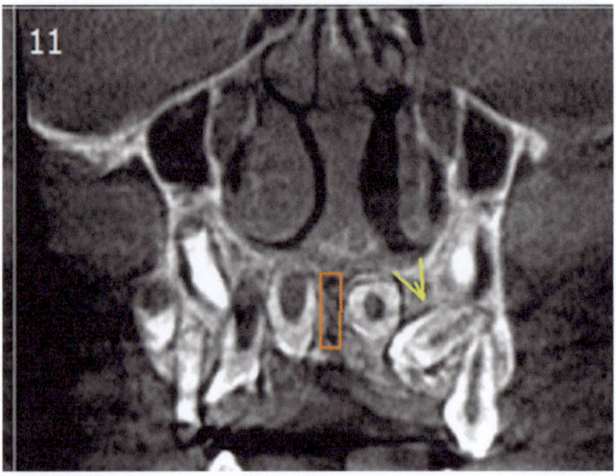

Fig. 14.40 The coronal cross section shows the mesiodistal position of the odontome and the relation with surrounding structures

14.7 Concluding Remarks

Cone Beam Computed Tomography (CBCT) has significantly advanced the diagnostic and treatment capabilities in Traumatic Dental Injuries. By providing three-dimensional imaging with precise anatomical detail, CBCT aids in detection of crown-root fractures, displacements, and root resorptions that may otherwise go unnoticed on conventional radiographs. However, its application must be judicious, particularly in children balancing the diagnostic benefit against the increased radiation. Patient selection according to age and cooperation, communicating the area of interest and findings of suspected pathology is essential for maximizing diagnostic yield while minimizing exposure. It is important to understand when and how to prescribe a CBCT to facilitate accurate diagnosis, provide evidence-based care, and patient safety in the management of Traumatic Dental Injury.

References

1. Oenning AC, Jacobs R, Pauwels R, Stratis A, Hedesiu M, Salmon B, on behalf of DIMITRA Research Group (http://www.dimitra.be). Cone-beam CT in pediatric dentistry: DIMITRA project position statement. Pediatr Radiol. 2018;48:308–16.
2. Cohenca N, Silberman A. Contemporary imaging for the diagnosis and treatment of traumatic dental injuries: a review. Dent Traumatol. 2017;33(5):321–8.
3. Patel S, Puri T, Mannocci F, Navai A. Diagnosis and management of traumatic dental injuries using intraoral radiography and cone-beam computed tomography: an in vivo investigation. J Endodont. 2021;47(6):914–23.
4. Sha X, Jin L, Han J, Li Y, Zhang L, Qi S. Comparison between periapical radiography and cone beam computed tomography for the diagnosis of anterior maxillary trauma in children and adolescents. Dent Traumatol. 2022;38(1):62–70.
5. Bourguignon C, Cohenca N, Lauridsen E, Flores MT, O'Connell AC, Day PF, Tsilingaridis G, Abbott PV, Fouad AF, Hicks L, Andreasen JO. International Association of Dental

Traumatology guidelines for the management of traumatic dental injuries: 1. Fractures and luxations. Dent Traumatol. 2020;36(4):314–30.
6. May JJ, Cohenca N, Peters OA. Contemporary management of horizontal root fractures to the permanent dentition: diagnosis–radiologic assessment to include cone-beam computed tomography. J Endodont. 2013;39(3 Suppl):S20–5.
7. Soares PB, Vilela AB, Moura CC, Estrela C, Bueno MR, Soares CJ. Lateral luxation of incisor-a case report of using a new cone-beam computed tomography software and reposition guideline. Braz Dent J. 2020;31:337–43.
8. Shokri A, Mortazavi H, Salemi F, Javadian A, Bakhtiari H, Matlab H. Diagnosis of simulated external root resorption using conventional film radiography, CCD, PSP, and CBCT: a comparison study. Biom J. 2013;36:18–22.
9. Cohenca N, Simon JH, Mathur A, Malfaz JM. Clinical indications for digital imaging in dento-alveolar trauma. Part 2: root resorption. Dent Traumatol. 2007;23:105–13.

Orofacial Trauma: Assessment and Emergency Management by the Pediatric Dentist

15

15.1 Introduction

While oral trauma in children most often affects the dentition, the damage can extend beyond to cause injury to the maxillofacial structures. In children below the age of 5, the midface is in a more retruded position in relation to the protective skull. This anatomical characteristic, the higher elasticity of bone and smaller sinuses contribute to a decreased incidence of midface and mandibular fractures in this age group. The midface becomes prominent with age making older children susceptible to fractures of the mid and lower face. Among mandibular fractures, the condylar region exhibits a higher prevalence, followed by fractures in the symphysis, angle, and body [1–4].

Alveolar bone fractures involve the labial or lingual bone plates of the tooth socket. Complete fractures extend all the way from the buccal to the palatal alveolar bone in the maxilla and from the buccal to the lingual bony surface in the mandible. They commonly occur in the anterior region, but the canine and premolar regions can also be involved. When the fracture line extends to the base of the mandible or maxilla it is defined as a ***jaw fracture*** of the concerned bone. These fractures may or may not involve the alveolar socket. Both ***alveolar bone fractures and jaw fractures*** are routinely associated with injuries to the soft tissues such as lacerations of gingiva, lips, tongue, and floor of the mouth [5, 6].

While alveolar fractures may be treated in a clinical setup, more complex alveolar and jaw fractures require an emergency medical facility. The scope of this chapter is to make the clinician aware of signs and symptoms of maxillofacial trauma to enable identification of the injury, provide initial management and advise appropriate referral.

H. Vyas et al., *Dental Caries and Traumatic Injuries in Pediatric Dentistry*,
https://doi.org/10.1007/978-3-031-98929-2_15

15.2 How Are Jaw Fractures in Children Examined?

First, an extraoral assessment of the patient is performed with special emphasis on assessing the jaw integrity and looking for bruises or edema on the face. Depending on the age of the child, cooperation, and severity of trauma, a detailed examination may need to be performed under sedation.

15.2.1 Extraoral Examination

- **Visual inspection**

A wet gauze soaked in saline is used to clean the face to remove debris and blood clots. An extraoral assessment should begin by examining the face for swelling/edema. Ecchymosis due to bruising must be noted. Any facial asymmetry should raise suspicion for the possibility of a jaw fracture.

- **Mouth opening**

In older children who are conscious and cooperate for initial examination, the mandibular range of motion must be examined on mouth opening and closure. Trismus or deviated mouth opening or difficulty in mouth closure indicates:

(a) Fracture of mandible/maxilla or both jaws
(b) Zygomatic bone
(c) Temporomandibular joint.

- **Palpation**

Gentle palpation should be done over all bony surfaces and temporomandibular joint to identify areas of tenderness, crepitation, and step defects.

(a) Bimanual palpation—The mandible is held such that the index finger of the operator lies on the occlusal surface of the teeth and the thumb on the inferior border of the mandible extraorally. The suspected fractured segment is moved supero-inferiorly and anteroposteriorly to assess mobility [7].
(b) The maxillary bone is held such that the thumb of the operator is in the vestibule and index finger on the palate. The suspected fragments are moved anteroposteriorly and supero-inferiorly to assess mobility.

15.2.2 Intraoral Examination

Intraoral examination must assess derangement of occlusion due to step defects or fractured teeth secondary to alveolar bone or jaw fracture.

(a) Mobility of multiple teeth in one segment indicates a dentoalveolar fracture.
(b) Degloving of gingiva may also be seen associated with a fracture of the alveolar plate.
(c) Ecchymosis in the vestibule along the zygomatic buttress is indicative of a maxillary or zygomatic bone fracture.
(d) A sublingual hematoma is indicative of a mandibular fracture [8].

15.3 What Are the Clinical Signs of Maxillofacial Injuries in Children?

While maxillofacial fractures need radiographic imaging to confirm the diagnosis, many of these fractures have a specific clinical presentation that can provide guidance for appropriate initial management.

15.3.1 Nasal Fractures

Nasal fractures are more commonly seen in slightly older children, where the soft cartilage has been replaced by bone. The presence of a deviated nasal septum, a depressed nasal bridge, and septal hematoma is indicative of a nasal fracture. More complex nasal fractures involve the turbinates or extend to the ethmoid bone or orbital floor. All the above injuries require immediate referral to an Ear Nose Throat (ENT) specialist for further investigations and treatment.

15.3.2 Mandibular Fractures

(a) A retruded chin and sublingual hematoma are indicative of *symphyseal and parasymphyseal fractures* in the canine region.
(b) An elongated face may be the result of *bilateral subcondylar, angle, or body fractures.*
(c) Trismus and deviation on opening may also be a sign *of fracture of the ramus, the coronoid process, and the mandibular condyle.*
(d) Inability to fully close and step deformity may signify *fracture of the dentoalveolar process, angle, ramus, or body of the mandible.*
(e) Temporomandibular joint (TMJ) must be evaluated for tenderness, movement restriction, and crepitus [9].

15.3.3 Maxillary Fractures

- Palatal or vestibular ecchymosis and edema, gingival or mucosal lacerations are seen in maxillary and zygomatic bone fracture.

- Mobility of bony segments on palpation of the maxilla is indicative of dentoalveolar or maxillary fracture.
- Severely luxated teeth are usually associated with fracture of the alveolar process.
- Premature posterior contacts preventing complete mouth closure can be also due to a displaced maxillary fracture [10].

While a complex maxillary fracture with involvement of the zygomatic process and orbital floor would rarely present in a dental clinic, any child showing the following symptoms should be referred to the emergency room.

15.3.4 Signs of Complex Maxillary Fractures

- Epistaxis.
- Orbital and midface ecchymosis.
- Swelling and flattening of the cheek due to fracture of the zygomatic bone.
- Subconjunctival hemorrhage and edema.
- Restricted eye movement, altered globe level, lowering of the pupil level, enophthalmos, reduced visual acuity.
- Pain on ocular movement, diplopia, blurred vision, and sensory abnormalities along the infraorbital nerve distribution.
- Step deformities and tenderness in the orbital rims or upper buccal sulcus.
- Mobility of maxillary bony segments along with the infraorbital rim and nasofrontal suture, or at the frontozygomatic sutures are indicative of more severe fractures.
- Trismus or pain and difficulty in mouth opening [11].

15.4 Radiographic Examination

For suspected alveolar fractures, a panoramic radiograph or a Cone Beam Computed Tomography (CBCT) scan is recommended to locate the fracture line and assess its direction and extent [12, 13]. For facial bone and TMJ fractures, extraoral radiographs advised are as follows:

(a) Orthopantomogram (OPG)
(b) Waters view (Posterior Anterior view for maxillary sinus)
(c) Caldwell view (Posterior Anterior view for frontal and ethmoid sinus)
(d) Lateral oblique view (TMJ, body and ramus of the mandible)
(e) Submentovertex view (Zygomatic arch and mandibular condyles)

Most children who have incurred maxillofacial injuries require sedation for investigations and treatment. They report to the emergency room in hospitals where advanced imaging techniques such as Computed Tomography (CT) and Magnetic Resonance Imaging (MRI) that possess a better diagnostic value are advised as a standard of care.

15.5 Management

The role of a Pediatric Dentist in maxillofacial injuries is to make a provisional diagnosis and perform emergency treatment if required. While certain injuries to the dentoalveolar process can be managed by the Pediatric Dentist, more severe maxillofacial injuries are best managed by an Oral and Maxillofacial surgeon, ENT surgeon, or Plastic surgeon. It is important for the clinician to have a basic understanding of the probable treatment to address the concerns of the anxious parents.

15.5.1 How Are Dentoalveolar Fractures Managed?

- In case where multiple teeth in a segment are mobile, and the fracture is limited to the dentoalveolar process, the alveolar bone must be repositioned back into its original anatomic position.
- Local anesthesia should be administered prior to repositioning. Repositioning may be performed under sedation based on the cooperation of the patient.
- Position yourself behind the patient and place your thumb intraorally at the apical part of the teeth/bone fractured unit and the index finger on the incisal or occlusal surface of the teeth (Fig. 15.1).
- On each side of the displaced segment, apply simultaneous bimanual downward and lingual pressure to disengage the apices from the labial plate allowing vertical seating of the displaced fractured segment.
- The occlusion should be checked as a guide to ensure successful reduction of the fracture.
- The teeth in the concerned segment should then be splinted with a stainless steel or titanium wire and composite splint or Biocryl® splint for 4 weeks.
- This must be followed by suturing of any gingival lacerations or extraoral soft tissue injuries [14, 15].

Follow-up Schedule

The child must be recalled after 4 weeks for splint removal. After this, recalls should be scheduled at 6–8 weeks, 4 months, 6 months, 1 year and yearly for at least 5 years.

The International Association of Dental Traumatology (IADT) recommends radiographs to be taken in the primary dentition at the 4-week and 1-year mark. In the permanent dentition, they recommend radiographs to be taken at every follow-up [12, 13].

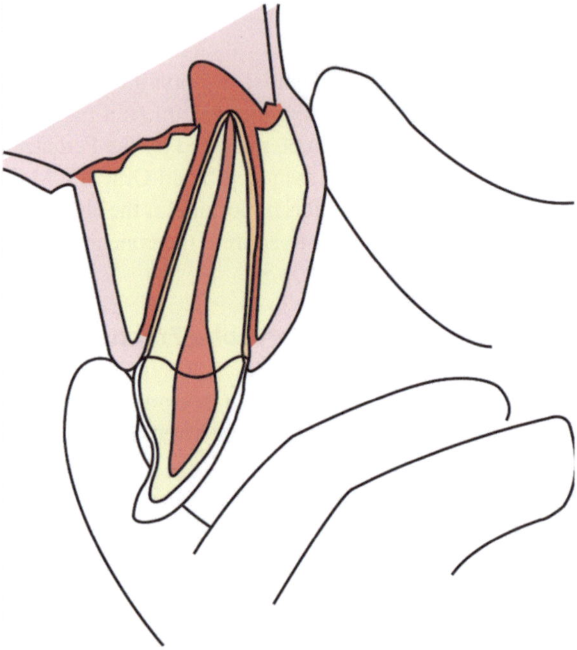

Fig. 15.1 Technique of repositioning a dentoalveolar fracture

15.5.2 How Are Jaw Fractures Managed?

Most jaw fractures in children are greenstick or incomplete fractures. They can be difficult to diagnose at times, due to their subtle clinical presentation. Symptoms include the presence of malocclusion, trismus, lacerations and soft tissue swelling, ecchymosis, limitations in mouth opening and lateral excursions, facial asymmetry, bleeding from the gingival sulcus, and sensory deficit of the inferior alveolar nerve. The child may not always complain of pain but may allude to difficulty in oral functions such as mastication and speech. A clinical diagnosis of a greenstick fracture must be confirmed with radiographic assessment using a CBCT or a Computed Tomography (CT) scan based on the severity of symptoms and the child's cooperation.

Greenstick fractures are managed conservatively and do not need active intervention. In younger children especially, the osteogenic capability of the developing craniofacial skeleton is very high and facilitates rapid healing even when there is imperfect apposition of the two fractured surfaces. Slight occlusal discrepancies resulting from lack of perfect reduction correct spontaneously as permanent teeth erupt and bone undergoes remodeling with function. The child should be advised to seek regular follow-up visits, follow a liquid-to-soft diet, and avoid strenuous physical activities for a few days. Analgesic and anti-inflammatory medication is prescribed based on the patient's degree of pain.

Conservative closed reduction is the recommended treatment for undisplaced favorable fractures. These fractures can be pushed back into the correct position and held in place by child's occlusion or a cap splint.

In case of severely displaced fractures of the maxilla or mandible, an open reduction approach maybe advised. This requires manual reduction with digital pressure and intermaxillary fixation by interdental wiring or arch bars in the permanent dentition. The patient is advised dietary restrictions and to avoid high physical contact sports. Management of displaced jaw fractures may require intervention by an Oral and Maxillofacial Specialist. Open reduction of jaw fractures is generally avoided in young children, as it can damage the developing tooth germs and the growth centers present in the jaw bones affecting physiological growth and development [16, 17].

Children who have suffered trauma to the chin should be screened for injury to the temporomandibular joint (TMJ) like condylar fractures. Symptoms include deviation of the chin to the affected side due to the shortening of ramal height on the ipsilateral side, flattening of the body of the mandible, and open bite can be appreciated on the contralateral side in such cases. Patients with bilateral condylar fractures may present with anterior open bite. The diagnosis is confirmed on an Orthopantomogram (OPG), CBCT, or a CT scan. An undiagnosed condylar fracture may lead to TMJ ankylosis.

Condylar fractures in children are often self-correcting. Nonoperative management includes liquid oral diet, aggressive physiotherapy exercises with ice-cream sticks, anti-inflammatory medication, and regular assessment of mouth opening. Functional appliances like a removable occlusal splint that reestablish the vertical dimension and encourage TMJ healing can be given for 1–3 months [18]. Open reduction may be performed in cases of severe injuries.

To perform the ice-cream stick exercise, patients are initially given a specific number of candy sticks to hold in the mouth depending on patient's current mouth opening. The sticks are to be held for at least 10–15 s and 10 repetitions of this exercise are to be performed 4–5 times a day. As the range of mouth opening improves, patients are asked to increase the number of sticks.

15.5.3 How Are Teeth in the Fractured Segment of a Jaw or Alveolar Fracture Managed?

Teeth in the line of fracture, interfering with reduction may need to be removed to avoid nonunion of the two segments or osteomyelitis. Permanent teeth retained in the fracture segment must be tested for pulp sensibility at periodic follow-up appointments for at least 1 year. In teeth with open apices, endodontic management should not be initiated unless multiple signs indicating non-vitality are observed. In mature teeth, if loss of pulp sensibility is seen during the follow-up coupled with other clinical or radiographic indications of necrosis, root canal treatment should be initiated. If any of these teeth have suffered concomitant traumatic dental injuries, treatment must be performed according to the IADT guidelines after initial stabilization of the alveolar or jaw fracture.

Erupting teeth in the line of fracture show aberrations in development like external root resorption, deficient root formation, abnormal bend of the root, nodule formation on the root, partial obliteration of the pulp cavity, impaction, and growth arrest [19]. Injury to the developing toothbud in the fracture line may develop aberrations such as hypoplasia, enamel defects, dilaceration of the root, odontome like malformation or even complete agenesis of the tooth bud. This depends on the severity and extent of injury, age of the child when trauma occurred, and the treatment rendered [20].

In the primary dentition, pulp testing is not accurate; but the teeth present in the fractured segment must be checked clinically and radiographically. These teeth often develop an abscess and require endodontic intervention or extraction.

Any child with history of maxillofacial trauma needs to be followed up for routine dental examination.

15.6 Concluding Remarks

Any child reporting to a dental operatory with orofacial trauma must undergo a comprehensive extra and intraoral examination. Children diagnosed with complex maxillary, mandibular, or nasal bone fractures may require treatment in hospital settings and must be immediately referred to the concerned specialist. Alveolar bone fractures may be reduced by a clinician with adequate training. Management of traumatic dental injuries should be done concurrently with the management of orofacial trauma and the clinician should work alongside with the referred specialist.

Children must be recalled to ascertain pulp vitality and monitor the eruption of succedaneous teeth in the region of trauma.

References

1. Gussack GS, Luterman A, Powell RW, Rodgers K, Ramenofsky ML. Pediatric maxillofacial trauma: unique features in diagnosis and treatment. Laryngoscope. 1987;97:925–30.
2. Haug RH, Foss J. Maxillofacial injuries in the pediatric patient. Oral Surg Oral Med Oral Pathol Oral Radiol Endod. 2000;90:126–34.
3. Baumann A, Troulis MJ, Kaban LB. Facial trauma I: midfacial fractures. In: Kaban LB, Troulis MJ, editors. Pediatric oral and maxillofacial surgery. Philadelphia: Saunders; 2004. p. 425–40.
4. Cole P, Kaufman Y, Hollier LH Jr. Managing the pediatric facial fracture. Craniomaxillofac Trauma Reconstr. 2009;2(2):77–83.
5. Andreasen JO, Andreasen FM, Andersson L. Chapter 21, Injuries to the supporting bone. In: Textbook and color atlas of traumatic injuries to the teeth. 5th ed. Copenhagen: Munksgaard; 2011. p. 529–55.
6. Lim L, Sirichai P. Bone fractures: assessment and management. Aust Dent J. 2016;61(Suppl 1):74–81.
7. Rai A. Fractures of the mandible. In: Bonanthaya K, Panneerselvam E, Manuel S, Kumar VV, Rai A, editors. Oral and maxillofacial surgery for the clinician. Singapore: Springer; 2021.
8. Panesar K, Susarla SM. Mandibular fractures: diagnosis and management. Semin Plast Surg. 2021;35(4):238–49.
9. Odono LT, Brady CM, Urata M. Mandible fractures. In: Facial trauma surgery. Thieme Medical Publishers; 2020. p. 168–85.

10. Jacob OA, Prathap A. Maxillary fractures. In: Bonanthaya K, Panneerselvam E, Manuel S, Kumar VV, Rai A, editors. Oral and maxillofacial surgery for the clinician. Singapore: Springer; 2021.
11. Zimmermann CE, Troulis MJ, Kaban LB. Pediatric facial fractures: recent advances in prevention, diagnosis and management. Int J Oral Maxillofac Surg. 2005;34(8):823–33.
12. Bourguignon C, Cohenca N, Lauridsen E, Flores MT, O'Connell AC, Day PF, Tsilingaridis G, Abbott PV, Fouad AF, Hicks L, Andreasen JO, Cehreli ZC, Harlamb S, Kahler B, Oginni A, Semper M, Levin L. International Association of Dental Traumatology guidelines for the management of traumatic dental injuries: 1. Fractures and luxations. Dent Traumatol. 2020;36(4):314–30.
13. Day PF, Flores MT, O'Connell AC, Abbott PV, Tsilingaridis G, Fouad AF, Cohenca N, Lauridsen E, Bourguignon C, Hicks L, Andreasen JO, Cehreli ZC, Harlamb S, Kahler B, Oginni A, Semper M, Levin L. International Association of Dental Traumatology guidelines for the management of traumatic dental injuries: 3. Injuries in the primary dentition. Dent Traumatol. 2020;36(4):343–59.
14. Burman S, Lal B, Alagarsamy R, Kumar J, Ankush A, Rai AJ, Yunus M. Evidence-based management of isolated dentoalveolar fractures: a systematic review. J Korean Assoc Oral Maxillofac Surg. 2024;50(3):123–33.
15. Venugopal P, Raj R, Kumaran P, Xavier AM. Custom splint: a conservative approach to pediatric mandibular dentoalveolar trauma. Sci Dent J. 2022;6(3):146–51.
16. López-Santacruz HD, Flores-Velázquez J, Rosales-Berber MÁ. Mandibular greenstick fracture healing: a conservative approach. Pediatr Dent J. 2019;29:146.
17. John B, John R, Stalin A, Elango I. Management of mandibular body fractures in pediatric patients: a case report with review of literature. Contemp Clin Dent. 2010;1(4):291–6.
18. Kamath AT, Roy S, Pai D. Paediatric condylar trauma – primary management considerations – a review. J Oral Biol Craniofac Res. 2023;13(2):236–42.
19. Kevci M, Lauridsen E, Andersson L. Risk of healing complications following alveolar process fractures in the primary dentition: a retrospective clinical cohort study. Dent Traumatol. 2025;41(1):29–36.
20. Suei Y, Mallick PC, Nagasaki T, Taguchi A, Fujita M, Tanimoto K. Radiographic evaluation of the fate of developing tooth buds on the fracture line of mandibular fractures. J Oral Maxillofac Surg. 2006;64(1):94–9.

FSC
www.fsc.org
MIX
Papier aus verantwortungsvollen Quellen
Paper from responsible sources
FSC® C105338

If you have any concerns about our products,
you can contact us on
ProductSafety@springernature.com

In case Publisher is established outside the EU,
the EU authorized representative is:
Springer Nature Customer Service Center GmbH
Europaplatz 3, 69115 Heidelberg, Germany

Printed by Libri Plureos GmbH
in Hamburg, Germany